Ambient Assisted Living

REHABILITATION SCIENCE IN PRACTICE SERIES

Series Editors

Marcia J. Scherer, Ph.D.

President
Institute for Matching Person and Technology

Professor
Physical Medicine & Rehabilitation
University of Rochester Medical Center

Dave Muller, Ph.D.

Executive
Suffolk New College

Editor-in-Chief
Disability and Rehabilitation

Founding Editor
Aphasiology

Published Titles

Forthcoming Titles

Ambient Assisted Living

Nuno M. Garcia
Joel J. P. C. Rodrigues

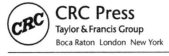

CRC Press
Taylor & Francis Group
Boca Raton London New York

CRC Press is an imprint of the
Taylor & Francis Group, an **informa** business

CRC Press
Taylor & Francis Group
6000 Broken Sound Parkway NW, Suite 300
Boca Raton, FL 33487-2742

First issued in paperback 2017

© 2015 by Taylor & Francis Group, LLC
CRC Press is an imprint of Taylor & Francis Group, an Informa business

No claim to original U.S. Government works

ISBN-13: 978-1-4398-6984-0 (hbk)
ISBN-13: 978-1-138-74774-6 (pbk)

Visit the Taylor & Francis Web site at
http://www.taylorandfrancis.com

and the CRC Press Web site at
http://www.crcpress.com

Because life is not only hard work, this book is dedicated to our families and all our friends.

Contents

Section III AAL Applications to Specific Areas

Section IV Business Models and Study Cases

Section V AAL Research Topics

Preface

The interest on the project for this book cannot be dissociated with the general interest on Ambient Assisted Living (AAL), especially in Europe. The European society is ageing, as other said western societies, and the consequences of this have to be foreseen in advance as to allow the elders that all of us will hopefully become, to live a life with quality in its many aspects. As recently heard in the corridors of a Personalized Medicine conference, if one is over 60 and knows no illnesses, this just means poor diagnostic. And yet we believe that physical senescence does not have to automatically imply loss of quality of life.

Personalized Medicine, Ambient Assisted Living and Enhanced Living Environments are often seen as the promise that, despite the inexorable advance of time, the science behind these technologies will allow us, future-to-be-elders (some sooner than others), to still enjoy a lifestyle that will not be impaired as a consequence of our loss of youth.

As AAL is such a broad area of interest that joins so many areas of science—from engineering to medicine, from business to psychology—it became a very complex task to focus the content of this book. Taking this into consideration, this volume arose from the interest in AAL and the willingness to bring together researchers with original work in this area of assisted living and to contribute to the enrichment of the state of the art, by helping disseminate good practices.

Our goal was to focus on the discussion of AAL technologies from its inception to implementation, creating a book whose content would be useful for students, practitioners, and users of AAL.

To achieve this, we included a comprehensive reference on methods, concepts, systems, devices, and services that provide unobtrusive support for the daily needs of an assisted person. This book also provides extensive coverage of applications, software, and information management for AAL, as well as coverage of the latest hardware and software for ergonomic design pertaining to AAL. Ambient intelligence is a covered key concept, which refers to electronic environments that are sensitive and responsive to the presence of people.

The hardest challenge was to get the right mix of researchers and authors who could contribute in for a well-balanced content. We believe that the goals we have defined at the beginning of this project were achieved and the book we now present will be a valuable tool for researchers and practitioners in the AAL area.

We would like to sincerely acknowledge all the contributors and specially thank CRC Press for coming forward to publish this volume. We appreciate the efforts of the reviewers and the editorial team for coming up with an excellent edition, in particular the work of Paula Sousa and Virginie Felizardo, whose organizational and scientific skills were essential to the closure of the project. We also want to acknowledge the contribution of COST Action IC1303 Architectures, Algorithms and Platforms for Enhanced Living Environments (AAPELE).

MATLAB® is a registered trademark of The MathWorks, Inc. For product information, please contact:

The MathWorks, Inc.
3 Apple Hill Drive
Natick, MA 01760-2098 USA
Tel: 508 647 7000
Fax: 508-647-7001
E-mail: info@mathworks.com
Web: www.mathworks.com

Contributors

Joaquim Alvarelhão
Higher School of Health
University of Aveiro
Aveiro, Portugal

Yacine Amirat
LISSI Laboratory
University of Paris-Est Créteil
Créteil Cedex, France

Pedro Araújo
Instituto de Telecomunicações
and
Department of Informatics
University of Beira Interior
Covilhã, Portugal

Artur Arsenio
Computer Science Department
Universidade da Beira Interior
Covilhã, Portugal

Oscar Alejandro Vásquez Bernal
Universidad Nacional Abierta y a
    Distancia
Bogotá, Colombia

Marta Díaz Boladeras
Technical Research Centre for Dependency
    Care and Autonomous Living
Universitat Politècnica de Catalunya
Barcelona, Spain

Maged N. Kamel Boulos
Faculty of Health
University of Plymouth
United Kingdom

Sarah Bourke
Skytek, Ireland

Kouamana Bousson
Laboratório Associado em Energia,
    Transportes e Aeronáutica (LAETA)/
    University of Beira Interior (UBI)-
    Aeronautics and Astronautics Group
    (AeroG)
and
Department of Aerospace Sciences
University of Beira Interior
Covilhã, Portugal

Luis M. Camarinha-Matos
Faculty of Sciences and Technology
    Campus de Caparica
Universidade Nova de Lisboa
Lisbon, Portugal

Carlos Abellán Cano
Facultat de Lletres
Universitat Rovira i virgili
Asociación de Investigadores de la
    Sociedad y la Cultura
Tarragona, Spain

Davide Carneiro
Department of Informatics
University of Minho
Braga, Portugal

Miguel Castelo-Branco
Health Sciences Faculty
University of Beira Interior
Covilhã, Portugal

Abdelghani Chibani
Laboratoire Images Signaux et Systèmes
    Intelligents (LISSI) Laboratory
University of Paris-Est Créteil
Créteil Cedex, France

Michał Choraś
ITTI Ltd.
Poznań, Poland

and

Institute of Telecommunications
UT&LS Bydgoszcz
Bydgoszcz, Poland

Bruno Colin
HOPES Project, Ambient Assisted Living
    Association (AAL) Call 2
and
Association JADES (Joindre les Arts au
    Développement, à l'Education et à la
    Santé)
Septfonds, France

Ângelo Costa
Computer Science and Technology Center
    (CCTC)–Department of Informatics
University of Minho
Braga, Portugal

Ricardo Costa
Escola Superior de Tecnologia e Gestão
Instituto Politécnico do Porto
Felgueiras, Portugal

Salvatore D'Antonio
University of Naples "Parthenope"
Naples, Italy

Ivo M. C. de M. Lopes
Instituto de Telecomunicações
University of Beira Interior
Covilhã, Portugal

Jorge Dias
Institute of Systems and Robotics
University of Coimbra
Coimbra, Portugal and Khalifa University
Abu Dhabi, United Arab Emirates

Liliana Dias
OUTCOME
Clínica Organizacional
Taguspark|Oeiras, Portugal

Miguel Sales Dias
Microsoft Language Development Center
Microsoft Portugal
Lisbon, Portugal

Pedro Dinis Gaspar
Electromechanical Engineering
    Department
Faculty of Engineering
and
Institute of Telecommunications
ALLab–Assisted Living Computing and
    Telecommunications Laboratory
University of Beira Interior
Covilhã, Portugal

Mari Ervasti
VTT Technical Research Centre of Finland
    Ltd.
Espoo, Finland

Susana Espadaneira
Comfort Keepers-Comforting Solutions for
    In-Home Care
Taguspark|Oeiras, Portugal

Miguel Martínez Espronceda
Departamento de Ingeniería Eléctrica y
    Electrónica
Universidad Pública de Navarra
Pamplona, Navarra, Spain

Francisco Falcone
Departamento de Ingeniería Eléctrica y
    Electrónica
Universidad Pública de Navarra
Pamplona, Navarra, Spain

Paulo Fazendeiro
Institute of Telecommunications
University of Beira Interior
Covilhã, Portugal

Virginie Felizardo
Instituto de Telecomunicações
ALLab–Assisted Living Computing and
  Telecommunications Laboratory
University of Beira Interior
Covilhã, Portugal

José Eduardo Fernandes
Bragança Polytechnic Institute
Bragança, Portugal

Carlos Fernández-Valdivielso
Departamento de Ingeniería Eléctrica y
  Electrónica
Universidad Pública de Navarra
Pamplona, Navarra, Spain

Filipa Ferrada
Faculty of Sciences and Technology
  Campus de Caparica
Universidade Nova de Lisboa
Lisbon, Portugal

Flávio Ferreira
Departamento Electrónica
  Telecomunicações e Informática
Instituto de Engenharia Electrónica e
  Telemática de Aveiro
Universidade de Aveiro
Aveiro, Portugal

Nuno Ferreira
I2S–Informática e Sistemas
Porto, Portugal

Paulo Freitas
Institute of Systems and Robotics
University of Coimbra
Coimbra, Portugal

César P. Gálvez-Barrón
Fundació Privada Sant Antoni Abat-
  Consorci Sanitari del Garraf
Barcelona, Spain

Nuno M. Garcia
Instituto de Telecomunicações
ALLab–Assisted Living Computing and
  Telecommunications Laboratory
Computer Science Department
and
Faculty of Engineering
University of Beira Interior
Covilhã, Portugal

and

Universidade Lusófona de Humanidades e
  Tecnologias
Lisbon, Portugal

Patrick Gatellier
Theresis Innovation Center
Thales, France

Hassan Ghasemzadeh
Washington State University
Pullman, Washington

Jordi Morales Gras
Technical Research Centre for Dependency
  Care and Autonomous Living
Universitat Politécnica de Catalunya
Barcelona, Spain

Marja Harjumaa
VTT Technical Research Centre of Finland
  Ltd.
Espoo, Finland

Victor Hernandez
Agencia Andaluza de Servicios Sociales de
  Andalucia (ASSDA)
Andalucia, Spain

Giulio Iannello
Centro Integrato di Ricerca
Universita Campus Bio-Medico di Roma
Rome, Italy

Roozbeh Jafari
The University of Texas at Dallas
Dallas, Texas

Andreas Jedlitschka
Fraunhofer Institute for Experimental
    Software Engineering
Kaiserslautern, Germany

Rüdiger Kays
Communication Technology Institute
Technische Universität Dortmund
Germany

Friedrich Köhler
Zentrum für kardiovaskuläre Telemedizin
    GmbH
Berlin, Germany

Rafał Kozik
Institute of Telecommunications
UT&LS Bydgoszcz
Bydgoszcz, Poland

Alain Krivitzky
Hospital Avicenne Bobigny
University Paris Seine Saint Denis
Assistance Publique Hôpitaux de Paris
Paris, France

and

HOPES Project, AAL Call 2
Septfonds, France

Nils Langhammer
Communication Technology Institute
TU Dortmund University
Dortmund, Germany

Santiago Led
Departamento de Ingeniería Eléctrica y
    Electrónica
Universidad Pública de Navarra
Pamplona, Navarra, Spain

Dominique Lemoult
Primary Care Practice
Cabinet Marcel Monny Lobe
Soisy sous Montmorency, France

Ana Lima
CCG–Centro de Computação Gráfica
University of Minho Guimarães
Guimarães, Portugal

Ralf Lindert
InWIS–Institute for Housing, Real Estate,
    Urban and Regional Development
EBZ Business School
Ruhr University of Bochum
Bochum, Germany

Antonio López-Martín
Departamento de Ingeniería Eléctrica y
    Electrónica
Universidad Pública de Navarra
Pamplona, Navarra, Spain

Ricardo J. Machado
Centro ALGORITMI
University of Minho
Guimarães, Portugal

Paulo Menezes
Institute of Systems and Robotics
University of Coimbra
Coimbra, Portugal

Klaus Miesenberger
Institut Integriert Studieren JKU
University of Linz
Linz, Austria

Marlou Min
ANBO
Woerden, The Netherlands

Gerard Nguyen
HOPES Project, AAL Call 2
Septfonds, France

and

Hospital Avicenne Bobigny
University Paris Seine Saint Denis
Assistance Publique Hôpitaux de Paris
and
Gerontology Coordinator ARPAD
Primary Care
Cabinet Marcel Monny Lobe
Soisy sous Montmorency, France

and

Institut du Bien Vieillir
Korian, Paris, France

Paulo Novais
Computer Science and Technology Center
(CCTC)–Department of Informatics
University of Minho
Braga, Portugal

Jorge Nunes Monteiro
Instituto Superior de Economia e Gestão
(ISEG)
Universidade Técnica de Lisboa
Lisbon, Portugal

Karol O'Donovan
National University of Ireland, Galway
(NUIG)
Galway, Ireland

Ana Inês Oliveira
Faculty of Sciences and Technology
Campus de Caparica
Universidade Nova de Lisboa
Lisbon, Portugal

André Oliveira
Departamento Electrónica
Telecomunicações e Informática
Instituto de Engenharia Electrónica e
Telemática de Aveiro
Universidade de Aveiro
Aveiro, Portugal

Henrique O'Neill
ISCTE
Lisbon University Institute
Lisbon, Portugal

António Pereira
CCG–Centro de Computação Gráfica
University of Minho Guimarães
Guimarães, Portugal

Carlos Pereira
Departamento Electrónica
Telecomunicações e Informática
Instituto de Engenharia Electrónica e
Telemática de Aveiro
Universidade de Aveiro
Aveiro, Portugal

Joaquim Sousa Pinto
Departamento Electrónica
Telecomunicações e Informática
Instituto de Engenharia Electrónica e
Telemática de Aveiro
Universidade de Aveiro
Aveiro, Portugal

Nuno Pombo
Instituto de Telecomunicações
and
Department of Informatics
University of Beira Interior
Covilhã, Portugal

Sandra Prescher
Charité-Universitätsmedizin Berlin
Berlin, Germany

Sharon Prins
The Netherlands Organisation for Applied
Scientific Research
Delft, The Netherlands

Alexandra Queirós
Higher School of Health
University of Aveiro
Aveiro, Portugal

Filipe Quinaz
Department of Informatics
University of Beira Interior
Covilhã, Portugal

José Duarte Realinho
ISCTE
University Institute of Lisbon
Lisbon, Portugal

Nelson Pacheco Rocha
Health Sciences Autonomous Section
University of Aveiro
Aveiro, Portugal

Joel J. P. C. Rodrigues
Instituto de Telecomunicações
University of Beira Interior
Covilhã, Portugal

Alejandro Rodríguez-Molinero
Fundació Privada Sant Antoni Abat-
   Consorci Sanitari del Garraf
National University of Ireland
Galway, Ireland

João Rosas
Faculty of Sciences and Technology
Campus de Caparica
Universidade Nova de Lisboa
Lisbon, Portugal

Lyazid Sabri
Le Laboratoire Images, Signaux et
   Systémes Intelligents (LiSSi)
University of Paris-Est Créteil
Créteil Cedex, France

Nuno Santos
CCG–Centro de Computação Gráfica
University of Minho Guimarães
Guimarães, Portugal

Antonio Sapuppo
Center for Communication, Media and
   Information Technologies
Aalborg University
Aalborg, Denmark

Katrin Schneiders
University of Applied Sciences of Koblenz
Koblenz, Germany

Boon-Chong Seet
Department of Electrical and Electronic
   Engineering
Auckland University of Technology
Auckland, New Zealand

Luis Serrano
Departamento de Ingeniería Eléctrica y
   Electrónica
Universidad Pública de Navarra
Pamplona, Navarra, Spain

François Sigwald
Primary Care Gerontology Coordinator
Soisy sous Montmorency, France

Anabela G. Silva
Higher School of Health
University of Aveiro
Aveiro, Portugal

Bruno M. C. Silva
Instituto de Telecomunicações
University of Beira Interior
Covilhã, Portugal

João C. Silva
Computer Science and Engineering
   Department
Instituto Superior Técnico
University of Lisbon
Lisbon, Portugal

Miguel Oliveira e Silva
Departamento Electrónica
   Telecomunicações e Informática
Instituto de Engenharia Electrónica e
   Telemática de Aveiro
Universidade de Aveiro
Aveiro, Portugal

Ricardo Simoes
Institute of Polymers and Composites IPC/
    I3N
University of Minho
Guimarães, Portugal

and

Life and Health Sciences Research Institute
    (ICVS)
University of Minho
Braga, Portugal

and

Polytechnic Institute of Cávado and Ave
Barcelos, Portugal

and

Institute of Telecommunications
ALLab–Assisted Living Computing and
    Telecommunications Laboratory
University of Beira Interior
Covilhã, Portugal

Paula Sousa
Institute of Telecommunications
ALLab–Assisted Living Computing and
    Telecommunications Laboratory
University of Beira Interior
Covilhã, Portugal

Marc Steen
TNO
Delft, The Netherlands

Emilio Suárez Ortega
Asociación de Investigadores de la
    Sociedad y la Cultura
Tarragona, Spain

António Teixeira
Departamento Electrónica
    Telecomunicações e Informática
Instituto de Engenharia Electrónica e
    Telemática de Aveiro
Universidade de Aveiro
Aveiro, Portugal

Cláudio Teixeira
Departamento Electrónica
    Telecomunicações e Informática
Instituto de Engenharia Electrónica e
    Telemática de Aveiro
Universidade de Aveiro
Aveiro, Portugal

Juliana Teixeira
CCG–Centro de Computação Gráfica
University of Minho Guimarães
and
Centro ALGORITMI
University of Minho
Guimarães, Portugal

Daniel Thiollier
HOPES Project, AAL Call 2
Septfonds, France

Ada Font Tió
Technical Research Centre for Dependency
    Care and Autonomous Living
Universitat Politècnica de Catalunya
Barcelona, Spain

Ricardo Vardasca
Institute of Polymers and Composites
    IPC/I3N
University of Minho
Guimarães, Portugal

Luca Vollero
Centro Integrato di Ricerca
Universita Campus Bio-Medico di Roma
Rome, Italy

Adam Wołoszczuk
Przemysłowy Instytut Automatyki i
    Pomiarów PIAP
Warsaw, Poland

Gian Piero Zarri
LISSI Laboratory
University of Paris-Est Créteil
Créteil Cedex, France

1

Ambient Assisted Living—From Technology to Intervention

Nuno M. Garcia, Paula Sousa, and Virginie Felizardo

ABSTRACT   This chapter introduces the contents of the book, presenting its goals and providing a brief description of structure and the chapters. The five sections containing the twenty-six chapters are presented and summarily described to allow a quick overview of the its content.

KEY WORDS: *ambient assisted living, book organization.*

The discussion about ambient assisted living (AAL) gained momentum when political players and governments could no longer ignore the fact that, in most developed countries, the demographic profile was changing, resulting in an inversion of the demographic pyramid. AAL encompasses technical systems to support people in their daily routines to allow an independent and safe lifestyle as long as possible. In particular, AAL may focus on the needs of special interest groups, such as the elderly, people with disabilities, or people who temporarily need assistance. For example, AAL aims at producing technological and media support to help elderly people to stay at their homes longer.

This book is focused on the discussion of AAL technologies from their inception to implementation and is aimed at students, practitioners, and users of AAL. This comprehensive reference covers methods, concepts, systems, devices, and services that provide unobtrusive support for the daily needs of an assisted person. This book also provides extensive coverage of applications, software, and information management for AAL, as well as coverage of the latest hardware and software for ergonomic design pertaining to AAL. A key concept covered is ambient intelligence, which refers to electronic environments that are sensitive and responsive to the presence of people.

Summarizing and highlighting the most relevant objectives in this book

- Covers the latest developments in AAL
- Provides extensive coverage of applications, software, and information management for AAL
- Includes coverage of the latest hardware and software for ergonomic design pertaining to AAL
- Offers extensive references at the end of each chapter for additional study

This book comprises five main parts, each one with a specific topic:

- Section I—"Review, State of the Art, and AAL Concepts"

    Often, the first step to achieve improvements in an area is to sharply assess what has been produced and researched so far, and to look for trends and clues on how the future will look. Section I contains Chapters 2 to 6, providing an overview of the concepts related to AAL.

- Chapter 2 describes a systematic review that summarizes and characterizes existing literature on AAL, making a survey of technology-oriented publications and others describing applications and scenarios.

- Chapter 3 presents a comprehensive review of the state of the art on pervasive and mobile health (m-health) applications. It presents the most important and significant work in the related literature and presents the top and most used m-health applications in the mobile market. New trends and insights for future research studies and new answers for emerging and challenging health care issues are also presented.

- Chapter 4 describes a set of projects and work with scientific relevance in AAL. The distribution of these publications was divided in two topics, home care technology and free living technology. The authors made a bibliographic collection that is the state of the art in monitoring and assisted therapeutic technology for AAL.

- In Chapter 5, the authors propose some recommendations for an evidence-based approach in gerontotechnology and information and communication technology (ICT) solutions, implementing knowledge and experiences from the medical research and health care fields.

- In Chapter 6, the authors present the results obtained when applying process-level modeling techniques to the derivation of the logical architecture for a real industrial AAL project, adopting a V-Model–based approach that expresses the AAL requirements from a process-level perspective, instead of the traditional product-level view. Additionally, they ensure the compliance of the derived logical architecture with the National Institute of Standards and Technology (NIST) reference architecture as a nonfunctional requirement to support the implementation of the AAL architecture in cloud contexts.

- Section II—"Communications in AAL"

  Communications in AAL are considered to be in the advanced research phase. These solutions include research in ubiquitous computing and sensing, ubiquitous communication, and intelligent user interfaces. The integration of ubiquitous computing and communication with intelligent interfaces significantly increases efficiency throughout AAL systems. Section II contains Chapters 7 to 10, on different aspects of communications applied to AAL.

  - Chapter 7 provides a background for the understanding of the lower layers of wireless home automation networks and the influence of important parameters, and describes and compares different solutions for the physical and medium access layer of a wireless data transmission.

  - Chapter 8 addresses research on context-aware systems for mobility and multihoming, in the scope of AAL, focusing on context-aware systems for mobility management, which are applied to aid the handover process.

  - Chapter 9 presents energy-efficient communication models for body area network (BAN) applications using buffers to limit communication to higher-rate short bursts, decreasing power usage and simplifying the communication.

  - Chapter 10 focuses on the optimal rollout of wireless sensor networks in terms of coverage/capacity relations, coexistence with other existing wireless networks, energy-efficient transceivers, and integration with building automation systems, with examples of operation of real telemonitoring devices.

- Section III—"AAL Applications to Specific Areas"

  This section is an overview of the development in pervasive health care systems and services developed for people with dementia, comorbidity, and memory and cognitive disabilities, and totally blind people, namely telemedicine, telehealth, or telecare, to provide support and medical care. Chapters 11 to 15 provide a non-exhaustive but comprehensive view of specific fields within AAL.

  - Chapter 11 presents the state of the art in terms of e-companionship and e-counseling solutions, particularly for elderly cognitively challenged people, and the major lessons learnt from previous projects using video technologies in health and social contexts.

  - Chapter 12 gives an analysis of the current scenario from the point of view of the different actors (patients, health care providers, and health care systems) aimed at identifying the needs to be covered by telemedicine systems that could contribute to overcoming several problems. This chapter provides a description and analysis of the specific scenario for a telemedicine application to monitor and provide health care to older people with comorbidity.

  - In Chapter 13, a framework focused on the monitoring and assistance of elderly persons living alone is presented, focusing on elderly persons with memory disabilities. The chapter describes the components of the framework directly related with the user: its architecture and functionalities, the simulation tool, the monitoring solution, and the personal memory assistant.

  - In Chapter 14, a prospective study on technological systems for people with cognitive disabilities is presented and discussed. The chapter provides an analysis of technological solutions for care of persons with dementia and of intelligent systems of assistance for improving quality of life in a preferred living environment.

  - Finally, Chapter 15 presents an innovative solution to support social inclusion of totally blind people. This chapter proposes the use of dedicated harnesses and mobile devices (e.g., smartphones) to support instrumentation for daily living activities and presents innovations in computer vision algorithms, multisensor data fusion, situational awareness, ontology, and risk assessment, as well as innovations in resilient personal telecommunications.

- Section IV—"Business Models and Study Cases"

  The implementation of solutions in real-life scenarios is often validated not only by the soundness of its technological innovations but also, to a larger extent, by the opportunity and expertise in the development and implementation of good business cases. Chapters 16 to 19 integrate this section.

  - In Chapter 16, a collaborative network business model is presented, with the aim of bringing together the distinct contributions of the different providers that are needed to offer AAL products and services.

  - Chapter 17 presents a case study, *service4home*, that can be seen as an attempt at a multidisciplinary social, technical, and economic innovation. The chapter also identifies a wide range of new possibilities of technologies and services based on AAL and many challenges in their implementation.

- Chapter 18 presents the conceptual architecture adopted for the living lab and the support architecture for the development of new and complex AAL services, aiming to create an environment where developers and care professionals are able to create innovative AAL applications and services.
- Chapter 19 presents the Ambient Assisted Living for All (AAL4ALL) project as a case study to analyze and illustrate the AAL developments for monitoring daily living activities, their roadmap with the expected technological development, and the impact of these developed solutions on end users.
- Section V—"AAL Research Topics"

  Chapters 20 to 26 discuss some of the most relevant research topics in AAL. The information provided by this section allows the reader to understand the current research lines in AAL, also giving an insight on the developments in this area for the next years.

  - Chapter 20 provides an overview of the machine learning (ML) concepts in the field of AAL. ML is described in terms of learning concepts, the principles of concept classification are explained, and the mathematical concepts of several methodologies are presented. Finally, an approach based on the fusion of several single methods is described for situations dealing with multiple learning models.
  - Chapter 21 presents an overview of soft computing techniques designed for automatic drug infusion and modeling of hypertensive patient response in the AAL environment. A brief description of the evolution of these systems, the identification of the most recent advances, and research trends are also provided.
  - In Chapter 22, a new semantic framework for monitoring the AAL heterogeneous ecosystems is presented. This framework deals with context awareness and closed-world assumption (CWA) semantic reasoning. It is capable of dynamically detecting real-world objects and capturing their contexts, in order to identify the specific changes that are happening in the environment, to infer the current situation, and to react accordingly.
  - Chapter 23 introduces a conceptual architecture to guide the development of a collaborative ecosystem of care services supporting active ageing. The notion of integrated care services, which are to be provided by multiple stakeholders through well-elaborated collaboration mechanisms, is explored.
  - In Chapter 24, the emerging concept of social ambient intelligence (socAmI) is discussed, as well as a review of the underlying methods and technologies to address the important challenges of socAmI: the acquisition of social context, enhancing ubiquitous social networking, and privacy protection.
  - Chapter 25 presents the WeCare project, focused on improving older people's well-being by enabling them to engage in online social networking and promoting social interaction and participation.
  - Chapter 26 conducts an analysis of human sensitivity-based project development from the perspective of design, project and development, functionality, and usability for the end customer.

The research and technological area of AAL will not lose its momentum in the following years. Increasingly, technology is seen as a tool that helps people achieve more and better in their daily lives, more so if the person has particular mobility or psychological issues or is otherwise impaired. The themes covered in this book do not exhaust the discussion on AAL, yet they provide a concise overview of what AAL is, from technology to intervention.

Section I

Review, State of the Art, and AAL Concepts

2

Characterization and Classification of Existing Ambient Assisted Living Systems: A Systematic Literature Review

Alexandra Queirós, Anabela G. Silva, Joaquim Alvarelhão, António Teixeira, and Nelson Pacheco Rocha

CONTENTS

ABSTRACT   This chapter describes a systematic review that summarizes and characterizes existing literature on ambient assisted living (AAL). This presents an added value for the future development in this area. To be included in this review, articles must have defined innovative concepts or characterized innovative technologies, products, or systems that can contribute to the development of the AAL paradigm, with the aim of enabling people with specific demands (e.g., elderly) to live longer in their natural environment. AAL could therefore be translated best as intelligent systems of assistance for a better and safer life.

Results indicate that most publications regarding AAL are technology-oriented with only a few articles found describing applications and scenarios. Another interesting finding is the effort made to adjust the technology to the characteristics and needs of the user considering the context in which the activity is taking place.

KEY WORDS: *ambient assisted living, elderly, intelligent systems systematic reviews.*

Introduction

The ambient assisted living (AAL) paradigm is very important nowadays, because it intends to develop innovative concepts or to integrate innovative technologies, products, systems, or services that can contribute to support a better and safer life. AAL was conceived as one strategy for addressing the difficulties that the forthcoming demographic shift will give rise to. It proposes the selective harnessing of information and communication technologies to deliver innovative systems and services that would enable the elderly to live independently for longer and reduce the need for long-term care (Steg et al. 2006). Despite being a new concept, the amount of literature in this area is substantial. This systematic literature review will provide a summary and characterization of the existing literature related to AAL. Studies were sought using health databases (PubMed, Web of Science, Academic Search Complete, and Science Direct) and engineering and technology databases (Cite Seer and IEEE Xplore). Two keywords were used without language restriction: ambient assisted living and ambient intelligence.

This chapter is divided into (1) a background section, where we contextualize the AAL technologies and define related concepts; (2) the methods, where the procedures used in this review are described; (3) the results and discussion sections; and (4) the conclusion, where the main issues are summarized and future research directions are suggested.

Background

A digital environment with a pervasive and unobtrusive intelligence able to proactively support people in their daily lives is the fundamental idea of the Ambient Intelligence (AmI) concept (Ramos 2007). AmI deals with new paradigms where computing devices are spread everywhere (ubiquity) to allow the people to have intelligent and natural interactions with the physical world environments.

Following the advice of the Information Society and Technology Advisory Group (ISTAG) (IST Advisory Group 2002, 2003), the European Commission used the AmI concept for the launch of the sixth framework (FP6) on Information, Society, and Technology (IST). The subsequent association of AmI with the European policies toward the knowledge society and the continued financial support in several research programs contributed to making AmI a very active research topic (Aarts and Grotenhuis 2009).

Prominent examples of AmI systems are smart homes. A smart home is a house equipped with a broad range of devices to provide advanced systems to its users (Augusto 2008). However, AmI environments may be so diverse, and other systems are also feasible and relevant. The use of sensors and smart devices can be found in different sectors—logistics and transportation, tourism, education, emergency, public surveillance, or health-related systems—allowing better support to the people and access to the essential knowledge to make better decisions (Aarts and Grotenhuis 2009; Augusto 2008).

Ambient Assisted Living

Within the AmI concept, AAL is currently one of the important development areas. The growing political importance of AAL is evident by the AAL Joint Programme, the initiative taken by the European Union with several Member States (July 2008) in order to obtain synergies in terms of management and financial resources by ensuring a single common evaluation mechanism with the assistance of independent experts (Decision No. 742/2008/EC).

The general goal of AAL solutions is to apply the AmI concept and technologies to enable people with specific demands (e.g., elderly) to live longer in their natural environment. In technological terms, the AAL comprises a heterogeneous field of systems ranging from quite simple devices such as intelligent medication dispensers, fall sensors, or bed sensors to complex systems such as networked homes and interactive systems.

Therefore, AAL solutions have high demands on the accessibility, usability, and suitability of the developed systems: user acceptance and support of natural user interfaces are absolute necessities (Kleinberger et al. 2007).

AAL systems can contribute to increase the performance of elderly people in a broad spectrum of activities and participation (PERSONA 2008): personal care, planning of the weekly menu, nutritional advisor, maintenance of house and garden, self-administration or agenda, support in finding and carrying out work, establishing and maintaining contacts with other people, and, in general, spending the day (through participation in different leisure activities) and social participation.

Finally, AAL systems can contribute to the reorientation in health systems that are currently organized around acute, episodic experiences of disease, allowing the development of a broad range of systems such as care prevention and care promotion and home-caregiver support.

AAL Technologies

The automation in an AAL environment, as in AmI environments, can be viewed as a cycle of perceiving the state of the environment, reasoning about the state together with task goals and outcomes of possible actions, and acting upon the environment to change the state (Cook and Das 2007).

Like all intelligent agents, a smart environment relies on sensory data from the real world. The perception of the environment needs devices embedded in the environment with the purpose to allow interaction of the occupants with the technology.

Using the sensory data, the technological structure is able to perform reasoning processes and select actions that can be taken to change the state of the environment. Therefore, the data resulting from the sensor activities must be transmitted by a communication network and preprocessed by a complex technological structure, which collates and harmonizes data from different devices (process the raw data into more useful knowledge such as models or patterns). To make that information beneficial to the occupants of the environment, AAL systems must have high-level reasoning and decision-making processes to accomplish diagnosis and advice or assist people (Cook and Das 2007).

Action execution flows top-down. The action is transmitted by the communication network to the physical actuators. These change the state of the surrounding environment.

Therefore, sensing, communicating, and acting are crucial issues within the AAL paradigm (Camarinha-Matos and Vieira 1999; Costa et al. 1999): (1) sensing—a sensorial network is indispensable for obtaining the correct information about the environment and its users; (2) communicating—all the components of an AAL environment must be interconnected in order to communicate with each other; and (3) acting—any AAL environment, in order to achieve its objective, must be able to act, through various types of actuators (Figure 2.1).

The sensing, communicating, and acting functions require a broad range of physical devices. Moreover, the technological structure of the AAL environment should have additional components (Camarinha-Matos and Vieira 1999; Costa et al. 1999): (1) using—the user interface is another important component of an AAL environment; (2) enjoying—an AAL environment is an extension of a conventional environment, making it appear as traditional as possible, but assisting its users in their daily activities, making their life more comfortable; and (3) involving—an AAL environment helps people to take part or participate in all areas of life and to be accepted, to be included, or to have access to the necessary resources.

Therefore, AAL systems must be able to properly distinguish the people present in the environment and what their roles, preferences, and limitations are. AAL systems must be

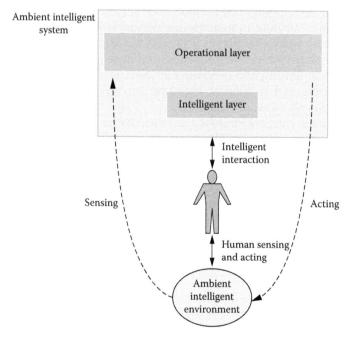

FIGURE 2.1
Automation in an AAL environment. (Adapted from Ramos, C. et al., *IEEE Intelligent Systems* 23:15–18, 2008.)

able to (1) recognize individual needs; (2) recognize situational context; (3) allow different answers according to personal needs and situational contexts; and (4) anticipate desires and needs without conscious mediation.

Having all this information about its users, the AAL technological structure will then be able to decide which systems to provide, when to provide, how to provide, and to whom to provide them. This means that the AAL technological structure should present a broad range of intelligent functions for the user management interface and context awareness (Hoareau and Satoh 2009).

The existence of all types of devices, such as sensors or video cameras, poses a set of complex problems in terms of privacy and security, which requires additional research and development effort.

An AAL environment comprises numerous invisible devices and ubiquitous systems. Effective architectures are required to mask the effects of heterogeneous physical devices, communication networks, and intelligent components and systems. Furthermore, the system's architectures must provide the availability of the devices and components needed for providing every system and must also know some other important characteristics about the systems it is providing (such as the geographic location, the cost, or the probable effects) so that when it suggests a specific system to a specific user, it is actually suggesting what it thinks is the most adequate system to that specific situation.

Last but not least, the acceptance of the AAL paradigm is, obviously, closely related with the quality of the available systems (e.g., private houses and home-care assistance in the presence of users with different abilities and needs).

Therefore, a brief description of intelligent components, architectures and frameworks, and system requirements of AAL environments will be presented in the following.

Architectures and Frameworks

As mentioned previously, an AAL environment comprises numerous invisible devices and ubiquitous systems. The development of effective architectures to mask the effects of heterogeneous devices and networks as well as mobility is a major challenge. A significant number of AAL general architectures follow the paradigm of system orientation, which allows developing software as systems that are delivered and consumed on demand. The benefit of this approach lies in the loose coupling of the software components that make up a system. Discovery mechanisms can be used for finding and selecting the functionality that a client is looking for. Many protocols already exist in the area of system orientation.

In general, the AAL architecture components can be divided into three macrolayers: the device compliant layer, the middleware layer, and the system layer: (1) the compliant device layer allows algorithms to access the different devices (such as sensors and actuators) by a single interface that abstracts from proprietary properties of the device wherever possible; (2) the middleware layer contains the functionality that is needed to facilitate the operation of the networked environment; and (3) the system layer allows the combination of different middleware systems to build domain-specific systems.

The existence of the middleware layer is justified due to the fact that many of AAL concerns (e.g., adaptability or heterogeneity) are common and, therefore, should be addressed by a common infrastructure (middleware) instead of each individual system (Bavafa and Navidi 2010).

Considering the complexity of the AAL principles, architectures, and devices, appropriate design methodologies are required to enable efficient engineering, deployment, and run-time management of reconfigurable AAL systems (Berger et al. 2008).

Physical Devices

An AAL environment is composed of a complex network of devices or subsystems work-ing together. All the devices must have communication capabilities for interaction with other devices (and also computational capabilities to implement the interaction protocols and to process information). Three generic classes based on device dimensions, power sources, and mobility factors can be considered (Snijders 2005): (1) autonomous micro-devices, (2) mobile mini devices, and (3) static devices.

The autonomous microdevice class includes small and simple actuators (e.g., on/off out-puts for signals) and a great variety of sensors. The sensors must collect and disseminate a range of environmental data (e.g., luminosity, temperature, or humidity). Networks of these devices are required for the implementation of user-friendly systems, such as environmen-tal control in homes and offices, person identification, health monitoring, home security, or robot control. Within the scope of an indoor environment, some examples of the types of sensors can be envisaged (IST Amigo Project 2005a): (1) comfort sensors related to the mea-sure of luminosity, temperature, humidity, CO_2, vibrations or pressure, inside or outside doors; (2) technical security detectors, such as water leakage in kitchens and bathrooms, gas leakage in the kitchen, or fire detectors; (3) security and safety detectors, including detectors of anti-intrusion, volumetric detectors, or gate detectors; (4) welfare and health devices to improve people's quality of life (e.g., a medical alarm medallion, blood pressure meters, heart frequency meters, or glucose meters); (5) voice capturing devices; and (6) sen-sors that are able to detect the presence of people and their activity inside the environment.

It is crucial that the sensors should be lightweight, extremely small, and very cheap. They are spread all around the environment, and therefore their appearance should be invisible to the users. They have to operate autonomously without any supervision over their entire lifetime, and they need to organize themselves in networks without any man-ual interaction and to be reliable (IST Amigo Project 2005a).

A broad range of portable mini devices can be found in AAL environments: infotain-ment pocket consoles, phones with built-in cameras and storage capacity, personal digital assistants, wireless tablets, or other portable access devices to audio and video informa-tion. All the portable mini devices have in common the characteristics of being battery-powered and small enough to be carried on the body.

The static maxi devices have neither power nor volume constraints, and consequently, they can have considerable processing and storage capacities. Examples of static maxi devices are as follows: visualization devices for systems related to entertainment, secu-rity, Internet access, information displays, or home decoration (e.g., TVs, different kinds of displays and wall panels, or smart displays); white goods appliances such as fridges, dishwashers, hobs, extractors, freezers, ovens, cookers, washing machines, microwaves, or a set of innumerable small devices dedicated to very specific and heterogeneous tasks (e.g., pressure cookers, coffee pots, toasters, mixers, hair dryers, deep fryers, or small electric heaters or radiators); comfort devices, such as air-conditioning or radiators; light genera-tors; or domotics components with new features in security, communication, power man-agement, comfort, and user interface.

Other classes of devices that are being included in AAL environments arose during the last few years. It is accepted that networked, ubiquitous robotic systems that convey data and physical actions (e.g., motion and forces) can pave the way to innovative prod-ucts. Based on analysis of the capabilities of various types of robots, enormous possibili-ties to use their capacity to interact with humans within AAL systems can be foreseen (ISTAG 2009).

Context Awareness

Context awareness is part of human nature. Consciously or unconsciously our actions and behaviors are dependent on a particular circumstance, the context, which is dependent on perceptual information (e.g., environmental, physical, or social) or nonperceptual information (e.g., memories of past experiences or emotional states) (Hoareau and Satoh 2009). The idea of context-aware computing is a fundamental topic in both the AAL and AmI paradigms.

Context is any information that can be used to characterize the situation of an entity. An entity is a person, place, or object that is considered relevant to the interaction between a user and a system, including the user and system themselves, such as contextual information related to devices (e.g., available memory, computation power, or communication quality), information that describes an individual (e.g., localization, personal, system, or social context), or contextual information related to the physical environment of an entity (e.g., device, room, building, or user) (IST Amigo Project 2005a).

The context should be abstracted, because it may depend on the sensors that acquire it, and it must be represented, managed, and used in relevant data structures and algorithms to be processed by context-aware systems. Therefore, currently, there are some interesting context modeling approaches being researched, which, when matured, may provide mechanisms to effectively model context (IST Amigo Project 2005a). Those mechanisms should constitute a central component of the context awareness management, which has to be shared by many systems and has to be understandable, unambiguous, and manipulated by various parties within a widely distributed system (Hoareau and Satoh 2009; IST Amigo Project 2005a).

In technological terms, context awareness is a property of a system that uses context to provide relevant information and/or systems to the user, where relevancy depends on the user's task. Therefore, the context awareness management should provide the basic functionality required to develop systems allowing people and other systems to stay aware of any significant change in context with minimal effort. As an example, the system should be able to keep track of changes in various types of context (e.g., activities or presence of people) or provide notifications with appropriate rendering of intensity, based on the user's preferences and current context (IST Amigo Project 2005b).

User Interaction

User modeling and profiling is essential for designing the user interaction management of AAL environments. User modeling and profiling provides the methodology to enhance the effectiveness and usability of systems and interfaces in order to (IST Amigo Project 2005b) (1) adapt interface features to the user and the context in which it is used; (2) tailor information presentation to the user and the context; (3) predict the user's future behavior; and (4) indicate interface and information presentation features for their adaptation to a multiuser environment.

User modeling is a very broad research area with decades of historical development. In general, the concept of user modeling addresses issues of understanding users in order to make a system useful and make user–system interactions user-friendly and universal. Different concepts of user modeling can be considered—including design-time adaptation of the system to dynamically respond in different ways depending on the user's behavior (IST Amigo Project 2005b), customization by the users who can select different options related with the functionality of the interaction, or user model-based adaptation—in which the system observes the user's behavior and adaptively modifies its interactive behavior online as a function of the data gathered (IST Amigo Project 2005b).

As a variety of users may operate the system, a user model is a representation of the properties of a particular user or group of users. More simply, user models serve as a description of the users of a system and a prediction of how they will behave and perform tasks. These goals are achieved by constructing, maintaining, and exploiting user models and profiles, which are explicit representations of an individual user's preferences.

AAL systems should be able to interact intelligently with humans. Through analogy with person-to-person communication, person-to-machine interaction modalities can be defined according to their relation with our five senses or their equivalent in existing technologies.

Some senses are poorly exploited by existing technologies, for example taste and smell, whereas other senses are very rich, like sight and touch. Some concrete examples for every possible sense and associated modality (IST Amigo Project 2005a) are as follows: (1) sound—any type of audible sound may be used for direct or implicit interactions; (2) sight—vision offers the widest range of possibilities concerning user interactions; (3) touch—the tactile sense can make information such as pressure level, temperature level, and recognition of surface textures available; and (4) combining modalities.

In an AAL environment, the user interface management encompasses several related systems, such as a multimodal dialogue manager and systems supporting interaction via specific modalities (including tangible user interfaces, natural anthropocentric input/output devices, natural language understanding, or augmented objects). The focus of the user interface components is to support the interaction on multiple smart artifacts with intuitive and natural interfaces that are multimodal and effectively humanized. Usability and comprehension by end users are crucial in order to create engaging and coherent experiences for the users (IST Amigo Project 2005b). Developing adaptive, natural, and multimodal human–computer interfaces is one of the main challenges of AAL (Kleinberger et al. 2007).

Privacy and Security

AAL environments are equipped with multimedia sensors such as cameras and microphones, and the users' activities are permanently monitored (Al Bouna et al. 2009). This presents several problems due to the fact that different networks (generally deployed and then left unattended) are mixed in order to provide such environments. All these aspects joined together make it unfeasible to directly apply the traditional security mechanisms, which means that the privacy and security components of AAL environments pose a heterogeneous set of new challenges (Bogdan et al. 2008).

Systems

Since as people age, their quality of life is largely determined by their ability to maintain autonomy and independence, the AAL concept intends to develop AAL systems to enable active aging at home, workplace, and community; to contribute to the autonomy, independence, and quality of life of elderly people; to improve the participation of the elderly in social activities; and to reduce the costs of health systems and social support systems.

The development of these systems demands definition of the requirements of different users' profiles (e.g., older adults, their relatives, and their formal and informal care

providers), different types of tasks, and different usage contexts. Furthermore, it is important to consider that assistive devices and human systems interactively work together to
express potentials from both sides providing high-quality systems to people with needs
(Sun et al. 2009). Effective and efficient solutions to meet the AAL challenges should combine forces from both the technological and societal parts. Although informal caregivers
are inherently very dynamic (their availabilities are continuously changing), they may
help fully express the potential of smart devices (reducing the needed social resources) but
maintain the social connections.

Methods

The objective of this chapter is to review the literature on AAL published since 2007 and
describe the main features and areas of products or systems that interlink and improve
new or existing technologies and systems. In the following, we will describe the methodology used to conduct this systematic review.

Data Sources and Searches

Studies were sought using health databases (PubMed, Web of Science, Academic Search
Complete, and Science Direct) and engineering and technology databases (Cite Seer and
IEEE Xplore). Two keywords were used without language restriction: *ambient assisted living*
as this was the main focus of this review and *ambient intelligence* because AAL is a subarea of AmI. This means that technologies such as user interaction or context awareness
that are classified as AmI technologies are also used in AAL. However, not all the AmI
systems are considered AAL systems. The search was performed on the 23rd of February
2011 and included all references published since 1st January 2007. This data limit, which
was established as 2007, was the year the Joint Programme *Ambient Assisted Living* from the
European Union was proposed (European Union 2007).

Study Selection

To be included in this review, studies must have defined innovative concepts or characterized innovative technologies, products, or systems, with the aim of enabling people with
specific demands to live longer in their natural environment. Therefore, for the purpose
of this review, AAL was defined as intelligent systems of assistance for a better and safer
life (Decision No. 742/2008/EC). Studies were excluded if they were concerned with legal
and ethical issues, market studies, or assessment of AAL systems that, albeit related with
AAL, did not meet the inclusion criteria. However, these articles were classified and their
references indicated for further reading. Titles and abstracts were screened by Alexandra
Queirós (AQ) and Anabela G. Silva (AGS) against eligibility criteria.

Study Characterization

After the initial screening, abstracts were subclassified by AQ, AGS, and Nelson Pacheco
Rocha (NPR) into one of seven areas: (1) architectures and frameworks, (2) physical
devices, (3) context awareness, (4) user interaction, (5) privacy and security, (6) systems,

and (7) conceptual papers. These areas are in accordance with the literature review in the "Background" section, and the operational definitions used in this review are as follows:

- *Architectures and frameworks*: Abstraction of the structure and rules needed to reason about AAL systems and how to implement them, including different middleware approaches. In this class, we also included all articles dealing with methodologies required to enable efficient, engineering, deployment, and runtime management of ALL systems (Bavafa and Navidi 2010).

- *Physical devices*: All the hardware components required for the implementation of an AAL system. In this review, the articles classified as dealing with physical devices are those that describe networks of sensors and actuators required to collect and disseminate a range of environment data (Snijders 2005).

- *Context awareness*: Includes all articles dealing with technologies and methodologies to abstract and model the situation of a person, place, or object considered relevant to the interaction between a user and a system (IST Amigo Project 2005a).

- *User interaction*: Articles dealing with technologies and methodologies to enhance the effectiveness and usability of a system and its interfaces (IST Amigo Project 2005a).

- *Privacy and security*: Articles dealing with the privacy and security challenges imposed by the AAL implementation, including those related to the continuous monitoring of users (despite their mobility) using a broad range of sensors (such as cameras and microphones) and whose gathered data are transmitted by various interlinked networks (Al Bouna et al. 2007; Bogdan et al. 2008).

- *Systems*: The articles classified in this class describe practical AAL systems applied in a specified context and with a well-defined aim (Sun et al. 2009).

- *Conceptual papers*: Articles describing innovative concepts related to the AAL or that may contribute to its development.

Considering that the final aim of AAL is to develop systems to enhance people's quality of life, it was decided to do a more detailed analysis of the articles classified as systems. These were characterized in terms of author, users, setting, objective, area of system, and project status.

Results and Discussion

The database searches resulted in 2427 references, of which 462 were duplicates and 1067 did not meet the inclusion criteria and were excluded. Thus, a total of 875 references were included in this review (Figure 2.2).

Excluded Articles

Among the excluded articles, there were 28 that, despite not meeting the previously defined inclusion criteria, were related to AAL and we decided to include their references for further reading. These were on topics concerning ethical and legal issues ($n = 18$), market studies ($n = 8$), and assessment of AAL systems ($n = 2$) (Table 2.1).

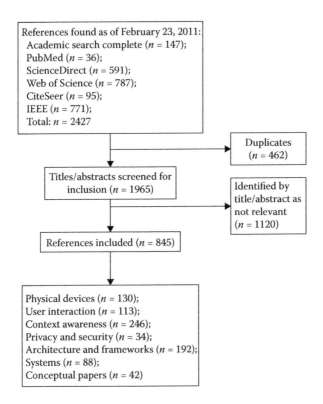

FIGURE 2.2
Flowchart for systematic review.

TABLE 2.1

Excluded Articles on AAL

Area	References of Articles That Did Not Meet the Inclusion Criteria but Are Related with AAL
Ethical and legal issues	Botella et al. 2009; De Hert et al. 2009; Fugger et al. 2007; Hildebrandt and Koops 2010; Kosta et al. 2008, 2010; Le Métayer and Monteleone 2009; Lehikoinen et al. 2008; Pedraza et al. 2010a,b; Poullet 2009; Remmers 2010; Rialle 2009; Soede et al. 2007; Spiru et al. 2009; van Dijk 2009, 2010; Wright et al. 2009
Market studies	Grauel and Spellerberg 2008; Gruber et al. 2009; Khan and Markopoulos 2009; Khan et al. 2010; Noh and Kim 2010; Rocker 2009, 2010; Ziefle and Rocker 2010
Assessment of AAL systems	Barbieri et al. 2010; Connelly et al. 2008

Included Articles

Of the 845 included studies, 192 (23%) were classified as architectures and frameworks, 130 (15%) as physical devices, 246 (29%) as referring to context awareness, 113 (13%) as user interaction, 34 (4%) as related to privacy and security, 88 (11%) as systems, and 42 (5%) as conceptual papers defining innovative concepts. The higher number of publications on context awareness may be related to the knowledge that individual performance is affected not only by individual abilities but also by the characteristics of the environment, which can either facilitate or hinder this performance (World Health Organisation 2001).

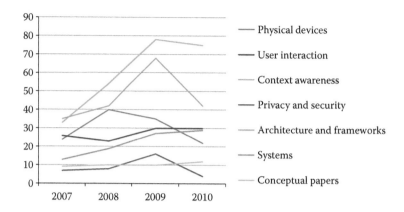

FIGURE 2.3
AAL articles output according to area of classification and year of publication.

When analyzing the publication output by year of publication, it increases from 2007 to 2009 and then decreases in 2010, with the exception of the number of publications on systems, user interaction, and conceptual papers, which are relatively stable or increase slightly from 2009 to 2010 (Figure 2.3). The decrease in the publication output from 2009 to 2010 may be related to the fact that there is usually a boom of researchers when a novel area of research appears. However, after a few years, the initial number of researchers tends to decrease. Another possible explanation is related to the need to rethink the approach regarding AAL research. For example, there is a lot of technology that needs to be reevaluated and the possible integration of the existing components needs to be assessed, instead of developing new components.

Architectures and Frameworks

Articles on architectures and frameworks covered topics such as (1) architecture ($n = 152$), (2) design and development methodologies ($n = 37$), and (3) safety ($n = 3$). Examples of the analyzed articles follow.

Architecture

The development of intelligent environments is a complex challenge. This complexity arises, in part, from the amount of different devices that need to be seamlessly integrated in a common and homogeneous environment, despite the fact of each device having its own characteristics. This represents a challenge and Carneiro et al. (2010) proposed a three-step approach to solve it in which components are used during all the development process, playing undoubtedly a much more preponderant role and making the path from specification to implementation a much easier and controllable one.

Another example is the work of Coronato and De Pietro (2010) whose article presents a system-oriented middleware architecture for safety critical AmI systems. This architecture provides systems that enable the designer to develop runtime verification mechanisms.

Design and Development Methodologies

Despite advances in software engineering methods and tools, understanding what software components do and ensuring that they work well together remains difficult. Examples of methodologies described in the revised articles included a model-driven development approach that combines unified modeling language (UML) and ontology techniques for the specification of component properties and development platforms that support component discovery, compatibility checking and deployment, and designing of digital ecosystems that integrate a number of different and complementary technologies, including agent-based and self-organizing systems, ontologies, swarm intelligence, AmI, data mining, and genetic algorithms (Floch et al. 2010; Hadzic and Chang 2010).

Safety

As we move to the age of smart homes, the more reliant an individual, for instance the elderly and ill, becomes on such environments, the more reliable the system must be. They must operate correctly 24/7. Sterritt and Nugent (2010) proposed an autonomic computing paradigm with its vision of creating self-managing (self-configuring, self-healing, self-optimizing, and self-protecting) systems to ensure that as components fail the system itself continues to operate, increasing the reliability of the system.

Physical Devices

The physical devices described included sensor networks ($n = 75$), robotics ($n = 32$), and new technologies ($n = 24$). In general, we could verify that there were only a few papers concerning the description of new technologies. Most papers described technologies that are already used in contexts other than the AAL and that are now being applied to the AAL context.

Sensor Network

Practical systems of AmI cannot leave aside requirements about ubiquity, scalability, and transparency to the user. An enabling technology to comply with this goal is represented by wireless sensor networks. However, although capable of limited in-network processing, they lack the computational power to act as a comprehensive intelligent system (De Paola et al. 2009).

Another question discussed was the relationship between autonomy and acquisition performance. The authors suggest that it may be worthless to design extremely low power acquisition electronics, sacrificing acquisition performance, when the main power consumption comes from the wireless subsystem, which is one order of magnitude higher (Figueiredo et al. 2010).

Robotics

One of the main challenges concerning robotics is to humanize the robots. Koch et al. (2008) conceptualize a system robot as a part of an intelligent environment where the robot not only offers its own features via natural speech interaction but also becomes a transactive agent featuring other systems' interfaces. Another example is the use of a social robot as a majordomo interface between users and smart environments, focusing on the need for the robot to plan its behavior by taking into account factors that are relevant in public environments in which the robot has a *social* role (De Carolis and Cozzolongo 2007).

New Technologies

This subclass refers to specialized components and features that are necessary for the development of AAL systems.

Intelligent environments employ electronics unobtrusively integrated with the ambient to predict and to respond to the needs of people, enhancing many aspects of everyday life.

This requires the use of wearable devices, which must be small, be lightweight, and have enough power autonomy for comfortable operation and wide acceptance. Articles dealing with these issues included the presentation of the smallest localization device known for using on localization systems, based on a Wi-Fi infrastructure (Silva et al. 2010), or the development of sensors energetically autonomous for long periods of time (Borca-Tasciuc and Kempitiya 2010).

Context Awareness

Abstracts describing context awareness technologies were subclassified into (1) environment (n = 18), (2) location/tracking (n = 32), (3) identity management (n = 12), (4) identity management and location (n = 8), (5) detection of specific events and situations (n = 18), (6) activity/interaction (n = 41), (7) human behavior (n = 25), (8) emotions (n = 10), and (9) reasoning (n = 82).

As an attempt to illustrate what is being done in the area of context awareness, we will give some examples from the analyzed articles.

Environment

Environment is considered a key determinant of human function as activities are determined by the context in which they take place. Work has been presented that considers the context information and uses it to inform technologies that can be dynamically enriched and extended by the discovered objects in the environment and able to reason over it (Almeida et al. 2009). Another example is the work of Cacciagrano et al. (2010) who proposed a ResourceHome, an innovative radio frequency identification (RFID) framework to locate objects in delimited environments and statically prevent/detect dangerous spatial/temporal configurations, i.e., configurations firing dangerous interactions of properties among objects.

Location/Tracking

Technologies regarding the location and tracking of individuals included a set of design structures for solving different problems related to mobility, such as location sensing and behavior adaptation, together with the design rationale underlying them (Fortier et al. 2010; Kohler et al. 2010).

Detection of Specific Events and Situations

Elderly people are at a higher risk of in-house accidents. Therefore, there is an increasing need for AAL systems, such as technologies that are capable of detecting falls and consequently of raising an alarm. Hartmann et al. (2010) built a robust and intelligent system that estimates the position of humans using only one camera. The position is used to detect falls and allows an immediate call for help. Other technological approaches integrate a fall detector prototype that includes two different sensors: a 3D time-of-flight range camera and a wearable micro-electro mechanical systems (MEMS) accelerometer (Siciliano et al. 2009).

Activity/Interaction

Activity/interaction included technologies related to instance-based algorithms to infer user activities on the basis of data acquired from body-worn accelerometer sensors (Bicocchi et al. 2010) and systems to recognize a whole sequence of activities with different durations (Mirarmandehi and Rabiee 2010), instead of the usual recognition of single activities with equal durations, among others.

Human Behavior

Ubiquitous computing research has extended traditional environments in the so-called intelligent environments. All of them use their capabilities for pursuing their inhabitants' satisfaction, but the ways of getting it are most of the time unclear and frequently unshared among different users. This last problem becomes obvious in shared environments in which users with different preferences live together. A possible way of helping to solve this is presented by Garcia-Herranz et al. (2009) who present a solution translating human hierarchies to the ubiquitous computing domain, in a continuing effort for leveraging the control capabilities of the inhabitants in their on-growing capable environments.

Emotions

The evidence suggests that human actions are supported by emotional elements that complement logic inference in our decision-making processes. However, this seems to be a new area of research and includes the use of technology (e.g., a context-aware yet situation-adaptive Bayesian inference framework) to predict human mental states in varying contexts (Abbasi et al. 2010). Evidence suggests positive effects of emotional information on the ability of intelligent agents to create better models of user actions inside smart homes (Leon et al. 2010).

Reasoning

Articles on reasoning technologies approached topics such as the combined use of different technologies to predict users' affective and cognitive states (Kapoor 2010) or the use of a reasoner at runtime to infer context knowledge that is not directly observable and that can be used by machine learning algorithms to give support to the system adaptation according to the contextual information (Serral et al. 2010).

User Interaction

The articles on user interaction included (1) new interfaces ($n = 53$), (2) personalized information ($n = 7$), (3) design ($n = 45$), and (4) evaluation ($n = 11$). The following topics present some examples illustrating this classification.

New Interfaces

Technology users are becoming more and more demanding, leading to the development of new ways of human–technology interaction. One of the user requirements is the use of interfaces that are embedded in the environment in a way that the technologies and systems are part of it. Examples of articles dealing with this issue include the use of tangible user interfaces to build a cognitive assistant for activities of daily living in the form of an interactive table in a kitchen. Interactions are modeled with token and constraints paradigm, which may allow the user to have a better experience and to be more independent (Boussemart and Giroux 2007). Other examples are the development of a perceived touch interaction through tagging context aiming to minimize the user's interactive effort (Chavira et al. 2010) and the speaker recognition and system in smart environments (Garipelli et al. 2008).

Personalized Information

New interfaces may be a means of adjusting the way information is presented to the characteristics and requirements of the user contributing to the personalization of the information. Mulvenna et al. (2011) illustrate how algorithms are required to contextualize and convey information across location and time, adjusting it to the needs of the differing end-user groups using work on nighttime AAL systems for people with dementia. Roa et al. (2009) personalize a system and a real-time knowledge generation from a distributed architecture including a sensor layer and computational models.

Design

Employing user-centered design principles along with systems engineering methodology to the development of smarter products has the potential of establishing a novel field of research. An example of this is a novel user-centered human factor knowledge management framework for collaborative design and modeling of the next generation of smarter products, introduced by Ahram et al. (2010).

Evaluation

Elderly people often experience difficulties in using modern information and communication technologies. Therefore, a key step in the development of any new technology is its evaluation that will inform on user acceptance and further development of the technology. Examples of technologies evaluated in the revised articles included an intuitive mobile environment controller, which aims to provide the user with mobile access to their physical environment and ambient media (Shirehjini 2007), and a touch screen–based Internet videophone (Oberzaucher et al. 2009).

Privacy and Security

AAL systems require that issues of security and privacy consider both the individual and the context to provide the user with adequate support. However, there were not clearly distinct areas of research within this topic. Thus, articles were not subclassified.

Articles included in this topic dealt with subjects such as multifold security challenges involved in the implementation of remote health care in smart homes (Busnel et al. 2008) or approaches to model dynamic changes in AmI scenarios using the Automated Validation of Internet Security Protocols and Systems model-checking tool suite (Munoz et al. 2009).

Systems

A total of 88 references were classified as systems. As AAL is related to the complex interaction of a variety of technology and system components with the aim of enhancing people's life, we decided to perform a more detailed analysis of the articles classified as systems as referred in the methodology.

The users were classified considering who will use the information provided by the system. For example, if the system provided information on patients' vital signs, this information was intended to be used by the health professional to improve the care delivered to the patient. Therefore, the user is the health professional. Who will use the information provided by the system was firstly classified into caregivers ($n = 24$), clients ($n = 59$), and caregivers/clients ($n = 5$).

The user was considered to be a caregiver if the system is to be used by anyone taking care of a patient such as a family member or any nonhealth professional ($n = 15$) or a health professional (i.e., medical personnel, including nurses, paramedics, and physicians) ($n = 9$).

Clients were classified into (1) a layperson if the article describes a system that is to be used by the individual in general independently of whether it is a patient with a specific medical condition or it belongs to a specific age group ($n = 37$), (2) elderly ($n = 16$), (3) patient ($n = 4$), and (4) people with disabilities ($n = 2$).

Considering the principles of the AAL, it is not surprising that most systems are intended to be used by the layperson, in particular, the elderly (Tables 2.2, 2.3, and 2.4). This is in line with the AAL solutions that claim to use the AmI concept and technologies to enable people with specific demands to live longer in their natural environment.

Considering the goal of the systems, the articles were classified into health, participation, participation/health, and security, as shown in Table 2.5.

TABLE 2.2

Articles Classified as Systems Where the Users Are Caregivers

Detailed User	Article
Health professionals	Alcaniz et al. 2009; Anmin et al. 2009; Bajo et al. 2009; Barcaro et al. 2007; Fanucci et al. 2009; Fernandes et al. 2010; Havasi and Kiss 2008; López-Matencio et al. 2010; Sehgal et al. 2007
Caregivers	Aung et al. 2010; Bono-Nuez et al. 2009; Bravo et al. 2008b, 2009a; Carneiro et al. 2009; Cascado et al. 2010; Chuan-Jun and Bo-Jung 2010; Corchado et al. 2008; Costa et al. 2007, 2009b,c; Grossi et al. 2009; Hui-Huang et al. 2009, 2010; Murgoitio and Fernandez 2008; Zaad and Allouch 2008

TABLE 2.3

Articles Classified as Systems Where the Users Are Caregivers and Clients

Detailed User	Article
Caregivers and clients	Valera et al. 2009
Caregivers and elderly	Boulos et al. 2007; Dohr et al. 2010a
Caregivers and people with disabilities	Kleinberger et al. 2009
Health professionals and patients with diabetes	Bal and Schwarz 2010

TABLE 2.4

Articles Classified as Systems Where the Users Are Clients

Detailed User	Article
Layperson	Ahn 2010; Arroyo et al. 2008a; Blesa et al. 2009; Borrego-Jaraba et al. 2010; Costa et al. 2010; Cui et al. 2009; Delgado et al. 2009; Dohr et al. 2010b; Fayn and Rubel 2010; Haosheng et al. 2009; Hopmann et al. 2008; Hossain et al. 2007; Iqbal et al. 2009; Kastner et al. 2010; Keegan et al. 2008; Knoll 2009; Krieg-Brückner et al. 2010; Kuhn et al. 2008; Kyung-Seok et al. 2010; Lazaro et al. 2010; Lee et al. 2010; Lindenberg et al. 2007; Maier and Kempter 2009; Martin et al. 2008; Mingjing and Yang 2008a,b; Paganelli et al. 2007; Pauws et al. 2008; Pawlowski et al. 2008; Pizzutilo et al. 2007; Schurmann and Volk 2008; Sparacino 2008; Torres-Solis and Chau 2007; Valiente-Rocha and Lozano-Tello 2010; Vansteenwegen et al. 2011; Yo-Ping et al. 2009; Yu et al. 2008
Patients	Costa et al. 2009a; Ferguson et al. 2010; Spanoudakis et al. 2010
Elderly	Aviles-Lopez et al. 2009; Boll et al. 2010; Busuoli et al. 2007; Costa et al. 2009b; Kantorovitch et al. 2009; Niemela et al. 2007; Plischke and Kohls 2009; Romero et al. 2010; Sun et al. 2007; Wei-Lun et al. 2007
Elderly and people with disabilities	Andrejkova et al. 2010; Casas et al. 2008; Falco et al. 2010; Huertas et al. 2010; Isomursu et al. 2009; Jingwen et al. 2009
Elderly and adults	Dadlani et al. 2011
People with disabilities	Alonso et al. 2009; Chang and Wang 2010

TABLE 2.5

Articles Classified as Systems by Area of Use

Area	Article
Health	Alcaniz et al. 2009; Anmin et al. 2009; Aung et al. 2010; Bajo et al. 2009; Bal and Schwarz 2010; Barcaro et al. 2007; Bono-Nuez et al. 2009; Boulos et al. 2007; Bravo et al. 2008b, 2009a; Carneiro et al. 2009; Cascado et al. 2010; Chuan-Jun and Bo-Jung 2010; Corchado et al. 2008; Costa et al. 1999, 2007, 2009a,b; Dohr et al. 2010a; Fanucci et al. 2009; Fernandes et al. 2010; Grossi et al. 2009; Havasi and Kiss 2008; Hui-Huang et al. 2009, 2010; Jingwen et al. 2009; Murgoitio and Fernandez 2008; Plischke and Kohls 2009; Sehgal et al. 2007; Spanoudakis et al. 2010; Valera et al. 2009; Wei-Lun et al. 2007; Zaad and Allouch 2008
Participation	Ahn 2010; Alonso et al. 2009; Andrejkova et al. 2010; Arroyo et al. 2008b; Aviles-Lopez et al. 2009; Borrego-Jaraba et al. 2010; Blesa et al. 2009; Boll et al. 2010; Casas et al. 2008; Chang and Wang 2010; Costa et al. 2010; Cui et al. 2009; Dohr et al. 2010b; Falco et al. 2010; Fayn and Rubel 2010; Ferguson et al. 2010; Guo and Zhao 2008; Haosheng et al. 2009; Hopmann et al. 2008; Hossain et al. 2007; Huertas et al. 2010; Iqbal et al. 2009; Isomursu et al. 2009; Kantorovitch et al. 2009; Kastner et al. 2010; Keegan et al. 2008; Knoll 2009; Krieg-Brückner et al. 2010; Kyung-Seok et al. 2010; Lazaro et al. 2010; Lee et al. 2010; Lindenberg et al. 2007; López-Matencio et al. 2010; Maier and Kempter 2009; Martin et al. 2008; Mingjing and Yang 2008a,b; Niemela et al. 2007; Paganelli et al. 2007; Pauws et al. 2008; Pawlowski et al. 2008; Pizzutilo et al. 2007; Romero et al. 2010; Sparacino 2008; Sun et al. 2007; Torres-Solis and Chau 2007; Valiente-Rocha and Lozano-Tello 2010; Vansteenwegen et al. 2011; Yo-Ping et al. 2009; Yu et al. 2008
Participation/health	Busuoli et al. 2007; Kleinberger et al. 2009; Tocino et al. 2009
Security	Dadlani et al. 2011; Delgado et al. 2009

Most systems were intended for use both indoors and outdoors in any environment (setting specified as anywhere; $n = 44$) or at home ($n = 30$). This may be related to an attempt to improve people's life in their natural environment. The system described by Chuan-Jun and Bo-Jung (2010) is to be used in an outdoor environment and allows the location of the elderly anywhere in the community. This system aims to provide more responsive and personalized care systems through the development of a Smart Community Care System based on the concept of AmI using RFID and mobile agent technologies. Caregivers may locate care receivers easily in a community with RFID while mobile agent furnishes timely and accurate information for the care provision. The Monitor de Salud Personal (Tocino et al. 2009) is one example of a system to be used indoors. It aims to explore various enabling technologies based on environmental intelligence by means of which the user interacts with his or her home in various scenarios: home assistance and well-being, entertainment, identity management, and location management.

Only a very small number of systems were designed to be used in both health care and care centers ($n = 9$). A possible explanation may be related to the European health directives, which highlight the need to empower patients on matters concerning their health through the promotion of self-care (Broek et al. 2008). Only one article referred to a system to be used at educational settings, and another system was to be used while driving a car.

Systems were conceived to be used in a variety of areas with the general aim of directly or indirectly improving people's quality of life. Most systems were conceived to help care delivery either by health professionals (health care delivery, $n = 14$) or by any formal or nonformal caregiver (care delivery, $n = 16$). Most of these aimed at monitoring and controlling biological signs and behaviors such as heart rate, electrocardiograph, or falls. The ultimate goal is to provide the caregiver with accurate, up-to-date information so that the right care can be delivered at the right time. The remaining systems are on very diverse areas with very diverse objectives such as education, physical activities, participation, participation and health, tourism, culture, self-care, shopping, mobility, and entertainment (Figure 2.4).

Regarding the scope of the systems, 53 were classified as participation, 33 as health, and 2 as security. Interestingly, the highest number of articles describes fundamental activities like participation in community events (15), self-care (8), or mobility (6). This may indicate that systems try to solve first the fundamental activities of an individual (Figure 2.4). However, a few studies also deal with other activities more related to quality of life (physical activities or tourism). These studies use technologies that take advantage of existing knowledge on context awareness. For example, considering the use of context awareness technology in shopping activities, the research presented by Ahn (2010) is a novel approach to evaluating customer aid functions with agent-based models of customer behavior and evolutionary strategies. Agent-based modeling is used to imitate users' rational behavior at Internet stores with regard to browsing and collecting product information. It is assumed that users evolve their browsing skill and strategy over time to maximize the efficiency and effectiveness of their shopping, and hence, evolutionary strategy, an optimization method, is combined with the agent-based model to find the rational behavior of each user.

Four stages of project status were distinguished: conceptualization, prototype, trial, and regular operation (Tables 2.6, 2.7, 2.8, and 2.9). As far as it was possible to tell from the articles' abstract, more than half ($n = 55$) are still in the conceptualization phase, 26 articles were classified as prototype, while only 5 were tested in a field trial, and 2 are in regular operation (Figure 2.5).

Of all the 88 abstracts classified as systems, 11 articles describe systems showing a higher level of complexity (Table 2.10) when compared to the systems described in the remaining 77 articles. The less complex systems included the reutilization of an existing technology or a new technology in order to create systems in a new field and with a very specific aim, for example the use of robotics to assist the elderly in daily activities. The more complex systems relate to the integration of several less complex systems or technologies applied in a specific field but with broader aims. One of the examples is the system described by Bravo et al. (2009a) that is to be used in a day center or at home to monitor the behavior and vital signs of a patient with Alzheimer's disease. This information is then sent to caregivers so that they are able to identify emergency situations and provide patients with the appropriate care. However, the system is also used to assist patients in daily activities in order to promote their autonomy.

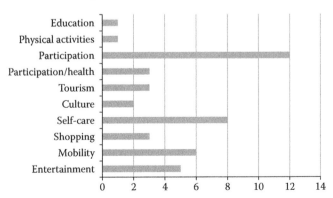

FIGURE 2.4
Distribution of articles by area.

TABLE 2.6

Articles Classified as Conceptualization Models by Setting

Setting	Article
Health and care centers	Cascado et al. 2010; Corchado et al. 2008; Costa et al. 2007, 2009b,c; Wei-Lun et al. 2007
Care centers/home	Bravo et al. 2008b, 2009b
Home	Alonso et al. 2009; Andrejkova et al. 2010; Anmin et al. 2009; Bal and Schwarz 2010; Blesa et al. 2009; Boll et al. 2010; Bono-Nuez et al. 2009; Busuoli et al. 2007; Casas et al. 2008; Dadlani et al. 2011; Delgado et al. 2009; Falco et al. 2010; Fanucci et al. 2009; Grossi et al. 2009; Haosheng et al. 2009; Havasi and Kiss 2008; Hopmann et al. 2008; Hui-Huang et al. 2009, 2010; Iqbal et al. 2010; Jingwen et al. 2009; Kastner et al. 2010; Kleinberger et al. 2009; Maier and Kempter 2009; Niemela et al. 2007; Spanoudakis et al. 2010; Torres-Solis and Chau 2007; Valera et al. 2009; Valiente-Rocha et al. 2010; Zaad and Allouch 2008
Anywhere	Ahn 2010; Alcaniz et al. 2009; Arroyo et al. 2008b; Aung et al. 2010; Aviles-Lopez et al. 2009; Borrego-Jaraba et al. 2010; Boulos et al. 2007; Carneiro et al. 2009; Chang and Wang 2010; Chuan-Jun and Bo-Jung 2010; Costa et al. 2009b, 2010; Cui et al. 2009; Dohr et al. 2010a,b; Fayn and Rubel 2010; Ferguson et al. 2010; Fernandes et al. 2010; Guo and Zhao 2008; Guo et al. 2010; Hossain et al. 2007; Huertas et al. 2010; Isomursu et al. 2009; Kantorovitch et al. 2009; Keegan et al. 2008; Knoll 2009; Krieg-Brückner et al. 2010; Kyung-Seok et al. 2010; Lazaro et al. 2010; Lee et al. 2010; Lindenberg et al. 2007; López-Matencio et al. 2010; Martin et al. 2008; Mingjing and Yang 2008a,b; Paganelli et al. 2007; Pauws et al. 2008; Pizzutilo et al. 2007; Plischke and Kohls 2009; Romero et al. 2010; Sparacino 2008; Sun et al. 2007; Vansteenwegen et al. 2011; Yo-Ping et al. 2009; Yu et al. 2008

TABLE 2.7

Articles Classified as Prototype by Setting

Setting	Article
Health care centers	Bajo et al. 2009; Barcaro et al. 2007; Sehgal et al. 2007
Home	Andrejkova et al. 2010; Anmin et al. 2009; Boll et al. 2010; Busuoli et al. 2007; Grossi et al. 2009; Havasi and Kiss 2008; Hui-Huang et al. 2010; Iqbal et al. 2010; Torres-Solis and Chau 2007
Anywhere	Borrego-Jaraba et al. 2010; Carneiro et al. 2009; Chang and Wang 2010; Dohr et al. 2010b; Ferguson et al. 2010; Keegan et al. 2008; Krieg-Brückner et al. 2010; Kyung-Seok et al. 2010; Lindenberg et al. 2007; Paganelli et al. 2007; Pauws et al. 2008
Car	Murgoitio and Fernandez 2008
School	Pawlowski et al. 2008

TABLE 2.8

Articles Classified as Being Tested in Field Trials by Setting

Setting	Article
Home	Dadlani et al. 2011; Kleinberger et al. 2009; Maier and Kempter 2009; Niemela et al. 2007; Zaad and Allouch 2008

TABLE 2.9

Articles Classified as Being in Regular Operation by Setting

Setting	Article
Care centers	Corchado et al. 2008
Anywhere	Vansteenwegen et al. 2011

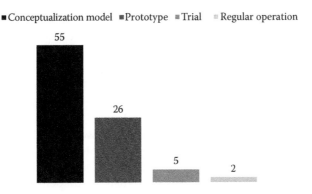

FIGURE 2.5
Four stages of project status.

TABLE 2.10

Articles Classified as AAL Systems

Objective	Article
Diagnose, prevent, and treat patients with diabetes mellitus	Bal and Schwarz 2010
Personal assistant	Boll et al. 2010
Complement and support daily activities	Casas et al. 2008
Promote well-being and health	Busuoli et al. 2007; Tocino et al. 2009
Monitor and collect vital signals	Dadlani et al. 2011
Promote autonomy	Niemela et al. 2007
Promote participation	Romero et al. 2010
Assist tourism	Vansteenwegen et al. 2011

Conceptual Papers

A total of 42 articles were classified as conceptual papers defining innovative concepts on the following areas: sensor networks ($n = 2$), user interaction ($n = 6$), technology development ($n = 6$), context awareness ($n = 2$), living lab ($n = 5$), and future challenges for the AAL systems ($n = 21$). The following topics present some examples illustrating this classification.

Sensor Networks

Bouet and Pujolle (2010) present the potential and challenges on the use of RFID in health care. Firstly, they state the required RFID infrastructure and its impact on the patient life cycle. Then, based on this description, they identify and discuss issues of large deployments, such as privacy, localization, and interference with medical devices, and also middleware systems to integrate this technology within multimedia and body area networks.

User Interaction

Bulut and Narayanan (2010) discuss implementation issues and challenges conducted in speech synthesis systems and the components necessary to incorporate AmI characteristics in them. Different and new interfaces, in combination with mobile technologies, can have tremendous implications for accessibility and can be of benefit for most people. An important issue is that interfaces must be accessible, useful, and usable (Holzinger et al. 2008).

Technology Development

New discoveries in materials of the nanometer-length scale are expected to play an important role in addressing ongoing and future challenges in the field of communication. Devices and systems for ultra-high-speed short- and long-range communication links, portable and power-efficient computing devices, high-density memory and logics, ultrafast interconnects, and autonomous and robust energy scavenging devices for accessing AmI and needed information will critically depend on the success of next-generation emerging nanomaterials and devices. Islam and Logeeswaran (2010) present some exciting recent developments in nanomaterials that have the potential to play a critical role in the development and transformation of future intelligent communication networks.

As data content mushrooms and becomes increasingly dispersed, the demand and need for bandwidth, both wired and wireless, continues to increase. Foty (2007) discusses the use of millimeter-wave radio as a way to transcend the *digital mindset* and addresses a wide variety of bandwidth challenges.

Context Awareness

Mastrogiovanni et al. (2008) elaborates on context assessment strategies for smart homes and, in a broader perspective, for context-aware cognitive systems. He proposes a framework, called functionalism, that aims at integrating ontology and logic approaches to context modeling.

Living Lab

Un and Price (2007) discuss AAL systems and the processes and practices regarding innovation within an organization, rather than the adoption of innovation by users or the rate of the adoption of a marketed solution. Panek and Zagler (2008) address the importance of taking into account the needs of future users of AAL systems that they suggest can be achieved by involving them right from the beginning of the process.

Future Challenges

Articles addressing the future challenges of AAL systems discuss the promises and possible advantages of AAL, indicate the challenges that need to be met in order to develop practical and efficient AAL systems for elderly people, or propose an approach to construct effective home-care system for the elderly people (Patkos et al. 2007; Sun et al. 2009).

Conclusion

The results of this systematic review indicate that there is a great amount of literature on AAL encompassing very diverse areas as illustrated in Figure 2.6.

Included articles were first classified into one of seven areas (architectures and frameworks, physical devices, context awareness, user interaction, privacy and security, systems, and conceptual papers), which are represented in Figure 2.6 according to the number of articles classified into each one of the areas. Each one of these areas was further specified into different subareas. The subareas with more articles are shown also in Figure 2.6 with empty circles.

Most of the literature on AAL is very technology-oriented, which is reflected in the huge number of articles on specific components (89%) when compared to only 88 articles (11%)

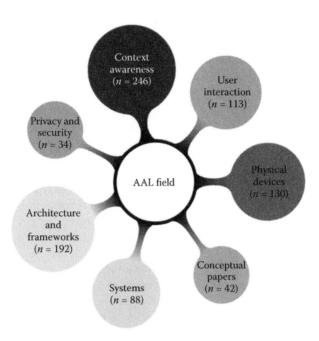

FIGURE 2.6
Included articles on AAL review.

related to complete systems. In addition, a considerable number of these 88 articles on systems focus on how technology can be used in the AAL context instead of looking at the users' needs and proposing ways in which the technology can be used to solve them. The focus is still on the technology rather than on the person. The results also show that different technologies come from different research groups with little interoperability between the AAL technologies. The environments where AAL can be used are very complex and can either use simple solutions or a combination of existing technologies. For this to happen, it is necessary that a bigger investment is made in the integration of existing technology and in their interoperability (Broek et al. 2008). This will not only provide a better answer to the existing needs but also save time and decrease costs. However, both these problems (focus on technology and lack of interoperability) require that research teams be composed of professionals with different backgrounds and skills such as health and social care professionals and engineers (transdisciplinary teams) and that all the stakeholders, including the future users, be actively involved in the process. This involvement of users will probably also facilitate the field testing of AAL technologies and promote their use, which is clearly a problem considering the small number of articles classified as describing technology tested in a trial field or already in regular operation. According to Broek et al. (2008, xiii) "common AAL platform based on selected standards which allow the interoperability of applications and services could be the basis for 3rd party services development and provision, and could stimulate the development of products at an early stage and the establishment of value chains that put into effect the business opportunities within AAL. The contradiction between user-centered system design and the need for a common application platform approach might turn out to be the central contradict and challenge for AAL in the years ahead."

A high number of systems were conceived to help care delivery either by health professionals or any formal or nonformal caregiver. This is probably related to the demographic changes occurring worldwide with the continuous aging of the population. With aging, there is a decrease in functioning associated with an increase in a variety of chronic diseases, which leads to a higher consumption of health care services (World Health Organisation 2002). This challenges the traditional health care system, and it is likely that the scarcity and costs of health resources compromise the ability of the health system to appropriately respond to a population that wants to not only live longer but also live with more autonomy and quality of life (Kairy et al. 2009). AAL technologies show promise in helping to minimize the pressure put on the health care system. It constitutes a means of providing quality health care services that reach a high number of individuals either in their natural environment or in care centers at a low cost and that are adjustable to the individual needs of each client (Kairy et al. 2009). Furthermore, AAL systems can contribute to the reorientation of health systems that are currently organized around acute, episodic experiences of disease, allowing the development of a broad range of systems such as care prevention and care promotion and home-caregiver support (PERSONA 2008). A considerable number of technologies/systems are developed for elderly users or users with disabilities, which may be related with the previously referred demographic changes and constitute an attempt to answer to the specific needs of these users. However, the emphasis probably needs to shift from specific groups of users to the general user/population by developing intelligent systems with the technology embedded in the environment that can automatically select the output and input information and mode according to the specific needs and characteristics of the users, in line with the principles of the Design for All (Bühler and Placencia-Porrero 2002). Therefore, AAL technologies would be usable by all people, regardless of their abilities, age, or health condition. This will contribute to the decrease in the price of this technology, which is one of the main barriers to its widespread use. Interestingly, an important step toward this direction is being given by using the intelligent AAL component (e.g., context awareness and user interaction) to develop technologies that consider not only the person but also the activity being performed and the context in which it is taking place. This is in line with the WHO International Classification of Functioning, which sees the environment as a crucial factor modulating the person's activity and participation as a member of the society (World Health Organisation 2001).

To summarize, this review of existing literature on AAL highlights the need to rethink the future research approach on the development of AAL systems in order to take advantage of already existing technologies and systems. The difficulty found when classifying the articles also suggests the need for a common classification that could be used to characterize existing AAL systems. Furthermore, according to what was described in the "Results and Discussion" section, the needed requirements to deliver viable, adaptive, and personalized AAL systems have still not been fulfilled. There is a general tendency to develop AAL systems from scratch with specific solutions. Therefore, there is a need for a normalized and coherent technological substratum over which AAL systems could be developed to answer the real demands of the users.

Acknowledgments

This work is part of the COMPETE—Operational Program of Competitive Factors and the European Union (FEDER) under QREN Living Usability Lab for Next Generation Networks (http://www.livinglab.pt) and QREN Primary Healthcare ALL Services (AAL4ALL).

References

Aarts, E., and F. Grotenhuis. 2009. Ambient Intelligence 2.0: Towards Synergetic Prosperity. *Ambient Intelligence, Proceedings* 5859:1–13.

Abbasi, A. R., A. Hussain, and N. V. Afzulpurkar. 2010. Towards Context-Adaptive Affective Computing. Paper read at Electrical Engineering/Electronics Computer Telecommunications and Information Technology (ECTI-CON), International Conference, 19–21 May.

Ahn, H. J. 2010. Evaluating Customer Aid Functions of Online Stores with Agent-Based Models of Customer Behavior and Evolution Strategy. *Information Sciences* 180:1555–1570.

Ahram, T. Z., W. Karwowski, and B. Amaba. 2010. User-Centered Systems Engineering Approach to Design and Modeling of Smarter Products. Paper read at System of Systems Engineering (SoSE), 5th International Conference, 22–24 June.

Al Bouna, B., R. Chbeir, and S. Marrara. 2007. A Multimedia Access Control Language for Virtual and Ambient Intelligence Environments. *SWS'07: Proceedings of the 2007 ACM Workshop on Secure Web Services*, 111–120.

Al Bouna, B., R. Chbeir, and S. Marrara. 2009. Enforcing Role Based Access Control Model with Multimedia Signatures. *Journal of Systems Architecture* 55:264–274.

Alcaniz, M., C. Botella, R. M. Banos, I. Zaragoza, and J. Guixeres. 2009. The Intelligent e-Therapy System: A New Paradigm for Telepsychology and Cybertherapy. *British Journal of Guidance and Counselling* 37:287–296.

Almeida, A., D. Lopez-de-Ipina, U. Aguilera, I. Larizgoitia, X. Laiseca, P. Orduna, and A. Barbier. 2009. An Approach to Dynamic Knowledge Extension and Semantic Reasoning in Highly-Mutable Environments. *3rd Symposium of Ubiquitous Computing and Ambient Intelligence 2008* 51:265–273.

Alonso, A. A., R. de la Rosa, L. del Val, M. I. Jimenez, and S. Franco. 2009. A Robot Controlled by Blinking for Ambient Assisted Living. *Lecture Notes in Computer Science* 5518:839–842.

Andrejkova, J., D. Simsik, and Z. Dolna. 2010. An Experience from Testing an Ambient Intelligence, Devices for Household. Paper read at Applied Machine Intelligence and Informatics (SAMI), IEEE 8th International Symposium, 28–30 January.

Anmin, J., Y. Bin, G. Morren, H. Duric, and R. M. Aarts. 2009. Performance Evaluation of a Tri-Axial Accelerometry-Based Respiration Monitoring for Ambient Assisted Living. Paper read at Engineering in Medicine and Biology Society, EMBC 2009, Annual International Conference of the IEEE, 3–6 September.

Arroyo, R. F., M. Gea, J. L. Garrido, and P. A. Haya. 2008a. Development of Ambient Intelligence Systems Based on Collaborative Task Models. *Journal of Universal Computer Science* 14:1545–1559.

Arroyo, R. F., M. Gea, J. L. Garrido, P. A. Haya, and R. M. Carro. 2008b. Authoring Social-Aware Tasks on Active Spaces. *Journal of Universal Computer Science* 14:2840–2858.

Augusto, J. C. 2008. Ambient Intelligence: Basic Concepts and Applications. *Software and Data Technologies* 10:16–26.

Aung, A. P. W., F. F. Siang, M. Jayachandran, J. Biswas, L. Jer-En, and P. Yap. 2010. Implementation of Context-Aware Distributed Sensor Network System for Managing Incontinence among Patients with Dementia. Paper read at Body Sensor Networks (BSN), International Conference, 7–9 June.

Aviles-Lopez, E., I. Villanueva-Miranda, J. A. Garcia-Macias, and L. E. Palafox-Maestre. 2009. Taking Care of Our Elders through Augmented Spaces. *La-Web: 2009 Latin American Web Congress*, 16–21.

Bajo, J., J. F. de Paz, Y. de Paz, and J. M. Corchado. 2009. Integrating Case-Based Planning and RPTW Neural Networks to Construct an Intelligent Environment for Health Care. *Expert Systems with Applications* 36:5844–5858.

Bal, N., and M. Schwarz. 2010. Ambient Assisted Living for Type 2 Diabetic Patients. Paper read at Pervasive Computing Technologies for Healthcare, 4th International Conference, 22–25 March.

Barbieri, T., P. Fraternali, A. Bianchi, and C. Tacchella. 2010. Autonomamente: Using Goal Attainment Scales to Evaluate the Impact of a Multimodal Domotic System to Support Autonomous Life of People with Cognitive Impairment. *Computers Helping People with Special Needs, Proceedings* 6179:324–331.

Barcaro, U., M. Righi, P. P. Ciullo, E. Palanca, K. Cerbioni, A. Starita, S. Di Bona, and D. Guerri. 2007. A Decision Support System for the Acquisition and Elaboration of EEG Signals: The AmI-GRID Environment. Paper read at Engineering in Medicine and Biology Society, EMBS 2007, 29th Annual International Conference of the IEEE, 22–26 August.

Bavafa, M., and N. Navidi. 2010. Towards a Reference Middleware Architecture for Ambient Intelligence Systems. Paper read at Knowledge Engineering, 8th International Conference on ICT, 24–25 November.

Berger, M., L. Dittmann, M. Caragiozidis, N. Mouratidis, C. Kavadias, and M. Loupis. 2008. A Component-Based Software Architecture—Reconfigurable Software for Ambient Intelligent Networked Services Environments. *ICSOFT 2008: Proceedings of the Third International Conference on Software and Data Technologies,* 174–179.

Bicocchi, N., M. Mamei, and F. Zambonelli. 2010. Detecting Activities from Body-Worn Accelerometers via Instance-Based Algorithms. *Pervasive and Mobile Computing* 6:482–495.

Blesa, J., P. Malagon, A. Araujo, J. M. Moya, J. C. Vallejo, J. M. de Goyeneche, E. Romero, D. Villanueva, and O. Nieto-Taladriz. 2009. Modular Framework for Smart Home Applications. *Distributed Computing, Artificial Intelligence, Bioinformatics, Soft Computing, and Ambient Assisted Living, Proceedings* 5518:695–701.

Bogdan, R., V. Ancusa, and M. Vladutiu. 2008. Fault Tolerance Issues in Non-Traditional Grids Implemented with Intelligent Agents. *ICCEE 2008: Proceedings of the 2008 International Conference on Computer and Electrical Engineering,* 912–917.

Boll, S., W. Heuten, E. M. Meyer, and M. Meis. 2010. Development of a multimodal reminder system for older persons in their residential home. *Informatics for Health and Social Care* 35:104–124.

Bono-Nuez, A., B. Martin-del-Brio, R. Blasco-Marin, R. Casas-Nebra, and A. Roy-Yarza. 2009. Quality of Life Evaluation of Elderly and Disabled People by Using Self-Organizing Maps. *Distributed Computing, Artificial Intelligence, Bioinformatics, Soft Computing, and Ambient Assisted Living, Proceedings* 5518:906–913.

Borca-Tasciuc, D. A., and A. Kempitiya. 2010. Micro-Power Generators for Ambient Intelligence Applications. Paper read at Soft Computing Applications (SOFA), 4th International Workshop, 15–17 July.

Borrego-Jaraba, F., I. L. Ruiz, and M. A. Gomez-Nieto. 2010. NFC Solution for the Development of Smart Scenarios Supporting Tourism Applications and Surfing in Urban Environments. *Trends in Applied Intelligent Systems, Proceedings* 6098:229–238.

Botella, C., A. Garcia-Palacios, R. M. Banos, and S. Quero. 2009. Cybertherapy: Advantages, Limitations, and Ethical Issues. *PsychNology Journal* 7:77–100.

Bouet, M., and G. Pujolle. 2010. RFID in eHealth Systems: Applications, Challenges, and Perspectives. *Annals of Telecommunications-Annales Des Telecommunications* 65:497–503.

Boulos, M. N. K., A. Rocha, A. Martins, M. E. Vicente, A. Bolz, R. Feld, I. Tchoudovski, M. Braecklein, J. Nelson, G. Laighin, C. Sdogati, F. Cesaroni, M. Antomarini, A. Jobes, and M. Kinirons. 2007. CAALYX: A New Generation of Location-Based Services in Healthcare. *International Journal of Health Geographics* 6:9–6.

Boussemart, B., and S. Giroux. 2007. Tangible User Interfaces for Cognitive Assistance. Paper read at Advanced Information Networking and Applications Workshops, AINAW '07, 21st International Conference, 21–23 May.

Bravo, J., R. Hervas, C. Fuentes, G. Chavira, and S. W. Nava. 2008a. Tagging for Nursing Care. *2008 2nd International Conference on Pervasive Computing Technologies for Healthcare,* 291–293.

Bravo, J., D. Lopez-de-Ipina, C. Fuentes, R. Hervas, R. Pena, M. Vergara, and G. Casero. 2008b. Enabling NFC Technology for Supporting Chronic Diseases: A Proposal for Alzheimer Caregivers. *Ambient Intelligence, Proceedings* 5355:109–125.

Bravo, J., C. Fuentes, R. Hervas, G. Casero, R. Gallego, and M. Vergara. 2009a. Interaction by Contact for Supporting Alzheimer Sufferers. *3rd Symposium of Ubiquitous Computing and Ambient Intelligence 2008* 51:125–133.

Bravo, J., R. Hervas, C. Fuentes, V. Villarreal, G. Chavira, S. Nava, J. Fontecha, G. Casero, R. Pena, and M. Vergara. 2009b. From Implicit to Touching Interaction by Identification Technologies: Towards Tagging Context. *Human-Computer Interaction* 5611:417–425.

Broek, G. V. D., F. Cavallo, L. Odetti, and C. Wehrmann. 2008. Ambient Assisted Living Roadmap, AALIANCE The European Ambient Assisted Living Innovation Alliance.

Bühler, C., and I. Placencia-Porrero. 2002. eEurope—Participation for All Action Line: Networking Centres of Excellence in Design-for-All and Developing an EU curriculum in Design for All—Final Report, edited by e. E. Group. Brussels: European Commission.

Bulut, M., and S. S. Narayanan. 2010. Speech Synthesis Systems in Ambient Intelligence Environments. In *Human-Centric Interfaces for Ambient Intelligence*, edited by A. Hamid, D. R. López-Cózar and A. Juan Carlos. Oxford: Academic Press.

Busnel, P., P. El-Khoury, S. Giroux, and K. Q. Li. 2008. Achieving Socio-Technical Confidentiality Using Security Pattern in Smart Homes. *FGCN: Proceedings of the 2008 Second International Conference on Future Generation Communication and Networking*, 1–2:925–930.

Busuoli, M., T. Gallelli, M. Haluzik, V. Fabian, D. Novak, and O. Stepankova. 2007. Entertainment and Ambient: A New OLDES' View. *Universal Access in Human-Computer Interaction: Applications and Services, Proceedings*, 511–519.

Cacciagrano, D., F. Corradini, and R. Culmone. 2010. ResourceHome: An RFID-Based Architecture and a Flexible Model for Ambient Intelligence. Paper read at Systems (ICONS), 2010 Fifth International Conference, 11–16 April.

Camarinha-Matos, L., and W. Vieira. 1999. Intelligent Mobile Agents in Elderly Care. *Robotics and Autonomous Systems* 27:59–75.

Carneiro, D., P. Novais, R. Costa, P. Gomes, and J. Neves. 2009. EMon: Embodied Monitorization. *Ambient Intelligence, Proceedings* 5859:133–142.

Carneiro, D., P. Novais, R. Costa, and J. Neves. 2010. Enhancing the Role of Multi-Agent Systems in the Development of Intelligent Environments. *Trends in Practical Applications of Agents and Multiagent Systems* 71:123–130.

Casas, R., R. B. Marin, A. Robinet, A. R. Delgado, A. R. Yarza, J. McGinn, R. Picking, and V. Grout. 2008. User Modelling in Ambient Intelligence for Elderly and Disabled People. *Computers Helping People with Special Needs, Proceedings* 5105:114–122.

Cascado, D., S. J. Romero, S. Hors, A. Brasero, L. Fernandez-Luque, and J. L. Sevillano. 2010. Virtual Worlds to Enhance Ambient-Assisted Living. Paper read at Engineering in Medicine and Biology Society (EMBC), 2010 Annual International Conference of the IEEE, August 31–September 4.

Chang, Y. J., and T. Y. Wang. 2010. Indoor Wayfinding Based on Wireless Sensor Networks for Individuals with Multiple Special Needs. *Cybernetics and Systems* 41:317–333.

Chavira, G., J. Bravo, S. W. Nava-Diaz, and J. C. Rolon. 2010. PICTAC: A Model for Perceiving Touch Interaction through Tagging Context. *Journal of Universal Computer Science* 16:1577–1591.

Chuan-Jun, S., and C. Bo-Jung. 2010. Ubiquitous Community Care Using Sensor Network and Mobile Agent Technology. Paper read at Ubiquitous Intelligence and Computing and 7th International Conference on Autonomic and Trusted Computing (UIC/ATC), 7th International Conference, 26–29 October.

Connelly, K., K. A. Siek, I. Mulder, S. Neely, G. Stevenson, and C. Kray. 2008. Evaluating Pervasive and Ubiquitous Systems. *Pervasive Computing, IEEE* 7:85–88.

Cook, D. J., and S. K. Das. 2007. How Smart are Our Environments? An Updated Look at the State of the Art. *Pervasive and Mobile Computing* 3:53–73.

Corchado, J. M., J. Bajo, and A. Abraham. 2008. GerAmi: Improving Healthcare Delivery in Geriatric Residences. *Intelligent Systems, IEEE* 23:19–25.

Coronato, A., and G. De Pietro. 2010. A Middleware Architecture for Safety Critical Ambient Intelligence Applications. *Smart Spaces and Next Generation Wired/Wireless Networking* 6294:26–37.

Costa, R., D. Carneiro, P. Novais, and L. Lima. 1999. Ambient Assisted Living. In *Proceedings of the 3rd Symposium of Ubiquitous Computing and Ambient Intelligence*, Salamanca, pp. 86–94.

Costa, R., J. Neves, P. Novais, J. Machado, L. Lima, and C. Alberto. 2007. Intelligent Mixed Reality for the Creation of Ambient Assisted Living. *Progress in Artificial Intelligence, Proceedings* 4874:323–331.

Costa, A., P. Novais, R. Costa, and J. Neves. 2009a. Memory Assistant in Everyday Living. *European Simulation and Modelling Conference 2009*, 269–273.

Costa, R., D. Carneiro, P. Novais, L. Lima, J. Machado, A. Marques, and J. Neves. 2009b. Ambient Assisted Living. *3rd Symposium of Ubiquitous Computing and Ambient Intelligence 2008* 51:86–94.

Costa, R., P. Novais, A. Costa, and J. Neves. 2009c. Memory Support in Ambient Assisted Living. *Leveraging Knowledge for Innovation in Collaborative Networks* 307:745–752.

Costa, A., P. Novais, R. Costa, J. M. Corchado, and J. Neves. 2010. Multi-Agent Personal Memory Assistant. *Trends in Practical Applications of Agents and Multiagent Systems* 71:97–104.

Cui, J., Y. Aghajan, J. Lacroix, A. van Halteren, and H. Aghajan. 2009. Exercising at Home: Real-Time Interaction and Experience Sharing Using Avatars. *Entertainment Computing* 1:63–73.

Dadlani, P., A. Sinitsyn, W. Fontijn, and P. Markopoulos. 2011. Aurama: Caregiver Awareness for Living Independently with an Augmented Picture Frame Display. *AI and Society* 25:233–245.

De Carolis, B., and G. Cozzolongo. 2007. Planning the Behaviour of a Social Robot Acting as a Majordomo in Public Environments. *Ai(Asterisk)Ia 2007: Artificial Intelligence and Human-Oriented Computing* 4733:805–812.

De Hert, P., S. Gutwirth, A. Moscibroda, D. Wright, and G. G. Fuster. 2009. Legal Safeguards for Privacy and Data Protection in Ambient Intelligence. *Personal and Ubiquitous Computing* 13:435–444.

De Paola, A., A. Farruggia, S. Gaglio, G. L. Re, and M. Ortolani. 2009. Exploiting the Human Factor in a WSN-Based System for Ambient Intelligence. Paper read at Complex, Intelligent and Software Intensive Systems, 2009, CISIS '09, International Conference, 16–19 March.

Decision No. 742/2008/EC. European Parliament and of the Council of 9 July 2008 on the Community's Participation in a Research and Development Programme Undertaken by Several Member States Aimed at Enhancing the Quality of Life of Older People through the Use of New Information and Communication Technologies.

Delgado, A. R., R. Blasco, A. Marco, D. Cirujano, R. Casas, A. R. Yarza, V. Grout, and R. Picking. 2009. Agent-Based AmI System Case Study: The Easy Line Plus Project. *Trends in Practical Applications of Agents and Multiagent Systems* 71:157–164.

Dohr, A., R. Modre-Opsrian, M. Drobics, D. Hayn, and G. Schreier. 2010a. The Internet of Things for Ambient Assisted Living. Paper read at Information Technology: New Generations (ITNG), 7th International Conference, 12–14 April.

Dohr, A., M. Drobics, E. Fugger, B. Prazak-Aram, and G. Schreier. 2010b. Medication Management for Elderly People. *Ehealth2010—Medical Informatics Meets Ehealth*.

European Union. 2007. Opinion of the European Economic and Social Committee on the Proposal for a Decision of the European Parliament and of the Council on the Participation by the Community in a Research and Development Programme Aimed at Enhancing the Quality of Life of Older People through the Use of New Information and Communication Technologies (ICT), Undertaken by Several Member States COM(2007) 329 final - 2007/0116 (COD).

Falco, J. M., M. Idiago, A. R. Delgado, A. Marco, A. Asensio, and D. Cirujano. 2010. Indoor Navigation Multi-Agent System for the Elderly and People with Disabilities. *Trends in Practical Applications of Agents and Multiagent Systems* 71:437–442.

Fanucci, L., G. Pardini, F. Costalli, S. Dalmiani, J. Salinas, J. M. De La Higuera, Z. Vukovic, and Z. Cicigoj. 2009. Health @ Home: A New Homecare Model for Patients with Chronic Heart Failure. *Assistive Technology from Adapted Equipment to Inclusive Environments* 25:87–91.

Fayn, J., and P. Rubel. 2010. Toward a Personal Health Society in Cardiology. *Information Technology in Biomedicine* 14:401–409.

Ferguson, G., J. Quinn, C. Horwitz, M. Swift, J. Allen, and L. Galescu. 2010. Towards a Personal Health Management Assistant. *Journal of Biomedical Informatics* 43:S13–S16.

Fernandes, M. S., N. S. Dias, A. F. Silva, J. S. Nunes, S. Lanceros-Méndez, J. H. Correia, and P. M. Mendes. 2010. Hydrogel-Based Photonic Sensor for a Biopotential Wearable Recording System. *Biosensors and Bioelectronics* 26:80–86.

Figueiredo, C. P., K. Becher, K. P. Hoffmann, and P. M. Mendes. 2010. Low Power Wireless Acquisition Module for Wearable Health Monitoring Systems. Paper read at Engineering in Medicine and Biology Society (EMBC), Annual International Conference of the IEEE, August 31–September 4.

Floch, J., C. Carrez, P. Cieslak, M. Rój, R. T. Sanders, and M. M. Shiaa. 2010. A Comprehensive Engineering Framework for Guaranteeing Component Compatibility. *Journal of Systems and Software* 83:1759–1779.

Fortier, A., G. Rossi, S. E. Gordillo, and C. Challiol. 2010. Dealing with Variability in Context-Aware Mobile Software. *Journal of Systems and Software* 83:915–936.

Foty, D. 2007. Next-Generation Wireless Networks: A New World, from Bottom to Top. Paper read at AFRICON, 26–28 September.

Fugger, E., B. Prazak, S. Hanke, and S. Wassertheurer. 2007. Requirements and Ethical Issues for Sensor-Augmented Environments in Elderly Care. *Universal Access in Human Computer Interaction: Coping with Diversity* 4554:887–893.

Garcia-Herranz, M., P. A. Haya, and X. Alaman. 2009. Easing the Smart Home: Translating Human Hierarchies to Intelligent Environments. *Bio-Inspired Systems: Computational and Ambient Intelligence* 5517:1098–1105.

Garipelli, G., F. Galan, R. Chavarriaga, P. W. Ferrez, E. Lew, and J. D. Millan. 2008. The Use of Brain-Computer Interfacing in Ambient Intelligence. *Constructing Ambient Intelligence* 11:268–285.

Grauel, J., and A. Spellerberg. 2008. Attitudes and Requirements of Elderly People Towards Assisted Living Solutions. *Constructing Ambient Intelligence* 11:197–206.

Grossi, F., V. Bianchi, G. Matrella, I. De Munari, and P. Ciampolini. 2009. Internet-Based Home Monitoring and Control. *Assistive Technology from Adapted Equipment to Inclusive Environments* 25:309–313.

Gruber, H. G., B. Wolf, and M. Reiher. 2009. Innovation Barriers for Telemonitoring. *World Congress on Medical Physics and Biomedical Engineering* 25:48–50.

Guo, B., D. Zhang, and M. Imai. 2010. Enabling User-Oriented Management for Ubiquitous Computing: The Meta-Design Approach. *Computer Networks* 54:2840–2855.

Guo, M. J., and Y. Zhao. 2008. An Extensible Architecture for Personalized Information Services in an Ambient Intelligence Environment. *2008 4th International Conference on Wireless Communications, Networking and Mobile Computing* 1–31:8344–8347.

Hadzic, M., and E. Chang. 2010. Application of Digital Ecosystem Design Methodology within the Health Domain. *Systems, Man and Cybernetics, Part A: Systems and Humans* 40:779–788.

Haosheng, H., G. Gartner, M. Schmidt, and Y. Li. 2009. Smart Environment for Ubiquitous Indoor Navigation. Paper read at New Trends in Information and Service Science, NISS '09, International Conference, June 30–July 2.

Hartmann, R., F. Al Machot, P. Mahr, and C. Bobda. 2010. Camera-Based System for Tracking and Position Estimation of Humans. Paper read at Design and Architectures for Signal and Image Processing Conference (DASIP), 26–28 October.

Havasi, F., and A. Kiss. 2008. Ambient Assisted Living in Rural Areas: Vision and Pilot Application. *Constructing Ambient Intelligence* 11:246–252.

Hildebrandt, M., and B. Koops. 2010. The Challenges of Ambient Law and Legal Protection in the Profiling Era. *Modern Law Review* 73:428–460.

Hoareau, C., and I. Satoh. 2009. Modeling and Processing Information for Context-Aware Computing: A Survey. *New Generation Computing* 27:177–196.

Holzinger, A., K. S. Mukasa, and A. K. Nischelwitzer. 2008. Introduction to the Special Thematic Session: Human-Computer Interaction and Usability for Elderly (HCI4AGING). *Computers Helping People with Special Needs, Proceedings* 5105:18–21.

Hopmann, M., D. Thalmann, and F. Vexo. 2008. Thanks to Geolocalized Remote Control: The Sound Will Follow. Paper read at Cyberworlds, International Conference, 22–24 September.

Hossain, M. S., M. A. Hossain, and A. El Saddik. 2007. Multimedia Content Repurposing in Ambient Intelligent Environments. Paper read at Data Engineering Workshop, IEEE 23rd International Conference, 17–20 April.

Huertas, S., J. P. Lazaro, S. Guille, and V. Traver. 2010. Information and Assistance Bubbles to Help Elderly People in Public Environments. Paper read at Engineering in Medicine and Biology Society (EMBC), Annual International Conference of the IEEE, August 31–September 4.

Hui-Huang, H., C. Zixue, T. K. Shih, and C. Chien-Chen. 2009. RFID-based Personalized Behavior Modeling. Paper read at Ubiquitous, Autonomic and Trusted Computing, UIC-ATC '09, Symposia and Workshops, 7–9 July.

Hui-Huang, H., C. Po-Kai, and L. Chi-Yi. 2010. RFID-Based Danger Prevention for Home Safety. Paper read at Aware Computing (ISAC), 2010 2nd International Symposium on, 1–4 November 2010.

Iqbal, M., H. B. Lim, W. Wenqiang, and Y. Yuxia. 2009. A Service Oriented Model for Semantics-Based Data Management in Wireless Sensor Networks. Paper read at Advanced Information Networking and Applications Workshops, WAINA '09, International Conference, 26–29 May.

Iqbal, M., L. Hock Beng, and N. Teng Jie. 2010. Ecosense: A Context and Semantics Driven Framework for Eco-Aware Ambient Environments. Paper read at Consumer Communications and Networking Conference (CCNC), 7th IEEE, 9–12 January.

Islam, M. S., and V. J. Logeeswaran. 2010. Nanoscale Materials and Devices for Future Communication Networks. *Communications Magazine, IEEE* 48(6):112–120.

Isomursu, M., M. Ervasti, and V. Tormanen. 2009. Medication Management Support for Vision Impaired Elderly: Scenarios and Technological Possibilities. Paper read at Applied Sciences in Biomedical and Communication Technologies, 2009, ISABEL 2009, 2nd International Symposium on, 24–27 November.

IST Advisory Group. 2002. Strategic Orientations & Priorities for IST in FP6, edited by E. Commission.

IST Advisory Group. 2003. Ambient Intelligence: From Vision to Reality, edited by E. Commission.

IST Amigo Project. 2005a. Deliverable D2.2—State of the Art Analysis Including Assessment of System Architectures for Ambient Intelligence.

IST Amigo Project. 2005b. Deliverable D2.3 Specification of the Amigo Abstract System Architecture.

ISTAG. 2009. Report on Orientations for Work Programme 2011–2013.

Jingwen, X., S. Boon-Chong, and J. Symonds. 2009. Human Activity Inference for Ubiquitous RFID-based Applications. Paper read at Ubiquitous, Autonomic and Trusted Computing, UIC-ATC '09, Symposia and Workshops, 7–9 July.

Kairy, D., P. Lehoux, C. Vincent, and M. Visintin. 2009. A Systematic Review of Clinical Outcomes, Clinical Process, Healthcare Utilization and Costs Associated with Telerehabilitation. *Disability and Rehabilitation* 31:427–447.

Kantorovitch, J., J. Kaartinen, L. C. Abri, R. D. Martin, J. A. M. Cantera, J. Criel, and M. Gielen. 2009. AmIE Towards Ambient Intelligence for the Ageing Citizens. *HEALTHINF 2009: Proceedings of the International Conference on Health Informatics*, 421–424.

Kapoor, A. 2010. New Frontiers in Machine Learning for Predictive User Modeling. In *Human-Centric Interfaces for Ambient Intelligence*, edited by A. Hamid, D. R. López-Cózar and A. Juan Carlos. Oxford: Academic Press.

Kastner, W., M. J. Kofler, and C. Reinisch. 2010. Using AI to Realize Energy Efficient yet Comfortable Smart Homes. Paper read at Factory Communication Systems (WFCS), 8th IEEE International Workshop, 18–21.

Keegan, S., G. M. P. O'Hare, and M. J. O'Grady. 2008. Easishop: Ambient Intelligence Assists Everyday Shopping. *Information Sciences* 178:588–611.

Khan, V. J., and P. Markopoulos. 2009. Busy Families' Awareness Needs. *International Journal of Human-Computer Studies* 67(2):139–153.

Khan, V. J., P. Markopoulos, B. Eggen, and G. Metaxas. 2010. Evaluation of a Pervasive Awareness System Designed for Busy Parents. *Pervasive and Mobile Computing* 6:537–558.

Kleinberger, T., M. Becker, E. Ras, A. Holzingerz, and P. Muller. 2007. Ambient Intelligence in Assisted Living: Enable Elderly People to Handle Future Interfaces. *Universal Access in Human-Computer Interaction: Ambient Interaction, Proceedings* 4555:103–112.

Kleinberger, T., A. Jedlitschka, H. Storf, S. Steinbach-Nordmann, and S. Prueckner. 2009. An Approach to and Evaluations of Assisted Living Systems Using Ambient Intelligence for Emergency Monitoring and Prevention. *Universal Access in Human-Computer Interaction, Proceedings* 5615:199–208.

Knoll, M. 2009. Diabetes City: How Urban Game Design Strategies Can Help Diabetics. *Electronic Healthcare* 1:200–204.

Koch, J., H. Jung, J. Wettach, G. Nemeth, and K. Berns. 2008. Dynamic Speech Interaction for Robotic Agents. *Recent Progress in Robotics: Viable Robotic Service to Human* 370:303–315.

Kohler, F., M. Thoss, and A. Aring. 2010. An Energy-Aware Indoor Positioning System for AAL Environments. Paper read at Indoor Positioning and Indoor Navigation (IPIN), 2010 International Conference, 15–17 September.

Kosta, E., O. Pitkanen, M. Niemela, and E. Kaasinen. 2008. Ethical-Legal Challenges in User-Centric AmI Services. Paper read at Internet and Web Applications and Services, ICIW '08, Third International Conference, 8–13 June.

Kosta, E., O. Pitkanen, N. Niemela, and E. Kaasinen. 2010. Mobile-Centric Ambient Intelligence in Health- and Homecare-Anticipating Ethical and Legal Challenges. *Science and Engineering Ethics* 16:303–323.

Krieg-Brückner, B., T. Röfer, H. Shi, and B. Gersdorf. 2010. Mobility Assistance in the Bremen Ambient Assisted Living Lab. *GeroPsych: The Journal of Gerontopsychology and Geriatric Psychiatry* 23:121–130.

Kuhn, T., T. Jaitner, and R. Gotzhein. 2008. Online-Monitoring of Multiple Track Cyclists during Training and Competition. *Engineering of Sport* 7 1:405–412.

Kyung-Seok, S., J. Yong-Hee, K. Yong-Jin, and L. Ryong. 2010. An Ambient Service Model for Providing Structured Web Information Based on User-Contexts. Paper read at Cyber-Enabled Distributed Computing and Knowledge Discovery (CyberC), International Conference, 10–12 October.

Lazaro, J. P., A. Fides, A. Navarro, and S. Guillen. 2010. Ambient Assisted Nutritional Advisor for Elderly People Living at Home. Paper read at Engineering in Medicine and Biology Society (EMBC), Annual International Conference of the IEEE, August 31–September 4.

Le Métayer, D., and S. Monteleone. 2009. Automated Consent through Privacy Agents: Legal Requirements and Technical Architecture. *Computer Law & Security Review* 25:136–144.

Lee, C. S., M. H. Wang, G. Acampora, C. Y. Hsu, and H. Hagras. 2010. Diet Assessment Based on Type-2 Fuzzy Ontology and Fuzzy Markup Language. *International Journal of Intelligent Systems* 25:1187–1216.

Lehikoinen, J., J. Lehikoinen, and P. Huuskonen. 2008. Understanding Privacy Regulation in ubicomp Interactions. *Personal and Ubiquitous Computing* 12:543–553.

Leon, E., G. Clarke, V. Callaghan, and F. Doctor. 2010. Affect-Aware Behaviour Modelling and Control Inside an Intelligent Environment. *Pervasive and Mobile Computing* 6:559–574.

Lindenberg, J., W. Pasman, K. Kranenborg, J. Stegeman, and M. A. Neerincx. 2007. Improving Service Matching and Selection in Ubiquitous Computing Environments: A User Study. *Personal and Ubiquitous Computing* 11:59–68.

López-Matencio, P., J. V. Alonso, F. J. Gonzalez-Castano, J. L. Sieiro, and J. J. Alcaraz. 2010. Ambient Intelligence Assistant for Running Sports Based on k-NN Classifiers. Paper read at Human System Interactions (HSI), 3rd Conference, 13–15 May.

Maier, E., and G. Kempter. 2009. AAL in the Wild—Lessons Learned. *Universal Access in Human-Computer Interaction, Proceedings* 5615:218–227.

Martin, S., E. Sancristobal, G. Temino, P. Losada, N. Oliva, A. Colmenar, M. Castro, and J. Peire. 2008. Interoperability and Integration of Context-Aware Services in an Ambient Intelligence Environment. Paper read at Internet and Web Applications and Services, ICIW '08, 3rd International Conference, 8–13 June.

Mastrogiovanni, F., A. Scalmato, A. Sgorbissa, and R. Zaccaria. 2008. An Integrated Approach to Context Specification and Recognition in Smart Homes. *Smart Homes and Health Telematics* 5120:26–33.

Mingjing, G., and Z. Yang. 2008a. An Architecture for Digital Library Information Service in an Ambient Intelligence Environment. Paper read at Computer Science and Software Engineering, International Conference, 12–14 December.

Mingjing, G., and Z. Yang. 2008b. An Extensible Architecture for Personalized Information Services in an Ambient Intelligence Environment. Paper read at Wireless Communications, Networking and Mobile Computing, WiCOM '08, 4th International Conference, 12–14 October.

Mirarmandehi, N., and H. R. Rabiee. 2010. An Asynchronous Dynamic Bayesian Network for Activity Recognition in an Ambient Intelligent Environment. Paper read at Pervasive Computing and Applications (ICPCA), 5th International Conference, 1–3 December.

Mulvenna, M., W. Carswell, P. McCullagh, J. C. Augusto, Z. Huiru, P. Jeffers, W. Haiying, and S. Martin. 2011. Visualization of Data for Ambient Assisted Living Services. *Communications Magazine, IEEE* 49:110–117.

Munoz, A., A. Mana, and D. Serrano. 2009. AVISPA in the Validation of Ambient Intelligence Scenarios. Paper read at Availability, Reliability and Security, ARES '09, International Conference, 16–19 March.

Murgoitio, J., and J. I. Fernandez. 2008. Car driver Monitoring by Networking Vital Data. *Advanced Microsystems for Automotive Applications 2008*, 37–48.

Niemela, M., R. G. Fuentetaja, E. Kaasinen, and J. L. Gallardo. 2007. Supporting Independent Living of the Elderly with Mobile-Centric Ambient Intelligence: User Evaluation of Three Scenarios. *Ambient Intelligence, Proceedings* 4794:91–107.

Noh, J. M., and J. S. Kim. 2010. Factors Influencing the User Acceptance of Digital Home Services. *Telecommunications Policy* 34:672–682.

Oberzaucher, J., K. Werner, H. P. Mairbock, C. Beck, P. Panek, W. Hlauschek, and W. L. Zagler. 2009. A Videophone Prototype System Evaluated by Elderly Users in the Living Lab Schwechat. *HCI and Usability for E-Inclusion, Proceedings* 5889:345–352.

Paganelli, F., G. Bianchi, and D. Giuli. 2007. Context Model for Context-Aware System Design Towards the Ambient Intelligence Vision: Experiences in the eTourism Domain. *Universal Access in Ambient Intelligence Environments* 4397:173–191.

Panek, P., and W. L. Zagler. 2008. A Living Lab for Ambient Assisted Living in the Municipality of Schwechat. *Computers Helping People with Special Needs, Proceedings* 5105:1008–1015.

Patkos, T., A. Bikakis, G. Antoniou, M. Papadopouli, and D. Plexousakis. 2007. Distributed AI for Ambient Intelligence: Issues and Approaches. *Ambient Intelligence, Proceedings* 4794:159–176.

Pauws, S., W. Verhaegh, and M. Vossen. 2008. Music Playlist Generation by Adapted Simulated Annealing. *Information Sciences* 178:647–662.

Pawlowski, J. M., M. Bick, and P. Veith. 2008. Context Metadata to Adapt Ambient Learning Environments. Paper read at Portable Information Devices, 2008 and the 7th IEEE Conference on Polymers and Adhesives in Microelectronics and Photonics, PORTABLE-POLYTRONIC 2008, 2nd IEEE International Interdisciplinary Conference, 17–20 August.

Pedraza, J. P., M. A. Patricio, A. De Asis, and J. M. Molina. 2010a. A Legal View of Ambient Assisted Living Developments. *Trends in Practical Applications of Agents and Multiagent Systems* 71:631–638.

Pedraza, J. P., M. A. Patricio, A. de Asis, and J. M. Molina. 2010b. Privacy and Legal Requirements for Developing Biometric Identification Software in Context-Based Applications. *International Journal of Bio-Science & Bio-Technology* 2:13–23.

PERSONA. 2008. PERceptive Spaces prOmoting iNdependent Aging, Deliverable 2.1.1—Report Describing Values, Trends, User Needs and Guidelines for System Characteristics in the AAL Persona Context.

Pizzutilo, S., B. Decarolis, G. Cozzolongo, V. Silvestri, and A. Petrone. 2007. An Active Environment to Manage User Adapted Interactions. *Proceedings of the 7th WSEAS International Conference on Applied Informatics and Communications*, 225–230.

Plischke, H., and N. Kohls. 2009. Keep It Simple! Assisting Older People with Mental and Physical Training. *Universal Access in Human-Computer Interaction: Addressing Diversity, Proceedings* 5614:278–287.

Poullet, Y. 2009. Data Protection Legislation: What is at Stake for Our Society and Democracy? *Computer Law & Security Review* 25:211–226.

Ramos, C. 2007. Ambient Intelligence—A State of the Art from Artificial Intelligence perspective. *Progress in Artificial Intelligence, Proceedings* 4874:285–295.

Ramos, C., J. C. Augusto, and D. Shapiro. 2008. Ambient Intelligence—The Next Step for Artificial Intelligence. *IEEE Intelligent Systems* 23:15–18.

Remmers, H. 2010. Environments for Ageing, Assistive Technology and Self-Determination: Ethical Perspectives. *Informatics for Health & Social Care* 35:200–210.

Rialle, V. 2009. La géolocalisation de malades de type Alzheimer: Entre urgence sociosanitaire et dilemme sociétal. *NPG Neurologie—Psychiatrie—Gériatrie* 9:101–105.

Roa, L. M., J. Reina-Tosina, and M. A. Estudillo. 2009. Virtual Center for the Elderly: Lessons Learned. *Distributed Computing, Artificial Intelligence, Bioinformatics, Soft Computing, and Ambient Assisted Living, Proceedings* 5518:722–726.

Rocker, C. 2009. Perceived Usefulness and Perceived Ease-of-Use of Ambient Intelligence Applications in Office Environments. *Human Centered Design, Proceedings* 5619:1052–1061.

Rocker, C. 2010. Information Privacy in Smart Office Environments: A Cross-Cultural Study Analyzing the Willingness of Users to Share Context Information. *Computational Science and Its Applications—ICCSA 2010, Proceedings* 6019:93–106.

Romero, N., J. Sturm, T. Bekker, L. de Valk, and S. Kruitwagen. 2010. Playful Persuasion to Support Older Adults' Social and Physical Activities. *Interacting with Computers* 22:485–495.

Schurmann, B., and R. Volk. 2008. Research Center Ambient Intelligence: Assisted Bicycle Team Training. *Ki 2008: Advances in Artificial Intelligence, Proceedings* 5243:399–401.

Sehgal, S., M. Iqbal, and J. Kamruzzaman. 2007. Ambient Cardiac Expert: A Cardiac Patient Monitoring System using Genetic and Clinical Knowledge Fusion. Paper read at Computer and Information Science, ICIS 2007, 6th IEEE/ACIS International Conference, 11–13 July.

Serral, E., P. Valderas, and V. Pelechano. 2010. Towards the Model Driven Development of Context-Aware Pervasive Systems. *Pervasive and Mobile Computing* 6:254–280.

Shirehjini, A. A. N. 2007. A Qualitative Usability Evaluation of a Mobile 3D-based Environment Controller. Paper read at Intelligent Environments, IE 07, 3rd IET International Conference, 24–25 September.

Siciliano, P., A. Leone, G. Diraco, C. Distante, M. Malfatti, L. Gonzo, M. Grassi, A. Lombardi, G. Rescio, and P. Malcovati. 2009. A Networked Multisensor System for Ambient Assisted Living application, 3rd International Workshop on Advances in Sensors and Interfaces, 132–136.

Silva, S., P. M. Mendes, and L. Domingues. 2010. Magtag—A Wearable Wrist Device for Localization Applications. Paper read at Pervasive Computing Technologies for Healthcare (PervasiveHealth), 4th International Conference, 22–25 March.

Snijders, F. 2005. Ambient Intelligence Technology: An Overview. In *Ambient Intelligence*, edited by W. Weber, J. Rabaey and E. Aarts. Berlin: Springer.

Soede, M., F. Vlaskamp, H. Knops, and R. Childs. 2007. Privacy Matters and Functionality in Ambient Supportive Technologies; Mobile Telephone Tased Activity Monitoring Systems. *Challenges for Assistive Technology* 20:615–619.

Spanoudakis, N., B. Grabner, C. Kotsiopoulou, O. Lymperopoulou, V. Moser-Siegmeth, S. Pantelopoulos, P. Sakka, and P. Moraitis. 2010. A Novel Architecture and Process for Ambient Assisted Living—The HERA Approach. Paper read at Information Technology and Applications in Biomedicine (ITAB), 2010 10th IEEE International Conference on, 3–5 November.

Sparacino, F. 2008. Natural Interaction in Intelligent Spaces: Designing for Architecture and Entertainment. *Multimedia Tools and Applications* 38:307–335.

Spiru, L., L. Stefan, I. Turcu, C. Ghita, I. Ioancio, C. Nuta, M. Blaciotti, M. Martin, U. Cortes, and R. Annicchiarico. 2009. Legal Concerns Regarding AmI Assisted Living in the Elderly, Worldwide and in Romania. *Bio-Inspired Systems: Computational and Ambient Intelligence* 5517:1083–1089.

Steg, H., H. Strese, C. Loroff, J. Hull, and S. Schmidt. 2006. Europe is Facing a Demographic Challenge: Ambient Assisted Living Offers Solutions. *IST Project Report on Ambient Assisted Living*.

Sterritt, R., and C. Nugent. 2010. Autonomic Computing and Ambient Assisted Living—Extended Abstract. Paper read at Engineering of Autonomic and Autonomous Systems (EASe), 7th IEEE International Conference and Workshops, 22–26 March.

Sun, H., V. De Florio, N. Gui, and C. Blondia. 2007. Towards Building Virtual Community for Ambient Assisted Living. *Proceedings of the 16th Euromicro Conference on Parallel, Distributed and Network-Based Processing*, 556–561.

Sun, H., V. De Florio, N. Gui, and C. Blondia. 2009. Promises and Challenges of Ambient Assisted Living Systems. Paper read at Information Technology: New Generations, ITNG '09, Sixth International Conference, 27–29 April.

Tocino, A. V., J. J. A. Gutierrez, I. A. Navia, F. J. G. Penalvo, E. P. Castrejon, and J. R. G. B. Giner. 2009. Personal Health Monitor. *New Directions in Intelligent Interactive Multimedia Systems and Services—2* 226:465–475.

Torres-Solis, J., and T. Chau. 2007. A Flexible Routing Scheme for Patients with Topographical Disorientation. *Journal of Neuroengineering and Rehabilitation* 4:44.

Un, S., and N. Price. 2007. Bridging the Gap between Technological Possibilities and People: Involving People in the Early Phases of Technology Development. *Technological Forecasting and Social Change* 74:1758–1772.

Valera, A. J. J., M. A. Z. Izquierdo, and A. F. G. Skarmeta. 2009. A Wearable System for Tele-Monitoring and Tele-Assistance of Patients with Integration of Solutions from Chronobiology for Prediction of Illness. *Ambient Intelligence Perspectives* 1:221–228.

Valiente-Rocha, P. A., and A. Lozano-Tello. 2010. Ontology-Based Expert System for Home Automation Controlling. *Trends in Applied Intelligent Systems, Proceedings* 6096:661–670.

Valiente-Rocha, P., J. L. Redondo-Garcia, and A. Lozano-Tello. 2010. Ambient Intelligence System for Controlling Home Automation Installations. Paper read at Information Systems and Technologies (CISTI), 5th Iberian Conference, 16–19 June.

van Dijk, N. 2009. The Legal Status of Profiles. *Intelligent Environments 2009* 2:510–516.

van Dijk, N. 2010. Property, Privacy and Personhood in a World of Ambient Intelligence. *Ethics and Information Technology* 12:57–69.

Vansteenwegen, P., W. Souffriau, G. V. Berghe, and D. Van Oudheusden. 2011. The City Trip Planner: An Expert System for Tourists. *Expert Systems with Applications* 38:6540–6546.

Wei-Lun, C., W. Shih-Hsiang, and Y. Soe-Tsyr. 2007. iCare Home Portal: Substitution-Based Case Adaptation CBR for Quality Aging in Place. Paper read at e-Health Networking, Application and Services, 9th International Conference, 19–22 June.

World Health Organisation. 2001. International Classification of Functioning, Disability and Health (ICF).

World Health Organisation. 2002. Active Ageing: A Policy Framework.

Wright, D., S. Gutwirth, M. Friedewald, P. De Hert, M. Langheinrich, and A. Moscibroda. 2009. Privacy, Trust and Policy-Making: Challenges and Responses. *Computer Law & Security Review* 25:69–83.

Yo-Ping, H., C. Yueh-Tsun, and F. E. Sandnes. 2009. QR Code Data Type Encoding for Ubiquitous Information Transfer Across Different Platforms. Paper read at Ubiquitous, Autonomic and Trusted Computing, UIC-ATC '09, Symposia and Workshops, 7–9 July.

Yu, Z., X. Zhou, Z. Yu, J. H. Park, and J. Ma. 2008. iMuseum: A Scalable Context-Aware Intelligent Museum System. *Computer Communications* 31:4376–4382.

Zaad, L., and B. S. Allouch. 2008. The Influence of Control on the Acceptance of Ambient Intelligence by Elderly People: An Explorative Study. *Ambient Intelligence, Proceedings* 5355:58–74.

Ziefle, M., and C. Rocker. 2010. Acceptance of Pervasive Healthcare Systems: A Comparison of Different Implementation Concepts. Paper read at Pervasive Computing Technologies for Healthcare (PervasiveHealth), 4th International Conference, 22–25 March.

3

Pervasive and Mobile Health Care Applications

Bruno M. C. Silva, Joel J. P. C. Rodrigues, and Ivo M. C. de M. Lopes

CONTENTS

ABSTRACT Health telematics is becoming a major source of improvement in patients' lives, especially for disabled, elderly, and chronically ill people. Information and communication technologies have rapidly grown along with the mobile Internet concept of anywhere and anytime connection. In this context, mobile health (m-health) proposes health care services delivery, overcoming geographical, temporal, and even organizational barriers. Pervasive and m-health services aim to respond to several emerging problems in health services, including the increasing number of chronic diseases related to lifestyle, high costs in existing national health services, the need to empower patients and families to self-care and manage their own health care, and the need to provide direct access to health services, regardless of the time and place. This chapter presents a comprehensive review of the state of the art on pervasive and m-health applications. It presents the most important and significant work in the related literature and presents the top and most used m-health applications in the mobile market. New trends and insights for future research studies and new answers to emerging and challenging health care issues are also presented.

KEY WORDS: *mobile health, m-health, e-health, ambient assisted living, pervasive computing, healthcare applications.*

Introduction

Health telematics, also known as electronic health (e-health), has in the last decade offered more accessible and affordable health care solutions to patients who live in remote rural areas, who travel constantly, or who are physically incapacitated (Moullee and Ray 2009; Akter et al. 2010). The introduction of information and communication technologies (ICTs) as home medical devices, such as blood pressure monitors, glucometers, and scales to connect with doctors/physicians, is already a success among common citizens. In the United States, three out of five patients with chronic diseases stated that the use of home medical devices really improved their health. Furthermore, three in four patients stated that computers help their doctors to deliver better care (Practice Fusion 2011a,b).

Mobile technologies and devices are in continuous evolution. The laptop is already becoming outdated compared to the emerging smartphones and tablets. According to Chilmark Research (2011), in the next 2 years, it is expected that about 50% of US physicians will have an Apple iPad (Apple 2011). Furthermore, Medtronic (2011), the world leader in medical technology, providing lifelong solutions for people with chronic pains, recently purchased 4500 iPads for its sales and marketing team (Kamp and Cheng 2011). Moreover, an online survey of 474 health professionals registered to practice in the United Kingdom found that 80% rely on a mobile phone at work (d4 2011). This mobile advent in the health environment creates innumerous possibilities for health professionals and patients. Physicians can easily download medical records, lab results, images, and drug information to handheld devices like personal digital assistants (PDAs) and smartphones. Patients could be aware of their diagnostics, disease control, and monitoring with comfortable mobile devices that accompany them everywhere. The actions required for these are so easy to perform and so intuitive that looking back to Mark Weiser's (1991) claim, "the most profound technologies are those that disappear," such technologic behaviors are indeed pervasive. The fact that wireless communications and mobile devices that provide access any time and anywhere are already pervasive in developed countries shows that pervasive and mobile systems will certainly have a strong technological impact on people's lives and daily routines (Schmidt 2010).

With the advent of mobile communications supported on smart mobile devices, mobile computing has been the main attraction of research and business communities, thus offering innumerous opportunities to create efficient mobile health (m-health) solutions. M-health is the new edge in health care innovation. It proposes to deliver health care anywhere and any time, surpassing geographical, temporal, and even organizational barriers (Tachakra et al. 2003; Akter and Ray 2010). Laxminarayan and Istepanian defined m-health for the first time in the year 2000, as *unwired e-med*. In 2003, the term *m-health* was defined as "emerging mobile communications and network technologies for healthcare systems" (Istepanian and Lacal 2003). Laxminarayan et al. presented in 2006 a comprehensive study on the impact of mobility on the existing e-health commercial telemedical systems. Furthermore, it served as the basis for future m-health technologies and services.

Pervasive m-health systems, and their inherent mobility functionalities, have a strong impact on typical health care monitoring and alerting systems, clinical and administrative data collection, record maintenance, health care delivery programs, medical information awareness, detection and prevention systems, drug counterfeiting, and theft (Zuehlke et al. 2009). M-health services and applications use the Internet and web services to provide an authentic pervasive interaction among doctors and patients. A physician or a patient can easily access the same medical record any time and anywhere through their personal

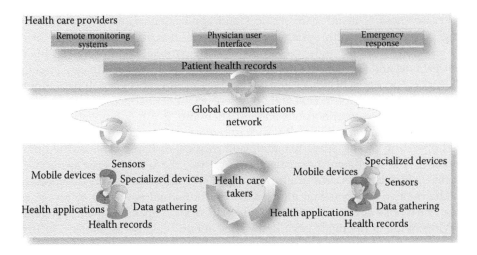

FIGURE 3.1
Illustration of a typical m-health service architecture.

computer, tablet, or smartphone. Figure 3.1 presents a typical m-health service architecture. Health care providers use remote monitoring systems; physician user interfaces and emergency response systems to provide and maintain patient health records. Through the global communication network, health care takers use several medical devices such as mobile devices, sensors, or specialized devices with embedded applications that allow health data gathering and the management of health records. The main objective of this review is to display the most important works and the major advances in the field.

The remainder of this chapter is organized as follows. The second section, entitled "Pervasive Health Care Services," elaborates on related work about the topic of pervasive health care services. The third section entitled "M-Health, the Health Care (R)Evolution," describes the m-health topic, and the m-health applications are presented in the fourth section, entitled "M-Health Application Awareness." The fifth section includes the "Current State of M-Health Applications Usage." Finally, this chapter ends with the "Conclusion and Future Trends," which also points out further research work.

Pervasive Health Care Services

Mark Weiser introduced to the world his vision of ubiquitous/pervasive computing at the beginning of the 90s, describing it as follows: "The most profound technologies are those that are invisible. They are woven in the manufacture of everyday life until they are indistinguishable from day to day."

Weiser presented a concept of a complete abstraction of technology where the machine interacts with man (Weiser 1991). However, Weiser's vision was too advanced for his time; it lacked the technological support that currently exists (Weiser 1994). The Internet as we know it today is a perfect example of a pervasive technology, where users focus only on the information and services rather than its intrinsic technology. Pervasive computing goes beyond the device, network, and protocol. The technology interacts with the user transparently without the user having requested it (Zhou et al. 2010a).

The pervasiveness of health care services and applications aims to respond to several emerging problems in health systems, including the increasing the number of chronic diseases related to lifestyle, high costs in the existing national health services, the need to empower patients and families to self-care and manage their own health care, and the need to provide direct access to health services, regardless of time and place. It uses innumerous technologies such as environmental and body sensors, or actuators to monitor and improve the physical or mental condition of patients. Therefore, it offers innovative services and applications in different areas of health, such as remote monitoring of elderly or sick people; advanced operating rooms; space for intelligent medical or home care, assisted intelligent environments, and intelligent hospitals; etc. However, the use of pervasive services and applications in health raises several ethical and professional issues. A key question concerns how much sensitive and personal information an individual is willing to reveal. Usually, people carry a mobile device (smartphone, tablet, iPod, etc.) capable of exchanging data with other devices, without having explicit knowledge about this process. Privacy, security, and reliability are issues of concern to end users; the exchange of personal data is always subject to unauthorized access by third parties. For example, in a ubiquitous environment, will the elderly be able to control information sharing? Another key issue relates to errors in information exchange or access (e.g., medical records), which can cause errors in diagnosis or disease prevention. Who will take responsibility for these errors? These and other important questions appear with inherent technological risks but need to be asked and answered to ensure the future of health services and applications, mainly for users, sake (Little and Briggs 2009).

There are, in the literature, several pervasive health services and applications related to health care. Graschew et al. (2007) presented a network of satellites that uses four satellite networks, GALENA, DELTA, MEDASHIP, and EMISPHER. The purpose of this project is to improve health services together on the same network for 14 clinics in 6 different countries supporting rapid care for emergency cases and cases on ships, and constant mobility as an online service for most countries of the Euro-Mediterranean. Furthermore, the literature presents systems for monitoring of electrocardiogram (ECG)/photoplethysmogram (PPG) signals (Cha et al. 2009; Rikitake et al. 2009; Shin et al. 2009; Sugano et al. 2010), monitoring drug dosage and quality of life of seniors (Lin et al. 2008; Suzuki and Nakauchi 2009), and monitoring of biological signals (Kwang 2009). Moreover, there are services for health care in cases of chronic diseases (Yoo et al. 2009); for data collection and monitoring of blood pressure, diabetes, blood sugar, and emergencies (Dong-Wook et al. 2007; Kwon et al. 2010); and for psychological care and therapy (Taleb et al. 2010).

M-Health, the Health Care (R)Evolution

In January 9, 2007, Steve Jobs, the CEO of Apple Inc. at that time (Apple Inc. 2011), presented to the world the iPhone 2G and its operating system (OS), the iOS (Apple Developer 2011). This event triggered a rapid evolution of smartphones and also the appearance of new mobile platforms, especially one that has proven to be market dominant: the Google Android (Android Developers 2011). Basically, four players dominate the mobile OS market: Google Android, Apple iOS, BlackBerry Research in Motion (RIM), and Microsoft Windows Phone. Figure 3.2 presents the number of worldwide mobile device sales to end users by vendor in the fourth quarter of 2012. Clearly, Samsung with the Google Android OS, Nokia with the Windows Phone OS and Apple, iOS dominated the market. The quality of the three OSs is unquestionable;

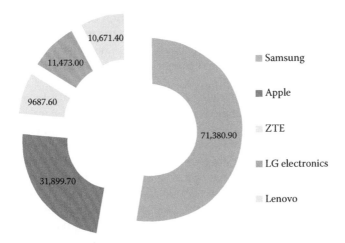

FIGURE 3.2
Worldwide smartphone sales to end users by vendors in 2013.

however, the success of both Google and Apple in the mobile market is sustained by their application markets, the Apple App Store and the Google Play Store (Gartner 2010).

Currently, there are several application online stores for different platforms such as Google Play Store, Blackberry App World, Apple App Store, Ovi Store, Samsung Apps, and Windows Marketplace, to name just a few. These market opportunities open new and potential areas of research, such as m-health applications. At the end of 2010, more than 200 million m-health applications were in use, and about 70% of citizens worldwide were interested in having access to at least one m-health application. Overall, smartphones' web browsers improved, making it easier to find free applications and information. In the fourth quarter of 2012, more than 168 million mobile units were sold to end users worldwide (Figure 3.3).

Most of the current market applications are directed toward patients, clinicians, and health care professionals. These applications are mainly suited for disease management, self-monitoring, and drug control as well as other clinical and educational applications. Excluding the free medical applications, the average price of consumer health and medical paid apps in 2010 in Apple's App Store was $3.63 and that of health care professional apps was $14.23. The Google Play Store's average prices are very similar to Apple's App

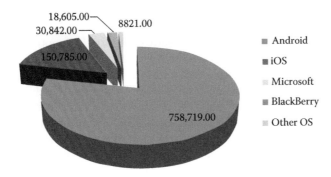

FIGURE 3.3
Worldwide smartphone sales to end users by operating system in 2013.

Store, with the average most expensive health application costing $13.11. Indeed, the most expensive market is the Blackberry App World, where the most expensive health application costs an average of $37.87 (Mobihealthnews 2010). The low cost of these health applications is an advantage and makes them potential investments for consumers and health care professionals.

According to the *Global Mobile Health Market Report 2010–2015* by research2guidance (2010), in 2015, about 500 million people will be using m-health applications. This raises several important and complex questions about these medical applications, such as security, reliability efficiency, and quality of service. Can these applications really perform a complete, secure, reliable, and efficient diagnostic? The fact is that there are already m-health services making claims, such as, "This app will lower your blood pressure" or "This app will help you to lose weight." Are these claims trustworthy? To protect users, the US Food and Drug Administration (FDA), from the Department of Health and Human Services (FDA—US Food and Drug Administration 2011), enforces regulations on medical device approval and clearance. Device manufacturers must first register and notify the FDA of their intent to market a medical device. This is known as 510(k) clearance and allows the FDA to determine if the device is valid and if it is equivalent to a device already in place in the market. The next step is premarket approval (PMA). PMA is the most rigorous approval of a request submitted to the FDA to market. This approval is based on valid scientific evidence that ensures that the proposed device is safe and effective for its intended use. FDA regulation also allows the submission of a Humanitarian Use Exception (HUE) approval. It applies to Humanitarian Use Devices (HUDs). HUDs are intended to care for patients by treating or diagnosing a disease that affects fewer than 4000 people in the United States per year. The HDE approval is very similar to PMA, except the effectiveness requirements (FDA—US Food and Drug Administration 2011). The FDA also defines in section 201(h) the term *device* as "…an instrument, apparatus, implement, machine, contrivance, implant, in vitro reagent, or other similar or related article, including any component, part, or accessory, which is … [either] intended for use in the diagnosis of disease or other conditions, or in the cure, mitigation, treatment, or prevention of disease, in man or other animals … [or] intended to affect the structure or any function of the body of man..."

The FDA regulations on devices are very clear. Analogously, the European Commission (EC) Medical Devices Directive (MDD) covers the regulatory requirements of the European Union for Medical Devices (Council Directive 93/42/EEC 1993). The MDD clears and places medical devices into one of four classes (I, IIa, IIb, and III). These classes concern the device increasing risk to the patient according to its characteristics, functions, and intended purposes. The MDD consists of 23 articles, 12 annexes, and 18 classification rules, and it is considerably more complex to read and understand than the FDA regulation. Recently, Ericsson Mobile Health (Ericsson 2010) was certified in accordance as a medical device of class IIa.

Although several medical devices have already been certified, both FDA and EC regulations on m-health software are yet to be well defined. Another important question that must be resolved is the definition of *medical device*. Does a device plus a health-related application result in a medical device? If so, can smartphones, which are already used by physicians for innumerous health purposes, be classified as medical devices?

Although m-health services and applications have several yet-unresolved issues, it is certain that m-health is more than another evolution in health care technologies. M-health is a revolution, the revolution of typical and old health care models based on the early twentieth century in hospitals and acute care.

M-Health Application Awareness

The study and development of m-health services and applications have been an important point of attention for the research community. Several research areas related to health have gathered important findings and contributions from m-health, such as cardiology (Morris and Guilak 2009; Scherr et al. 2009; Chin-Teng et al. 2010; Fayn and Rubel 2010; Paré et al. 2010), diabetes (Kollmann et al. 2007; Preuveneers and Berbers 2008; Mougiakakou et al. 2010; Paré et al. 2010; Zhou et al. 2010b), obesity (Joo and Kim 2007; Tsai et al. 2007; Khalil and Glal 2009; Patrick et al. 2009; Pollak et al. 2010; Zhu et al. 2010; Rodrigues et al. 2013), smoking cessation (Whittaker et al. 2011), and elderly care and chronic diseases (Giuli and Paganelli 2007; Benlamri and Docksteader 2010; Vergara et al. 2010). These different medical topics make use of m-health essentially for monitoring, prevention, and detection of diseases, and, in more advanced services, present basic diagnosis. Besides all medical applications, m-health services are even becoming popular in developing countries (Akter et al. 2010; Vatsalan et al. 2010), where health care facilities are frequently remote and inaccessible.

Several countries, governments, and health care–related institutions are already improving their health care services and also offering m-health solutions. In July 2010, the federal government's USA.gov website presented a mobile app store (U.S. Mobile Apps 2011a). This store contains five health-related applications. Most of the available mobile applications have a fee, while the health-related apps are free to use. The five health-related applications available are the following:

- *MyDS—My Dietary Supplements*: This iPhone application is an easy way to keep track of vitamins, minerals, herbs, and other product intake (U.S. Mobile Apps 2011b).
- *MedlinePlus Mobile*: A mobile web interface that browses health information to find important drug information and other health related topics (U.S. Mobile Apps 2011c).
- *Find a Health Center*: This iPhone application finds federally funded health centers near the user's current location (U.S. Mobile Apps 2011d).
- *AIDSinfo HIV/AIDS Glossary*: Designed only for iOS, this application helps health care providers, caseworkers, community-based organization professionals, and people living with HIV/AIDS or even their families and friends to help understand the complex HIV/AIDS terminology (U.S. Mobile Apps 2011e).
- *BMI calculator*: This iPhone application is one of the most popular tools from the National Heart, Lung, and Blood Institute (NHLBI) website. BMI is an indicator of total body fat, which is related to the risk of disease and death. It receives 1.6 million visitors a month and ranks #1 on Google (U.S. Mobile Apps 2011f).

Harvard Medical School (HMS) is encouraging students to buy a mobile device of their choice (iPhone, iPad, Android, Blackberry, etc.). The school provides for those devices software licenses and controlled host applications for medical education purposes (Halamka 2011). According to the chief information officer (CIO) and dean for Technology at HMS, Dr. John Halamka, the top five mobile applications downloaded from the HMS mobile resources web page are the following:

- *Dynamed*: A clinical reference tool created by physicians for point-of-care situations. It is designed for physicians and other health care professionals, with clinically organized summaries for more than 3200 topics. *Dynamed* is updated daily and monitors the content of over 500 medical journals (Calabretta and Fitzpatrick 2005).
- *Unbound Medicine uCentral*: Unbound Medicine delivers a wide range of medical customizable solutions for nursing schools, publishers/associations, medical schools, residency programs, departments, pharmaceutical or medical device companies, and hospitals or health systems. These health-related solutions are available for almost all mobile platforms and also the web. uCentral is a completely customizable mobile and web application that delivers answers about clinical references to the point of need. Clinicians, students, and researchers, through their mobile devices, can easily answer clinical questions (Unbound Medicine 2011).
- *VisualDx Mobile*: VisualDx provides physician-reviewed clinical information with thousands of medical images. It is the only medical application showing the variation of disease presentation through age, stage, and skin type. This application allows a visual validation of a diagnosis by comparing medical images, allows a quick search by disease for next steps in patient care, and provides on-the-spot patient education with real medical images (VisualDx 2011).
- *Epocrates Essentials*: Epocrates is the #1 mobile medical application among US physicians. More than 1.3 million health care professionals, including 45% of physicians, use Epocrates to improve patient care and efficiencies with its drug reference and clinical/educational applications. Basically, the application is a mobile guide to drugs and disease, with an integrated and comprehensive search tool for diseases, infectious diseases, medications, diagnosis, laboratory tests, and resource centers. Epocrates is available for almost every mobile platform but also for the desktop market and the web (Epocrates 2011).
- *iRadiology*: This iPhone/iPad application is a free learning tool for medical students and residents. iRadiology provides quick reviews of classic radiology cases and images, including more than 500 radiology cases, to improve skills to interpret plain film, computed tomography (CT), and MRI readings (Liberman 2011).

The University of California, Los Angeles (UCLA) School of Nursing, also makes a stand and clearly moves interests toward m-health. The nursing school equipped its third-year undergraduate students and first-year master's entry clinical nursing students with iPod touch devices. Dr. Courtney Lyder, dean of the UCLA School of Nursing, stated, "We want to make sure that we provide them with the tools to be successful and prepare them for 21st-century healthcare" (UCLA Newsroom 2011). The mobile devices provide students with the following preloaded health-related applications.

- *Nursing Central*: This application provides information about diseases and drugs and test information for nurses. It includes top trusted references such as the Davis Drug Guide, Davis's lab and diagnostic tests, a disease and disorder reference, and Taber's Medical Dictionary. There is also a MEDLINE journal citation and study-abstract explorer. *Nursing central* is an *unbound medicine* solution that is available for almost all mobile platforms (Nursing Central 2011).
- *Medical Spanish*: The Hispanic community is now nearly half the population in Southern California. Proper communication between health care providers and

patients is essential to deliver the proper care. Medical Spanish is designed to support Spanish-speaking patients. It translates more than 3000 English questions and phrases into Spanish (Medical Spanish 2015).

The US Army is also adhering to m-health evolution. The Army's Medical Communications for Combat Casualty Care (MC4) is testing electronic medical record (EMR) applications running on Apple iOS and Android devices in the field. The goal is to upgrade the existing EMR systems to include better methods for documenting mild traumatic brain injury (mTBI) data. The MC4 is already performing field tests in Iraq and Afghanistan and is planning to conduct future pilots in Southwest Asia and 12 other countries (Federal Telemedicine News 2011). It is also planning a mobile version of the Transportation Regulating and Command and Control Evacuation System (TRAC2ES) application (Kott et al. 1999), which tracks the movement of sick and injured soldiers in transit.

Current State of M-Health Application Usage

As mentioned, the two main online stores for mobile applications are the Apple App Store (2011) and Google Play Store (2011). Both online stores provide to end users and health professionals a vast number of m-health applications. This section presents and briefly describes the top paid applications related to health services in both online stores and by category.

Apple Store, Health Care and Fitness Category

- *Nike+ GPS*: This application maps user runs, tracks progress, and provides the motivation that a user needs to go even further (e.g., midrun cheers every time a friend likes or comments on the run status, or outrunning them in a game of Nike+ Tag).
- *iMuscle*: iMuscle is a sophisticated workout aid that can be taken anywhere. It allows a user to identify the muscle or muscles to be worked out. It also presents the respective and adequate physical exercises.
- *Sleep Cycle alarm clock*: The Sleep Cycle alarm clock is a bioalarm clock that analyzes sleep patterns and wakes the user in the lightest sleep phase. It is a natural way to wake up that helps the user to feel rested and relaxed. Sleep Cycle has become a huge success and has a #1 paid app position in many countries, including Germany, Japan, and Russia.
- *All-in Fitness*: This is a very polished fitness app that is very easy to get around. The main screen is laid out in four sections, My Workouts, Exercise Base, Food & Calories, and Body Tracker. Exercise Base and Body Tracker are fairly straightforward, with Exercise Base showing how to do just about every exercise on the planet, including the exercise history and a video. Body Tracker tracks body measurements over time.
- *White Noise*: This provides ambient sounds of the environment to help the user to relax or sleep. It includes high-quality looping noises such as ocean waves crashing, hard rain pouring, and stream water flowing.

Apple Store, Medical Category

- *Medical Calculator*: Medical Calculator is an iPhone and iPod touch app that helps doctors and nurses compute useful formulas and equations. With more than 250,000 installs worldwide, this is the most popular medical calculator for the iPhone.
- *MedCalc*: Very similar to Medical Calculator. This application also helps doctors and nurses compute useful formulas and equations. The main difference is that this one contains a vast encyclopedia with detailed information concerning each formula.
- *WebMD*: This application helps the user to make decisions to improve his/her health. It provides mobile access 24/7 to mobile-optimized health information and decision-support tools, including WebMD's Symptom Checker, Drugs & Treatments, First Aid Information, and Local Health Listings. WebMD also gives access to first-aid information without the need of an Internet connection.
- *Epocrates*: Epocrates is the #1 mobile drug reference resource used by health care providers at the point of care. Trusted for accurate content and innovative offerings, Epocrates is chosen by physicians 3 to 1 as their point-of-care drug reference of choice.

Google Play Store, Medical Care Category

- *Menstrual Calendar*: This application tracks one's period, ovulation, temperature, and more. It includes a customizable calendar with icons, customizable symptoms, cycle Report + Weight Chart + Basal Body Temperature Chart, and smart forecast (using historical data to forecast menstruation and ovulation), desktop widget, password protection, and notifications.
- *ICE: In Case of Emergency*: ICE stores important information for first responders and hospital staff to use in case of an emergency. It includes a list of people to call, insurance information, primary doctor's name and number, allergies, medical conditions, medications, and any special instructions or other information.
- *EMS Advanced Life Support (ACLS)*: The EMS ACLS app puts critical information at the fingertips of an emergency medical technician (EMT). It includes quick navigation to critical information, custom bookmarks, search capability, capability to add notes to a page, and medical calculators.
- *AmbiScience—Pure Sleep*: This application combines ambient electronic sounds and a variety of effective programs that attune the brain to desired states of mind using entrainment frequencies. The main objective of this application is to resolve sleeping problems.

Google Play Store, Health Care and Fitness Category

- *Endomondo sports tracker*: This application is a trainer for running, cycling, walking, etc. It includes real-time GPS tracking of time, distance, speed, and calories, and audio feedback for every mile or kilometers. It also includes real-time pep talks from friends, who can follow live runs; a workout route on a map; a history with lap times and a music playlist; and competition between friends, connected through the social network Facebook.

- *JEFIT Pro—Workout & Fitness*: An app designed by bodybuilders for bodybuilders or for those who aspire to be in top physical condition. It is an app designed to help you keep track of the progress you are making—find out how well in today's review.
- *Calorie Counter PRO MyNetDiary*: MyNetDiary is a diet application with 1.4 million downloads. This application provides a diet plan including 40 screens and a 416,000-plus food database, and website access for online food entry and backup.

Conclusion and Future Trends

This chapter studied and reviewed the current state of the art in m-health services and applications and also in ubiquitous technologies applied to health care. This chapter began by introducing the concept of m-health and pervasive health. Next, it described and presented how pervasiveness responds to several health care problems. This section included the relevant literature and market approaches. The following section reflected upon m-health regulation and legislation issues. The next section discussed the awareness of several governmental and public institutions of m-health, and the last section briefly described the top paid applications on the mobile market.

Based on this study, we believe that pervasive and m-health services and applications propose to deliver health care services any time and anywhere, overcoming geographical, temporal, and even organizational barriers. They will have a very important and determinant role in restructuring the *old* health care services and systems that are still based on the physical relationship between patient and doctor. Besides that, m-health applications will have a strong impact on all health care services, such as hospitals, care centers, emergency attendance, etc.

Future Trends

Based on this review of the state of the art and market research on pervasive and m-health applications, we believe that the future of both areas will bypass the transpositions of services and applications based on the individual to services that involve groups and social networks related to health. Nowadays, social networks are playing an important role in people's daily lives. Pervasive and m-health solutions may enable social networking to promote healthy behaviors and awareness among patients involved in network groups and communities.

The cooperation between m-health applications is another future challenge that needs more comprehensive study. Patients or doctors who use the same or different services must be able to cooperate in sharing medical information to accomplish common objectives. Cooperation methods also aim at better efficiency and performance of mobile devices (for example, a device battery).

An important growing aspect of m-health systems is the usability and embedded ubiquitous technology. However, these characteristics raise several security issues concerning private and sensitive medical information. Privacy is a major issue in information management for public health needs. Until now, the focus of pervasive and m-health research has been on services and applications, more than evaluating their impacts. A study related to the impact of mobile communication technologies for health on patients and health professionals must be preformed. This study should include questionnaires to collect data related to the influence of m-health applications on end users'/patients' daily routine. Furthermore, questions to inquire how m-health applications can reduce financial costs to end users/patients and how the health care public system is affected by m-health may be included.

Acknowledgments

This work has been partially supported by Instituto de Telecomunicações, Next Generation Networks and Applications Group (NetGNA), Portugal; by national funding from Fundação para a Ciência e a Tecnologia (FCT) through the UID/EEA/50008/2013 Project; and by the Ambient Assisted Living for All (AAL4ALL) project cofunded by COMPETE under FEDER via the QREN program.

References

Akter, S. and Ray, P. 2010. mHealth—An ultimate platform to serve the unserved. In *International Medical Informatics Association (IMIA), Year Book*, 75–81.

Akter, S., D'Ambra, J. and Ray, P. 2010. User perceived service quality of mHealth services in developing countries: Research paper. In *European Conference on Information Systems (ECIS 2010)*. Pretoria, South Africa, June 6–9.

Android Developers. 2011. What is android. Available at http://developer.android.com/guide /basics/what-is-android.html (Accessed: December 2010).

Apple. 2011. iPad. Available at http://www.apple.com/ipad/ (Accessed: April 2011).

Apple App Store. 2011. Available at http://www.apple.com/iphone/apps-for-iphone/ (Accessed: September 2011).

Apple Developer. 2011. Develop for iOS. Available at http://developer.apple.com/technologies /ios/ (Accessed: July 2011).

Apple Inc. 2011. Available at http://www.apple.com/ (Accessed: September 2011).

Benlamri, R. and Docksteader, L. 2010. MORF: A mobile health-monitoring platform. *IT Professional*, Vol. 12, no. 3, 18–25.

Calabretta, N. and Fitzpatrick, R. B. 2005. DynaMed at the point of care. In *Journal of Electronic Resources in Medical Libraries*, Vol. 2, 55–64.

Cha, Y. D. and Yoon, G. 2009. Ubiquitous health monitoring system for multiple users using a ZigBee and WLAN dual-network. In *Telemedicine Journal and e-Health the Official Journal of the American Telemedicine Association*, Vol. 15, 891–897.

Chilmark Research. 2011. Providing perspective on key IT trends in the healthcare sector. Available at http://chilmarkresearch.com/ (Accessed: April 2011).

Chin-Teng, L., Kuan-Cheng, C., Chun-Ling, L., Chia-Cheng, C., Shao-Wei, L., Shih-Sheng, C. et al. 2010. An intelligent telecardiology system using a wearable and wireless ECG to detect atrial fibrillation. In *IEEE Transactions on Information Technology in Biomedicine*, Vol. 14, no. 3, 726–733. doi:10.1109/TITB.2010.2047401.

Council Directive 93/42/EEC of June 14, 1993, Concerning Medical Devices. 1993. In *Official Journal of the European Communities*, Vol. 36, no. L169, July 12.

d4—Better Communication Means Better Care. 2011. New data show mobile devices increase productivity in everyday clinical practice and support patient care. Available at http://blog.d4.org.uk/2010/12/new-data-show-mobile-devices-increase-productivity-in-everyday-clinical-practice.html (Accessed: April 2011).

Dong-Wook, J., BokKeun, S., Sang-Yeon, C., Surgwon, S. and Kwang-Rok, H. 2007. Implementation of ubiquitous health care system for active measure of emergencies. In *Sixth International Conference on Advanced Language Processing and Web Information Technology (ALPIT 2007)*, 420–425.

DynaMed. Available at http://www.ebscohost.com/dynamed/default.php (Accessed: April 2011).

Epocrates. 2011. Available at http://www.epocrates.com/company/ (Accessed: April 2011).

Ericsson. 2010. Live smart mobile health. Available at http://www.ericsson.com:80/hr/ict_solutions/e-health/emh/index.shtml (Accessed: April 2011).

Fayn, J. and Rubel, P. 2010. Toward a personal health society in cardiology. In *IEEE Transactions on Information Technology in Biomedicine*, Vol. 14, no. 2, 401–409. doi:10.1109/TITB.2009.2037616.

FDA—U.S. Food and Drug Administration. 2011. Device approvals and clearances. Available at http://www.fda.gov/MedicalDevices/ProductsandMedicalProcedures/DeviceApprovalsandClearances/default.htm (Accessed: April 2011).

Federal Telemedicine News. 2011. Mc4 testing apps. Available at http://telemedicinenews.blogspot.com/2010/12/mc4-testing-apps.html (Accessed: July 2011).

Gartner. 2010. Available at http://www.gartner.com/it/page.jsp?id=1529214 (Accessed: December 2010).

Giuli, D. and Paganelli, F. 2007. An ontology-based context model for home health monitoring and alerting in chronic patient care networks. In *Proc. IEEE 21st Int'l Conf. Advanced Information Networking and Applications Workshops (AINAW 07)*, Vol. 2. IEEE CS Press, 838–845.

Google Play Store. 2011. Available at https://play.google.com/store (Accessed: July 2012).

Graschew, G., Roelofs, T. A., Rakowsky, S. and Schlag, P. M. 2007. Design of satellite-based networks for u-Health—GALENOS, DELTASS, MEDASHIP, EMISPHER. In *9th International Conference on e-Health Networking, Application and Services*, June 19–22, 168.

Halamka, J. D. 2011. Mobile applications for medical education. Available at http://geekdoctor.blogspot.com/2011/04/mobile-applications-for-medical.html (Accessed: April 2011).

Istepanian, R. and Lacal, J. 2003. Emerging mobile communication technologies for health: Some imperative notes on m-Health. In *The 25th Silver 59 Anniversary International Conference of the IEEE Engineering in Medicine and Biology Society*. IEEE, Cancun, Mexico.

Joo, N. S. and Kim, B. T. 2007. Mobile phone short message service messaging for behaviour modification in a community-based weight control programme in Korea. In *Journal of Telemedicine and Telecare*, Vol. 13, no. 8, 416–420.

Kamp, J. and Cheng, R. 2011. IPads are Latest Weapon in Medical Sales. The Wall Street Journal 2011 [online]. Available at http://online.wsj.com/article/SB10001424052748703493504576007723119984758.html?mod=WSJ_Tech_LEFTTopNews (Accessed: April 2011).

Khalil, A. and Glal, S. 2009. StepUp: A step counter mobile application to promote healthy lifestyle. In *International Conference on the Current Trends in Information Technology (CTIT)*, December 15–16, 1–5.

Kollmann, A., Riedl, M., Kastner, P., Schreier, G. and Ludvik, B. 2007. Feasibility of a mobile phone–based data service for functional insulin treatment of type 1 diabetes mellitus patients. In *Journal of Medical Internet Research*, Vol. 9, no. 5, e36. Available at http://www.jmir.org/2007/5/e36/.

Kott, A., Saks, V. and Mercer, A. 1999. A new technique enables dynamic replanning and rescheduling of aeromedical evacuation. In *Artificial Intelligence Magazine*, Vol. 2, no. 1, 43–54.

Kwang, S. P. 2009. Nonintrusive measurement of biological signals for ubiquitous healthcare. In *Annual International Conference of the IEEE Engineering in Medicine and Biology Society*, 6573–6575.

Kwon, O., Shin, S. and Kim, W. 2010. Design of U-health system with the use of smart phone and sensor network. In *Proceedings of the 5th International Conference on Ubiquitous Information Technologies and Applications*, 1–6.

Laxminarayan, S. and Istepanian, R. S. 2000. UNWIRED E-MED: The next generation of wireless and internet telemedicine systems. In *IEEE Transactions of Information Technology and Biomedicine*, Vol. 4, no. 3, 189–193.

Laxminarayan, S., Istepanian, R. and Pattichis, C. S. (Eds.). 2006. *M-Health: Emerging Mobile Health Systems.* Springer, New York.

Liberman, G. 2011. iRadiology. Available at http://itunes.apple.com/us/app/iradiology /id346440355?mt=8 (Accessed: April 2011).

Lin, C., Lee, R. and Hsiao, C. 2008. A pervasive health monitoring service system based on ubiquitous network technology. In *International Journal of Medical Informatics*, Vol. 77, 461–469.

Little, L. and Briggs, P. 2009. Pervasive healthcare: The elderly perspective. In *Proceedings of the 2nd International Conference on Pervasive Technologies Related to Assistive Environments.* New York, 1–5.

Medical Spanish: Healthcare Phrasebook with Audio. 2015. *Batoul Apps.* Available at https://itunes .apple.com/us/app/medical-spanish-healthcare/id301655973?mt=8.

Medtronic. 2011. Available at http://www.medtronic.com/ (Accessed: April 2011).

Mobihealthnews. 2010. The fastest growing and most successful health & medical apps. In *Mobihealthnews 2010 Report.*

Morris, M. and Guilak, F. 2009. Mobile heart health: Project highlight. *In IEEE Pervasive Computing*, Vol. 2, 57–61.

Mougiakakou, S. G., Bartsocas, C. S., Bozas, E., Chaniotakis, N., Iliopoulou, D., Kouris, I. et al. 2010. SMARTDIAB: A communication and information technology approach for the intelligent monitoring, management and follow-up of type 1 diabetes patients. In *IEEE Transactions on Information Technology in Biomedicine*, Vol. 14, no. 3, 622–633.

Moullee, B. L. and Ray, P. 2009. Issues in e-Health cost impact assessment. In *IFMBE Proceeding of the World Congress on Medical Physics and Biomedical Engineering.* Munich, Germany, September 7–12, 223–226.

Nursing Central. 2011. Available at http://www.unboundmedicine.com/nursingcentral/ub (Accessed: June 2011).

Paré, G., Moqadem, K., Pineau, G. and St-Hilaire, C. 2010. Clinical effects of home telemonitoring in the context of diabetes, asthma, heart failure and hypertension: A systematic review. In *Journal of Medical Internet Research*, Vol. 12, no. 2, e21. Available at http://www.jmir.org/2010/2/e21/.

Patrick, K., Raab, F., Adams, M. A., Dillon, L., Zabinski, M., Rock, C. L. et al. 2009. A text message–based intervention for weight loss: Randomized controlled trial. In *Journal of Medical Internet Research*, Vol. 11, no. 2, e1. Available at http://www.jmir.org/2009/1/e1/.

Pollak, J. P., Gay, G., Byrne, S., Wagner, E., Retelny, D. and Humphreys, L. 2010. It's time to eat!—Using mobile games to promote healthy eating. In *IEEE Pervasive Computing*, Vol. 9, 21–27.

Practice Fusion—Free, Web-based Electronic Health Records. 2011a. Survey: Three in five Americans with chronic disease say using home medical devices would improve their health. Available at http://www.practicefusion.com/pages/pr/many-americans-with-chronic-disease-say-using -medical-devices-would-improve-health.html (Accessed: April 2011).

Practice Fusion—Free, Web-based Electronic Health Records. 2011b. Survey: 3 in 4 patients say computers help their doctors deliver better care. Available at http://www.practicefusion.com /pages/pr/survey-3-in-4-patients-say-computers-help-their-doctors-deliver-better-care.html (Accessed: April 2011).

Preuveneers, D. and Berbers, Y. 2008. Mobile phones assisting with health self-care: A diabetes case study. In *Proceedings of the 10th International Conference on Human Computer Interaction with Mobile Devices and Services.* NY, 177–186.

Research2guidance—The Mobile Research Specialists. 2010. The impact of smartphone applications on the mobile health industry. In *Mobile Health Market Report 2010–2015.*

Rikitake, K., Araki, Y., Kawahara, Y., Minami, M. and Morikawa, H. 2009. NGN/IMS-based ubiquitous health monitoring system. In *6th IEEE Consumer Communications and Networking Conference (CCNC 2009).* Las Vegas, NV, January 10–13.

Rodrigues, J. J. P. C., Lopes, I. M. C., Silva, B. M. C., and de la Torre, I. 2013. A new mobile ubiquitous computing application to control obesity: SapoFit. In *Informatics for Health and Social Care*, Vol. 38, no. 1, 1–29. doi:10.3109/17538157.2012.674586.

Scherr, D., Kastner, P., Kollmann, A., Hallas, A., Auer, J., Krappinger, H. et al. 2009. Effect of home-based telemonitoring using mobile phone technology on the outcome of heart failure patients after an episode of acute decompensation: Randomized controlled trial. In *Journal of Medical Internet Research*, Vol. 11, no. 3, e34. Available at http://www.jmir.org/2009/3/e34/.

Schmidt, A. 2010. Ubiquitous computing: Are we there yet? In *IEEE Computer*, Vol. 43, 95–97.

Shin, W., Dae Cha, Y. and Yoon, G. 2009. ECG/PPG integer signal processing for a ubiquitous health monitoring system. *In Journal of Medical Systems*, Vol. 34, 891–898.

Silva, B. M. C., Rodrigues, J. J. P. C., Lopes, I. M. C., Machado, T. M. F. and Zhou, L. 2013. A novel cooperation strategy for mobile health applications. In *IEEE Journal on Selected Areas in Communications (JSAC), Special Issue on Emerging Technologies in Communications – eHealth*, IEEE Communications Society, Vol. 31, no. 9, 28–36, doi:10.1109/JSAC.2013.SUP.0513003.

Sugano, H., Tsujioka, T., Inoue, T., Nakajima, S., Hara, S., Nakamura, H. et al. 2010. Clinical tests and evaluations of a wireless ECG sensor for realization of ubiquitous health care systems. In *32nd Annual International Conference of the IEEE EMBS*. Buenos Aires, Argentina, August 31–September 4.

Suzuki, T. and Nakauchi, Y. 2009. Dosing monitoring system using iMec and ubiquitous sensors. In *2009 Annual International Conference of the IEEE Engineering in Medicine and Biology Society*, 6163–6166.

Tachakra, S., Wang, X., Istepanian, R. and Song, Y. 2003. Mobile e-Health: The unwired evolution of telemedicine. In *Telemedicine Journal and e-Health*, Vol. 9, 247–257.

Taleb, T., Bottazzi, D. and Nasser, N. 2010. A novel middleware solution to improve ubiquitous health-care systems aided by affective information. In *IEEE Transactions on Information Technology in Biomedicine*, Vol. 14, 335–349.

Tsai, C. C., Lee, G., Raab, F., Norman, G. J., Sohn, T., Griswold, W. G. and Patrick, K. 2007. Usability and feasibility of PmEB: A mobile phone application for monitoring real time caloric balance. In *Journal of Mobile Networks and Applications*, Vol. 12, 173–184.

U.S. Mobile Apps. 2011a. Available at http://apps.usa.gov/ (Accessed: April 2011).

U.S. Mobile Apps. 2011b. My Dietary Supplements (MyDS). Available at http://apps.usa.gov/my-dietary supplements-myds/ (Accessed: April 2011).

U.S. Mobile Apps. 2011c. MedlinePlus mobile. Available at http://apps.usa.gov/mobile-medline-plus/ (Accessed: April 2011).

U.S. Mobile Apps. 2011d. Find a health center. Available at http://apps.usa.gov/find-a-health-center/ (Accessed: April 2011).

U.S. Mobile Apps. 2011e. AIDSinfo HIV/AIDS glossary. Available at http://apps.usa.gov/aidsinfo-hivaids-glossary/ (Accessed: April 2011).

U.S. Mobile Apps. 2001f. BMI calculator. Available at http://apps.usa.gov/bmi-app/ (Accessed: April 2011).

UCLA Newsroom. 2011. Keeping nursing students in touch. Available at http://newsroom.ucla.edu/portal/ucla/keeping-nursing-students-in-touch-187148.aspx (Accessed: July 2011).

Unbound Medicine. 2011. Available at http://www.unboundmedicine.com/ (Accessed: April 2011).

Unbound Medicine—uCentral. 2011. Available at http://www.unboundmedicine.com/solutions/ucentral (Accessed: April 2011).

Vatsalan, D., Arunatileka, S., Chapman, K., Senaviratne, G., Sudahar, S., Wijetileka, D. et al. 2010. Mobile technologies for enhancing eHealth solutions in developing countries. In *2010 Second International Conference on eHealth, Telemedicine, and Social Medicine (ETELEMED)*. St. Maarten, Netherlands Antilles, February 10–16, 84–89.

Vergara, M., Díaz-Hellín, P., Fontecha, J., Hervás, R., Sánchez-Barba, C., Fuentes, C. and Bravo, J. 2010. Mobile prescription: An NFC-based proposal for AAL. In *2010 Second International Workshop on Near Field Communication*. Monaco, April, 27–32.

VisualDx. 2011. Visual diagnostic decision support—VisualDx mobile. Available at http://www.visualdx.com/mobile/ (Accessed: April 2011).

Weiser, M. 1991. The computer for the twenty-first century. In *Scientific American*, September, 94–104.

Weiser, M. 1994. The world is not a desktop. In *ACM Interactions*, Vol. 1, no. 1, 7–8.

Whittaker, R., Dorey, E., Bramley, D., Bullen, C., Denny, S., Elley, C. R. et al. 2011. A theory-based video messaging mobile phone intervention for smoking cessation: Randomized controlled trial. In *Journal of Medical Internet Research*, Vol. 13, no. 1, e10. Available at http://www.jmir.org/2011/1/e10/.

Yoo, H. J., Park, M. S., Kim, T. N., Yang, S. J., Cho, G. J., Hwang, T. G. et al. 2009. A ubiquitous chronic disease care system using cellular phones and the internet. *In Diabetic Medicine*, Vol. 26, 628–635.

Zhou, J., Gilman, E., Ylianttila, M. and Riekki, J. 2010a. Pervasive service computing: Visions and challenges. In *2010 IEEE 10th International Conference on Computer and Information Technology (CIT)*, 1335–1339.

Zhou, F., Yang, H., Álamo, J. M. R., Wong, J. S. and Chang, C. K. 2010b. Mobile personal health care system for patients with diabetes. In *Proceedings of International Conference on Smart Homes and Health Telematics*. Seoul, Korea, 94–101.

Zhu, F., Bosh, M., Woo, I., Kim, S., Boushey, C. J., Ebert, D. S. et al. 2010. The use of mobile devices in aiding dietary assessment and evaluation. In *IEEE Journal of Selected Topics in Signal Processing*, Vol. 4, 756–766.

Zuehlke, P., Li, J., Talai-Khoei, A. and Ray, P. 2009. A functional specification for mobile eHealth (mHealth) systems. In *IEEE 11th International Conference on e-Health Networking, Application & Services (HEALTHCOM 2009)*. Sydney, Australia, December 16–18.

4

A Review of Monitoring and Assisted Therapeutic Technology for AAL Applications

Pedro Dinis Gaspar, Virginie Felizardo, and Nuno M. Garcia

CONTENTS

ABSTRACT This chapter describes a set of technologies (projects and scientific works) with relevance in care and medical monitoring for application outside the clinical context. The number of older people continues to increase and with it the increase in the number of people with chronic diseases. In order to reduce costs in health care, solutions emerged such as information and communication technologies (ICTs). All these solutions, in the context presented here, can come together in an area called ambient assisted living (AAL).

This area presents innovative solutions that improve the quality of life of these people. In this chapter, we have collected together projects and works with scientific relevance in this application area. The distribution of these publications was divided into two topics: home care technology and free living technology.

KEY WORDS: *monitoring devices, assisted therapeutic devices, ambient assisted living, home care technology, free living technology.*

Introduction

Worldwide, there are around 600 million people aged 60 and over. This number will double by 2025 and will reach virtually 2 billion by 2050 [1,2].

Many individuals will face, as they age, the risk of having at least one chronic disease, such as hypertension, diabetes, and osteomuscular conditions.

Increased longevity is a triumph for public health. However, the majority of older people will be living in developing countries that are often the least prepared to face the challenges of rapidly ageing societies.

All countries need to be prepared to address the consequences of demographic trends [2]. Recent advances in telecommunications, medical devices, and technology in the home environment have enabled elderly people to live independently for longer. However, integrated systems targeting health monitoring in the home environment are at best scarce. The use of these systems would enable medical practitioners to perform an early diagnosis of potential issues, which in turn would result in a better chance of recovery and lower hospitalization costs [2,3].

The ageing of population and the increasing risk of developing chronic diseases enhance the demand for a better available health care system. Additionally, today's lifestyle is synonymous with stress, that in conjunction with an unbalanced food intake increases disease risks in middle-aged and younger populations. Therefore, the need for developing technological solutions for monitoring and therapy increased in order to improve the quality of life as well as to reduce health care costs by providing as many services as possible at home [1,4–6].

A large number of new medical devices had to be designed, tested, and adopted for health monitoring and therapy, home care, wellness promotion, and gerontotechnology, among others, to meet the special needs and demands of different population groups [6].

The aim of the new approach in ambient assisted living (AAL) is not only to monitor and improve health of individuals but also to increase their independence, mobility, safety, and social contact through increased communication, inclusion, and participation using available technologies [6,7].

The level of daily physical activity has a strong effect on a person's health. During the last decades, sedentary and inactive lifestyles have raised serious concerns regarding public health, with diseases such as cardiac illnesses, diabetes, obesity, and others receiving a strong concern focus, since it is estimated that obesity alone is responsible for 6% of the health budget of the World Health Organization (WHO) in European nations [8,9].

Over the last decades, manufacturers of medical equipment kept pace with the demand for reliable, lightweight, and easy-to-operate medical devices for home and ambulatory use [10].

Five system blocks are commonly used when designing health care devices (Figure 4.1): (1) power/battery management; (2) sensor interface, signal conditioning, and analog-to-digital

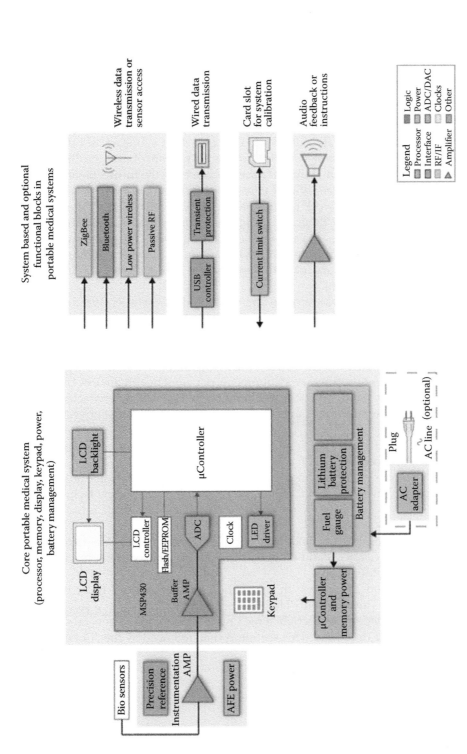

FIGURE 4.1

System blocks for health care technologies. Product availability and design disclaimer—The system block diagram depicted above and the devices recommended are designed in this manner as a reference. Please contact your local TI sales office or distributor for system design specifics and product availability. (From *Medical Applications Guide*. 2010. Courtesy of Texas Instruments.)

conversion; (3) control and data processing; (4) user interface and display; and (5) wireless connectivity [11]. In this type of system, the block that greatly differs between devices is the sensor block. The block implementation topology depends on the sensing, processing, and information demands of the meter type and feature set. Connectivity for portable medical applications has become critical as consumers require data to move from medical devices to other devices such as computers and mobile phones [11].

Characteristics such as portability, energy autonomy, accuracy and measuring frequency, feature customization, and others will be taken into account.

The connection between personal health devices, aggregation manager, and the health care center can be wired or wireless. Their interoperability is now based on Bluetooth® and universal serial bus (USB) as standard interfaces; however, in the future, Bluetooth low energy (BLE) technology and ZigBee® will be considered for the low-power personal area network (PAN) and local area network (LAN) interfaces, respectively [12]. Today, health care devices use a combination of Ethernet, Wi-Fi, and cellular interfaces, such as GSM for the aggregation manager wide area network (WAN) interface. The Continua Health Alliance, which comprises a group of health device original equipment manufacturers, service providers, and silicon vendors, is defining guidelines in order to provide interoperability between medical devices [13].

Wireless standards used in PAN are operating in the industrial, scientific, and medical (ISM) bands. The personal health devices that connect to the aggregation manager usually operate in the 2.4 GHz frequency and in most cases use Bluetooth classic, Bluetooth low energy, or ANT protocol (an open access multicast wireless sensor network technology) [3]. In other cases, standards such as ZigBee/IEEE 802.15.4 are being used. It is also common to find a few proprietary solutions for personal health devices that operate in sub-1 GHz frequency band. The devices operating in the PAN are characterized by low power, long battery life, and short range with a typical range varying between 10 and 100 m.

The ageing combined with an increasing burden of chronic, concurrent diseases threatens to make the current models of health care unsustainable [14].

Information and communication technology (ICT) can support older people only if they understand its *helping role*. However, old habits, and a reluctance to try new technologies, ingrained ways of thinking, and insistence on the accustomed way of life all act to perpetuate the shortage of ICT services [15].

AAL, as a specific user-oriented type of ambient intelligence, may greatly help in this situation. Recent European projects and other scientific works are focused on improving the independent living of older people.

This chapter is organized as follows: In the section "Methodology," the criteria for collecting bibliography are presented. In "Home Care Technologies," several solutions for home health care are exposed. In the section "Free Living Technologies," several solutions for outdoor applications are described. This section is then followed by the "Conclusion."

Methodology

The criteria used for the collection of scientific papers and projects are given by the following: (1) the relevance of application to AAL, (2) relation to medical applications, and (3) date of publication between 2004 and 2012 included. Some of the projects and scientific

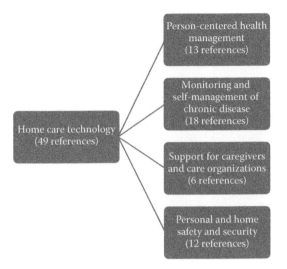

FIGURE 4.2
Collection of scientific papers and projects for home care technology.

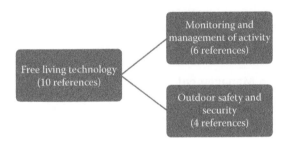

FIGURE 4.3
Collection of scientific articles and projects for free living technology.

papers obtained in this collection belong to the Ambient Assisted Living Joint Programme (AALJP). The AALJP is an activity of the Ambient Assisted Living Association.

In order to organize the information obtained, this chapter is divided into two main topics: (1) home care technology and (2) free living technology. Each of these topics is divided into subtopics, and the projects and scientific papers are distributed among them (see Figures 4.2 and 4.3).

Home Care Technologies

The home care devices can be divided into several groups of applications for AAL: (1) person-centered health management, (2) monitoring and self-management of chronic disease, (3) support for caregivers and care organizations, and (4) personal and home safety and security [16].

Stationary and portable medical devices as well as biotelemetry systems are devices that can be found most commonly in the home environment. These devices are more

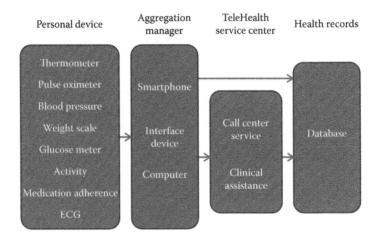

Personal device	Aggregation manager	TeleHealth service center	Health records
Thermometer	Smartphone	Call center service	Database
Pulse oximeter			
Blood pressure	Interface device		
Weight scale			
Glucose meter			
Activity	Computer	Clinical assistance	
Medication adherence			
ECG			

FIGURE 4.4
Basic home care technologies.

comfortable and easier to use at home in order to facilitate patient-centered care and to enable communication with a medical center (Figure 4.4).

Table 4.1 shows several physiological parameters and signals of great importance in medical monitoring and therapeutic, which require the intervention of simple technology with high reliability.

Person-Centered Health Management

This subsection addresses the systems and devices that will adapt themselves to the needs of a person during their life and that relate to their conditions using their personal health profile.

The applications can be a coach for health-conscious people who want to avoid becoming ill in order to help them to follow a healthy lifestyle. This type of application can be a disease management application for a chronically ill person who needs extensive monitoring, guidance, and help to maintain medication compliance [16].

Hope (Smart Home for Elderly People) is a project of the AALJP. It consists of a solution that is installed in the home and provides services for care management, health support, self-monitoring, and decision making [17,18].

The system is divided into two main blocks: the server block and the home block. The home block covers functionalities associated to each person's environment monitoring, indicating alarms when necessary. The server block is responsible for decision-making functionalities of the system, including storage of all information and alarm service [17,18].

Decision Support System

There have been attempts to develop agent-based medical decision support systems to minimize the diagnosis error rate and to conduct effective diagnosis on the basis of real-time data of the patient [19].

One of the approaches considers a diagnosis support system based on the smart medical home station where a patient already owns several monitoring devices [19].

In this type of a system, it is important to define the following: (1) input parameters (e.g., Jung and Wang [19] considered SaO_2, HR, BP, temperature, and respiratory rate); (2) clusters

TABLE 4.1

Physiological Parameters and Signals in Home Care Technologies Context

Physiological System	Monitoring/Therapeutic	Physiological Parameter/Signals
Cardiovascular system	Monitoring	Electrocardiogram (ECG)
		Blood pressure (BP)
		Heart rate (HR)
	Therapeutic	Increase blood flow
Cerebral system	Monitoring	Electroencephalography (EEG)
		Electrodermal activity (EDA)
		Sleep activity
	Therapeutic	Cognitive games
Orthopedic system	Monitoring	Continuous step activity
	Therapeutic	Reduce pain caused by arthritis
Muscular system	Monitoring	Electromyography (EMG)
	Therapeutic	EMG (biofeedback)
Respiratory system	Monitoring	Respiratory rate
		Cough frequency
		Hemoglobin oxygen saturation
	Therapeutic	Continuous positive airway pressure (sleep apnea)
Circulatory system	Monitoring	Metabolites (glucose, cholesterol, others)
		Blood coagulation
	Therapeutic	Glucose (insulin pump)
Reproductive system	Monitoring	Ovulation
Sensory system	Monitoring	Temperature
Biomechanical system	Monitoring	Activity (position, motion, others)
	Therapeutic	Activity games

of the patient level (e.g., Jung and Wang [19] considered regular, careful, serious, and dangerous); and (3) standard values and levels risk of each of the input parameters (Table 4.2).

Based on these definitions, the system will determine the patient risk level. The main advantage of screening from home is to prevent the person from going to a hospital unnecessarily.

For example, in regular and careful level situations, patients do not need to go to the hospital. They just need to take some medicines and follow prescriptions at home. However, in serious situations, patients require first aid and to be readily in contact with their private doctor. When a patient's level is dangerous, the agent computes the location for the nearest hospital to call an ambulance [19].

A commercial example of medical decision support system is the health buddy system, which connects patients in their homes to their care providers. What sets the health buddy system apart is its ability not only to communicate historical patient information for patients with chronic conditions but also to facilitate patient education and encourage medication and lifestyle compliance [20].

Each day, patients answer a series of questions about their health and well-being. The data are sent over a telephone line or Ethernet connection to a secure data center. The data are then available for review on the web-based Health Buddy Desktop. The application is designed to quickly risk-stratify and present patient results, enabling proactive providers to intervene before a patient's condition becomes acute. Patient responses are color-coded

TABLE 4.2

Standard Values and Risk Levels

Physiological Data	Standard Values and Risk Levels	
SaO$_2$	Normal	>90%
	Mild	90%–94%
	Moderate	75%–90%
	Severe	<75%
Heart rate (HR)	Normal	60–100/min
	Tachycardia	>100/min
	Paroxysmal tachycardia	150–250/min
	Flutter	250–350/min
	Fibrillation	350–450/min
Blood pressure (BP)	Normal	120/80 mmHg
	Hypertension	>140/90 mmHg
	Danger hypertension	>200/140 mmHg
	Hypotonic	>100/60 mmHg
	Danger hypotonic	<80/60 mmHg
Respiration rate	Normal	12–20/min (adult)
	Tachypnea	>20/min
Temperature	Normal	36.5°C–37°C
	Slight fever Morning	>37.2°C
	Afternoon	>37.7°C
	High fever >38.3°C	

Source: Jung, I. and G.-N. Wang, User pattern learning algorithm based MDSS (Medical Decision Support System) framework under ubiquitous. In *World Academy of Science, Engineering and Technology*, 2007.

by risk level as high (red), moderate (yellow), and low (green) based on symptoms, patient behaviors, and self-care knowledge [20].

Drug Delivery Systems

If medicines are taken irregularly, incorrectly, or even not at all, physicians and pharmacists assume it as a lack of compliance. This phenomenon increases with age, duration of medicine consumption, and the number of prescribed drugs—with negative consequences for individual therapy success and considerable costs for the social security system [21].

Goals for the use of automated dispensing devices in the medication-use process should focus on improving patient care and resource use. Specific objectives related to these goals may include the following [22]:

- Information necessary for appropriate medication management and patient care is accurate, accessible, and timely.
- Appropriate medications are readily available and accessible to meet patient needs within safety and security controls.
- Vulnerabilities to medication errors are minimized, and those that remain are identified, documented, and mediated.
- Patients are satisfied with the quality and delivery of care.

In order to demonstrate the requirements of this type of equipment, the operation of the Vitality's GlowCap is presented.

Inside the GlowCap is a wireless chip that enables four services: (1) personal reminders; (2) social network support (each week, a report summarizing progress is e-mailed); (3) pharmacy coordination (refill reminders and connect the patient to their pharmacy as pills deplete); and (4) doctor accountability (each month, a report may also be sent to the patient doctor). Collectively, the services help people stick with their prescription regimen [23].

GlowCap uses light and sound to signal when it is time to take a pill. This device is used when the bottle is opened and wirelessly relays their status to Vitality's secure network. If the bottle is not opened 2 h after a scheduled dose, the user is automatically reminded with a telephone call [23].

Brandherm et al. [21] presented a prototypical implementation of an authorized access to a digital product memory (DPM) by means of a role and right management concept with identification by the electronic identity (eID) card. This approach is demonstrated as an example on an instrumented medicament blister (individualized weekly blister), a solution for the oral intake of tablets, capsules, and pills.

According to the German Medicines Act, the content of the blister is imprinted. These data could be made electronically accessible, achieved by the DPM (a product item-centric storage), or can be realized by a smart label attached to the item. Smart labels range from radio-frequency identification (RFID) tags to sensor nodes, which differ not only in the computational capabilities but also in the size of available memory where data can be stored in the item. Digital assistants are required, which translate and visualize memory contents tailored to the user's abilities and goals. One possibility to identify authorized persons is given by the eID card. It has the following three main applications: (1) the ePass application, (2) the mutual online identification, and (3) the qualified electronic signature.

As a future work, the authors propose to equip the blister with certain sensors such that it would be possible to record the actual timestamps of the prescription drug use or data concerning the storage conditions like temperature, humidity, and shocks or damage.

Cognitive and Physical Activities Management

Insufficient social inclusion and isolation often leads to depression. Affected persons tend to be less active and inattentive concerning their own health, with considerable consequences for their well-being and physical and mental health [24,25].

AGNES (User-Sensitive Home-Based Systems for Successful Ageing in a Networked Society), a project of the AALJP, is motivated by relationships between levels of social integration and mental stimulation and the maintenance of cognitive functioning and psychological well-being [24].

Peter et al. [25] described their work within the frame of the project AGNES, introducing an implementation of the Affect- and Behaviour-Related Assistance (ABRA) system, a modular system comprising components for assessing a person's mental and physical state. For assessing a person's mental and physical state, physiological sensors and off-the-shelf motion sensors are used.

Sensing and recognizing emotional and other mental states is a challenging task and requires the integration of sensors and algorithms for data enhancement and processing [25]. In this work, the system consists of a sensor glove (heart rate, skin temperature, and electrodermal activity) and a small wrist pocket that carries the sensor electronics. The three parameters measured by the sensor glove are understood to be key indicators for emotional as well as cognitive processes [25].

Assessing activity patterns allows analyzing a person's behavior. Atypical activity patterns might be indicators for inappropriate lifestyle, insufficient social inclusion, or generally disadvantageous life conditions. For the activity assessment, the system uses acceleration sensors integrated in smartphones.

Muuraiskangas et al. [26] describe a work part of Ambient Intelligence for the Elderly Project (AmIE), which is related to an application for instructing and monitoring exercise. The application was designed for untrained computer users with possible physical constraints, and it was realized with touch-screen computers.

Hendeby et al. [27] describe a technical assistance system, PAMAP, which can monitor the physical activity both in a clinical setting and in the subject's home environment. The goal is to provide physicians with the means to encourage people to a healthy activity level and also to diagnose problems at an early stage.

The PAMAP system has two separate conceptual parts: the information management and the underlying information acquisition system. The body area network (BAN) consists of the PAMAP sensor network and a control unit that links the sensors and several different I/O devices. Each sensor module comprises accelerometers, gyroscopes, and magnetometers capable of measuring in three dimensions.

An interactive TV (i-TV) is used for communication between different system users. The i-TV solution is used to increase the acceptance and ease the learning among elderly users, who generally are not very familiar with computers.

The PAMAP system is still at an early stage of development, and there is ongoing work to improve and extend the quality of the information delivered.

Recently, new tools in neurorehabilitation based on virtual reality (VR) technologies have appeared. These have the advantage of flexibly deploying scenarios that can be directed toward specific needs [28].

Cameirão et al. [28] describe the key components of the Rehabilitation Gaming System (RGS), another project of the AALJP, and the psychometrics of one rehabilitation scenario called Spheroids. The RGB is a VR-based system. In this work, a personalized training module (PTM) for online adjustment of task difficulty is developed.

According to the authors, the RGS scenario (Spheroids) consists of a green landscape populated with a number of trees against the background of a mountain range. Integrated in the virtual world, it is a model of a human torso with arms positioned in such a way that the user has a first-person view of the upper extremities.

In this RGS scenario, spheres move toward the user, and these are to be intercepted through the movement of the virtual arms. The authors describe that each time a sphere is intercepted, the user obtains a number of points that accumulate toward a final score.

They also describe that arm movements are tracked by the camera mounted on top of the display and that the tracking system determines in real time the position of the color patches positioned at wrists and elbows.

The authors showed that the PTM implemented in RGS allows one to effectively adjust the difficulty and the task parameters to the user by capturing specific features of arm movements. The usability assessment showed that the RGS is highly accepted by stroke patients as a rehabilitation tool.

Cameirão et al. [29] investigated the clinical impact of RGS on the recovery time course of acute stroke. The results suggest that rehabilitation with the RGS facilitates the functional recovery of the upper extremities and that this system is therefore a promising tool for stroke neurorehabilitation.

RFID technologies are highly reliable, are very unobtrusive, and have quite low cost. The strong advantage of RFID over comparative technologies is the ever-growing level of standardization of protocols in use and, of course, its wireless communication between small embeddable units and readers. RFID devices are easy to use and usable both outdoors and indoors. Furthermore, they have good endurance with respect to damage or environmental factors [30].

Marcellini et al. [30] present the *HAPPY AGEING* project, in the framework of the AALJP, developing a new device, the HAPPY AGEING system, for the support of older people's daily activities, following the user-centered design paradigm.

The HAPPY AGEING system will be composed of three main modules: a lifestyle monitor (capable of recording main activities that take place in the home and comparing them with the habits of the monitored subject), a navigation assistant to support user mobility in close environment, and a personal assistant.

The main technology on which the system is based is the RFID.

Peter et al. [31] describe part of the work within the framework of project AGNES, presenting a user-sensitive ICT-based home environment that supports a personalized and person-centric care process by detecting, communicating, and meaningfully responding to relevant states taking into account that the users did not want too much information of them being captured and relayed to the social network.

Thus, the following states or situations can be detected:

1. Well-being: is the person happy or sad?
2. Activity: is the person physically active or not?
3. Presence: is the person at home?

For this, a suitable collection of sensors were chosen. On the computer, a webcam was placed that was used for observing the person's face as he or she is using the computer (well-being); for observing activity (interaction); and for observing the room in which the PC is located, usually the living room (presence). Accelerometers included in smartphones or smartwatches were used for detecting the physical activity of a person.

Monitoring and Self-Management of Chronic Disease

Chronic diseases are diseases of long duration (or recurring) and generally with slow progression: Alzheimer's disease and other dementias, arthritis, cardiovascular disease, chronic kidney disease, chronic respiratory disease, diabetes, hypertension, Parkinson's disease, and others.

Individualized therapies and care lead to high success rates, which results in a better quality of life for those people accessing the service [16].

Medical devices are more and more designed and geared toward the needs and experience of the actual user [32]. However, much of the equipment available on the market still requires the intervention of a clinician.

Throughout this section, we will address the AAL perspective, giving some examples of devices and solutions for the home care application.

Boulos [14] developed a project within the framework of AALJP, the Enhanced Complete Ambient Assisted Living Experiment (eCAALYX), that comprises the following objectives: (1) health monitoring of older and elderly persons with multiple chronic conditions (at home and outdoors); (2) improving the quality of life of elderly persons by increasing their freedom and safety; and (3) preventing the deterioration of the patient's condition by providing continuous support, guidance, and relevant health education.

The eCAALYX system is composed of three main interconnected subsystems. The home subsystem includes customer-premises equipment, a set top box, and an interactive TV (to deliver health education and other functions). The home subsystem also has additional home sensors that are stationary and not continuously worn on the body or included in the smart garment. The mobile subsystem includes a smart garment, with vital sign sensors integrated into a wireless BAN of wearable body sensors, and a mobile phone; the caretaker subsystem/ site includes the remote caretaker server and the autoconfiguration server.

The eCAALYX is a great example of contemporary technological infrastructure inserted in homes of aging people with chronic diseases.

Additional examples of works and projects targeted at some chronic diseases are presented in the following.

Cardiovascular Disease

Arrhythmias are often limited in duration and occurrence and cannot be detected during ECG hospital routine. To diagnose the arrhythmia and to assess its relationship with the patient's symptoms, or to assess the effectiveness of a medication, it is necessary to record ECG while the patient continues with their normal routine (long period of time).

Currently, the Holter device is used for recording 24 h of continuous ECG during normal daily activity. The classical ECG home care system consists of an ECG recorder (3–12 leads), and the employed recorder is developed for use inside of a clinic or hospital; thus the use is complicated for a home user [33]. This type of equipment is used as a complementary test to diagnose and not for prevention monitoring.

ECG systems with centralized data management expand the classic type with an option to store and access the ECG data on a central server [33]. In this sense, it is an AAL solution that brings advantages to users.

Korsakas et al. [34] developed a mobile wireless ECG and motion activity recording device, software for real-time signal analysis, and a warning system based on ordinary or pocket PC and designed for home care patients with cardiac risk. The monitoring system makes a decision about patient state changes from the calculated parameters using the convolution of Mealy and Moore automata, and in case of appearance of dangerous situation sends the warning signal to the patient and analysis results to the physician on duty.

Vergari et al. [35] developed a portable, wireless ZigBee-based ECG monitoring device prototype, which is able to acquire, sample, and communicate over the air a single lead ECG signal to a remote base station in real time.

According to these authors, ZigBee is a prominent wireless protocol that offers an efficient relay protocol, good transmission range, and flexible network structure (allowing various network topologies) with emphasis on power consumption efficiency, supporting several *low-power* transmission modes that allow for higher autonomy and battery life. These characteristics influenced the choice of transmission wireless protocol.

D'Angelo et al. [33] presented a system for Internet-based, automated home care ECG upload and prioritization. This system consists of three components: ECG recording (commercial ECG recorder), web application, and prioritization algorithm.

The user connects the ECG electrodes to himself or herself, when he or she wants to record an ECG. The computer application establishes a wireless connection to the ECG recorder and checks whether all the electrodes are connected correctly. The user can click on the *start measurement* button. After 10 s, ECG recording is done and the data are sent onto the web server; the user gets a notice about the successful transmission and can remove the ECG electrodes and see their data and diagnosis online.

Additionally, the web application running on the web server uses the Hospital Episode Statistics (HES) algorithm to analyze the incoming ECGs and a serial ECG comparison to prioritize the ECGs automatically according to their clinical urgency.

There are currently numerous medical applications for smartphones. The big news is the iPhoneECG, developed by AliveCor Company. It has the functionality to perform electrocardiograms using just an iPhone and an iPhone case. AliveCor installed two electrodes in a case for iPhone 4, and as the patient holds the appliance, it communicates, wirelessly or not, the heart activity reading to iPhone. The electrodes are placed either on the hands or on the chest. The iPhoneECG also monitors the heart rate [36]. This product is not yet cleared for sale in the United States as a medical device.

Silva et al. [37] developed a mobile platform based on Android OS. This platform is developed by Plux (a Portuguese company). The proposed platform was used in the context of a continuous real-time monitoring of the ECG signal.

Blood pressure changes throughout the day, and it is influenced by various stimuli [38]: activity, posture, location (home or work), food and fluid intake, psychological state, and medication, among others. Some people, especially the mild hypertensive, have tension rises caused by the presence of doctors (alarm reaction) [38]. During the rest of the day, these individuals may have blood pressure values within normal limits. In selected cases, it is therefore advantageous for doctors to decide on diagnosis and treatment based on measurements performed by the patient at home. This is particularly important in individuals with suspected light hypertension, in which decisions are sometimes more difficult.

A variety of models with different features manufactured by different companies are available. Most of the pieces of equipment are based on the conventional method: the oscillometric method.

Texas Instruments offers a solution to monitor blood pressure using Korotkoff, oscillometry, or pulse transit time methods to measure blood pressure. The system blocks include (Figure 4.5) (1) sensor interface, (2) user interface, (3) processor/memory, and (4) power management.

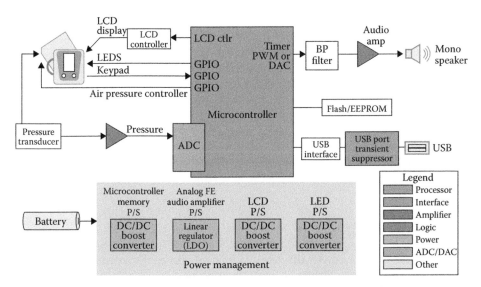

FIGURE 4.5
Blood pressure monitor application block diagram. (From *Medical Applications Guide*. 2010. Courtesy of Texas Instruments.)

Medical portable devices for the twenty-first century and beyond have increasing needs for higher speeds, higher precision, lower power, and smaller dimensions, while maintaining or increasing the high standards for quality and reliability. The development of medical embedded systems is driven by characteristics such as extended battery life, ultralow power, and fast response times imposed by users' desire to quickly know their health status. Requirements such as historical profiling, data upload or access to the sensor, and detailed user interface that drive the development of battery-operated, microcontroller-managed handheld medical devices with more available memory, several cabled or wireless interfaces, and a feature set besides intuitive and detailed user interface ensuring low-power consumption are a significant challenge for researchers and device designers [11]. The goal is to provide innovative medical electronics that are more flexible, affordable, and accessible for the consumer.

PULSE CASPro®, developed by HealthSTATS International, is a simple and yet revolutionary device for the measurement of central aortic systolic pressure (CASP) in clinical environment or home setting. It is empowered by evidence-based blood pressure (EVBP) technology, an FDA listed and patented technology using modified applanation tonometry on the radial artery at the wrist. It is completely noninvasive, painless, and easy to operate (HealthSTATS International, 2011). The system consists of four main elements: (1) A-PULSE CASPro® monitor; (2) wrist sensor module; (3) A-PULSE CASP® software; and (4) integrated oscillometric blood pressure module for calibration [39].

Saponara et al. [40] proposed a telecare system that has been developed in the framework of the Health at Home (H@H) project of the AALJP. The project aims at solving societal problems related to the provision of health care services for elderly citizens affected by chronic heart failure, providing them with wearable sensor devices for monitoring pathophysiological cardiovascular and respiratory parameters and, at the same time, enabling the medical staff to monitor the elderly citizens' situations at a distance and to take action in case of necessity by the involvement of public and private health organizations.

The H@H system has the typical client/server architecture. The platform for home vital signs acquisition and processing directly integrated with the usual hospital information system (HIS) by means of a specific module that allows the management of patients since their enrollment in the system.

The H@H system comprises a set of Bluetooth sensing devices for measuring the main vital parameters and a home gateway that centralizes all needed computation and communication resources. The home gateway receives data from sensors and processes them to detect critical alterations. Then all data are forwarded to the remote server, using one of the transmission channels, to be further analyzed and made available in the existing HIS.

The home monitoring sensor system is designed for the acquisition of patients' electrocardiographic signals (ECG), oxygen saturation (SpO_2) data, arterial blood pressure, and body weight.

The blood pressure measuring device, based on the oscillometric method, is already used in various telemedicine systems as it is certified for medical use and can also be employed at home.

Respiratory Disease

Chronic obstructive pulmonary disease (COPD) is the major cause of mortality and increased levels of disability, particularly in the elderly.

Martins et al. [41] developed and tested a sound platform for remote auscultation, Look4MySounds, that is able to automatically classify respiratory sounds by means of a new robust detection algorithm.

AMICA, or the Autonomy Motivation and Individual Self-Management for COPD patients, a project of the AALJP, tries to emulate the medical consultation at home: auscultation and interview. To achieve this, a series of physiological signals are obtained daily by means of an *ad hoc* sensor. This information is then provided by the patient that interacts with a mobile device and combines this information coming from sensors. This system is able to set off medical alarms, is able to modify small aspects of the patients' treatment program or lifestyle, or even suggest hospitalization [18].

AMICA provides disease management and medical care to patients suffering from COPD by means of an integrated telemedicine system. A multifunctional biomedical sensor records breathing and monitors the heart rate, physical activity, and tracheal sounds. It also displays variables and physiological parameters relevant to COPD and respiratory-related dysfunctions. AMICA service includes using a telemedicine platform especially adapted for disease management and also to fit with the needs of older people [42,43].

Akker et al. [44] presented a dataset consisting of multiple wireless sensors that monitor movement and various types of bio signals, recorded from patients that suffer from COPD. This work is a part of the Inertial Sensing Systems for Advanced Chronic Condition Monitoring and Risk Prevention (IS-ACTIVE) project of the AALJP. The resulting dataset is included in sensor data outputs captured while performing a wide range of movements like walking, nordic walking (with sensors on the sticks), cycling, and any physiotherapy exercises that are commonly prescribed to COPD patients. The use of multiple movement sensors, such as the inertia sensor, which will feature 9 degrees of freedom from three sensors—3D accelerometer, 3D magnetic compass, and 3D gyroscope—will result in a dataset comprising as many as 40–50 layers of data.

According to authors, the feedback device will have some sort of PDA charged with the task of collecting relevant features from the nodes and doing the actual activity recognition.

This feedback allows the patients to be as active as possible, while preventing attacks of breathlessness and giving motivational feedback. In order to provide each patient with the optimal feedback, the system will adapt to the behavior and health status of the user: (1) warn a patient in time to lower his/her activity level and (2) aid patients in performing their daily physiotherapy exercises in a correct way.

Diabetes

New solutions that combine the psychological knowledge on elderly users' requirements for sustained behavior change are necessary for the prevention and management of two of the most prevalent chronic diseases in the elderly, thus resulting in a higher quality of life.

The physical activity is recognized as a crucial element for the prevention, cure, and management of many chronic illnesses including diabetes type II and cardiovascular diseases and directly related to physical and mental health and hereby substantially contributing to the well-being and quality of life.

A²E² (Adaptive Ambient Empowerment for the Elderly), a project of the AALJP, is a tool that alerts and is oriented through lifestyle changes that are essential for the prevention and management of diabetes type II and cardiovascular diseases in elderly individuals [18,45]. This tool stimulates beneficial levels of exercising in elderly individuals who are at risk to come down with diabetes type II and cardiovascular diseases, and it supports exercise behavior changes in patients who have already been diagnosed with these diseases by stabilizing or even reversing their condition [18,45].

A sensor platform is built and integrated to the virtual coach system platform. These personal virtual coaches are created in order to help to find the right balance between activity and rest throughout each day. The coach is connected to several biosensors including activity sensors, blood pressure, and weight sensors for interaction and adaptive feedback [18,45].

This daily organizational structure is designed by a care program manager and researchers through a simple interface to create and arrange events for the client [18,45].

Alzheimer's Disease and Other Dementias

Increasing life expectancy is accompanied by an increasing prevalence of health impairments, mental health problems, as well as dementia, e.g., Alzheimer's disease [16].

Elderly people often suffer from the effects of social and physical isolation. According to a research team, AGNES focuses on improving the mental and physical well-being of elderly people living alone at home [18,46].

The project started with a basic ICT platform to create and maintain an easy-to-use web-based social network, and thus used to stimulate elderly persons [18,46].

The in-home system is enhanced with technology to assess the subjective and objective states of the elderly persons along carefully selected parameters. Timely information on the activities and subjective state of the elderly persons will be passed to the network (e.g., presence, state of wellness, etc.) [18,46].

Xefteris et al. [47] present a reconfigurable event detection mechanism used in the ALADDIN (A Technology Platform for the Assisted Living of Dementia Elderly Individuals and Their Carers) platform for risk assessment and analysis (a project of the AALJP).

The authors describe that the risk assessment and analysis component (RAAC) is based on an existing set of *rules* and processes both physical data input and answers to cognitive and behavioral evaluation tests to produce its warnings.

The architecture of the ALADDIN platform is organized according to the service-oriented architecture (SOA) principles and consists of three main parts: the caregiver's client application, server application, and external services.

The caregiver's client application is an application used by caregivers and patients to access the services of the platform. With the help of this application, the caregiver can answer the questionnaires about the patient's mental health condition. The information about the physiological measurements of the patient's condition can be submitted by the caregiver using the application, which is then analyzed by the clinicians, enabling a caregiver to send a warning message to the clinician.

The server application is the core of the platform, implementing the basic functionalities, providing secure communication with client applications, storing the information about patients and caregivers, providing the possibility to exchange information with external HIS, and providing the graphical user interface for clinicians and platform administrators to interact with the system. The section on "Support for Caregivers and Care Organizations" discusses in more detail the RAAC, which is a component of the server application.

The third part of the platform are external services provided by external web portals. There are two types of services involved: cognitive games and a social network.

Active living for Alzheimer's patients (ALFA) is a project of the AALJP, which aims to develop a platform and a set of tools to enable people with dementia to interact with their environment, make their own choices, stay active, and work on their cognitive and physical health in their own home.

According to the research team, ALFA works by means of three technologies: (1) visual stimulation of mirror neurons in Alzheimer's patients, (2) an interactive agenda or diary, and (3) a movement monitoring system; people with dementia will be able to improve or sustain their cognitive functions [18,48].

By using ICT, people with dementia can (1) be visually stimulated to walk and eat better than before; (2) plan, perform, and control daily activities; and (3) be monitored in their movement patterns. This platform intends to preserve and improve their cognitive functions as long as possible and stay in control of their lives with the help of informal and formal care when needed [18,48].

Parkinson's Disease

Without treatment, Parkinson's disease progresses over 5–10 years to a disability status in which patients are incapable of caring for themselves. Death frequently results from complications of immobility, including aspiration pneumonia or pulmonary embolism [16].

Home-based empowered living for Parkinson's disease patients (HELP), another project of the AALJP, proposes a body sensor and actuator network made up of portable/wearable and home devices to monitor health parameters (e.g., blood pressure) and body activity (e.g., to detect gait, absence of movement), and to release a controlled quantity of drugs in an automated fashion. It also includes a remote point-of-care unit to supervise the patients under clinical specialist control [18,49].

Support for Caregivers and Care Organizations

A vital part of home care is the use of highly trained personnel and experts. Since they are alone at the home of the client, they must cope with any situation that arises on their own. This responsibility and solitary decision making are a major strain on caregivers such as in expert interviews.

The project AGNES will develop innovative applications to support the needs of families and caregivers, and to reduce health care costs by improving care provision and extending the period of independent and successful living of older persons in their own home [50].

Hoshi et al. [50] describe the combination and integration of home-based ICT and social networks, connecting elderly persons living at home with their families, friends, and caregivers.

The user-sensitive home environment will support a personalized and human-centered care process by detecting, communicating, and meaningfully responding to relevant states, situations, and activities of elderly persons with regard to mild cognitive impairment.

This system is composed of ambient displays, tangible interaction objects, and interaction mechanisms and protocols, including gesture detection, which makes for easy-to-use and natural interaction.

Xefteris et al. [47] describe a system that has a basic component of the server application, the RAAC. This component provides functionality for the analysis of patients' and caregivers' measurement data. The RAAC receives as input the data from physiological measurements, as well as the results from Cognitive and Behavioural Assessment Questionnaires, and processes them in order to evaluate the patient's status and produce a warning for the clinician. The list of functionalities includes warning the clinician for situations where the patient's physiological and/or psychological measurements indicate an alarming condition for the patient's health and for situations where the caregiver's psychological measurements indicate an alarming condition for the caregiver's health, and presenting evidence for the produced warning.

The following physiological parameters will be monitored: (1) nutritional state (weight control) and (2) arterial pressure. A clinical warning (mail warning) is generated if >1 kg is lost in a week and/or if the systolic arterial pressure is <80 or >150 mmHg or the diastolic arterial pressure is <50 or >90 mmHg.

Several parameters will be monitored in order to assess and slow down the patient cognitive decline. These items for cognitive decline and cognitive stimulation status assessment are temporal and spatial orientations. The patient answers the questions given by the caregiver about temporal and spatial orientations on a daily basis, at the same time, and in their home (with the support of the caregiver); to assess the patient's adequate adherence to the pharmacological treatment in order to avoid side effects, the caregiver will post on the monitor (daily) some questions.

REMOTE (Remote Health and Social Care for Independent Living of Isolated Elderly with Chronic Conditions) is a project of the AALJP in which one of the objectives is to support professionals to identify and react collaboratively to health risks by monitoring real-time activity, and medical data of isolated elderly at any time and from anywhere. The project introduces an open reference architecture and platform that will enable interoperability, seamless connectivity, and data sharing among different services [18,51].

Sousa et al. [52] developed a new wireless biosignal system that monitors on a long-term basis users at their homes (pilot phase) within the Portuguese company, Plux. The system consists of wearable sensors that measure heart rate, blood oxygen saturation, and physical activity levels, sending data to a mobile phone and from this to a remote monitoring station located in a clinical facility (Figure 4.6). Whenever an abnormal situation occurs, an alarm is triggered and caregivers can provide assistance.

The results so far are very positive and demonstrate that, according to requirements, it has good usability and portability and is able to enhance the caregivers' quality of work [52].

CARE@HOME (Care Services Advancing the Social Interaction, Health Wellness, and Well-being of Elderly People at Home), a project of the AALJP, aims at creating an open platform that is able to provide services to the elderly who choose to live independently while enjoying the assurance of timely access to caregivers when needed, and thereby offer better living.

According to the research team, the project activities can be summarized as follows: (1) system analysis and evaluation; (2) sensor requirement collection and analysis, design, development, and adaptation for bathroom and other indoor applications (e.g., immunize

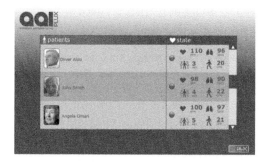

FIGURE 4.6
Schematic representation of the web interface of aal@home. (From Sousa, J. et al., aal@home: A new home care wireless biosignal monitoring tool for ambient assisted living, In *Proc. INSTICC International Living Usability Lab Workshop on AAL Latest Solutions, Trends and Applications—AAL*, Rome, Italy, 2011.)

against bathroom conditions like moisture and higher temperature); (3) data analysis and interpretation by making use of pattern recognition and unsupervised learning; (4) embedded processing for real-time data interpretation and software development; and (5) sensor integration in the monitoring and alarming system [18,53].

The MyGuardian (A Pervasive Guardian for Elderly with Mild Cognitive Impairments) project from the AALJP provides the following technologies: easy-to-use communication between the mobile senior and the caregivers (communication messages with contextual data on the senior's psychological state); remote tracking and assistance that will enable the monitoring of senior physiological state and behavior (detect risk situations and offer appropriate and personalized intervention); and coordination between caregivers that will improve awareness within their group (distribution and delegation of care tasks) [18,54].

Personal and Home Safety and Security

Staying well and comfortable, and feeling safe and secure within a person's own home, is an important part of and plays a central role in life. Many technologies may offer an enhanced sense of security, prolonged independence, and an improved perceived quality of life for seniors; these technologies also help the informal caregivers to experience less strain and provide an improved quality of service [16].

Fall Detection System

In elderly people, a simple fall can have devastating consequences without immediate help. They may suffer pain or emotional distress, or may experience serious secondary medical problems such as dehydration, hypothermia, or pneumonia. Thus, the need to develop early warning systems arose for people who live alone or are debilitated.

The main challenge in installing ICT-based monitoring systems is the balance between surveillance and privacy, i.e., home safety versus ethics.

Bourke et al. [55] describe a part of work developed in the eCAALYX project, evaluating a variety of existing and novel fall detection algorithms for a waist-mounted accelerometer-based system. Three different parameters associated with falls were examined: velocity, impact, and posture.

The results of this study demonstrated that algorithms that take into account the three parameters (velocity, impact, and posture) are the most suitable methods for fall detection, when tested using continuous unscripted activities performed by elderly healthy volunteers, which is the target environment for a fall detection device.

Gamboa et al. [56] describe a work of Plux (Portuguese enterprise) regarding a system that continuously monitors health parameters and location of its users inside a building, such as assisted living facilities (Figure 4.7). The system is designed to be worn by each patient as a necklace (Figure 4.7a) that senses heart rate, involuntary falls, and location. It automatically generates alarms when some abnormality in these variables is detected. The sensors integrated on the necklace communicate wirelessly to a central monitoring station, which in turn communicates with a portable device (Figure 4.7b) that the caregivers wear. The ultimate goal of the system is to detect early the critical situations and facilitate an early intervention. The patient monitoring device has the form of a necklace with a pendant that integrates three different sensors: an ECG sensor, a triaxial accelerometer, and a localization module. Fall events are identified when sudden changes in the magnitude of the acceleration signal are detected. This triggers an alarm, ensuring that adequate

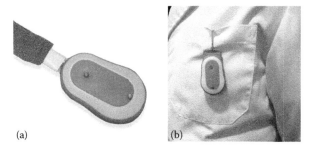

(a)   (b)

FIGURE 4.7
Patient tracking system. (a) Neklace and (b) caregiver device. (From Gamboa, H. et al., Patient tracking system—Continuous monitoring and location solution for ambient assisted living facilities, In *Proceedings of ICST International Conf. on Pervasive Computing Technologies for Healthcare*, Munich, Germany, 2010; *Plux*, Available from http://www.plux.info/frontpage, cited March 23, 2011.)

assistance is rapidly provided to the patient. The fall detector is included on the pendant part of the device and integrates one ADXL330 ±3G MEMS® triaxial accelerometer [56].

Leone et al. [57] present an automated monitoring system for the detection of dangerous events that might happen to elderly people (such as falls) in AAL applications. This paper presents a method for fall detection in a 3D range image that combines information about the 3D position of the centroid of the elderly people with the detection of inactivity.

Elderly people are observed through a nonwearable device (a time-of-flight [TOF] camera), which allows to implement more efficient vision algorithms, overcoming the well-known drawbacks of the passive vision systems such as time-varying light conditions, shadows, occlusion presence, etc. The approach searches for human silhouettes in the 3D point cloud by applying segmentation methods and metric filtering. The height of the 3D human centroid is evaluated by using the previously estimated calibration parameters, and the related trend is used as a feature in a thresholding-based clustering for fall detection.

The system shows high performance in terms of efficiency and reliability on a large real dataset of falls acquired in different conditions.

Cardile et al. [58] propose a computer vision-based wireless sensor system for remote tracking and monitoring of elderly people based on low-cost embedded systems that are able to visually track a patient and detect critical motion and posture patterns associated with dangerous situations. This system is based on a network of wireless sensors in which each node is equipped with an embedded video camera (camera sensor network). Based on video analysis, dangerous actions are detected (behavior analysis), and warning signals to the caregivers are wirelessly generated.

The network of camera sensors is composed of a set of autonomous and compact devices called camera sensor nodes. The IEEE 802.15.4 radio protocol is used to communicate with all the nodes in the system. The system is controlled using a custom graphical user interface. This graphical user interface is split into two sections: the first is devoted to displaying (and interacting with) the video streams acquired by the cameras distributed in the regions under control, and the second is devoted to configuring the sensor nodes.

The user can select a camera of interest and set some parameters: the view angle of the onboard camera, the type of processing, and face blurring (on/off)—required for privacy reasons in some applications.

The CARE (Safe Private Homes for Elderly Persons) project is an R&D activity running under the AALJP, which aims to realize an intelligent monitoring and alarming system for independent living of elderly persons.

According to the research team, this project targets the automated recognition and alarming of critical situations (like fall detection) using a visual sensor and real-time processing while preserving the privacy and taking into account system dependability issues, especially ensuring reliability, availability, security, and safety.

A biologically inspired neuromorphic vision sensor will be integrated into the system (alarm, security, and monitoring) for seamless analysis and tracking of elderly persons at home. This real-time information can be exploited for incident detection (e.g., fall detection, immobilized person) and instantaneous alarming of the concerned parties [18,59].

The SOFTCARE project (unobstrusive plug-and-play kit for chronic condition monitoring based on customized behavior recognition from wireless localization and remote sensoring), within the framework of the AALJP, developed a prototype of a monitoring system for seniors that allows caregivers (formal and informal) and senior users to get real-time alarms in dangerous or potentially dangerous situations and warnings on long-term trends that could indicate a future problem. According to the research team, this objective is achieved by the implementation of the designed artificial intelligence techniques that allow the recognition of daily activities based on the data obtained from an accelerometer (bracelet device) and location information. Users need to wear a bracelet containing a 3D accelerometer and a Zigbee module that will make the bracelet communicate (mobile node) with the rest of the static devices on the user's home (one per room) [18,60].

Brulin et al. [61] proposed a computer vision-based posture recognition method for home monitoring of the elderly. The proposed system performs human detection prior to the posture analysis; posture recognition is performed only on a human silhouette. The human detection approach has been designed to be robust to different environmental stimuli. According to the authors, the posture is analyzed with simple features that are not designed to manage constraints related to the environment but are only designed to describe human silhouettes and to identify four static postures.

Planinc and Kampel [62] developed part of the work of the FEARLESS (Fear Elimination As Resolution for Losing Elderly's Substantial Sorrows) project within the framework of the AALJP, in which three different noninvasive technologies are used: audio, 2D sensors (cameras), and introducing a new technology for fall detection: the Kinect as a 3D depth sensor. The fall detection algorithms using the Kinect are evaluated on 72 video sequences, containing 40 falls and 32 activities of daily living. The evaluation results are compared with state-of-the-art approaches using 2D sensors or microphones.

Home Embedded Devices

Embedded devices certainly provide more comfort to users than wearable devices. As development of the home care concept is related to care for elderly people, highly accurate automatic fall detectors are important for their care.

Sensors are incorporated into furniture, e.g., into beds, in order to follow parameters during sleep [63–65]. Postolache et al. [66] proposed a multisensing system with wireless communication capabilities embedded on a smart wheelchair that can measure physiological parameters such as heart rate and respiratory rate in an unobtrusive way.

Monitoring physiological signals in an unobtrusive way can significantly reduce stress impact of apparatus utilization on patients, particularly to those with a certain degree of physical limitation. However, such built-in devices can produce data on a very limited number of patient-related information and therefore can be taken only as part of an intelligent environment [6].

Free Living Technologies

The free living devices can be divided into two groups for AAL: (1) monitoring and management of physical activities and (2) outdoor safety and security.

Devices are being developed to identify movement and physiological variables outside the laboratory and home environment.

Monitoring and Management of Activity

Taken to the next stage, the evaluation of the physical activity level of a person has its roots in the need to determine if their physical activity behavior falls within an interval or profile defined by appropriate criteria, determined as essential to their good health status. This condition is based on the fact that physical activity reduces the risk of various diseases and brings several benefits, including improved glucose metabolism, reduced body fat, and lower blood pressure [67].

The goals and expected benefits of physical activity monitoring underline the importance of the acquisition of physiological parameters during exercise. This chapter provides an insight on the autonomous and portable monitoring devices suited for physiological variable monitoring without weight and energy constraints to the user.

Heart Rate Monitoring Devices

Some heart rate monitors measure the electrical activity of the heart, which reflects the number of heart contractions per minute. Several companies sell this type of equipment such as Polar Electro Inc., Sensor Dynamics, Inc., and Acumen Inc.

Continuous Step Activity Monitoring

A pedometer or step counter is a device, usually portable and electronic or electromechanical, that counts each step a person takes by detecting the motion of the person's hips. Because the distance of each person's step varies, an informal calibration performed by the user is required if a standardized distance (such as in kilometers or miles) is desired.

The technology for a pedometer includes a mechanical sensor and software to count steps. Today advanced step counters rely on microelectromechanical system (MEMS) inertial sensors and sophisticated software to detect steps. These MEMS sensors have either 1-, 2-, or 3-axis detection of acceleration. The use of MEMS inertial sensors allows more accurate detection of steps and fewer false positives.

Often worn on the belt and kept on all day, it can record how many steps the wearer has walked that day. Several companies sell this type of equipment such as Omron, Apple Inc., and Nike Inc.

Wearable Sensors Embedded in Clothes

Great strides have been made in the category of capturing vital signals with wearable systems, especially in a system integrated into textiles. There are a number of commercial projects in this area such as LifeShirt Chest Strap (RAE Systems) and VitalJacket® (Biodevices).

The Department of Textile Science and Technology (University of Beira Interior, Portugal) developed an armband made of plain weave fabric (Figure 4.8), integrating embroidery textile electrodes of stainless steel (SS) and elastics to conform to human forearms [68].

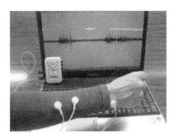

FIGURE 4.8
Armband integrating textile electrodes. Sleeve knit with elastic textile sensors signals electromyography surface and handheld *bioPlux* processing and transmission of wireless signal. (From Trindade, I.G. et al., Light-weight portable sensors for health care, In *12th IEEE International Conference on e-Health Networking Applications and Services [Healthcom]*, 2010.)

The fabric integrates stitched conductive threads of SS/cotton and snaps fasteners inter-connecting the textile electrodes to a bioPlux signal processing electronic module [68].

The electronic module connects through shielded cables to a portable unit, which can be held in a pocket and can wirelessly transmit to a PC located anywhere in the room where the person is, for real time monitoring and recording of the processed signals [68].

EMG signals obtained with an armband integrating textile electrodes, worn by a vol-unteer and processed by a wireless portable unit, exhibited comparable quality to those obtained with bipolar Ag/AgCI electrodes [68].

Activity Monitoring

Typically the activity monitor contains an accelerometer, which measures acceleration. Acceleration measurements are converted into units of movement intensity and fre-quency. All activity monitors contain a microprocessor and onboard memory so that data can be downloaded to either a microcomputer or a PC for offline processing and display [10].

Several companies sell this type of equipment such as Stayhealthy, Inc. (RT3 Triaxial Research Tracker), CamNtech Ltd. (Actiwatch AW7), and Siemens HealthCare (*Smart Senior* Project).

The eZ430-Chronos software development tool developed by Texas Instruments is a highly integrated, wearable, wireless development system that is based on MCU CC430F6137. It may be used as a reference platform for watch systems, a personal display for PANs, or a wireless sensor node for remote data collection [69]. Based on the MCU CC430F6137 sub-1-GHz RF SoC, the eZ430-Chronos is a complete development system featuring a 96-segment LCD display, an integrated pressure sensor, and a three-axis accelerometer for motion-sensitive control. The integrated wireless interface allows the eZ430-Chronos to act as a central hub for nearby wireless sensors such as pedometers and heart rate monitors. The eZ430-Chronos offers temperature and battery voltage measure-ment and is complete with a USB-based CC1111 wireless interface to a PC [69].

The sports watch firmware (default) provides a broad set of features. Besides basic watch functions such as time, date, alarm, and stopwatch, advanced sports watch features such as an altimeter, heart rate monitor, calorie, vertical speed, and distance information are available. The internal accelerometer provides acceleration data on the watch LCD and allows controlling a PC by transferring the sensor's measurements [69].

The Smart Senior is the latest research and development project of Siemens HealthCare. Managed to senior population, this remote diagnostic system consists of a portable device that transmits information to a medical center. The equipment allows the elderly to feel safe while parameters such as movement, blood oxygen levels, and heart rate are measured providing in-house monitoring. The first prototypes became available in 2011. Researchers and doctors are working on a device that can be used in the pulse and measures, for example, the heart rate. The device can also recognize the absence of micro-movements characteristic of sleep, or detect whether the user has collapsed, and is programmed to trigger an alarm to provide assistance at the place of residence. For patients suffering from chronic pain, a kind of *smart adhesive patches* that measures temperature, pulse, and blood oxygenation is being developed. This device is used in the upper arm and consists of a flexible band that integrates a transmitter, a receiver circuit, and an intelligence assessment battery. The radio chip in the wrist device sends all information to a communication node, which in turn sends information via Internet to a medical center [70].

The bioPlux system is related to physical activities because it has great potential for free-living applications. The bioPlux is a device that collects and digitizes signals from sensors, transmitting them via Bluetooth (connectivity: 10 m range with a standard adapter, >100 m with a high-range adapter) to a computer, where they are viewed in real time. The analog-to-digital converter channels have 12 bits, and its sampling frequency is 1 kHz. The bioPlux also has a digital port, a terminal for connecting the AC adapter and charge the internal battery (allows a lifespan of approximately 12 h), and a channel to connect the reference electrode, which is essential for the proper monitoring of the electromyography signal [71].

Plux has several sensors that can be linked to bioPlux (see Figure 4.9) such as respiration sensor respPlux, single button resistive sensor forcePlux, air pressure airPlux, angle measurement tool anglePlux, ambient luminosity lightPlux, triaxial accelerometer xyzPlux,

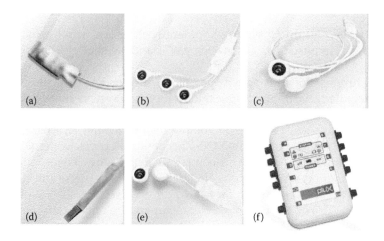

FIGURE 4.9
Wireless physiological data acquisition system bioPlux and sensors. (a) Triaxial accelerometer xyzPlux, (b) ECG sensor (ECG triodes) ecgPlux, (c) electrodermal activity edaPlux, (d) temperature sensor tempPlux, (e) electromyography sensor emgPlux, and (f) bioPlux acquisition system. (From *Plux*, Available from http://www.plux .info/frontpage, cited March 23, 2011.)

ECG sensor (ECG triodes) ecgPlux, electrodermal activity sensor edaPlux, peripheral temperature sensor tempPlux, and electromyography sensor emgPlux [71].

Bieber et al. [72] developed part of the work of the AGNES project, addressing the methodology of mobile physical activity recognition of transitions between sitting and standing by using only one 3D acceleration sensor. The recognition task is performed using a synthetic kernel signal and a correlation of the measurement signal. For the evaluation, a detection application has been developed, which uses the built-in sensors of a standard mobile phone.

The presented algorithm for feature extraction and transition classification was implemented on a standard mobile phone, which is equipped with a 3D acceleration sensor. The phone, a Sony Ericsson w715, sampled movements with a frequency of 20 Hz by 6 bit resolution per G (samples/second). The phone was equipped with WiFi connectivity, so a control of a WiFi switch by the detection of movements such as standing up or sitting down was possible. The features and classification were generated in real time on the device.

Health and Health Care Smartphone Applications

The latest generation of smartphones is increasingly viewed as handheld computers with onboard computing capability, capacious memories, large screens, and open operating systems that encourage application development. Platforms available today include Android, Apple iOS, RIM BlackBerry, Symbian, and Windows (Windows Mobile 6.x and the emerging Windows Phone 7 platform) [73].

Boulos et al. [73] cover applications targeting both patients and health care professionals in various scenarios, e.g., health, fitness, and lifestyle education and management applications; AAL applications; continuing professional education tools; and applications for public health surveillance.

The paper describes in detail the development of a smartphone application within the eCAALYX project. The eCAALYX Android smartphone app receives input from a BAN (a patient-wearable smart garment with wireless health sensors) and the Global Positioning System (GPS) location sensor in the smartphone, and communicates over the Internet with a remote server accessible by health care professionals who are in charge of the remote monitoring and management of older patients with multiple chronic conditions.

According to the authors (Boulos et al. [73]), the technological platform in the current prototype is the Google Nexus, which is running the Android 2.1 platform, with 1 GHz processor and 512 MB RAM memory. From a software point of view, the internal structure follows a blackboard architecture, in which several concurrent processes share information using the SQLite database provided in the Android platform. Access to necessary resources, such as GPS, Bluetooth, and the Internet, is also provided through the Android platform. The interface with the caretaker/clinicians' site is accomplished using the W3C Web Services technology, while the interface with the health sensors (in a *smart garment* worn by the patient) is realized using the Bluetooth wireless technology.

Outdoor Safety and Security

Cavallo et al. [74] provide a first preliminary characterization of a ZigBee pervasive sensor network for localization of people and objects in indoor environments.

It was composed of several miniaturized ZigBee boards and was conceived to have three typologies of nodes: coordinator node, mobile node, and anchor node. The coordinator node was USB-connected to a personal computer and was used to create and hold the network, and acquire and process data; the mobile node was conceived to be worn by the user and endowed a triaxial accelerometer; the anchor nodes were placed in fixed and known positions in the environment. In this work, four anchor nodes were used for localization of one mobile node in one of the meeting rooms of our laboratory, and one coordinator node was used to hold the network and collect data. A plastic support was used to keep the anchor nodes 60 cm from the ground. The coordinator was connected to a USB port of a notebook, and an opportune graphical interface developed in C# was used for network management and data saving.

Gustarini et al. [75] present the work developed for the Way Finding Seniors (WayFis) project from the AALJP, which describes the first route planning service for elderly people that considers both the pedestrian and public transportation mobility issues and that is based on a wide range of personalization features, building up user profiles that include the health state of the person and his or her common behaviors and needs. WayFiS also includes localization and positioning features for both indoor and outdoor environments that will guide the elderly along complex paths.

Dossy (Digital Outdoor and Safety System) is a project of the AALJP that supports outdoor activities, which is a fast-growing and important field in the area of software and hardware development. Taking into account that outdoor activities become a more and more important part of the lives of elderly people, the project stands for a self-determined life to be able to practice outdoor activities irrespective of one's age and constitution. Furthermore, outdoor activities contribute largely to the health and well-being of the elderly and improve their quality of life. A commercial roll-out of the system can contribute to better health, enabling elderly people to keep up their mobility. The solution will be evaluated by end users during the development process using an appropriate mobile device and an application to improve its usability by receiving consumer feedback [18,76].

E-mossion (Elderly Friendly Mobility Services for Indoor and Outdoor Scenarios) is a project from the AALJP that is based on a combination of existing and future open mobile platforms, an IP connected server platform, and a home security sensor network. An accessory portable easy-to-wear device will allow easy control of the main functionalities of the service to interface with the mobile phone. The development and analysis of applications consist of two parts: the identification of services and features to be exploited and/or offered, and the development of a user-friendly graphic interface. This methodology allows the exploitation of services developed by applications from other platforms by eliminating duplication and ensuring interoperability, scalability, and easy development of new features [18,77].

Conclusion

Through this literature review, it is possible to verify that the AAL area has many applications in the context of health care.

This very diverse set of solutions continues to expand, putting together a very comprehensive set of knowledge. A problem that arises in some countries regarding the use of these technologies is acceptance by users.

The success and development of this area are undoubtedly based on the cooperation of various scientific areas. The creation of multidisciplinary teams and cooperation between companies, universities, and health care organizations are some of the strategies.

The main focus of this area is to provide a higher quality of life for the elderly and people with special needs, allowing for increased independence and confidence.

Acknowledgments

The authors acknowledge the contribution of the Instituto de Telecomunicações, R&D Unit 50008, financed by the applicable financial framework (FCT/MEC through national funds and, when applicable, cofunded by FEDER—PT2020 partnership agreement). The authors also acknowledge the contribution of COST Action IC1303—AAPELE—Algorithms, Architectures and Platforms for Enhanced Living Environments.

References

1. O'Donovan, T. et al. A context aware wireless body area network (BAN). In *3rd International Conference on Pervasive Computing Technologies for Healthcare*. 2009, London.
2. WHO. WHO age-friendly environments programme. (cited May 2011); Available from: http://www.who.int/ageing/age_friendly_cities/en/.
3. Yao, J., R. Schmitz, and S. Warren. A wearable point-of-care system for home use that incorporates plug-and-play and wireless standards. *IEEE Transactions on Information Technology in Biomedicine*, 2005. 9(3): pp. 363–71.
4. Scanaill, C.N.I. et al. A review of approaches to mobility telemonitoring of the elderly in their living environment. *Annals of Biomedical Engineering*, 2006. 34(4): pp. 547–63.
5. Koch, S. Home telehealth—Current state and future trends. *International Journal of Medical Informatics*, 2005. 75(8): pp. 565–76.
6. Magjarevic, R. Home care technologies for ambient assisted living. In *IFMBE Proceedings, Medicon 2007: XI Mediterranean Conference on Medical and Biological Engineering and Computing*. 2007, Ljubljana, Slovenia.
7. Haux, R. et al. The Lower Saxony research network design of environments for ageing: Towards interdisciplinary research on information and communication technologies in ageing societies. *Informatics for Health & Social Care*, 2010. 35(3–4): pp. 92–103.
8. WHO. Diet and physical activity for health. 2006. (cited May 2011); Available from: http://www.euro.who.int/__data/assets/pdf_file/0006/96459/E90143.pdf.
9. Chen, M. et al. Body area networks: A survey. *Mobile Networks and Applications*, 2011. 16: pp. 171–93.
10. Moore, J., and G. Zouridakis, eds. *Biomedical Technology and Devices Handbook*. CRC Press LLC. Boca Raton, FL, 2004.
11. *Medical Applications Guide*. 2010, Texas Instruments. Available from: http://www.ti.com/lit/sg/sszb143a/sszb143a.pdf.
12. Huang, A. et al. *Aggregation Managers for the Connected Health System*. 2010, Texas Instruments. Available from: http://www.ti.com/pdfs/wtbu/agg_mgr_swpy026.pdf.
13. Altuna, A. et al. OPENHEALTH ASSISTANT: The OpenHealth FLOSS implementation of the ISO/IEEE 11073-20601 standard. In *AALIANCE Conference*. 2010, Malaga, Spain.
14. Boulos, M.N. An enhanced ambient assisted living experiment for older people with multiple chronic conditions. In *2nd International Symposium on Applied Sciences in Biomedical and Communication Technologies (ISABEL 2009)*. 2009, Bratislava.

15. Szeman, Z., and C. Kucsera. Happy ageing- users' expectations. In *PETRA '11 Proceedings of the 4th International Conference on PErvasive Technologies Related to Assistive Environments*. 2011, New York.
16. Broek, G.v.d. et al. *Ambient Assisted Living Roadmap*. 2009, AALIANCE—The European Ambient Assisted Living Innovation Platform. Available from: http://www.aaliance2.eu/sites/default/files/RM2010.pdf.
17. HOPE (Smart Home for Elderly People). (cited November 5, 2012); Available from: http://www.hope-project.eu/.
18. Catalogue of Projects 2012. 2012, Ambient Assisted Living Joint Programme.
19. Jung, I., and G.-N. Wang. User pattern learning algorithm based MDSS (Medical Decision Support System) framework under ubiquitous. *World Academy of Science, Engineering and Technology*, 2007. 1(12): pp. 175–179.
20. Bosch Healthcare. (cited May 2011); Available from: http://www.bosch-telehealth.com/en/us/products/health_buddy/health_buddy.html.
21. Brandherm, B. et al. Roles and rights management concept with identification by electronic identity card. In *8th IEEE International Conference on Pervasive Computing and Communications Workshops (PERCOM Workshops), 2010*. 2010, Mannheim.
22. American Society of Health-System Pharmacists. ASHP guidelines on the safe use of automated dispensing devices. *American Journal of Health-System Pharmacists* 2010. 67: pp. 483–90.
23. VITALITY, Inc. (cited June 2010); Available from: http://www.vitality.net/.
24. Waterworth, J.A., S. Ballesteros, and C. Peter. User-sensitive home-based systems for successful ageing. In *Proceedings of HSI 2009—2nd International Conference on Human System Interaction*. 2009, Catania, Italy.
25. Peter, C., G. Bieber, and B. Urban. Affect- and behaviour-related assistance for families in the home environment. In *The 3rd ACM International Conference on Pervasive Technologies Related to Assistive Environments: PETRA 2010*. 2010, New York.
26. Muuraiskangas, S., J. Tiri, and J. Kaartinen. Easy physical exercise application for the elderly. In *AALIANCE Conference*. 2010, Malaga, Spain.
27. Hendeby, G. et al. Healthy aging using physical activity monitoring. In *AALIANCE Conference*. 2010, Malaga, Spain.
28. Cameirão, M.S. et al. Neurorehabilitation using the virtual reality based Rehabilitation Gaming System: Methodology, design, psychometrics, usability and validation. *Journal of NeuroEngineering and Rehabilitation*, 2010. 7: p. 48.
29. Cameirao, M.S. et al. Virtual reality based rehabilitation speeds up functional recovery of the upper extremities after stroke: A randomized controlled pilot study in the acute phase of stroke using the Rehabilitation Gaming System. *Restorative Neurology and Neuroscience*, 2011. 29: pp. 287–98.
30. Marcellini, F., R. Bevilacqua, and V. Stara. HAPPY AGEING (AAL-2008-1-113) project overview. Solutions for independent living and technology acceptance. In *PETRA'11—4th International Conference on Pervasive Technologies Related to Assistive Environments*. 2011, Crete, Greece.
31. Peter, C. et al. The AGNES system for ambient social interaction. In *PETRA 2012: 5th Workshop on Affect and Behaviour Related Assistance*. 2012, Crete, Greece.
32. Asveld, L., and M. Besters. The personalization of care technology. In *AALIANCE Conference*. 2010, Malaga, Spain.
33. D'Angelo, L.T. et al. A system for intelligent home care ECG upload and priorisation. In *32nd Annual International Conference of the IEEE EMBS*. 2010, Buenos Aires, Argentina.
34. Korsakas, S. et al. The mobile ECG and motion activity monitoring system for home care patients. *Computers in Cardiology*, 2006. 33: pp. 833–6.
35. Vergari, F. et al. A ZigBee-based ECG transmission for a low cost solution in home care services delivery. *Mediterranean Journal of Pacing and Electrophysiology*, 2009. 3(4): pp. 181–6.
36. AliveCor Company. (cited May 2011); Available from: http://alivecor.com/.

37. Silva, H., A. Lourenço, and N. Paz. Real-time biosignal acquisition and telemedicine platform for AAL based on Android OS. In *AAL 2011—Proceedings of the 1st International Living Usability Lab Workshop on AAL Latest Solutions, Trends and Applications*. 2011, Rome, Italy.

38. Jobbágy, Á., P. Csordás, and A. Mersich. Accurate blood pressure measurement at home. In *IFMBE Proceedings*. 2007.

39. HealthSTATS International. (cited June 2001); Available from: http://www.healthstats.com/.

40. Saponara, S. et al. Remote monitoring of vital signs in patients with chronic heart failure. In *Sensors Applications Symposium (SAS), 2012 IEEE*. 2012, Brescia.

41. Martins, A.M. et al. Look4MySounds: A remote monitoring platform for auscultation. In *AALIANCE Conference*. 2010, Malaga, Spain.

42. Foix, L.F.C. et al. AMICA telemedicine platform: A design for management of elderly people with COPD. In *Proceedings of the 9th International Conference on Information Technology and Applications in Biomedicine, ITAB 2009*. 2009, Larnaca, Cyprus.

43. Crespo, L.F. et al. Telemonitoring in AMICA: A design based on and for COPD. In *10th IEEE International Conference on Information Technology and Applications in Biomedicine (ITAB)*. 2010, Cadiz, Spain.

44. Akker, H.o.d., V. Jones, and H. Hermens. Personalized feedback based on automatic activity recognition from mixed-source raw sensor data. In *International Workshop on Intelligent Data Analysis in Biomedicine and Pharmacology*. 2009, Verona, Italy.

45. A²E² (Adaptive Ambient Empowerment of the Elderly). (cited November 6, 2012); Available from: http://www.a2e2.eu/.

46. AGNES (User-Sensitive Home-Based Systems for Successful Ageing in a Networked Society). Available from: http://www.agnes-aal.eu/site/.

47. Xefteris, S., A. Androulidakis, and M. Haritou. Enabling risk assessment and analysis by event detection in dementia patients using a reconfigurable rule set. In *PETRA'11—4th International Conference on PErvasive Technologies Related to Assistive Environments*. 2011, Crete, Greece.

48. ALFA (Active Living for Alzheimer-Patients). (cited November 6, 2012); Available from: http://www.aal-alfa.eu/.

49. HELP (Home-Based Empowered Living for Parkinson's Disease Patients). (cited November 6, 2012); Available from: http://www.help-aal.com/.

50. Hoshi, K., A. Nyberg, and F. Öhberg. Bridging the contextual reality gap in blended reality space: The case of AGNES. In *6th International Conference on Inclusive Design*. 2011, London.

51. REMOTE (Remote health and social care for independent living of isolated elderly with chronic conditions). (cited November 7, 2012); Available from: http://www.remote-project.eu/.

52. Sousa, J. et al. aal@home: A new home care wireless biosignal monitoring tool for ambient assisted living. In *Proc INSTICC International Living Usability Lab Workshop on AAL Latest Solutions, Trends and Applications—AAL*. 2011, Rome, Italy.

53. CARE@HOME (CARE services advancing the social interaction, health wellness and well-being of elderly people AT HOME). (cited November 7, 2012); Available from: http://www.careathome-project.eu/.

54. MyGuardian (A Pervasive Guardian for Elderly with Mild Cognitive Impairments). (cited November 7, 2012); Available from: http://www.aal-europe.eu/projects/myguardian/.

55. Bourke, A.K. et al. Evaluation of waist-mounted tri-axial accelerometer based fall-detection algorithms during scripted and continuous unscripted activities. *Journal of Biomechanics*, 2010. 43: pp. 3051–7.

56. Gamboa, H., F. Silva, and H. Silva. Patient tracking system—Continuous monitoring and location solution for ambient assisted living facilities. In *Proceedings of ICST International Conference on Pervasive Computing Technologies for Healthcare*. 2010, Munich, Germany.

57. Leone, A., G. Diraco, and P. Siciliano. A 3D range vision system for abnormal behavior monitoring of elderly people in ambient assisted living applications. In *AALIANCE Conference*. 2010, Malaga, Spain.

58. Cardile, F., G. Iannizzotto, and F.L. Rosa. A vision-based system for elderly patients monitoring. In *3rd Conference on Human System Interactions (HSI), 2010*. 2010, Rzeszow, Poland.
59. CARE (Safe Private Homes for Elderly Persons). (cited November 7, 2012); Available from: http://care-aal.eu/.
60. SOFTCARE (Unobtrusive plug and play kit for chronic condition monitoring based on customized behaviour recognition from wireless localization and remote sensing). (cited November 7, 2012); Available from: http://www.softcare-project.eu/.
61. Brulin, D., Y. Benezeth, and E. Courtial. Posture recognition based on fuzzy logic for home monitoring of the elderly. *Posture Recognition Based on Fuzzy Logic for Home Monitoring of the Elderly*, 2012. 16(5): pp. 974–82.
62. Planinc, R., and M. Kampel. Introducing the use of depth data for fall detection. *Personal and Ubiquitous Computing*, 2013. 17(6): pp. 1063–1072.
63. Spillman, W.B. et al. A 'smart' bed for non-intrusive monitoring of patient physiological factors. *Measurement Science and Technology*, 2004. 15(8): p. 1614.
64. Jones, M.H., R. Goubran, and F. Knoefel. Identifying movement onset times for a bed-based pressure sensor array. In *IEEE International Workshop on Medical Measurement and Applications*. 2006.
65. Choi, B.H. et al. Nonconstraining sleep/wake monitoring system using bed actigraphy. *Medical and Biological Engineering and Computing*, 2007. 45(1): pp. 107–17.
66. Postolache, O.A. et al. Physiological parameters measurement based on wheelchair embedded sensors and advanced signal processing. *IEEE Transactions on Instrumentation and Measurement*, 2010. 59(10): pp. 2564–74.
67. Choi, J.H. et al. Estimation of activity energy expenditure: Accelerometer approach. In *27th Annual Conference, Proceedings of the 2005 IEEE Engineering in Medicine and Biology*. 2005.
68. Trindade, I.G. et al. Lightweight portable sensors for health care. In *12th IEEE International Conference on e-Health Networking Applications and Services (Healthcom)*. 2010.
69. eZ430-Chronos™ Development Tool—User's Guide. 2009–2010, Texas Instruments Incorporated.
70. Smart Senior—Siemens HealthCare. (cited March 2011); Available from: https://www.swe.siemens.com/portugal/web_nwa/pt/PortalInternet/QuemSomos/negocios/Healthcare/Noticias_Eventos/noticias/Pages/Siemens_desenvolve_sistema_de_diagnostico_remoto.aspx.
71. Plux. (cited March 23, 2011); Available from: http://www.plux.info/frontpage.
72. Bieber, G. et al. Mobile physical activity recognition of stand-up and sit-down transitions for user behavior analysis. In *3rd International Conference on Pervasive Technologies Related to Assistive Environments*. 2010, Samos, Greece.
73. Boulos, M.N.K. et al. How smartphones are changing the face of mobile and participatory healthcare: An overview, with example from eCAALYX. *BioMedical Engineering OnLine*, 2011. 10: p. 24.
74. Cavallo, F. et al. Preliminary characterization of an indoor localization system using a ZigBee-based sensor network and a triaxial accelerometer. In *AALIANCE Conference*. 2010, Malaga, Spain.
75. Gustarini, M. et al. WayFiS: From geospatial public transport information to way finding seniors. In *Workshop on User Issues in Geospatial Public Transport Information, co-located with 25th Conference of the International Cartographic Association*. 2011, Paris, France.
76. Dossy (Digital Outdoor and Safety System). (cited November 8, 2012); Available from: http://dossy.iwi.unisg.ch/the-project/.
77. E-mossion (Elderly friendly MObility Services for Indoor and Outdoor sceNarios). (cited November 8, 2012); Available from: http://www.emotion-project.eu/.

5

Implementing Best Evidence-Based Practice into Ambient Assisted Living Solutions: From User Outcome Research to Best Social Practices

Gerard Nguyen, Bruno Colin, Dominique Lemoult,
François Sigwald, Daniel Thiollier, and Alain Krivitzky

CONTENTS

ABSTRACT The evidence-based approach derived from the health care and medicine disciplines is the explicit and rational use of current best evidence in making decisions about the care of individuals and the population. At present, new technology may enter directly into the people care service without evaluation and without the evidence-based approach. Knowledge and evaluation bypasses will delay the time to market for a rapid and systematic routine use of innovations. Decision making about the purchase of equipment is more problematic when there is less evidence available or when this evidence is of poor quality, because there is no demonstration of efficacy and cost-effectiveness before the introduction of new technology. Information and communication technology (ICT) solutions aim to improve health care providers, professional and informal carers, decision makers, and all stakeholders in the field of elderly care. Implementing knowledge and experiences from the medical research and health care fields, we propose some recommendations for an evidence-based approach in *gerontotechnology* and ICT solutions. The final outcomes of any intervention in the elderly population would ensure well-being and good health and the improvement of quality of life by respecting the autonomy of a potentially frail and vulnerable population. Besides the technology development of ICT solutions, an evidence-based approach including a clinical research–like program would be necessary. Translational research using models from the health care and medicine disciplines will provide added value and also help to spread the use of cost-effective ICT solutions in the elderly. A call to action implementing evidence-based practice into ambient assisted living (AAL) organization and call procedures may be challenging.

Let us hope that our desire to use it for the good of the person is stronger than the temptation to use it for our own convenience.

Richard Fleming

KEY WORDS: *evidence-based practice, evidence-based health care, evidence-based medicine, gerontology outcomes, elderly ecosystem, cost-effectiveness, guidelines, best-practice recommendations.*

Introduction

Population ageing will have major implications for Organization for Economic Co-operation and Development (OECD) economies and societies over the next few decades, and many of these implications have been analyzed in depth (Jacobzone et al. 1999). The area in which the implications are obviously important is long-term care for the frail elderly. The results from research on the impact of age-specific disability trends have important implications in several areas but are specially relevant for the health and ageing dimensions of social policies, particularly with regard to long-term care policies. In pure financial terms, such trends suggest that caution is needed in inferring links between improvements in health and health care spending. It seems that better health can be acquired through better lifestyles and through appropriate access to new technologies like ICT.

We should always refer back to the double objective of the ambient assisted living (AAL) program to enhance the quality of life of older people and to strengthen the industry and the use of ICT in Europe (Cullen and Kubitshk 2008). The concept of AAL has to be understood as follows:

- To extend the time people can live in their preferred environment by increasing their autonomy, self-confidence, and mobility
- To support maintaining the health and functional capability of elderly individuals
- To promote a better and healthier lifestyle for individuals at risk
- To enhance security, to prevent social isolation, and to support maintaining the multifunctional network around the individual
- To support carers, families, and care organizations
- To increase the efficiency and productivity of used resources in ageing societies

Thus, one may implement into practice the ambition of the AAL program in two opposite directions: to focus on the development of ICT for the elderly considering that the field is naive or to have a person-centered approach to the elderly and ICT development as part of the ecosystem. We will discuss the following key challenges of ICT for the elderly by considering

- The person-centered approach
- The evidenced-based practice methodology
- The application of evidence-based practice to AAL
- The strategies to implement best practices

Implementing knowledge and experiences from the medical research and health care fields, we will propose some recommendations for an evidence-based approach in *geronto-technology* and ICT solutions. The final outcomes of any intervention in the elderly population will ensure well-being and good health and the improvement of quality of life by respecting the autonomy of a potentially frail and vulnerable population.

Rationale for an Elderly-Centered ICT Evidence-Based Practice

The Concept of Ageing

The classical vision of ageing via the decline status, overestimated the burden of ageing and limited ICT development to compensation for deficiencies. Healthy ageing is likely to be of importance for the global cost of ageing.

The concept of ageing must be viewed from three dimensions: decline, change, and development.

- The term *ageing* can connote decline, and decline is not successful. After age 20, our senses slowly fail us. By age 70, we can identify only 50% of the smells that we could recognize at 40. Our vision in dim light declines steadily, until, by age 80, few of us can drive safely at night; by age 90, 50% of us can no longer use public transportation.
- The term *ageing* also conveys development and maturation. Analogous to a grand cru wine evolving from bitterness to perfection, at 70, we are often more patient, more tolerant, and more accepting of affect (ours and that of others). We are more likely to tolerate paradox, to appreciate relativity, and to understand that every present has both a past and a future. Finally, like age itself, experience can only increase with time.

The Berlin Aging Study (Baltes and Mayer 2001) recently concluded, "Old age is not foremost a negative and problem-ridden phase of life." The MacArthur study of ageing (Seeman et al. 2001) also provided excellent support for the finding that our greater longevity is resulting in fewer, not more, years of disability. On one hand, after age 70, almost all of the subjects suffered at least one serious (chronic but treatable) illness, and many suffered up to five. Fifty percent had painful arthritis; after age 95, 50% experienced significant dementia. On the other hand, before age 95, less than 10% manifested dementia; 9 out of 10 still retained life goals.

When we look at mental functioning, first, the bad news is that the Berlin Aging Study's old-old subjects (aged 85–100 years) resembled humans coping with severe stress. They experienced fewer positive emotions, more emotional loneliness, and a feeling that others controlled their lives. After age 90, only 50% felt they had a confidante.

The good news was that with the exception of dementia, there was not more mental illness among the elderly, even among the old-old. Like arthritis and hip fractures, even dementia should be viewed as a common, but not inevitable, consequence of longevity.

With increasing age, spirituality and serenity increase. By *serenity*, we mean faith, acceptance, and allowing someone else to take over (Berlin study). The strategies of *giving up* or of information seeking were more common among the young-old, whereas the more *Buddhist* strategy of perceiving life as *being without meaning* was preferred by the old-old. Coping strategies that did not change between ages 70 and 90 were humor and comparing oneself with others more severely afflicted. The two most important psychosocial predictors of successful ageing were high level of education and having an extended family network. In a hierarchical regression model, the important correlates of poor ageing (defined as dependence, dissatisfaction with living, and being bedridden) were trouble walking (mobility), poor vision, age per se, depression, and dementia.

Integration of these three ageing dimension concepts into ICT solutions would be the cornerstone of a development framework with a person-centered approach and also of an evidence-based approach. Implementing the third dimension, development, one could expect to have a positive health approach, described by Martin Seligman (2008), contrasting with the classical assistive ICT solutions focusing on deficiencies of the older person.

Concept of the Person-Centered Approach

The person-centered approach was developed by Carl Rogers (1902–1987), who proposed new humanistic psychotherapy. Rogers trusted in people and believed that if a safe psychological environment existed, then all people would naturally move toward greater awareness and better fulfillment of their potentials.

The following potentials are within all of our actions in the field of ICT development for the elderly:

1. Sociability: the need to be with other human beings and a desire to know and be known by other people
2. Being trusting and trustworthy
3. Being curious about the world and open to experience
4. Being creative and compassionate

Today, there are many applications of Carl Rogers's approach in child care, patient care, elderly care, and relationship development that use his three guiding principles or *core conditions*, empathy, unconditional positive regard, and congruence. Patient- and family-centered care is an approach to the planning, delivery, and evaluation of health care that is grounded in mutually beneficial partnerships among patients, families, and health care practitioners. It is founded on the understanding that the family plays a vital role in ensuring the health and well-being of patients of all ages. The ultimate goal of patient- and family-centered care is to create partnerships among health care practitioners, patients, and families that will lead to the best outcomes and enhance the quality and safety of health care (Mead and Bower 2000).

The person-centered approach applied to the elderly is defined as services, solutions, treatment, care, and ICT applications provided by caregiver services that place the person at the center of their own care and consider the needs of the older person's carers.

Person-centered care is about a collaborative and respectful partnership between the service provider and the service user:

1. Getting to know the service user as a person
2. Sharing of power and responsibility between the service user and service provider
3. Accessibility and flexibility of both the service provider as a person and of the services provided
4. Coordination and integration of care for the service user
5. Having an environment that is conducive to person-centered care for both service providers and service users

Bridging the ambition of AAL program objectives and the elderly-centered approach should be the framework of our ICT assistive technology development, aiming to maintain the autonomy and empowerment of the elderly and to leave the old paternalistic model of care. ICT development would not create a *new numeric control* of dependence.

Elderly Ecosystem

There are some common approaches to ecological interdependence. Any change in one component of a natural ecosystem influences the other components.

Human development is the result of continual and reciprocal interactions between the organism and its environment. The body and its environment influence each other, and constantly, each adapts in response to changes in the other. The adaptation is the balance between the strengths and weaknesses of the individual, and the risks and opportunities encountered in the environment. Urie Bronfenbrenner (1979) described the human environment as a set of five systemic levels, which are concentric structures that are included into each other and that hold each other within their functional relationships to varying degrees (Figure 5.1):

- The ontosystem is the body itself, with its innate or acquired characteristics, the physical, emotional, intellectual, and behavioral.
- The exosystem is the social environment, the place or context in which the individual is not directly involved but which nevertheless influences their lives. It refers to physical locations but also to people and objects they contain, activities and roles that take place, and very often, the decisions made there.
- The microsystem is the place or immediate context in which the individual has an active and direct participation (family, clubs, social groups, etc.). It refers to physical locations but also to people and objects they contain, activities and role of tension there (the environment).
- The mesosystem is a set of links, relationships, and processes that take place between two or more microsystems.
- The macrosystem is a set of beliefs, ideologies, values, and way of life of a culture or subculture. This is the background that encompasses and influences all other systemic levels.

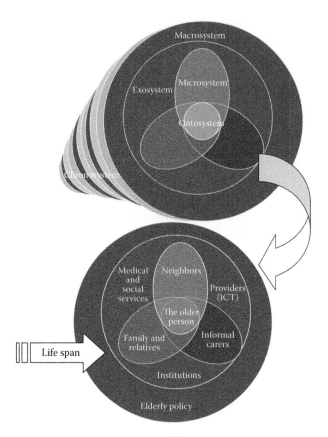

FIGURE 5.1
The elderly ecosystem.

Bronfenbrenner introduced also the concept of the chronosystem (Figure 5.2) to refer to models that examine the developmental change and the cumulative influence of environments over time (years).

The chronosystem applied to the elderly ecosystem is the life span and represents functional and physiological evolution with age.

The model proposes a perspective on the life cycle that allows taking into account the history, development, and interplay of environments. It refers to the influences arising from the

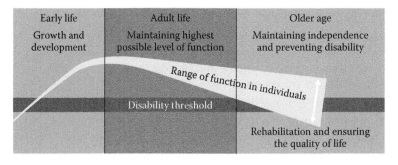

FIGURE 5.2
The chronosystem (or the life span): physiological and functional evolution with age.

passage of time. The individual is presented in a context through which different parts of evolution interact with various socioeconomic and cultural organisations and institutions.

This reading ecosystem with the vision of implementing ICT has the advantage of cross-matching the interaction of biogenetic factors, psychological resources, and lifestyle habits developed by the individual, the various organizations and social institutions, social and cultural values and economic conditions, and the social communities in web social media with on-demand add-on extensions. With the elderly-centered approach putting the elderly in the center of the human ecology concept as the ontosystem, one will see the necessity of a *social network* development of elderly care. The microsystem population represents *natural carers or helpers*.

Many innovative services and technical solutions, including assistive living environments, are brought to the market highly fragmented and do not adapt to the person's needs. This is due to an isolated business perspective without a thorough methodological framework to investigate the person's environment as an ecosystem.

One of the important impacts of an assistive living ecosystem approach is the systematic integration of a user interface requirement protocol according to impairments (Table 5.1).

The assistive living ecosystem is considered a paradigm that stimulates ICT innovation in favor of the elderly. An assistive living ecosystem ICT platform will aim to satisfy some of the primary needs of elderly people, such as alerts and control of basic vital parameters, and to satisfy some of the secondary needs, such as social interactions (Newell et al. 2006). The lack of web accessibility (easy to use, properly designed) will create an overexclusion (Fleming and Sum 2010).

An assistive living ecosystem ICT development designed for all should also be easy to use for operators and carers. Robotic products designed for an elder ecology must be conceived as part of a larger system of existing products and environments that serve elders and others in the ecology. When designing, first-order effects (such as fit) and second-order effects (such as social and cultural implications) must be considered (Forlizzi et al. 2004). Familiar

TABLE 5.1

Ambient Assisted Living User Interface Requirements

Impairments	Interface Standards
Visual	Use of colors
	Large text size
	Background color of text
	Background designs
	Audio description of visual part
Hearing	Volume control
	Signing videos or animations
	Subtitles/captioning of videos
Cognitive	Headings and subheadings
	Scroll bars
	Image/icons/graphs to illustrate textual content
	Use of icons associated with buttons and pages
Dexterity	Big-size buttons/menu items
	Allowing users to control size and formatting of elements
	Keyboard shortcuts
Low literacy	Labels familiar to users
	Explanation of descriptions

product forms with augmented product functionality will fit the system and maximize early product adoption.

The ecology of ageing in the design and the development of assistive technologies for the elderly has to be considered a framework toward best evidence practice.

Evidence-Based Practice

Appraisal of Evidence-Based Practice

During the last decades, the concepts of evidence-based practice have stimulated wide-ranging interest among health professionals as one of the central foundations underpinning the organization and provision of care services (Grol and Grimshaw 2003). The core of the evidence-based approach is decision making (between a patient and a doctor or a caregiver). This first concept concerning decision making for individual patients is named evidence-based medicine (EBM). EBM is the conscientious, explicit, and judicious use of current best evidence in making decisions about the care of individual patients. The practice of EBM means integrating individual clinical expertise with the best available external clinical evidence from systematic research. By *individual clinical expertise*, we mean the proficiency and judgment that individual clinicians acquire through clinical experience and clinical practice. Increased expertise is reflected in many ways but especially in more effective and efficient diagnosis and in the more thoughtful identification and compassionate use of individual patients' predicaments, rights, and preferences in making clinical decisions about their care.

By *available evidence* we mean clinically relevant research, often from the basic sciences of medicine but especially from patient-centered clinical research, into the accuracy and precision of diagnostic tests (including the clinical examination), the power of prognostic markers, and the efficacy and safety of interventions (therapeutic, rehabilitative, preventive, and assistive regimens).

In contrast, a wider approach called evidence-based health care (EBHC) incorporates approaches to understanding the target population's and practitioners' beliefs, values, and attitudes. This approach also takes account of evidence at a population level, such as the burden of disease and implications for resource utilization including delivery of care.

Considering that ICT solutions for the elderly population have somewhere a link to and an impact on health status from a population and individual perspective, evidence-based practice will include EBM and EBHC.

Evidence-Based Approach

Decisions about groups or populations are a combination of three factors: evidence, values, and resources. Most of the time, many decisions (i.e., health care decisions) are driven by values and resources, as opinion-based decision making. Little attention has been given or is paid to applying any evidence from research. Even in cases for which the evidence is low or lacking, the decision made in the context of increasing pressure on resources has to follow the transition from opinion-based to evidence-based decision making (Corring and Cook 1999).

ICT solutions developed in the elderly may be considered as decision-making systems or processes. Besides the technology framework, every ICT solution development in the elderly must be based on a systematic appraisal of the best evidence available. A critical

TABLE 5.2

Skills for Evidence-Based Decision-Making Management

Skills
To ask the *right* questions (research, use, population, outcomes, etc.)
To define a priori criteria such as effectiveness, safety, and acceptability
To track down the evidence (to find articles and validated information, to have expert opinions, etc.)
To assess the quality of evidence (what is the available level of evidence?)
To assess whether the results of existing research are generalizable or applicable to the target population (to define the experimental population [study sample] among the final users)
To define an experimental plan including a cost-effectiveness approach
To publish the results in peer-reviewed journals
To define an implementation plan for the population
To test the use and to measure best use and misuse
To define a risk management plan
To define a reevaluation of evidence

pathway of questions may help every project leader find and apply the best evidence available (Green and Kreuter 2005). This requires the development of evidence management skills (Table 5.2).

Tracking Down the Evidence: The Value of Information

The evidence-based approach consists of three key stages: producing evidence, making evidence available, and using evidence (Figure 5.3).

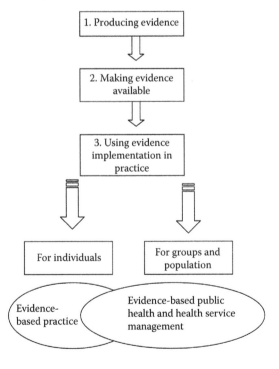

FIGURE 5.3
The three stages of the evidence-based approach.

Evidence comes from research. There are over 2 million research articles in the world's health care literature each year. One could add hundreds of thousands of scientific publications on ICT. The challenge is to be able to access effectively the information required to address the specific decision-making needs and to be able to use the information appropriately. Making the evidence available is valuable. In the era of Web 2.0, access to information has changed the scene and the scenario. In the era of Web 2.0, patients and final users have access to similar professional information, which forms the basis of discussion and negotiation. They also produce information via social media, blogs, tweets, etc. Access to information also increases the patient's and user's sense of autonomy and ability to take responsibility for their health.

However, not all sources provide information of equal quality or relevance.

ICT solutions should nowadays include options on information analysis, knowledge organization, and management. Portals must define the information production sources, the links with relevant libraries and scientific databases (such as MEDLINE, Embase, PASCAL, Cochrane Collaboration, etc.), and undergo some certifications. Health on the net (HON) certification has to be a prerequisite, and a conflict-of-interest policy has to be transparent. Quality of information, specifically information in the field of gerontology and gerontotechnology, will be the key challenge of the AAL evaluation policy.

Levels of Evidence

It is possible to conceptualize a hierarchy of evidence (Muir Gray 2001). This particular hierarchy is used to prepare guidelines of good practice in medicine in order to give some idea of the *grade of evidence* (Table 5.3).

Example of Low Evidence: Do We Answer to Carers' Unmet Needs?

Caring for others is a human value. Caring is everybody's task during the life cycle as life expectancy has been extended. It generates financial, health, and social activities and

TABLE 5.3

Grades of Evidence: Grading of Recommendations Assessment, Development, and Evaluation (GRADE)

Code	Quality of Evidence	Definition
A	High	Further research is very unlikely to change our confidence in the estimate of effect. • Several high-quality studies with consistent results • In special cases: one large, high-quality multicenter trial
B	Moderate	Further research is likely to have an important impact on our confidence in the estimate of effect and may change the estimate. • One high-quality study • Several studies with some limitations
C	Low	Further research is very likely to have an important impact on our confidence in the estimate of effect and is likely to change the estimate. • One or more studies with severe limitations
D	Very low	Any estimate of effect is very uncertain. • Expert opinion • No direct research evidence • One or more studies with very severe limitations

Source: Grading of Recommendations Assessment, Development and Evaluation (GRADE) Working Group 2007.

penalties. Care of older persons by family and friends, defined as *informal carers*, has provided the nutshell of home care and will continue to do so in the future everywhere across Europe.

In the European Union of 27 members (EU 27), it was estimated that there were more than 19 million carers and that the numbers would increase by 13% by 2030 to 21.5 million providing at least 20 hours of care a week and 10.9 million providing at least 35 hours of care a week (source, European Quality of Life Survey [EQLS] described by Anderson et al. 2009). Recalculation to include only those who report they are involved in caring on a daily basis leads to an estimate that 32 million people care on a daily basis.

The gendered nature of informal care is clearly evident, with more women than men. According to EUROFAMCARE, 76% of those caring for an older person were found to be women. Women were also predominately found to be the main older person cared for (68%). Carers of older people were children of the older persons. There may be a care gap in the years ahead with the demand of informal carers outweighing the needs. There is a growing concern that the reliance on family carers in Europe in the future will not be sustainable. The concentration of carers in the age group of 50–64 reflects the prevalence of older people as the recipients of care.

The Eurofamcare study reported by Triantafillou et al. (2006) on older peoples' needs for care and help reported by family carers across Europe:

- Domestic needs, household: 92%
- Emotional/psychological/social needs, companionship, reassurance: 89%
- Mobility needs, inside or outside; transport: 82%
- Financial management, paying bills from the older person's money: 80%
- Organizing and managing care support, contacting services: 79%
- Health care needs, assistance with medication, medical treatment, rehabilitation: 79%
- Physical/personal care needs, washing, dressing, eating, going to the toilet: 66%
- Financial support: 36%

Caring for others is an enriching and rewarding experience when the expectations placed on carers are reasonable and adequate support is provided. Caring can also be a source of burden and stress, with costs to many aspects of the carers' life—emotionally, physically, socially, and financially.

User-friendly ICT has a vital part in facilitating care by family members and in supporting care providers to enable them to do so. Therefore, ICT should respond to the service provisions made by carers and also should aim to relieve the burden of caring. The highest quality of life reported may reflect the availability of support services and the policies for carers.

Example of High Evidence: Preventing Falls

Falls in the elderly are a public health problem. Falls occur in 30–60% of older adults each year, and 10–20% of these result in injury, hospitalization, and/or death. Most falls are associated with identifiable risk factors. Fall prevention has been an area of active research over the past 20 years. There is evidence that multifactorial interventions reduce falls and the risk of falling in hospitals and may do so in nursing care facilities. Vitamin D supplementation is effective in reducing the rate of falls in nursing care facilities. Exercise in hospital settings appears effective, but its effectiveness in nursing care facilities remains uncertain.

Recent research shows that detection and amelioration of risk factors can significantly reduce the rate of future falls. Other evidence-based fall reduction methods include systematic exercise programs and environmental inspection and improvement programs. Those combining all these approaches seem to have the strongest effects on the consequences of falls (hip fracture, hospitalization, loss of autonomy, etc.).

Recent international groups have developed useful clinical guidelines for reducing the risk of falls.

Contrary to this evidence, ICT solutions or assistive technology has been developed over time mainly for the detection of falls and not for fall prevention.

Evidence-Based Practice for AAL Solutions

ICT or assistive technologies could be considered as interventions aiming somehow to increase the autonomy and the quality of life of elderly people. Keep in mind that these interventions are for a frail population with a high prevalence of *gerontology diseases*. Implementation of an evidence-based approach in the development of ICT solutions is the best value for money.

Few data existed to build research (external) evidence in the field of ICT for the elderly. A number of generalizations can be made on the basis of the literature:

1. The technology studied to date is often unreliable.
2. There is marked resistance to the acceptance of most of the technologies available.
3. The available technologies are no substitute for supportive human contact.
4. The technology should be tailored to the needs of the person.
5. The simpler the technology, the more likely it is to have a beneficial effect.
6. There is a great need for better-designed studies with larger samples.

Within the context of low external evidence, with the lack of convincing research published studies, a review of all sources of information, experts' opinions in both fields of ICT and gerontology, and users' qualitative and quantitative evaluation of unmet needs is mandatory.

TABLE 5.4

The PRECEDE–PROCEED Model

PRECEDE Phases	PROCEED Phases
Phase 1—Social diagnosis	**Phase 5**—Implementation
Phase 2—Epidemiological, behavioral, and environmental diagnosis	**Phase 6**—Process evaluation
Phase 3—Educational and ecological diagnosis	**Phase 7**—Impact evaluation
Phase 4—Administrative and policy diagnosis	**Phase 8**—Outcome evaluation

Users' evaluations and opinions on a web-based platform or social media or by interviews are possible approaches to increase the level of evidence and to certify or validate ICT solutions. In the field of health care the predisposing, reinforcing and enabling constructs in educational diagnosis and evaluation-policy, regulatory and organizational constructs in educational environmental development (PRECEDE–PROCEED) (Table 5.4) model of health planning and evaluation could be adapted in the assessment phase of high-health-care-impact ICT solutions.

Implementing Best Evidence Practices in AAL Solutions: Guidelines Needed

Designing guidelines of evidence-based practice in the field of AAL solutions is challenging. One may remember the conclusion of Richard Grol and Jeremy Grimshaw (2003): "If you would like to start tomorrow to change practice and implement evidence, prepare well: involve the relevant people; develop a proposal for change that is evidence-based, feasible, and attractive; study the main difficulties in achieving the change, and select a set of strategies and measures at different levels linked to that problem; of course, within your budget and possibilities. Define indicators for measurement of success and monitor progress continuously or at regular intervals. And, finally, enjoy working on making patients' care more effective, efficient, safe, and friendly."

Guidelines could be developed on different aspects:

1. The development of ICT solutions in the elderly would be done on the model of LivingLab based on coconception with users supported by the European Network of Living Labs (EnoLL).
2. AAL projects will include
   a. The review of existing data and information on unmet needs
   b. The description of the ecosystem of the final users
   c. The description of the target population with at least the *autonomy* status with the use of validated scales (activities of daily living [ADL], instrumental activities of daily living [IADL], etc.)
   d. The territory or the perimeter of action
   e. The definition and the metrology of the primary global public health indicators or use benefits indicators
      i. Quality-of-life scales
      ii. Autonomy grids
      iii. Acceptability
      iv. Medicoeconomics
   f. The comparative study versus nonintervention
3. AAL projects will have a risk management plan including the follow-up of the elderly abuse (weakness abuse) risks.

TABLE 5.5

Design Guidelines and Example of Design Recommendations

Design Guideline	Recommendations
Robotic products must fit the ecology as part of a system.	Consider scale and footprint.
	Consider placement in the home environment.
	Make the product portable and usable beyond a home context.
	Use familiar product forms to inspire early adoption.
Robotic products must support the migrating values of the elderly and others within the ecology.	Provide a natural, "walk-up-and-use" interface.
	Allow the user to initiate product interactions.
	Provide more than one choice to complete any given task.
	Provide options for aesthetic appearance.
Robotic products must be functionally adaptive.	Provide multimodal input and consistent lightweight output.
	Support universal access and use by the largest number of people in the ecology.
	Provide mutable functionality for different users and contexts.

4. AAL projects will comply regarding the respect of autonomy of the subject, which means that an informed consent form has to be signed.

5. Web accessibility and interfaces responding to impairments are the minimum required. A design guideline is part of development (Table 5.5).

6. Web-based platform services should have a description of the data warehouse, data management, and data analysis.

7. A quality process has to be defined and followed.

8. Audits have to be performed.

Elderly ICT Ecosystem: An Evidence-Based Approach Proposal for the Future

Coming back to the two most important unanswered questions of the AAL program, we are convinced that ICT solutions to elderly care are innovative interventions

- To support maintaining the health and functional capability of elderly individuals
- To increase the efficiency and productivity of used resources in ageing societies

These two objectives are the background of a framework focused on an evidence-based practice. We will propose an evidence-based stepwise approach and an evidence-based organization within the elderly ecosystem. ICT solutions and assistive technology should integrate some evidence from the gerontology and geriatric disciplines to become innovative gerontotechnology as interventions to address the two remaining AAL objectives (Figure 5.4).

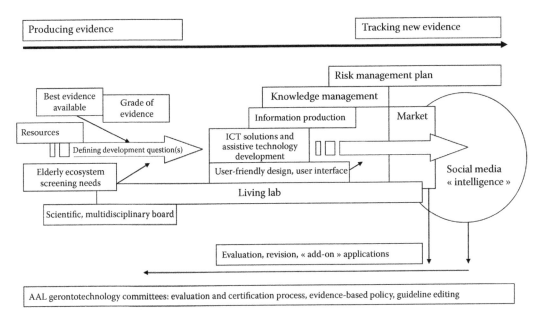

FIGURE 5.4
Elderly ICT ecosystem and evidence-based approach: a certification pathway.

Conclusion

The realities of health care complexity, the frail status of our final user population together with masked or visible impairments adding to the *invasive* intervention nature of any ICT solutions or assistive technologies in daily life, led us to rethink our practice. A minimum set of best-practice guidelines may be welcome. The ambition of all ICT in the elderly is, besides the economical development of ICT solutions, services, tools, or equipment, an improvement of some global health indicators and the quality of life of the elderly. A minimum level of evidence is needed. A culture of research and evaluation complying with scientific research methodology should be boosted. The line between ICT solutions or assistive technologies and medical devices is blurred and, in some cases, is nonexistent. Many ICT solutions are models of web-based services; added value created by the data analysis via data mining and new approaches of data analysis in the era of Web 2.0 has to become a standard. The challenge in the near future will be to transform patient-related information into patient-related outcomes with appropriate tools and methodology.

ICT could be the key to progress, or it could be harmful to a frail population. An evidence-based approach, which is good value for money, will help ICT solution providers to reach the market with a sustainable business by responding to unmet needs and also to the cost-effectiveness vision of decision-making stakeholders and public buyers of innovative equipment.

References

Anderson, R. et al., European Foundation for the Improvement of Living and Working Conditions (Eurofound), Second European Quality of Life Survey: Overview, Luxembourg, Office for Official Publications of the European Communities, 2009.

Baltes, P.B., and Mayer, K.U. (Eds.), *The Berlin Aging Study: Aging from 70 to 100*. New York: Cambridge University Press, 2001.

Bronfenbrenner, U., *The Ecology of Human Development, Experiments by Nature and Design*. Cambridge: Harvard University Press, 1979.

Corring, D., and Cook, J., Client-centered care means that I am a valued human being. *Canadian Journal of Occupational Therapy*, 66(2): 71–82, 1999.

Cullen, K., and Kubitshk, L., EC Report: Europe(s) Information Society, Study of accessibility of ICT products and services to disabled and older people, November, 2008.

Fleming, R., and Sum, S., A review of the empirical studies on the effectiveness of Assistive Technology in the care of people with dementia, 2010. UNSW as part of the Australian government's Dementia.

Forlizzi, J., DiSalvo, C., and Gemperle, F., Assistive robotics and an ecology of elders living independently in their homes. *Human-Computer Interaction*, 19: 25–59, 2004.

Green, L.W., and Kreuter, M.W., *Health Program Planning*, 4th edition. New York; London: McGraw Hill, 2005.

Grol, R., and Grimshaw, J., From best evidence to best practice: Effective implementation of change in patients' care. *Lancet*, 362: 1225–1230, 2003.

Jacobzone, S., Cambois, E., Chaplain, E., and Robine, J.M., The Health of Older Persons in OECD Countries: Is It Improving Fast Enough to Compensate for Population Ageing? Directorate for Education, Employment, Labour and Social Affairs Employment, Labour and Social Affairs Committee, OECD, Paris, 1999.

Mead, N., and Bower, P., Patient-centeredness: A conceptual framework and review of the empirical literature. *Social Science and Medicine*, 51(7): 1087–1110, 2000.

Muir Gray, J.A., *Evidence-Based Healthcare, How to Make Health Policy and Management Decision*. Churchill Livingstone, London, 2001.

Newell, A.F., Dickinson, A., Smith, M.J., and Gregor, P., Designing a portal for older users: A case study of an industrial/academic collaboration. *Transactions on Computer-Human Interaction (TOCHI)*, 13(3): 347–375, 2006.

Seeman, T.E., Lusignolo, T.M., Albert, M., and Berkman, L., Social relationships, social support, and patterns of cognitive aging in healthy, high-functioning older adults: MacArthur studies of successful aging. *Health Psychology*, 20(4): 243–255, 2001.

Seligman, M., Positive health. *Applied Psychology*, 57: 3–18, 2008.

Triantafillou, J., Mestheneos, E., Bien, B., Döhner, H., Krevers, B., Lamura, G., and Nolan, M., Summary of main findings from the Trans-European Survey Report (TEUSURE) and their implications for policy and practice in the support of family carers. In: *EUROFAMCARE Consortium* (eds). Services for Supporting Family Carers of Elderly People in Europe: Characteristics, Coverage and Usage. Trans-European Survey Report. Hamburg: Hamburg University Medical Centre of Hamburg-Eppendorf, 2006.

6

A Demonstration Case on the Derivation
of Process-Level Logical Architectures for
Ambient Assisted Living Ecosystems

Nuno Santos, Juliana Teixeira, António Pereira, Nuno Ferreira,
Ana Lima, Ricardo Simoes, and Ricardo J. Machado

CONTENTS

ABSTRACT   When representing the requirements for an intended software solution during the development process, a logical architecture is a model that provides an organized vision of how functionalities behave regardless of the technologies to be implemented. If the logical architecture represents an ambient assisted living (AAL) ecosystem, such representation is a complex task due to the existence of interrelated multidomains, which, most of the time, results in incomplete and incoherent user requirements. In this chapter, we present the results obtained when applying process-level modeling techniques to the derivation of the logical architecture for a real industrial AAL project. We adopt a V-Model–based approach that expresses the AAL requirements in a process-level perspective, instead of the traditional product-level view. Additionally, we ensure compliance of the derived logical architecture with the National Institute of Standards and Technology (NIST) reference architecture as nonfunctional requirements to support the implementation of the AAL architecture in cloud contexts.

KEY WORDS: *logical architectures, requirements engineering, AAL multidomains, interoperability standards for AAL.*

Introduction

The information and communication technologies (ICTs) can contribute to an improved quality of life by supporting persons with special needs (for instance, elderly people), contributing to a healthier and independent life, and opposing the most common difficulties in this age group. Therefore, this is the starting point for the concept of ambient assisted living (AAL). The concept of AAL is perceived to extend the time people can live in their environment by increasing their autonomy, self-confidence, and mobility [1]. AAL refers to electronic environments that are sensitive and responsive to the presence of people and provide assistive solutions for maintaining their lifestyle. AAL is primarily concerned with the individual in his/her immediate environment by offering user-friendly interfaces for all sorts of equipment in the home and outside, taking into account that many older people have impairments in vision, hearing, mobility, or dexterity [2]. AAL focuses on supporting persons with special needs and is viewed as one of the most promising areas of ambient intelligence (AmI). AmI incorporates sensitive, adaptive electronic environments that respond to the actions of persons and objects [3].

Several segmentations have been proposed for the main actors in the AAL, i.e., the stakeholders [4,5]. The European Ambient Assisted Living Innovation Alliance (AALIANCE) project [6] divides the stakeholders into four distinct groups:

1. The main users who can benefit from AAL technology are the elderly and people with limited abilities and their caregivers. The private users of ICT for ageing solutions such as senior and impaired citizens and private caregivers (usually family members or relatives) represent the primary stakeholders. This category can include senior citizens (those with limited abilities), their family members, and any caretakers. They are also separated into *living persons* and *healthy persons*, where living persons require help with day-to-day activities and healthy persons need ICT to ensure continued good health.

2. The professional users of ICT, such as medical professionals, other service providers, and *mobility providers*, represent the secondary stakeholders. The role of secondary stakeholders is taken by organizations that provide services to the main target group (i.e., security-service providers, care-service organizations, shopping services, transport services, delivery services, social services, community centers, etc.).

3. The tertiary stakeholders are represented by suppliers of ICT ageing solutions and are all industries and companies that supply goods and services to the secondary stakeholders.

4. Finally, the quaternary stakeholders are the supporters of ICT: policy makers, social (and private) insurance companies, public administrations, civil society organizations, etc.

In practical terms, AAL systems help in prevention and classification of situations such as falls and physical immobility, monitoring activities of daily living, behavior analysis, and other possibilities. To achieve these objectives, it is necessary to consider the development of several distinct areas. Mobile devices, including sensors, are of high importance to provide the ability to perceive the environment. Another area of great importance is ubiquitous computing, where it is expected that mobile devices may evolve towards greater mobility and autonomy, making them easier and more comfortable to carry. In terms of human–machine interaction, it is essential to further develop natural interfaces to humans, such as speech, gestures, or even thoughts. The elderly population of today is faced with highly complex systems that do not present intuitive interfaces, which makes their use difficult. A user interface based on virtual characters can improve the accessibility of technical devices to the elderly.

The area of artificial intelligence has contributed at various levels. Specifically, there is interest in adaptation tools and learning environments that can provide technology with the ability to learn the routines and user preferences in a noninvasive way to adjust their actions. The European Union (EU), through the Healthy Ageing initiative [7], promotes active ageing and encourages the use of technology within elders' lives. The EU commission strategy implies a rise in employability through the greater participation of older workers and the promotion of social inclusion, in particular, through the reduction of poverty. It was suggested through the Healthy Ageing project [8] that the EU and the Member States have to develop research to assess the effectiveness and the cost-effectiveness of health-promoting interventions and interventions for the prevention of disease or ill health throughout the life course and especially in later life; strengthen research to find ways of motivating and changing the lifestyles of older people, especially the *hard-to-reach* groups, paying special attention to environmental and cultural aspects; strengthen research to develop indicators of healthy ageing; include data on the very old in health-monitoring statistics and research; and disseminate research findings and promote their practical applications among all stakeholders.

This has resulted in the development of AAL-related projects and solutions. One of the first approaches in the development of an integrated AAL system and teleassistance was developed in the Multiagent Telesupervision System for Elderly Care (TeleCARE) project [9]. More recently, Hristova et al. [10] presented a prototype system integrating a set of health care services, such as heart rate monitoring, prescription medication, generating schedule reminders, and emergency notifications. O'Flynn [11] developed a wireless biomonitor, which integrated wearable sensors: blood volume pulse and electrocardiogram (ECG). Moreover, Stelios [12] developed a system capable of providing location data of people with associated tools, notifications, and alarms.

The ALLIANCE project [6] has elaborated a roadmap of AAL research challenges based on the identification of the needs of elderly people and the necessary technological support. Three principal application domains are considered: (1) AAL for home and mobile support, including AAL for health, rehabilitation and care, personal and home safety and security, etc.; (2) AAL in the community, addressing social inclusion, entertainment, and mobility; and (3) AAL at work, addressing the needs of older people in the workplace.

The Universal Open Platform and Reference Specification for Ambient Assisted Living (UniversAAL) project [13] intends to reduce barriers to adoption and to promote the development and widespread uptake of innovative AAL solutions. The project will produce a platform providing the necessary technical support and acting as an open, common basis for both developers and end users and will carry out support activities promoting widespread acceptance and adoption of the platform.

The Bridging Research in Ageing and ICT Development (BRAID) project [14,15] aims developing a comprehensive Research and Technological Development (RTD) roadmap for active ageing by consolidating existing roadmaps and by describing and launching a stakeholder coordination and consultation mechanism. The project characterized key research challenges and produced a vision for a comprehensive approach in supporting the well-being and socioeconomic integration of increasing numbers of senior citizens in

Europe. The objectives of BRAID included the development of a consensus on requirements for active ageing and ageing well, a vision of a desirable future for older people, a research and technology roadmap, a strategic research agenda, and the development of a self-sustaining stakeholder coordination mechanism.

Extending Professional Active Life (ePAL) [16], Common Awareness and Knowledge Platform for Studying and Enabling Independent Living (CAPSIL) [17], Social ethical and privacy needs in ICT for older people (SENIOR) [18], and Accessibility and Usability Validation Framework for AAL Interaction Design Process (VAALID) [19,20] are other examples of research projects engaged to address the challenges enunciated by the EU Commission guidelines for the AAL area.

Current worldwide works for AAL provide architectures, roadmaps, standards, and technological solutions that aim to assist in elders' well-being. It is a big challenge when eliciting functional requirements for AAL ecosystem concerns, which brings many difficulties for properly specifying the requirements for the intended solution at a product-level perspective, because the inherent complexity results in incoherent and misaligned information.

Thus, we propose adopting a requirements elicitation approach that starts by eliciting requirements at a process level, based on the needs of the intended AAL domain, and then eliciting requirements at a product-level perspective aligned with the process-level requirements. The adopted approach (which we call the V+V process [21]) is composed of two V-Models [22] that are executed in both process- and product-level perspectives and whose resulting requirements are aligned with each other. Requirements are expressed by a composition of models—logical architectural models and stereotyped sequence diagrams [23]—derived in successive executions and iterations. The adopted V+V process acts in the analysis phase and enables the transition to the design phase, by using the Four-Step-Rule-Set (4SRS) method [24,25] for model transformation.

In this chapter, we conduct a demonstration case analysis on how the first V-Model execution within the V+V process (the process-level one) required some changes in executing some of its parts, due to some constraints regarding the AAL multidomain context. The initial information refinement could not be gathered like in the typical process-level V-Model execution, such as described in Ref. [26]. Alongside an overview of the typical process-level V-Model execution, we present the main implications of this specific AAL context within the modeling and derivation of artifacts in order to provide a process-level logical architectural model for the AAL context that enables creating context for product-level requirements elicitation. It should be ensured that the process-level logical architecture complies with some interoperability issues (and, in the specific case of this project, cloud computing). Thus, as an example, we demonstrate how a process-level logical architecture based on domain scenarios did not deal with some issues suggested by the NIST reference architecture for cloud computing and how a new iteration of the derivation of the logical architecture was promoted.

This chapter is structured as follows: in the "Requirements Elicitation" section, we present some related work and definitions that allow us to understand the context in which this demonstration case is conducted and the context itself (AAL ecosystems); in the "Derivation of Logical Architectures" section, we focus on the demonstration case for eliciting process-level requirements for the Ambient Assisted Living for All (AAL4ALL) project, by presenting the V-Model execution and the obtained artifacts; in the "Interoperability and Cloud Issues" section, we address interoperability and cloud issues and how they can be aligned with the modeled process-level logical architecture; and in the "Conclusions" section, we present the conclusions of the conducted analysis.

AAL4ALL Project

We demonstrate the applicability of the proposed approach by using a case study that results from the process-level requirements elicitation in a real project: the AAL4ALL project [27]. The AAL4ALL project brought together all relevant stakeholders, such as public institutions, industry, user organizations, and RTD institutions, in the discussion and definition of the basic AAL services of general interest for a Portuguese nationwide solution. The analysis of already existing standards and other international activities is also a key aspect of this project, which aims capitalizing on existing knowledge, avoiding redundant development, with a clear focus only on the missing pieces to achieve optimum solutions in this area. Thus, the main objective of the AAL4ALL project is the development of a standard ecosystem of products and services for AAL, associated with a business model and validated through a large-scale trial [28]. The AAL4ALL project focuses on providing health care services and products to the elderly community, and it implements the base structure to the foundations of the work presented. The objective is to present a roadmap and initial structures of an AAL project, focusing on the defined personas and a mobile solution to these personas. The current AAL projects lack a real user guidance structure, aiming at a broad area where every user has different needs and limitations.

The AAL4ALL project, similar to the recommendations of the BRAID roadmap [15], adopts a holistic perspective of ambient assisted living, i.e., life settings. Taking into account typical lifestyles of different users, different life settings are considered, corresponding to the main areas of a person's life, and will need to be supported in the ageing process. Therefore, four life settings defined in the BRAID project [14] describe different aspects of either interest or necessity for persons of every age. The AAL4ALL project considered that those four settings should be directly addressed by the adopted scenarios for the development of AAL4ALL products and services [29]:

1. *Independent living*: The individual would be safe and have all the care needed at home. Their activities would be managed, and they would have support for physical mobility in terms of localization, positioning, and mobility assistance.

2. *Health and care in life*: The subject would be sensorial monitored. If affected by a chronic disease, it would be monitored; and the subject would have assistance in medication, would be assisted in lifestyle intervention and in health care management, would be compensated in the physical and neurocognitive aspects, and would be assisted in rehabilitation in the case that it is needed.

3. *Occupation in life*: The individual's workplace would be adjusted in order to have a minimal effect on their ageing by adjusting the work space and establishing intergenerational relations. In order to facilitate the extension of professional life, links with former employers would be kept and the subject placed to work in professional communities. Aid for freelancing and entrepreneurship could also be provided if it was the subject's intention to do such work.

4. *Recreation in life*: The person would be encouraged to socialize through real-world and virtual communities and through the management of social events. They would be requested to participate in entertainment such as games, online and remote cultural activities, and remote recreation activities. They would be required to engage in learning activities like remote learning or experience exchange and knowledge sharing.

These settings can demonstrate how technology can assist in normal daily-life activities and includes services such as living status monitoring, with connection to care providers in case of any emergency; an agenda manager to compensate for memory losses; companion and service robots; and integration of intelligent home appliances. There is also support outside the home in terms of mobility assistance, shopping assistance, and other daily-life activities. Monitoring includes rehabilitation and disability compensation, caring, and assistance regarding health-related interventions. Also, technology can assist in health-related activities like emergency assistance, sensing environments, prescription reminders, and remote health monitoring; support the continuation of professional activities; and facilitate socialization and participation of ageing citizens in social, leisure, learning, and even religious, cultural, and political activities.

In order to be able to fully execute within the presented life settings and, mainly, within the several environments, the AAL4ALL ecosystem will be composed of several devices and systems, from different vendors and service providers. Additionally, the platform to be developed should follow the evolution of technological developments in the AAL domain. The heterogeneity of devices and systems makes it impossible to adopt a single technological approach and requires the definition of interoperability mechanisms, as well as the use of interoperability standards to enable consistent interoperability between products (software components, systems, devices).

Regarding technological development, the AAL4ALL project will result in the development of a core platform that allows an aggregation of all stakeholders' systems to enable the composition of the AAL services that will be provided to end users in both home and in mobility environments, where several types of devices are installed to gather data from user environments and to provide AAL services. Thus, we consider that AAL4ALL platform development should aim at providing a service-oriented architecture (SOA) and a cloud-based solution, capable of ensuring a set of services for the AAL4ALL ecosystem, such as (1) AAL services to the end user, (2) services to support AAL business activities, (3) services to support the service provisioning, and (4) services that ensure the systems' interoperability.

Requirements Elicitation

Requirements elicitation is concerned with where software requirements come from and how they are collected [30] within the requirements engineering area. The objective of a requirements elicitation task is to communicate the needs of users and project sponsors to system developers. When eliciting process-level requirements, it is expected that the result is a characterization of the domain in question. Some elicitation tasks may thus include domain engineering tasks. Domain engineering focuses on finding common and variable parts of a domain in order to support reuse in that domain. In order to achieve reuse in a domain, domain knowledge must be captured in terms of commonalities and variability. Commonalities allow reuse of software components in a domain; they result from domain features that are common. Therefore, the variability [31] enables the differentiation of applications in a domain. Arango [32] argues that a domain engineering process should incorporate three main activities: domain analysis, infrastructure specification, and infrastructure implementation.

An important view considered in our approach is regarding the architecture. The literature encompasses a plethora of definitions, and most agree that architecture concerns both structure and behavior. There are several views regarding architectures, ranging from reference architectures to technological architectures. Some of these views and concerns were first observed by Parnas [33]. Later, Kruchten, in 1995 [34], defined four main views and a fifth that tied the previous four together. A logical architecture can be considered a view of a system composed of a set of problem-specific abstractions supporting functional requirements [35]. The logical architecture acts as a common abstraction of the system providing a representation of the system able to be understood by all the stakeholders regardless of their background. IEEE 1471 [36] defines software architecture as the "fundamental organization of a system embodied in its components, their relationships to each other, and to the environment, and the principles guiding its design and evolution."

There are several approaches, from a product-level perspective, to support the design of software architectures, like Reuse-Driven Software Engineering Business (RSEB) [37], Family-oriented Abstraction, Specification and Translation (FAST) [38], Feature-Oriented Reuse Method (FORM) [39], Komponentenbasierte Anwendungsentwicklung (KobrA) [40], and Quality-driven Architecture Design (QADA) [41]. Tropos [42] and 4SRS [25] are process-level requirement modeling methods that allow the derivation of logical architectures. Our approach is based on the 4SRS method to derive a process-level logical architecture for creating context for product design. The 4SRS method ensures the transition from the problem to the solution domain by transforming process-level use cases into process-level logical architectures, allowing the uncovering of hidden requirements. The adopted process level is related to real-world activities, includes domain (business) requirements, and supports the evolution into the typical software development life cycle by next executing the product-level version of the 4SRS method [24] that allows the functional decomposition of software systems. The multidomain characteristic of AAL projects justifies the adoption of process-level approaches as a way to control the complexity of dealing with simultaneous domains during requirements elicitation and modeling.

Derivation of Logical Architectures

In this section, we present our approach, based on successive and specific artifact derivation. We use ageing scenarios [43], *A-type* and *B-type* sequence diagrams [26], use-case models, and a process-level logical architecture diagram. The original V-Model approach as presented in [26] starts with organizational configuration (OC) modeling. An OC model is a high-level representation of the activities (interactions) that exist between the business-level entities of a given domain. In the AAL4ALL project, the first information regarding the high-level business activities to be described in our V-Model is ageing scenarios.

V-Model Process and 4SRS Method

The original V-Model is a variation of Royce's waterfall model [44], in a *V* shape folded in half and having in the vertex the lowest level of decomposition. The V-Model's left side represents the decreasing abstraction from user requirements into components by a process of decomposition and definition. The right side of the V-Model represents the integration and verification of the previous components into greater levels of implementation and assembly, by realizing them and thus decreasing the abstraction level. The V-Model representation [22] provides a balanced process representation and, simultaneously, ensures that each step is verified before moving onto the next. In our V-Model approach (Figure 6.1), the generated artifacts are based on the information existing in previously defined artifacts, i.e., A-type sequence diagrams are based on scenarios, the use-case model is based on A-type sequence diagrams, the logical architecture is based on the use-case model, and B-type sequence diagrams comply with the logical architecture.

Scenarios are textual descriptions of a possible execution or interaction between a set of users of the system. In the AAL4ALL project, we have used the template of Table 6.1 for capturing the first scenario information. They promote simple textual descriptions, but they can also be graphically modeled by using, for instance, Business Process Model and Notation (BPMN) [45] or stereotyped sequence diagrams, like the ones we present in our V-Model approach. We have adopted Unified Modeling Language (UML) instead of BPMN because UML takes an object-oriented approach to design applications, focusing on software. BPMN takes that approach to systems modeling, focusing on the business process. The two are complementary views on systems. Nevertheless, it is possible to map between BPMN constructs and UML use-case and sequence diagram constructs. The A-type sequence diagrams used in our V-Model are composed of use cases, so we consider them a feasible graphical representation for modeling the scenarios. Additionally, the 4SRS method takes as input use-case models that capture the intended system requirements, making their adoption mandatory in our specifications.

Our approach uses a UML stereotyped sequence diagram representation to describe interactions in the early analysis phase of system development. These diagrams are called A-type sequence diagrams. Another stereotyped sequence diagram, called B-type sequence diagrams, allows for deriving process sequences represented by the sequence flows between the architectural elements (AEs; depicted in the logical architecture). One must ensure that process sequences modeled in B-type sequence diagrams depict the same flows as the ones modeled in A-type sequence diagrams, as well as being in conformity with the interactions between AEs depicted in the logical architecture associations. An AE is a representation of the pieces from which the final logical architecture can be built. This

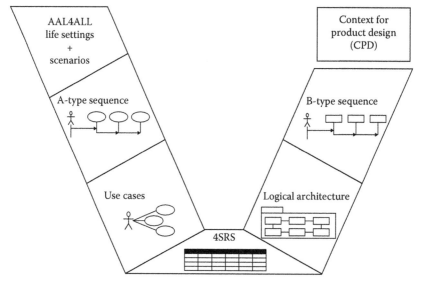

FIGURE 6.1
V-Model adaption from Ref. [26] for the AAL4ALL project.

TABLE 6.1

Scenario Description Template

ID
Name
Actors
Stakeholders
Personas
Trigger
Scenario description
Persona characterization
Functional requirements
Nonfunctional requirements
Performance
Reliability
Security
Configuration
Portability
Legal requirements
Usability
Design
Communication protocol
Availability
Business rules
Special requirements

term is used to distinguish those artifacts from the components, objects, or modules used in other contexts, like in the UML structure diagrams. An example of A-type and B-type sequence diagrams can be found in Figure 6.2.

The generated models and the alignment between the domain-specific needs and the context for product design can be represented by the V-Model depicted in Figure 6.1. A-type sequence diagrams can be gathered and afterwards used as an elicitation technique for modeling the use cases. It can be counterintuitive to consider that use-case diagrams can result from refinement efforts of sequence diagrams. This is possible, if we take into consideration that the scenarios expressed in the A-type sequence diagrams are built using the use-case candidates in the form of activities that will be executed and must be computationally supported by the system to be implemented. These activities in the form of use cases are placed in a stereotyped sequence diagram and associated with the corresponding actors and other use cases. These use cases are later arranged in use-case diagrams after

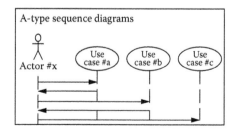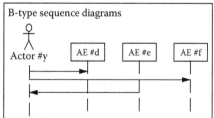

FIGURE 6.2

A- and B-type sequence diagram examples.

redundancy is eliminated and proper naming is given. The flow expressed by the sequences creates the rationale for discovering the necessary use cases to complete the process.

In the V-Model represented in Figure 6.1, the artifacts placed on the left-hand side of the path representation are properly aligned with the artifacts placed on the right side, i.e., B-type sequence diagrams are aligned with A-type sequence diagrams, and the logical architecture is aligned with the use-case model. Alignment between the use-case model and the logical architecture is ensured by the correct application of the 4SRS method. The resulting sets of transformations along our V-Model path provide artifacts properly aligned with the organization's business needs, which, in the AA4ALL project, are formalized through ageing scenarios.

The 4SRS method allows for the transformation of user requirements into an architectural model representation and is traditionally applied in a product-level perspective [24] including variability and recursive mechanisms [24,35]. The method is organized into four steps to transform use cases into AEs: Step 1 (AE creation) automatically creates three kinds of AEs for each use case: *i-type* (interface), *c-type* (control), and *d-type* (data). Step 2 (AE elimination) removes redundancy in the requirements described in the use case's textual descriptions and promotes the discovery of hidden requirements. Step 3 (AE packaging and aggregation) groups AEs in semantically consistent packages and also allows the representation of aggregations (of, for instance, existing legacy systems). Step 4 (AE association) has the goal of representing associations between the remaining AEs. According to what has been described, the 4SRS method takes use-case representations (and corresponding textual descriptions) as input and (by recurring in tabular transformations) creates a logical architectural representation of the system. We present a subset of the tabular transformations in Figure 6.3. In these tabular transformations, each column has its own meaning and rules. They ensure traceability between the derived logical architecture diagram and the initial use-case representations. At the same time, they make possible to adjust the results of the transformation to changing requirements. Tabular transformations are thoroughly described [24,25].

When traditional product-level requirements elicitation fails due to insufficient information, we propose an approach that begins with eliciting process-level requirements and later evolves to properly aligned product-level requirements. Our proposal, a V+V process [21], is based on the execution of two V-Model–based approaches, one executed in a process-level perspective and the other executed in a product-level perspective. In this chapter, we present only the process-level V-Model execution, which allows for creating context for later execution of product-level efforts.

As stated before, our approach is based on the premise that there is no clearly defined context for directly eliciting product requirements. The initial request for the AAL4ALL project requirements resulted in mixed and confusing sets of misaligned information. The discussions inside the project consortium relative to (1) the multidomains considered to be covered; (2) the technologies, solutions, and devices to be adopted; as well as (3) the uncertainty relative to interoperability issues (among others) resulted in a lack of consensus for the definition of product-level requirements. Adopting a process-level perspective allows the eliciting of requirements in multidomain ecosystems, as well as dealing with interoperability issues. The fact that the AAL4ALL platform is intended to execute in a cloud-based context does not bring more complexity to the adoption of this approach, since [25] presents the execution of the process-level 4SRS in order to derive a logical architecture to execute in a cloud environment. The rationale for the design of the models proposed in the approach, in the case of the AAL4ALL project, is based on specifying processes that intend to fulfill the previously presented issues, i.e., (1) to execute in a cloud-based software solution, (2) to deal with several AAL multidomains, and (3) to support interoperability between solutions and devices.

Step 1—Architectural element creation	Step 2—Architectural element elimination									Step 3—Packaging and aggregation	Step 4—Architectural element association	
	2i—Use case classification	2ii—Local elimination	2iii—Architectural element naming	2iv—Architectural element description	2v—Architectural element representation (Represented by)	2v—Architectural element representation (Represent)	2vi—Global elimination	2vii—Architectural element renaming	2viii—Architectural element specification		4i—Direct associations	4ii—UC associations
{0b.1.2} Check health values	ci											
{AE0b.1.2.c}		T	Health monitoring decisions	Makes decisions on how the measured information from {AE0b.1.2.i} is used within the AAL4ALL Node. The information can be used by the platform for preventing abnormalities	{AE0b.1.2.c}	{AE0b.3.3.1.c}	T	Health monitoring decisions	Makes decisions on how the measured information from {AE0b.1.2.i} is used within the AAL4ALL Node. The information can be used by the platform for preventing abnormalities in user's wellbeing ...The Information is also used by the formal caretaker (doctor) to have...	{P1} Activity monitoring	{AE0b.1.2.i}	{AE0b.1.1.i} {AE0b.5.2.c} {AE0b.4.2.i} {AE0b.4.3.5.i}
{AE0b.1.2.d}		F										
{AE0b.1.2.i}		T	Receive current vital signs information	Receives the current values for vital signs (e.g., blood pressure, heart rate, etc.) measured by the health monitoring devices.	{AE0b.1.2.i}	{AE0b.1.3.i} {AE0b.1.4.i} {AE0b.3.3.1.i}	T	Receive current information	This AE is responsible for receiving all monitoring-related information from the several monitoring devices...	{P8} System interoperability	{AE0b.1.2.c} {AE0b.1.3.c} {AE0b.1.4.c}	{AE0b.3.2.i} {AE0b.3.3.2.d} {AE0b.3.4.i}

FIGURE 6.3
Process-level 4SRS tabular transformations.

AAL4ALL Examples

In this subsection, we describe the execution of the process-level V-Model presented in the previous subsection and the modeling of its composing artifacts for the AAL4ALL project. Our purpose is not to thoroughly describe the artifacts and their alignment with each other but, instead, to explain the rationale and demonstrate the implications of the specific AAL4ALL context encountered in the V-Model execution.

The AAL4ALL Scenarios for Ageing

The first step in the scenario specification regards a general identification of a user's functional limitations and level of dependency on basic and instrumental daily activities [28]. The analysis supported by questionnaires allows the identification of a set of personas and their characterization. These personas represent typical users of the AAL4ALL solution within the scenarios to be developed.

Having in mind the four life settings previously presented for the AAL4ALL project, scenarios were developed in order to describe possible interactions between users and the several solutions (most of them based on active ageing scenarios [43]), as well as the interaction between these solutions and the future AAL4ALL platform. These scenarios are built upon the conception of the availability of technology to the user in a form of set-and-forget. An easy setup and full integration of the devices are a key requirement.

The AAL scenarios were developed in consensus with the expected results and the typical users who can benefit from the devices and services. An extensive search and compilation of data, acquired through inquiries to the caretakers, experts, and common population, served as the initial conceptualization base for the construction of actors that represent an unbiased user. The scenario detailed in Table 6.2 considers the user's common

TABLE 6.2

Scenario Description Regarding Daily Routine Monitoring

ID	Independent living #1
Name	Daily routine monitoring
Actors	
Stakeholders	User, formal caretaker (call center); informal caretaker (family, girlfriend)
Personas	Manuel
Trigger	Manuel executes daily routines.
Scenario description	A system installed in his house provides an environment with a range of interconnected sensors, devices, and smart appliances working together to provide a safe and secure place to live. Several video cameras distributed along the house allow observing Manuel's daily routines (by authorized people) and, at the same time, maintain his privacy. The system is capable of interpreting the situation from the captured images and can react in order to provide assistance to Manuel in case of need. ...
Persona characterization	Manuel, 76 years old, lives in the city's outskirts and is retired. ...
Functional requirements	• The system is composed of body motion sensors. • Additionally, it is composed of fire, flood, and gas sensors. • If an abnormal situation occurs, a call center is notified. • The call center calls and asks user if everything is okay, and may call emergency units. • Etc.

...

and everyday problems, providing technological solutions that can have an impact on the user's life.

A-Type Sequence Diagrams

In an early analysis phase, we need to define the relations between activities and actors, defined through interactions in our approach. Interactions are used during the more detailed design phase, where the precise interprocess communication must be set up according to formal protocols [46]. An interaction can be displayed in a UML sequence diagram. Traditional sequence diagrams involve system objects in the interaction. Since modeling structural elements of the system is beyond the scope of the user requirements, Machado et al. [23] propose the usage of a stereotyped version of UML sequence diagrams that only includes actors and use cases to validate the elicited requirements at the analysis phase of system development. We also use such diagrams in our work and define them as A-type sequence diagrams, as shown in Figure 6.4.

Use Cases

Gathering A-type sequence diagrams can be used as an elicitation technique for modeling the use cases. All use cases defined in the A-type sequence diagrams must be modeled and textually described in the use-case artifact. For the textual descriptions, we strongly recommend that they comply with the templates proposed by the Rational Unified Process (RUP) [47] as well as incorporate any design decisions, if applicable. Use cases, in the process-level perspective, portray the activities (processes) executed by persons or machines in the scope of the system, instead of the characteristics (requirements) of the intended products to be developed. An actor, like in the product level, represents a user that interacts with the AAL4ALL system.

Regarding the use-case modeling, issues concerning the multidomains in the AAL4ALL project (i.e., the four life settings) brought more complexity in achieving a unified view of the system. At first sight, one could elicit requirements for each of the domains. The problem is that the execution of a domain analysis task would result in one use-case model for

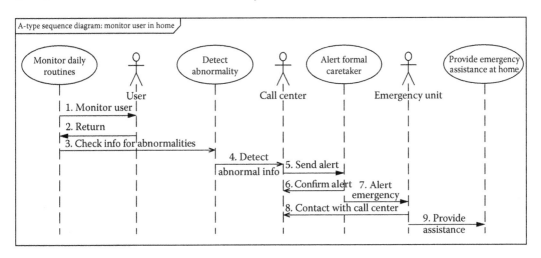

FIGURE 6.4
A-type sequence diagram.

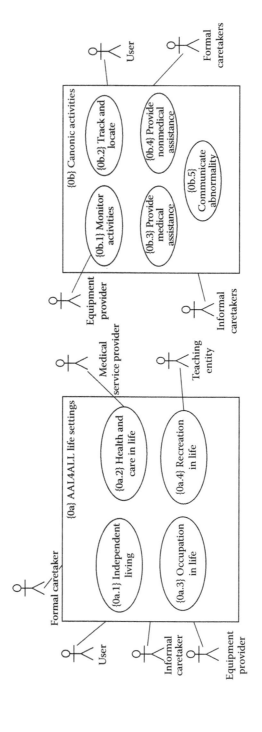

FIGURE 6.5
The use-case model composed of two orthogonal views.

each of the four domains, and the following 4SRS method execution would result in four independent logical architectures. By analyzing the ageing scenarios and A-type sequence diagrams, we concluded that some of the domains *share* common activities; although very different, domains present some interrelations.

Thus, we decided to use two orthogonal views from the system under analysis: the {0a} *AAL4ALL Life Settings* and the {0b} *Canonic Activities*. The existence of two orthogonal views in user requirements' higher abstraction level (level 0 of use-case diagrams) has enabled us to cope with the inherent complexity when dealing with both Canonic Activities and AAL4ALL Life Settings. Both views are depicted in Figure 6.5.

Using an orthogonal view allows us to optimize use-case representation, since requirements for all domains are easily captured and the final use-case model is composed of fewer use cases than a typical requirements elicitation approach. The orthogonal view {0a} *AAL4ALL Life Settings* regards the specific requirements for each one of the four considered life settings. The {0b} *Canonic Activities* orthogonal view is composed of common activities regardless of the domain. The aim is to represent requirements intentionally generic, so they are applicable in every domain. Such information is provided by the ageing scenarios and A-type sequence diagrams. These use cases can be functionally refined and still represent a common activity. Such refinement can be modeled until a point is reached where it is impossible to be independent from the domain. This was the case, for instance, for the activity {0b.1} *Monitor Activities*, used in this chapter as an example and depicted in Figure 6.6. In the AAL4ALL project, generic characterization of requirements was not applicable to all use cases. Use cases {0b.2} *Track and Locate* and {0b.3} *Provide Medical Assistance* are not applicable to the orthogonal use cases {0a.2} *Health and Care in Life* and {0a.3} *Recreation in Life*. These restrictions are also reflected in refinements of these use cases. After common activities are refined, these restrictions are taken into account.

In Figure 6.6 we depict a subset of the use-case model regarding the refinement of {0b.1} *Monitor Activities*. This use-case model concerns activities for monitoring a user's steps, allowing some independence in the user's (elderly or citizens with limited abilities) performed activities and responding in case of need. The intended system will be composed of a set of interconnected devices that continuously monitor the user's steps, monitoring health parameters, recognizing the user's daily routines, and assisting the user in performing them (by using *intelligent* equipment, as well as ensuring energy saving). Devices publish the monitored information in the AAL4ALL platform.

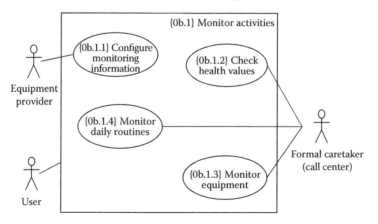

FIGURE 6.6
Refinement of use case {0b.1}.

Execution of the Process-Level 4SRS Method

The process-level 4SRS method is thoroughly described [25]. Here, our purpose is to focus on how AAL concerns are treated during the execution of the four steps of the 4SRS method. We present some examples on how to derive a logical architecture that acts as a basis for the requirements elicitation of a solution that enables interoperability between products/services for the AAL4ALL project.

Step 1: AE Creation

This step regards the creation of AEs. Interface, data, and control AEs are created for each use case. I-type, d-type, or c-type stereotypes, respectively, are added to each AE (Table 6.3). No particular rationale or decision is required at this step, since it concerns mainly the transformation of one use case into three specific AEs. Preconditions or post-conditions require the creation of glue elements, having the c-type stereotypes since they require decisions to be made with computational support.

Step 2: AE Elimination

In this step, AEs are submitted to elimination actions according to a set of predefined rules. At this moment, the system architect decides which of the original three AEs and which of the eventual glue AEs created during step 1 are maintained or eliminated, taking into account the entire system.

- *Microstep 2i: Use-Case Classification.* In this step, each use case is classified according to the nature of its AEs, previously created in step 1. The nature of an AE is defined according to the suffix the AE was tagged with. There are three stereotyped AEs: d-type, which refers to generic decision repositories (data), representing decisions not supported computationally by the system under design; c-type, which encompasses all the processes focusing on decision making that must be supported computationally by the system; and i-type, which refers to a process' interfaces with users, software, or other processes.

  In the AAL4ALL project, d-type AEs refer to noncomputational decisions executed by the AAL4ALL stakeholders (e.g., users, formal caretakers, other entities, etc.); c-type AEs refer to computationally supported decisions to be made by the AAL4ALL platform; and i-type AEs refer to interfaces with users or with software/devices and are responsible for dealing with interoperability issues (Table 6.4).

- *Microstep 2ii: Local Elimination.* This microstep refers to the determination of which AEs must be eliminated in the context of a use case, guaranteeing its full representation. This is required since microstep 2i disregards any representativeness concerns.

- *Microstep 2iii: AE Naming.* In this microstep, AEs that survived the previous microstep are given a name. The name must reflect the role of the AE within the entire

TABLE 6.3

Step 1 of the 4SRS Method

Step 1—Architectural Element Creation	
{0b.1.2} Check Health Values	
{AE0b.1.2.c}	Generated AE
{AE0b.1.2.d}	Generated AE
{AE0b.1.2.i}	Generated AE

TABLE 6.4

Microsteps 2i to 2iv of the 4SRS Method

	Step 2—Architectural Element Elimination			
	2i—Use Case Classification	2ii—Local Elimination	2iii—Architectural Element Naming	2iv—Architectural Element Description
{0b.1.2}	cd			
{AE0b.1.2.c}		T	Health Monitoring Decisions	Makes decisions on how the measured information from {AE0b.1.2.i} is used within the AAL4ALL platform. The information can be used by the platform for preventing abnormalities in user's wellbeing. This AE defines for whom the values are sent.
{AE0b.1.2.d}		F		
{AE0b.1.2.i}		T	Receive Current Vital Signs Information	Receives the current values for vital signs (e.g., blood pressure, heart rate, etc.) measured by the health monitoring devices. The information is published in the AAL4ALL Node.

use case, in order to semantically give hints on what it represents and not just copy the original use-case name. Usually, the AE name also reflects the use case from which the AE originated.

- *Microstep 2iv: AE Description.* The resulting AEs that were named in the previous microstep must be described, and the requirements that they represent must be addressed in the process-level perspective. This microstep is where the transition is made from the problem domain to the solution domain, so the descriptions must detail, in process terms, *how, why, when,* and *by whom* that AE is going to be executed. This microstep must explicitly describe the expected behavior of the AE execution, including which decisions will be made and how they will be supported. For instance, the {AE0b.1.2.i} *Receive Current Vital Signs Information* description contains the following: "This AE is responsible for receiving all monitoring-related information from the several monitoring devices. This AE is also responsible for assuring the interoperability between the devices and the AAL platform. Receives the current values for vital signs (e.g., blood pressure, heart rate, etc.) measured by the health monitoring devices..."

- *Microstep 2v: AE Representation.* The purpose of this microstep is to eliminate redundancy in the global process, ensuring a semantic coherence of the logical architecture and discovering anomalies in the use-case model. In this microstep, all AEs are considered and compared in order to identify if one AE is represented by any other one. The identification of redundancy takes into consideration issues like the execution context, actors involved, used artifacts, and activities and tasks, among others. If all of these factors are similar, though the AEs are originated by different use cases, one given AE can be considered to represent another. In the AAL4ALL project, the four i-type AEs representing data publication concerning monitoring of a user's steps, vital signs, and routines were represented by a single i-type AE, since the publication task is similar in those four cases and would result in redundancy in the global model. Thus, a single i-type AE was considered to represent those four AEs, resulting in the elimination of three AEs and maintaining one AE (Table 6.5).

- *Microstep 2vi: Global Elimination.* This microstep refers to determining which AEs must be eliminated in the context of the global model, similar to microstep 2ii, since its execution is automatic. Each AE that is represented by itself or represents another AEs is maintained. All the other AEs (i.e., AEs that are represented by other AEs) are eliminated. This is a fully *automatic* microstep, since it is based totally on the results of the previous one.

- *Microstep 2vii: AE Renaming.* In this microstep, AEs that have not been eliminated in microstep 2vi may have to be renamed. When one AE under analysis results in the representation of more than one AE, the new name must reflect the global execution of the AE in the final system context. In the AAL4ALL project, the *new* AE described in the previous example was renamed {AE0b.1.2.i} *Receive Current Information.*

- *Microstep 2viii: AE Specification.* Though it is similar to microstep 2iv, this microstep intends to describe AEs that, in microstep 2v, are considered to represent other AEs. The execution of this microstep is only applicable to define the behavior of the new AEs in a way that is clear to system architects. The specification must also include references to an execution sequence of AEs. The specification information produced in this microstep is crucial to support the transition from the process-level approach to the product-level approach after the execution of the first V-Model. In the AAL4ALL project, the new AE is specified in this microstep as follows: "This AE is responsible for receiving all monitoring-related information from the several monitoring devices. Receives the current values for vital signs

TABLE 6.5

Microsteps 2v to 2viii of the 4SRS Method

	Step 2—Architectural Element Elimination				
	2v—Architectural Element Representation		2vi—Global Elimination	2vii—Architectural Element Renaming	2viii—Architectural Element Specification
	Represented by	Represent			
{0b.1.2}					
{AE0b.1.2.c}	{AE0b.1.2.c}		T		
{AE0b.1.2.d}					
{AE0b.1.2.i}	{AE0b.1.2.i}	{AE0b.1.3.i} {AE0b.1.4.i} {AE0b.3.3.1.i}	T	Receive Current Information	This AE is responsible for receiving all monitoring-related information from the several monitoring devices. Receives the current values for vital signs (e.g., blood pressure, heart rate, etc.) measured by the health monitoring devices, the current information regarding equipment usage and the currente information regarding user's steps. The information is published in the AAL4ALL platform. ...

(e.g., blood pressure, heart rate, etc.) measured by the health monitoring devices, the current information regarding equipment usage and the current information regarding User's steps. The information is published in the AAL4ALL platform."

Step 3: Packaging and Aggregation

In this step, the remaining AEs (those that were maintained after executing step 2), for which there is an advantage in being treated in a unified process, should give the origin to aggregations or packages of semantically consistent AEs. This step supports the construction of a truly coherent process-level model (Table 6.6).

Step 4: AE Association

Decisions on the identification of associations between AEs can be based on information contained in the use-case model and in microstep 2i. Thus, as an addition to the original 4SRS, step 4, was divided in microsteps 4i, direct associations, and 4ii: use-case associations, with the purpose of identifying unnecessary direct associations and to help reflect, in the model, changes made in the previous steps (Table 6.7). It must also be noted that any textual reference to eliminated AEs in microstep 2vi must be included in microstep 2viii, making it another source of information for step 4.

Derivation of Process-Level Logical Architectures

The 4SRS method execution ends with the construction of a logical diagram, which represents the logical architecture of the process-level AAL4ALL system. The architecture is

TABLE 6.6

Step 3 of the 4SRS Method

	Step 3—Packaging and Aggregation
{0b.1.2}	
{AE0b.1.2.c}	{P1} Activity Monitoring
{AE0b.1.2.d}	
{AE0b.1.2.i}	{P7} System Interoperability

TABLE 6.7

Step 4 of the 4SRS Method

	Step 4—Architectural Element Association	
	4i—Direct Associations	4ii—UC Model Associations
{0b.1.2}		
{AE0b.1.2.c}	{AE0b.1.2.i}	{AE0b.1.1.i} {AE0b.5.2.c} {AE0b.4.2.i} {AE0b.4.3.5.i}
{AE0b.1.2.d}		
{AE0b.1.2.i}	{AE0b.1.2.c} {AE0b.1.3.c} {AE0b.1.4.c}	{AE0b.3.2.2.i} {AE0b.3.3.2.d} {AE0b.3.4.i}

composed of the AEs that survived after the execution of step 2. The packaging activity performed in step 3 allows the identification of major processes. The associations identified in step 4 are represented in the diagram by the connections between the AEs (for readability purposes, the *direct associations* are represented in dashed lines, and the *use case model associations*, in straight lines).

Figure 6.7 depicts the process-level logical architecture for the AAL4ALL system and contains more than 70 AEs. This figure is intentionally not zoomed in (and, thus, also not readable), just to show the complexity of the AAL4ALL project that has justified the adoption of process-level techniques to support the elicitation efforts. A proper zoom of the architecture can be found in Figure 6.8, where some of its constructors are detailed, in this case, a subset of AEs regarding the package {P1} *Activity Monitoring*.

There is a noticeable interdependency between the macropackages of the presented logical architecture. Looking at the logical diagram in Figure 6.7—for the packages and associations—it is possible to identify that there are three groups of packages and AEs, located at the top, middle, and the bottom of the logical architecture diagram. The upper package is composed of the AEs that represent decision-making processes executed by the human actors (d-type AEs), which are the input for the process execution. The packages in the middle regard the processes to be executed within the AAL4ALL platform. These packages concern the activities that enable the execution of the products and services that

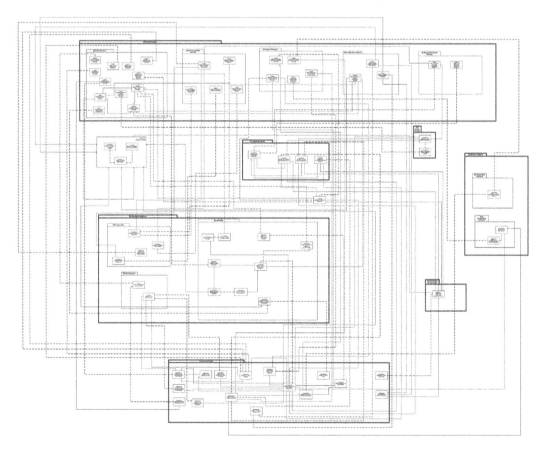

FIGURE 6.7
AAL4ALL process-level logical architecture.

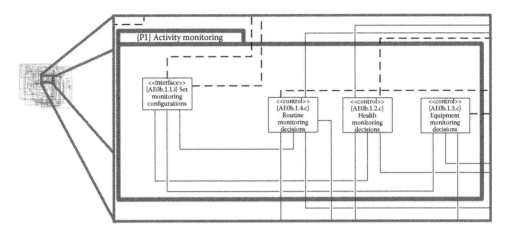

FIGURE 6.8
Subset of the AAL4ALL process-level logical architecture.

belong to the AAL4ALL ecosystem (e.g., activity monitoring, home care, socialization, mobility, medication assistance, and abnormality communication, among others).

The lower package is composed of the AEs whose activities regard communication with the systems that compose the AAL4ALL ecosystem (i-type AEs) and that are required to deal with interoperability issues. These AEs typically represent the process output.

The most typical process execution starts with an input from an AE belonging to the upper package; the information flow is treated in the AAL4ALL platform-related packages (middle packages) and is finalized with an output in an AE belonging to the lower package, which enables communication with the other systems. Some processes start from the upper package and go directly to the lower package because there is no need for any decision within the AAL4ALL platform at a process-level perspective.

B-Type Sequence Diagrams

One of the purposes of creating a software logical architecture is to support the system's functional requirements [34]. It must be ensured that the derived logical architecture is aligned with the business needs. On one hand, the execution of a software architecture design method (e.g., 4SRS) provides an alignment of the logical architecture with user requirements. On the other hand, it is necessary to validate whether the behavior of the logical architecture is as expected. So, at a later stage, after deriving a logical architecture, to analyze the sequential process flow of AEs, we construct B-type sequence diagrams (stereotyped UML sequence diagrams), where interactions between AEs (presented in the logical architecture), actors, and packages (if justifiable) are modeled. In Figure 6.9, we present the same scenario as in Figure 6.4 concerning user monitoring at home but at a lower level of abstraction.

The B-type sequence diagram modeling and the inherent validation efforts of the process-level logical architecture promote a new iteration into the modeling process, and new requirements may be included [26].

In Figure 6.10, we represent the four iterations performed of the process-level V-Model for the AAL4ALL project. Each iteration into the V-Model process also embeds one iteration of the process-level 4SRS method to promote new undiscovered requirements and to derive a new version of a more robust logical architecture.

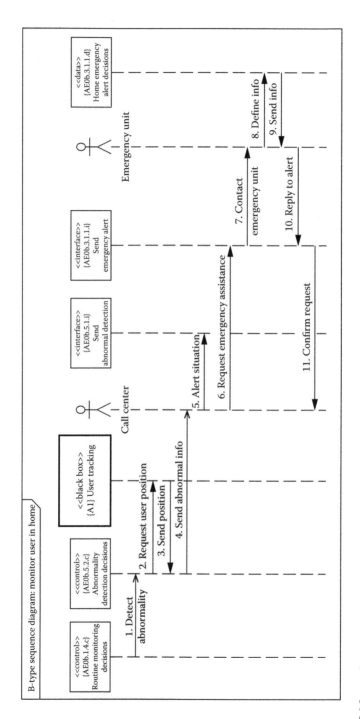

FIGURE 6.9
B-type sequence diagram.

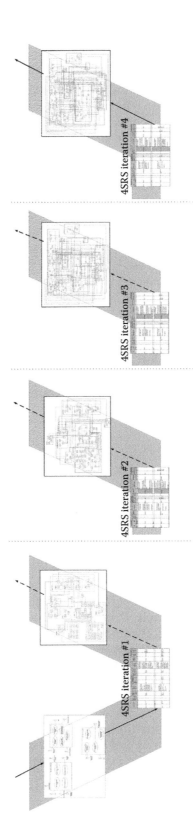

FIGURE 6.10
The four V-Model iterations performed in the AAL4ALL project.

Interoperability and Cloud Issues

Since the AAL4ALL project aims at developing a unified AAL ecosystem, by using a single platform for integrating and orchestrating the products, services, and devices, the product-level requirements should reflect the integration of legacy systems, instead of a typical approach that elicits product-level requirements that reflect applications to be developed and their functionalities. The process-level requirements include all activities performed in the ecosystem, regardless of whether they are executed within the platform or in any already existing application. In opposition, the product-level requirements only regard interoperability needs.

If, on one hand, the resulting complexity regarding the multidomains drove our first approach to base the requirements elicitation on the life setting scenarios (described in the previous sections) and the logical architecture provided a specification of how activities from the life settings interact with each other, on the other hand, issues like security and privacy must be considered critical when developing AAL solutions. Thus, it is advisable that developed platforms comply with those issues as recommended by domain reference architectures.

There are some widely accepted standards and reference architectures that deal with nonfunctional issues, such as interoperability for AAL and cloud computing, that provide best practices for any AAL project. Thus, those standards should also be considered in requirements elicitation. Typically, these standards are only applicable to technological decisions, which regard the elicitation of product-level requirements. Here, we will be considering them in our process-level elicitation process.

Reference Architectures and Standards

Taking into account the four life setting scenarios, the demonstration case conducted in this chapter provides a specification of the activities that will be supported by the AAL4ALL platform. However, the deployment of the services that compose the AAL4ALL ecosystem cannot be completely derived from those scenarios, since some technical issues regarding the final software deployment and distribution are out of the scope of the logical architecture. This is one of the issues to be considered when designing the technical architecture of the system [48]. A reference architecture can be used to support those decisions, since it is a framework in which system-related concepts are organized taking into account application domain characteristics or cross-cutting concerns [49–51]. In contrast with the technical architecture, the implementation architecture shows a system's physical layout, revealing which pieces of software run and what pieces of hardware are used [52]. In this section, we will not deal with implementation issues. We will focus on cloud computing and interoperability in AAL. The widely used architectures and standards for our analysis purpose regards the NIST cloud computing reference model and Continua Health Alliance, respectively.

The NIST [53] Cloud Computing reference architecture is the most known and used by the ICT industry for cloud-based architectures. NIST defines cloud computing as a computing model that allows ubiquitous and on-demand access to a set of configurable computing resources available on the network, such as communications networks, servers, storage, applications, and services that can be rapidly provisioned and updated with minimal management effort or service provider interaction [54]. According to NIST, this computing model is characterized by its five main features: (1) on-demand self-service, (2) broad network access, (3) resource pooling and rapid elasticity, (4) three possible service models (software as a service [SaaS], platform as a service [PaaS], and infrastructure as a service [IaaS]), and (5) four possible deployment models (private cloud, public cloud, hybrid cloud, community cloud). NIST has developed a logical extension of their cloud definition by the development of a NIST cloud computing reference architecture (Figure 6.11). This generic high-level conceptual model constitutes an effective tool for discussing the requirements, structure, and operation of cloud computing; defines a set of actors, activities, and functions that can be used in the process of developing cloud computing architectures; and relates to a companion cloud computing taxonomy.

In the AAL domain, Continua [55] interoperability architectures are the most widely used due to their maturity and completeness for technical interoperability approaches. Continua is an international open alliance for the health industry that develops interoperability guidelines for personal telehealth ecosystems. They have identified some barriers that typically occur during the implementation of such systems: the lack of data and system interoperability. To overcome these barriers, Continua has defined interfaces for local area network (LAN) and wide area network (WAN) to enable end-to-end interoperability [56]. For promoting the adoption of existing standards in the creation end-to-end interoperable solutions, Continua has developed a guideline that specifies the requirements for the connectivity interfaces of personal health system (PHS) devices at the communications transport network and the message and data format layers.

The Continua end-to-end (E2E) reference architecture provides a high-level architectural view of the AAL ecosystem, including its topological constraints (Figure 6.12). The distributed system architecture breaks down its functionalities into five reference device classes and four network interfaces that connect the devices to a reference topology. The network interfaces are at the center of Continua's interoperability goals [56]. Additionally, it defines three kinds of elements [56,57]: (1) components (a model's logical entities, such as services); (2) devices (physical entities); and (3) interfaces (communication between components). Depending on the implemented interfaces, devices are classified as follows: (1) application hosting devices (such as personal computers and smartphones); (2) personal area network (PAN) devices (either sensors or actuators); (3) LAN devices

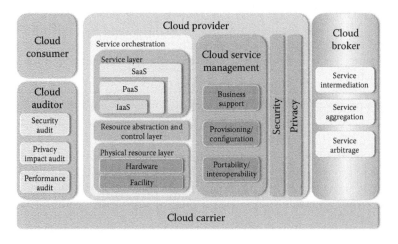

FIGURE 6.11
NIST cloud computing reference model [54].

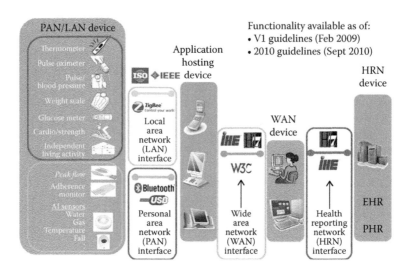

FIGURE 6.12
Continua end-to-end reference architecture with interfaces and standards [56].

(aggregate and share [though a network] the bound PAN devices information); (4) WAN device (implements a managed-network-based service, using IP communication capabilities); and (5) health record network (HRN) devices (implement a health care record). Figure 6.12 provides an overview of the Continua E2E reference architecture and the specification of interfaces and standards [58].

Interoperability in the AAL4ALL Project

The context in which the AAL4ALL platform must operate requires that the product-level (software) requirements comply with cloud and interoperability issues. Existing reference architectures provide best practices for implementing those issues. In our case, we have mapped the AEs of the derived AAL4ALL logical architecture with the components of the NIST reference architecture. This mapping classifies the process-level AEs with cloud and interoperability issues. The results of the mapping can be used for preparing the transition to the technical architecture. Product-level requirements should reflect these results, so we ensure that business needs are fulfilled and that the requirements comply with technological best practices.

The NIST cloud computing reference architecture does not represent the system architecture of a specific cloud computing system; rather, it is a tool for describing, discussing, and developing a system-specific architecture using a common framework of reference for cloud computing that can be used for designing architectures. In our analysis, the NIST reference model was used to study the suitability of our logical architecture for cloud computing environments. This study has allowed an understanding of which of the various cloud services should be considered in the AAL4ALL system, as well as the identification of the candidate standards for dealing with interoperability and reference implementations.

The AEs from the process-level logical architecture (from Figure 6.7) have been mapped onto the functional block architectural components of the NIST cloud reference model in

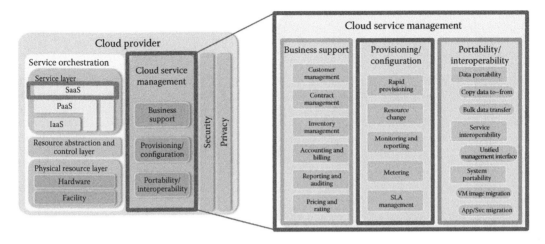

FIGURE 6.13
Focused layers of NIST cloud reference model in the mapping.

order to verify which AEs comply with the NIST reference model and discover lacking requirements for supporting cloud contexts within the AAL4AL logical architecture. In Figure 6.13, we depict the main layers of the NIST cloud reference model that were considered: the service layer (focused on the SaaS layer), the functional blocks from the cloud service management layer, security, and privacy.

The result of the overall mapping is presented in Figure 6.14. In Figure 6.15, we depict a zoom of the mapping result. The mapping task was executed so that each AE of the AAL4ALL logical architecture was affected with the NIST layer that best complies with its functionality. This execution of this mapping task allowed us to find some limitations of the AAL4ALL logical architecture relative to the NIST cloud reference model: (1) the lack of AEs related to business support (mainly justified by the naive elicitation process adopted in the AAL4ALL project); (2) the lack of AEs related to security and privacy (mainly justified by design decisions that will occur only when deciding about the technical architecture; up to now, security and privacy issues have been considered nonfunctional requirements and were not included in the initial requirements; they are addressed in future tasks); and (3) AEs with semantics not fully compatible with the NIST cloud reference model—for instance, {AE0b.4.3.2.c1} *Verify Systems Interoperability* and {AE0b.2.1.c1} *Validate User Indoor Position* (Figure 6.15) were affected as monitoring activities in the NIST reference model, but the monitoring activities are unclear in these AEs names.

These results have justified performing a new iteration of the V-Model process. This fifth iteration of our derivation of the AAL4ALL logical architecture allowed us to complement the elicitation efforts of the project and to align the logical architecture with cloud concepts. The fifth version of the AAL4ALL logical architecture (Figure 6.16) is more prepared to support the design of the AAL4ALL technical architecture. Although it is not the intention to present the new added AEs in this new iteration, we depict new AEs and packages when comparing to the fourth iteration. This new iteration (Figure 6.17) has allowed the depiction of an overview of the AAL4ALL cloud-based services, providing a global overview of the AAL4ALL ecosystem.

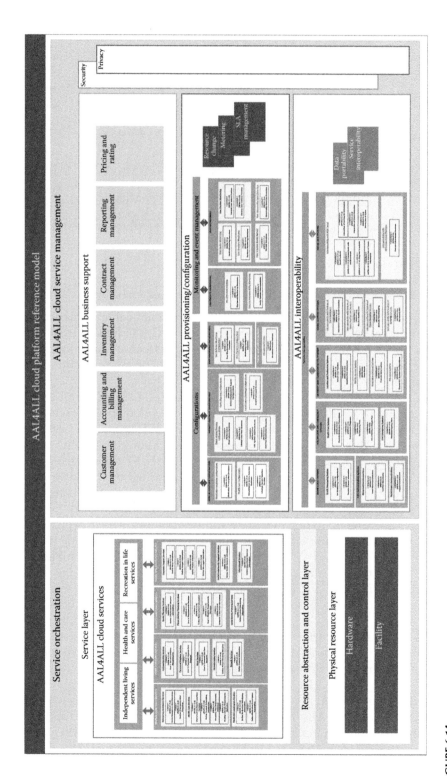

FIGURE 6.14
AE affection in the NIST reference model.

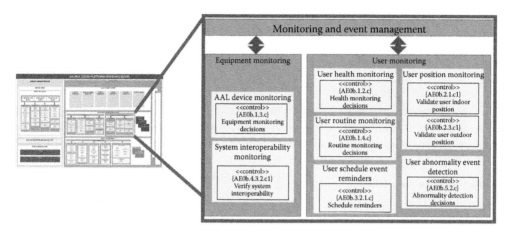

FIGURE 6.15
Architectural elements adapted to NIST cloud reference.

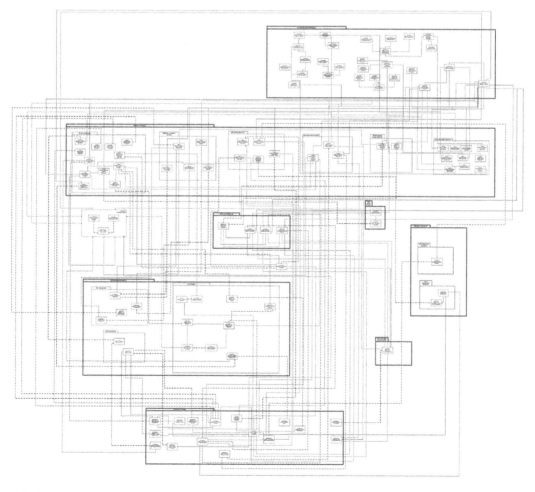

FIGURE 6.16
Fifth version of the AAL4ALL logical architecture.

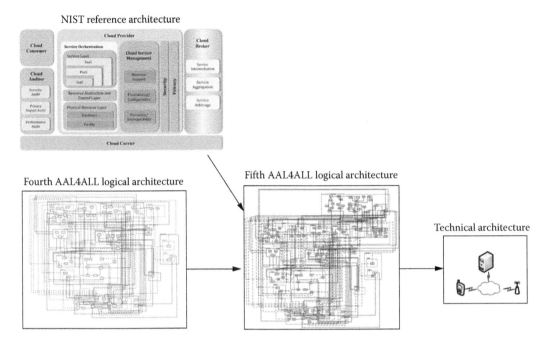

FIGURE 6.17
Derivation of the fifth version of the AAL4ALL logical architecture.

At a high-level perspective, six clouds could be considered to compose the whole eco-system (Figure 6.18): (1) AAL4ALL cloud services—to support the AAL4ALL cloud-based services provided to end users and AAL service providers; (2) AAL devices cloud—composed of local devices; (3) events and transport private cloud—composed of systems that ensure reservations for events and transport tickets; (4) social support private cloud—composed of systems of entities that provide social support services, such as personal hygiene care and housekeeping services; (5) health care private cloud—composed of entities that provide health care and emergency support services, such as health care centers, hospitals, and fire brigades; and (6) social web public cloud—composed of social web platforms. These clouds represent functional modules depicted from our logical architecture that work together to ensure interoperability between AAL4ALL systems. The arrows between clouds represent the interoperability and communication between clouds. The AAL4ALL cloud services and AAL devices cloud are now detailed, and their cloud representation is properly zoomed into. For the scope of this chapter, we do not consider it relevant to detail and zoom the rest of the clouds that compose the AAL4ALL ecosystem.

The central cloud (designated as AAL4ALL cloud services) is the core of the AAL4ALL system, functioning as a central node where different services (provided by several service providers) that will compose the AAL4ALL ecosystem are aggregated, composed in new services, processed, and delivered to the final users. Figure 6.19 depicts the four different types of services to be supported: (1) end-user services—to support end users, covering independent living, health and care, and recreating in life; (2) business support services—considering all business-related services with the clients and supporting process; (3) operation support services—to handle all aspects of provisioning, configurations, and monitoring; and (4) interoperability services—to support interoperability of services and data between clouds.

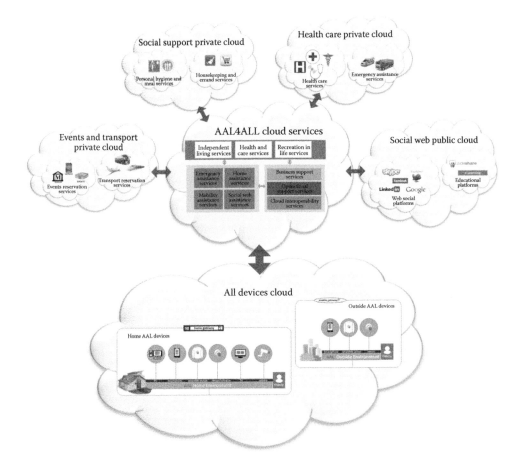

FIGURE 6.18
Cloud-based services for the AAL4ALL ecosystem.

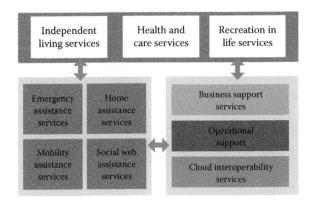

FIGURE 6.19
AAL4ALL cloud-based services.

The AAL devices cloud represents the second cloud layer responsible for integrating local devices. Each device should be directly connected to a gateway, which provides interoperability, establishing the connection with the AAL4ALL core platform to send and receive interesting data that support the AAL services, such as data related to users and systems to support the AAL services that are also provided through the gateway. For home environments (inside), it should be considered a home gateway. On the other hand, in mobile environments (outside), it should be considered a mobile gateway, as represented in Figures 6.20 and 6.21. AAL4ALL platform configuration and monitoring, including AAL local system gateways, are ensured by the *operational support services*.

The fifth version of the AAL4ALL logical architecture is prepared to support business functionalities that enable service providers to manage their business processes related to AAL4ALL services offers, such as customer management, billing and accounting, and contract management. These functionalities are supported by *business support services* that ensure the management of the AAL4ALL customer's life cycle.

Based on the Continua reference architecture, Figure 6.22 depicts a high-level diagram that characterizes the functional block *cloud interoperability services*. It is composed of the clouds, functional blocks, and components from Figure 6.18, and proposes interoperability standards to promote communication between them.

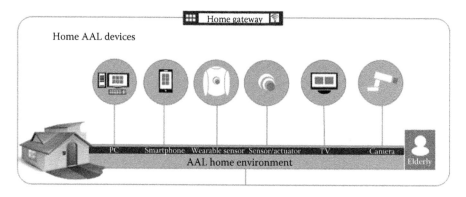

FIGURE 6.20
High-level diagram: AAL logical diagram for home environment.

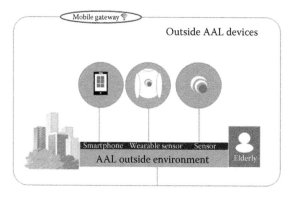

FIGURE 6.21
High-level diagram: AAL logical diagram for mobility environment.

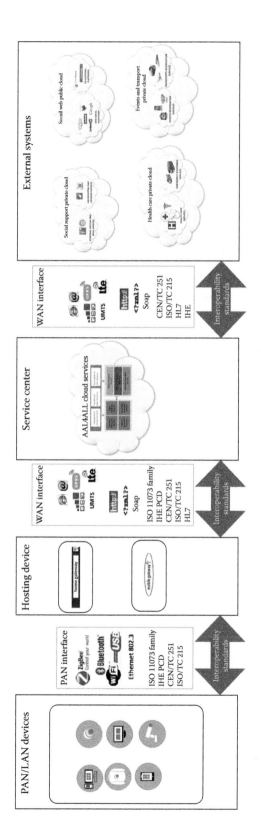

FIGURE 6.22
End-to-end interoperability architecture for AAL4ALL ecosystem.

Conclusions

In this chapter, we have demonstrated how a process-level requirements elicitation approach—a V-Model approach for requirements elicitation—was executed in order to derive a process-level logical architecture diagram for an AAL platform. The intended AAL platform supports interoperability needs between AAL software solutions to cover the four AAL life settings that were identified in a roadmap for ageing and ICT development.

The derived process-level logical architecture is compliant with the Active Reviews for Intermediate Designs (ARID) [58] method, which was used for ensuring that the attained logical architecture representation is tenable. The approach ensures that validation tasks are performed continuously along the modeling process. It allows for validating the following: (1) the final information technology (IT) solution according to the initial expressed requirements; (2) the B-type sequence diagrams according to A-type sequence diagrams; (3) the logical diagram by traversing it with B-type sequence diagrams according to ARID specifications; and (4) multiple refinements of the logical architecture trough iterations of the 4SRS method, promoted by issues raised during ARID application.

The fifth iteration of the AAL4ALL logical architecture, promoted by the mapping with the NIST reference model, allowed us to achieve an architecture more robust and complete that complies with cloud computing requirements to support the delivering of cloud-based services capable of implementing the AAL4ALL ecosystem: (1) AAL services provided to end users; (2) business support services; (3) operation support services; and (4) system services that ensure system interoperability. The main identified interoperability scenarios regard (1) interoperability between gateways and devices; (2) interoperability between the AAL4ALL platform and gateways; and (3) interoperability between the AAL4ALL platform and external systems.

Acknowledgments

Project AAL4ALL was cofinanced by the European Community Fund (FEDER) through COMPETE—Programa Operacional Factores de Competitividade (POFC), Foundation for Science and Technology, Lisbon, through project PEst-C/CTM/LA0025/2011.

References

1. AAL Europe. Ambient Assisted Living Joint Programme website. 2012. Available from: http://www.aal-europe.eu/ (accessed December 27, 2012).
2. Pieper, M., M. Antona, and U. Cortes. Ambient Assisted Living, in *ERCIM News*. 2011, ERCIM EEIG, pp. 18–64. Available from: http://ercim-news.ercim.eu/en87/special/introduction-to-the-special-theme-ambient-assisted-living.
3. Aarts, E., and R. Wichert. *Ambient Intelligence Technology Guide*, H.-J. Bullinger, Editor. 2009, Springer, Berlin/Heidelberg, pp. 244–249.

4. Bridging Research in Ageing and ICT Development (BRAID). Report on mechanisms for stakeholder co-ordination. October 2010.

5. Wright, D. Structuring stakeholder e-inclusion needs. *Journal of Information, Communication and Ethics in Society.* 2010. **8**(2): pp. 178–205.

6. AALIANCE Project. Ambient Assisted Roadmap. 2010. Available from: http://www.aaliance2 .eu/sites/default/files/RM2010.pdf. 2010 (accessed December 27, 2012).

7. Healthy Ageing Project. Available from: http://www.healthyageing.eu/ (accessed December 27, 2012).

8. Stegeman, I., T. Otte-Trojel, C. Costongs, and J. Considine. Healthy and Active Ageing. 2012. EuroHealthNet: A report commissioned by Bundeszentrale für gesundheitliche Aufklärung (BZgA).

9. Telecare Project. Available from: http://www.uninova.pt/~telecare/.

10. Hristova, A., A.M. Bernardos, and J.R. Casar. Context-aware services for ambient assisted living: A case-study, in *Applied Sciences on Biomedical and Communication Technologies, 2008. ISABEL '08. First International Symposium on.* 2008.

11. O'Flynn, B. et al. Wireless bi monitor for ambient assisted living, in *Oral Presentation at ICSES 2006 (International Conference on Signals and Electronic Systems).* Lodz, Poland, September 17–20, 2006.

12. Stelios, M.A. et al. An indoor localization platform for ambient assisted living using UWB, in *Proceedings of the 6th International Conference on Advances in Mobile Computing and Multimedia.* 2008, ACM, Linz, Austria, pp. 178–182.

13. UniversALL Project. Universal open platform and reference Specification for Ambient Assisted Living. 2010. Available from: http://universaal.org/ (accessed December 27, 2012).

14. BRAID Project. Bridging Research in Ageing and ICT Development (BRAID). 2010. Available from: http://braidproject.eu/ (accessed December 27, 2012).

15. Camarinha-Matos, L.M., and J. Rosas. BRAID D6.1 Interim Roadmap for ICT and ageing. 2011.

16. Camarinha-Matos, L.M. et al. ePAL roadmap for active ageing—A collaborative networks approach to extending professional life, in *Proceedings of AGEmap Workshop/Pervasive Health 2010 Conference.* Munich, Germany. Springer Berlin Heidelberg, 2010. 46–59.

17. Capsil Project. Roadmap document. 2010. Available from: http://capsil.org/capsilwiki/index .php/File:CAPSIL_Roadmap_Document.pdf (accessed December 27, 2012).

18. Senior Project. Roadmap. Available from: http://www.ifa-fiv.org/wp-content/uploads/2012 /12/059_Report-on-good-practices-ethical-guidance-15-Nov-09.pdf.2009.

19. VAALID Project. Accessibility and usability validation framework for AAL interaction design process. 2008. Available from: http://www.vaalid-project.org (accessed December 27, 2012).

20. Naranjo, J.-C. et al. A modelling framework for ambient assisted living validation, in *Universal Access in Human-Computer Interaction. Intelligent and Ubiquitous Interaction Environments*, C. Stephanidis, Editor. 2009, Springer, Berlin/Heidelberg, pp. 228–237.

21. Ferreira, N. et al. Transition from process- to product-level perspective for business software, in *6th International Conference on Research and Practical Issues of Enterprise Information Systems (CONFENIS'12).* 2012. Ghent, Belgium.

22. Haskins, C., and K. Forsberg. *Systems Engineering Handbook: A Guide for System Life Cycle Processes and Activities; INCOSE-TP-2003-002-03.2. 1.* 2011, INCOSE, San Diego, CA.

23. Machado, R. et al. Requirements validation: Execution of UML models with CPN tools. *International Journal on Software Tools for Technology Transfer (STTT)*, 2007. **9**(3): pp. 353–369.

24. Machado, R.J. et al. Refinement of software architectures by recursive model transformations, in *Product-Focused Software Process Improvement*, J. Münch, and M. Vierimaa, Editors. 2006, Springer, Berlin/Heidelberg, pp. 422–428.

25. Ferreira, N. et al. Derivation of process-oriented logical architectures: An elicitation approach for cloud design, in *13th International Conference on Product-Focused Software Development and Process Improvement—PROFES 2012*, A.J.O. Dieste, and N. Juristo, Editors. 2012, Springer-Verlag, Berlin/Heidelberg, pp. 44–58.

26. Ferreira, N. et al. Aligning domain-related models for creating context for software product design, in *Proceedings of the 5th Software Quality Days Conference—SWQD'2013*, G. Berlin Heidelberg, Editor. 2013 (accepted for publication), Springer-Verlag, Vienna, Austria.

27. AAL4ALL. AAL4ALL (Ambient Assisted Living for All) project. 2011. Available from: http://www.aal4all.org/ (accessed December 27, 2012).

28. Vardasca, R., L. Ferreira, and R. Simões. Needs and opportunities in Assisted Ambient Living in Portugal, in *Proceedings of the 2nd International Living Usability Lab Workshop on AAL Latest Solutions, Trends and Applications AAL 2012*, M.S. Dias, A. Teixeira, and D. Braga, Editors. 2012, In conjunction with BIOSTEC 2012: Vilamoura, Algarve, Portugal.

29. Camarinha-Matos, L.M. et al. ICT & Ageing Scenarios. Available from: http://www.braid project.eu/sites/default/files/Ageing_scenarios.pdf.

30. Abran, A. et al. Guide to the Software Engineering Body of Knowledge (SWEBOK), 2004 ed., P. Bourque, R. Dupuis, A. Abran, and J.W. Moore, Editors. IEEE Press, Los Alamitos, CA, 2001.

31. Azevedo, S. et al. Support for variability in use case modeling with refinement, in *Proceedings of the 7th International Workshop on Model-Based Methodologies for Pervasive and Embedded Software*. 2010, ACM: Antwerpen, Belgium, pp. 1–8.

32. Arango, G. Domain analysis: From art form to engineering discipline, in *ACM Sigsoft Software Engineering Notes*. 1989, ACM, New York.

33. Parnas, D.L. On the criteria to be used in decomposing systems into modules. *Communications of the ACM*, 1972. **15**(12): pp. 1053–1058.

34. Kruchten, P. The 4+1 view model of architecture. *IEEE Software*, 1995. **12**(6): pp. 42–50.

35. Azevedo, S. et al. Refinement of software product line architectures through recursive modeling techniques, in *On the Move to Meaningful Internet Systems: OTM 2009 Workshops*, R. Meersman, P. Herrero, and T. Dillon, Editors. 2009, Springer, Berlin/Heidelberg, pp. 411–422.

36. IEEE Computer Society. *IEEE Recommended Practice for Architectural Description of Software Intensive Systems—IEEE Std. 1471-2000*. 2000. Available from: http://standards.ieee.org/findstds /standard/1471-2000.html.

37. Jacobson, I., M. Griss, and P. Jonsson. *Software Reuse: Architecture, Process and Organization for Business Success*. 1997, Addison-Wesley Longman, Harlow, UK.

38. Weiss, D.M., and C.T.R. Lai. *Software Product-Line Engineering: A Family-Based Software Development Process*. 1999, Addison-Wesley Professional, Boston.

39. Kang, K.C. et al. FORM: A feature-oriented reuse method with domain-specific reference architectures. *Annals of Software Engineering*, 1998. **5**(1): pp. 143–168.

40. Bayer, J., D. Muthig, and B. Göpfert. The library system product line. A KobrA case study. Fraunhofer IESE, 2001.

41. Matinlassi, M., E. Niemelä, and L. Dobrica. *Quality-Driven Architecture Design and Quality Analysis Method, A Revolutionary Initiation Approach to a Product Line Architecture*. 2002, VTT Tech. Research Centre of Finland, Espoo.

42. Castro, J., M. Kolp, and J. Mylopoulos. Towards requirements-driven information systems engineering: the Tropos project. *Information Systems*, 2002. **27**(6): pp. 365–389.

43. Camarinha-Matos, L.M. et al. BRAID active ageing scenarios. 2011. Available from: http://www.braidproject.eu/sites/default/files/Ageing_scenarios.pdf (accessed June 5, 2012).

44. Ruparelia, N.B. Software development lifecycle models. *SIGSOFT Software Engineering Notes*, 2010. **35**(3): pp. 8–13.

45. OMG. Business Process Model and Notation (BPMN) v2.0. Available from: http://www.omg .org/spec/BPMN/2.0.

46. OMG. Unified Modeling Language (UML) Superstructure Version 2.4.1. 2011. Available from: http://www.omg.org/spec/UML/2.4.1/ (accessed January 27, 2012).

47. Kruchten, P. *The Rational Unified Process: An Introduction*. 2004, Addison-Wesley Professional, Boston.

48. Chen, D., G. Doumeingts, and F. Vernadat. Architectures for enterprise integration and interoperability: Past, present and future. *Computers in Industry*, 2008. **59**(7): pp. 647–659.

49. Browning, T.R., and S.D. Eppinger. Modeling impacts of process architecture on cost and schedule risk in product development. *IEEE Transactions on Engineering Management*, 2002. **49**(4): pp. 428–442.
50. Zwegers, A.J.R. *On Systems Architecting: A Study in Shop Floor Control to Determine Architecting Concepts and Principles*. 1998, Technische Universiteit Eindhoven, Eindhoven, Netherlands.
51. Wyns, J. et al. Workstation architecture in holonic manufacturing systems, in *Proceedings of the 28th CIRP International Seminar on Manufacturing Systems*, Z. Katz, Editor. 1996. Rand Afrikaans University, Johannesburg, South Africa.
52. Fowler, M. *UML Distilled: A Brief Guide to the Standard Object Modeling Language*. 2004, Addison-Wesley Professional, Boston.
53. NIST (National Institute of Standards and Technology). 2010. Available from: http://www.nist.gov/index.html (accessed December 27, 2012).
54. Bohn, R.B. et al. NIST cloud computing reference architecture, in *Services (SERVICES), 2011 IEEE World Congress on*. 2011.
55. Continua Health Alliance. 2006. Available from: http://www.continuaalliance.org/ (accessed December 27, 2012).
56. Carroll, R. et al. Continua: An interoperable personal healthcare ecosystem. *Pervasive Computing, IEEE*, 2007. **6**(4): pp. 90–94.
57. HearthCycle Deliverable D19.7. Personalized health certification procedure. 2011.
58. Clements, P.C. *Active Reviews for Intermediate Designs*. 2000, Technical Note CMU/SEI-2000-TN-009. Carnegie Mellon University. Pittsburgh, PA.

Section II

Communications in AAL

7

Enabling AAL Wireless Data Transmission in Home Automation Networks

Nils Langhammer and Rüdiger Kays

CONTENTS

ABSTRACT   This chapter gives an overview on the physical characteristics of wireless data transmission in the field of ambient assisted living (AAL). The evaluations focus on wireless home networks that can be used for transmission of sensor and control data for AAL applications. In this field, several technologies compete with each other, and a trend to a *de facto* standard is not noticeable.

All wireless technologies differ in their characteristics and have specific advantages and disadvantages regarding the physical data transmission in the wireless indoor channel. Therefore, an objective of this chapter is to describe and compare different solutions for the physical and medium access layer of wireless data transmission. It also examines how transmission parameters influence the performance of an AAL wireless network.

The mission of this chapter is to provide background for understanding the lower layers of wireless home automation networks and influence of important parameters. Thereby the reader is enabled to decide which wireless technology or system is most suitable for a certain AAL application.

KEY WORDS: *wireless home network, WHAN, evaluation, coverage range, energy consumption, IEEE 802.15.4, Bluetooth Low Energy, Konnex-RF.*

Introduction

Wireless home automation networks (WHANs) have been an actual research topic during the last few years. Nonetheless, they are not widespread in practice so far, but this will most likely change in the near future because of the introduction of ambient assisted living (AAL) services. Currently, multiple WHAN technologies and standards exist. This variety makes it difficult to decide which solution is best suited for a certain AAL application. Therefore, this chapter presents a methodology that can be used to evaluate the performance of WHANs in realistic scenarios. This serves to compare different wireless technologies, which are often regarded as a good basis for AAL.

This chapter is organized as follows: the section "Basic Aspects of Wireless Data Transmission" describes the building blocks and parameters of a wireless data transmission chain. Starting from an examination of the general link budget calculation, additional evaluation parameters are derived and mathematically described. Examples of the derived evaluation parameters are the expected coverage range as well as the required transmission energy and the relationship between these parameters. The section concludes with a description of mathematical representations covering all important parameters that are involved in wireless data transmission.

The section "Building Blocks and Parameters" describes the impact on the performance of wireless data transmission caused by the elements and parameters of the data transmission chain. Therefore, the elements and parameters of the transmission chain are varied, and the resulting coverage range and the energy demand are investigated. First, the impact caused by the physical parameters of wireless transmission is evaluated, and the influence of the modulation and coding are discussed. Next, different concepts for multiplexing and spectrum usage are classified and explained in detail. Besides that, principal pros and cons of these concepts are investigated, and the performance in wireless indoor channels is compared.

Afterwards, the section "System Examples for AAL-WHANs" gives an overview on current and evolving WHAN systems and technologies relevant to AAL. The characteristics of selected technologies are investigated in detail and compared by applying the methods described in the first sections with respect to the requirements of AAL applications.

The "Conclusion" summarizes this chapter's main points.

Basic Aspects of Wireless Data Transmission

This section presents the basic aspects of wireless data transmission and the interrelationship between all involved physical parameters and building blocks. At first, the generic data transmission chain is presented, and the function and characteristics of individual building blocks are briefly summarized. In the next step, the general link budget is calculated, and the physical parameters are described in detail. Finally, useful evaluation metrics are derived from the link budget calculation. These evaluation metrics can be used to compare the performance of wireless home networks for AAL applications.

Generic Data Transmission Chain

The generic data transmission chain comprising a transmitter and a receiver of a wireless communication link is visualized in Figure 7.1. The image contains the main building blocks that have an impact on the performance of a wireless link. This generic transmission chain will be used as a reference model that will be applied to the description of the system examples in the last section of this chapter.

Starting from the data source located at the transmitter, data are protected by using a channel code, which adds redundancy to the data bits in order to perform forward error

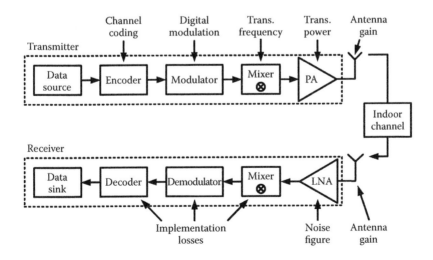

FIGURE 7.1
Generic data transmission chain.

correction (FEC) or error detection. Then the encoded bits are forwarded to the digital modulator that maps them according to the applied digital modulation scheme and performs pulse forming. The output is analog, and analog components are used for the following processing steps. The next building block comprises one or more mixers depending on the applied modulation, which finally outputs the resulting radio frequency (RF) signal at the desired transmission frequency. Moreover, this analog signal is amplified by a power amplifier (PA) according to the selected transmission power, and it is fed into the transmitter antenna, which can provide an additional gain for the radio link.

The radiated signal is transmitted over the wireless indoor channel, which is mainly characterized by the attenuation originating from the physical environment. This attenuation is constant if the location of the devices and their environment do not change. If the attenuation is constant within the occupied frequency range, this is referred to as flat fading. This quite favorable situation may be disturbed by effects caused by multipath propagation, which occur due to reflection, diffraction, and scattering of radio waves. The effects resulting from multipath propagation are summarized as frequency selective fading. The transmission chain adds noise to the signal. Besides that, in case an interferer is active on the wireless channel, additional interference power is added to the signal.

The receiver antenna captures the signal and forwards it to the low noise amplifier (LNA). The receiver antenna may have an additional gain, while the LNA further degrades the signal-to-noise ratio (SNR). The additional noise can be described by the so-called noise figure. The output of the LNA is down-converted by one or multiple mixers and forwarded to the demodulator, which demaps the received signal according to the used modulation. Finally, the demapped symbols are processed in the decoder that outputs the received data bits and forwards them to the data sink. In practical systems, these remaining parts are also characterized by additional losses, which are called implementation losses.

Link Budget Calculation

The general link budget that describes the SNR at the receiver for a certain wireless link is described in logarithmic representation as

$$\mathrm{SNR}|_{dB} = P_S|_{dBm} + G_S - L_B + G_R - P_T|_{dBm} - F - I. \tag{7.1}$$

Here, parameter P_S is the transmission power at the antenna connector of the transmitter, and parameters G_S and G_R represent the gain of the transmitter and receiver antenna, respectively. Parameter L_B describes the static attenuation of the link caused by the physical characteristics of the building. In addition to that, parameters F and I are the noise figure and the implementation losses of the receiver, respectively. Both values strongly depend on the hardware implementation. For evaluation purposes, they have been set to realistic values of $F = 7$ dB and $I = 10$ dB in all following evaluations to allow for a fair comparison. Accordingly, the antenna gain of the receiver antenna has been set to $G_R = 0$ dBi.

The logarithmic sum of parameters P_S and G_S represents the equivalent isotropically radiated power (EIRP) that is defined as

$$\mathrm{EIRP}|_{dBm} = P_S|_{dBm} + G_S. \tag{7.2}$$

The EIRP describes the amount of power in the direction of the maximum antenna gain that is equivalent to an isotropically radiating transmitter. This radiated transmission power is limited by the regulations of the responsible authorities, which specify rules for each frequency band.

Finally, parameter P_T describes the thermal noise at the receiver input that can be calculated from

$$P_T|_{dBm} = 10 \log_{10}(k \cdot T \cdot B_{eff}). \tag{7.3}$$

Within this equation, parameter B_{eff} denotes the effective bandwidth of the evaluated technology in hertz. Parameter T is the noise temperature that has been set to a fixed value of $T = 290$ K for all further evaluations. Additionally, k represents the Boltzmann constant, which has a given value of $k = 1.38 \times 10^{-23}$ J/K. In case T differs from $T = 290$ K, Equation 7.1 is only an approximation, which will lead to small deviations in practice.

Useful Evaluation Parameters

In general, the transmission energy in joules that has to be applied by the transmitter is defined as

$$E_S = \int_0^{T_S} (P_S + P_{SO}) \cdot dt = \int_0^{T_S} P_S \cdot dt + \int_0^{T_S} P_{SO} \cdot dt. \tag{7.4}$$

Within this equation, parameter T_S is the time span of a transmission procedure and parameter P_S denotes the power at the output of the PA. Also, P_{SO} represents additional offset power, which must be applied in order to run the wireless transceiver. The transceiver comprises both the *transmitter* and the *receiver*. The resulting energy E_S that is needed to perform this transmission procedure is determined by integrating the transmission powers P_S and P_{SO} over the time interval T_S.

If a constant transmission power is assumed and parameter T_S represents the time that is required to transmit a packet, the transmission energy per packet E_{Packet} in joules can be derived as

$$E_{Packet} = \int_0^{T_S} P_S \cdot dt = P_S \cdot T_S = P_S \cdot \frac{pl}{R}. \tag{7.5}$$

Here, the transmission time T_S is calculated from the packet length pl and the data rate R, which is assumed constant during the transmission of a packet. The packet length pl represents the length of the PHY protocol data unit (PPDU).

The second term from Equation 7.4 can be modeled as an additional offset energy E_O that is needed to operate the wireless transceiver. If the overall energy consumption has to be evaluated, this parameter has to be taken into account, as E_O can cause significant additional losses depending on the hardware implementation. In addition, the energy efficiency of the transmission procedure for a certain transceiver can be calculated from

$$\eta_{EnergyT} = \frac{E_{Packet}}{E_S} = \frac{E_{Packet}}{E_{Packet} + E_O} = \frac{P_S}{P_S + P_{SO}}. \tag{7.6}$$

Equations 7.1 and 7.5 can be reorganized, resulting in a description of the required transmission energy per packet in joules for a certain link as

$$E_{\text{Packet}}(L_B) = \frac{k \cdot T \cdot B_{\text{eff}}}{R} \cdot pl \cdot 10^{\left(\frac{\text{SNR}|_{\text{dB}}}{10}\right)} \cdot 10^{\left(\frac{L_B}{10}\right)} \cdot 10^{\left(\frac{-G_S - G_E + F + I}{10}\right)}.$$ (7.7)

Herein, the static attenuation of a link is characterized by parameter L_B, which significantly varies among different transmission frequency bands. Furthermore, parameter SNR has to be set according to the receiver requirements of the applied technology in order to achieve the target packet error rate (PER). Since this parameter depends on the performance of modulation and coding within the evaluated channel model, impacts caused by frequency selective fading are also covered by this parameter.

Within Equation 7.6, the term

$$\eta_B = \frac{R}{B_{\text{eff}}}$$ (7.8)

denotes the bandwidth efficiency. This is a measure that describes how much bandwidth B_{eff} is required to transmit at a certain data rate R. It can be seen that η_B has a strong impact on the transmission energy per packet, since E_{Packet} is linearly dependent on η_B.

Another important aspect regarding E_{Packet} is the maximum transmission energy per packet, since E_{Packet} depends on the transmission power P_S and the resulting EIRP. In general, the combination of transmission power P_S and transmitter antenna gain G_S has to fulfill

$$P_S|_{\text{dBM}} + G_S \leq \text{EIRP(max)}|_{\text{dBM}}$$ (7.9)

because transmission power is limited due to requirements of the regulatory authorities and the guidelines of the individual specifications. Therefore, it is possible to derive the corresponding maximum transmission energy $E_{\text{Packet}}(\text{max})$ per packet from Equation 7.5 as

$$E_{\text{Packet}}(\text{max}) = P_S(\text{max}) \cdot \frac{pl}{R}.$$ (7.10)

In this equation, parameter $P_S(\text{max})$ represents the maximum transmission power in the current regulatory domain, which depends on the transmitter antenna gain and the maximum EIRP according to Equation 7.9.

In terms of the following evaluations, parameter $E_{\text{Packet}}(\text{max})$ is of prime importance, since it indicates whether a link is capable to operate within the regulatory limitations. This relationship between the required transmission energy per packet for a given building attenuation L_B and $E_{\text{Packet}}(\text{max})$ can be summarized as

$$\begin{aligned} E_{\text{Packet}}(L_B) \leq E_{\text{Packet}}(\text{max}) &\quad \text{link can operate within limitations} \\ E_{\text{Packet}}(L_B) > E_{\text{Packet}}(\text{max}) &\quad \text{link cannot operate within limitations} \end{aligned}$$ (7.11)

In addition to this formulation, which focuses on required transmission energy, it is also possible to derive the maximum coverage range for a given EIRP. If the EIRP is set to the maximum applicable value, Equation 7.1 can be reorganized to

$$L_B(\text{max}) = \text{EIRP}(\text{max})|_{\text{dBm}} + G_R - P_T|_{\text{dBm}} - \text{SNR}|_{\text{dB}} - F - I. \tag{7.12}$$

Within this equation, $L_B(\text{max})$ describes the maximum attenuation within the building that can be overcome by a certain wireless technology. Since SNR covers impacts caused by the wireless channel, $L_B(\text{max})$ is also the theoretical lower bound of the coverage range. Consequently, this lower bound is the communication range that can be reliably achieved, if additional effects caused by interference are not taken into account.

Building Blocks and Parameters

This section investigates the impacts on the coverage range and the energy demand caused by the functional blocks and parameters of the data transmission chain. Starting with the analog part of the wireless link, the impact of transmission frequency and transmission power is evaluated. Regarding the transmission power, a model will be presented that describes the energy consumption of the transmitter by taking the efficiency of the PA into account. Afterward, the impacts caused by modulation and channel coding are briefly summarized. Finally, the characteristics and parameters of transmission technologies are described, which are used in state-of-the-art WHANs. Here, a realistic indoor channel model will be applied in order to show the resulting system performance for a certain technology.

Physical Parameters

This section gives an overview on the physical parameters of a wireless link and how they interact with each other. As depicted in Figure 7.1, the data transmission chain comprises several blocks, which depend on different physical parameters. Among the physical parameters, the transmission frequency and the transmission power have a key role regarding the coverage range and the required transmission energy per packet. Therefore, further evaluations in this section investigate the role of these two parameters in detail.

Transmission Frequency

Among all physical parameters, the transmission frequency f is of great importance regarding the resulting indoor coverage range, as the attenuation within the building L_B for a given scenario depends on this parameter. In general, a wireless link is described by the distance between the transmitter and the receiver, which leads to the so-called path loss. The path loss describes the attenuation caused by the distance for a given transmission frequency. Moreover, the number of intersecting walls and floors between the receiver and the transmitter has to be taken into account, as they add significant additional attenuation. This attenuation depends on the building materials and their characteristics regarding the transmission frequency. Additionally, the attenuation of floors and walls is influenced by further parameters, e.g., the angle of intersection. In order to define a pragmatic model, the further parameters are neglected. Hence, it is possible to calculate the building attenuation for a given scenario by evaluating

$$L_B = \eta(f) \cdot 10 \cdot \log_{10}\left(\frac{d}{d_0}\right) + 2 \cdot 10 \cdot \log_{10}\left(\frac{4\pi \cdot f \cdot d_0}{c_0}\right)$$

$$+ \sum_{i=0}^{n_{walls}} L_{wall}(i,f)|_{dB} + \sum_{i=0}^{n_{floors}} L_{floor}(j,f)|_{dB}.$$

(7.13)

The first part of this equation represents the path loss that is characterized by the path loss exponent η that is dependent upon the transmission frequency f. Parameter d is the distance between the devices of the wireless link given in meters. d_0 is a reference distance up to which quadratic power decay is assumed. The given models assume that $d_0 = 1$ m, and constant c_0 represents the speed of light. The remaining parts describe the attenuation of the intersecting walls and floors. Here, $L_{wall}(i,f)$ describes the individual attenuation of the ith wall at the current transmission frequency, while $L_{floor}(j,f)$ represents the attenuation of the jth floor. Since the attenuations depend on the building materials, it must be noted that it is very difficult to determine the exact attenuation of an individual wall or floor. The same applies for the path loss exponent. Therefore, it is suitable to determine representative mean values that can be applied to estimate the resulting building attenuation for a given scenario. If mean values are assumed for the attenuation of walls and floors, Equation 7.13 can be simplified to

$$L_B = \eta(f) \cdot 10 \cdot \log_{10}\left(\frac{d}{d_0}\right) + 20 \cdot \log_{10}\left(\frac{4\pi \cdot f \cdot d_0}{c_0}\right)$$

$$+ n_{walls} \cdot L_{wall}(f)|_{dB} + n_{floors} \cdot L_{floor}(f)|_{dB}.$$

(7.14)

Here, $L_{wall}(f)$ is the mean attenuation per wall, and $L_{floor}(f)$ describes the mean attenuation per floor for the applied transmission frequency.

In order to determine representative mean values for these parameters, the results published in Wiesbeck et al. (2006) are taken into account in the following. Here, more than 2000 measurements were carried out in residential indoor environments in order to determine the parameters mentioned above. The results are summarized in Table 7.1.

With the help of these parameters, it is possible to show the impact on the building attenuation caused by the transmission frequency. Figure 7.2 shows the attenuation for a certain indoor scenario. The scenario comprises a wireless link between two devices that are separated by a distance of 7 m. Furthermore, one additional wall and a floor obstruct the direct path between them, which are intersected after 3 and 5 m, respectively. Figure 7.2 shows the resulting building attenuation for transmission frequencies of 868 MHz and 2.45 GHz. It is evident that the lower transmission frequency results in a lower overall building attenuation. If both attenuation values are compared at a distance of 6 m, the usage of the lower frequency would result in about 17.4 dB less attenuation. According to Equation 7.7, this reduction of the building attenuation would reduce the required energy per packet E_{Packet} by a factor of 55, which would be a very significant saving. Furthermore, the lower attenuation at lower frequencies could also be utilized to reduce the transmission power.

TABLE 7.1

Measured Building Attenuation Parameters

Parameter	Frequency	
	Sub GHz	2.4 GHz
$\eta(f)$	2	2.3
$L_{wall}(f)$	3 dB	6 dB
$L_{floor}(f)$	12 dB	15 dB

Source: Wiesbeck, W. et al., Minimizing the Exposure of Future Communication Systems—miniWatt II— Final Project Report. miniWatt II. Available at http://www.ihe.kit.edu/download/miniWatt _II_ web_version.pdf, 2006.

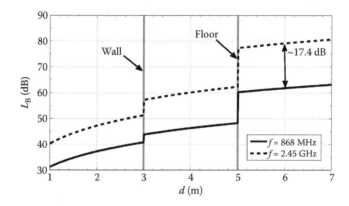

FIGURE 7.2
Resulting building attenuation for different transmission frequencies.

Transmission Power

The transmission power P_S has a significant impact on the resulting coverage range of a wireless link according to Equation 7.12. If this relationship between the building attenuation and P_S is further investigated, it is evident that a doubling of P_S will result in an increased coverage range equivalent to 3 dB. This will lead to 3 dB additional building attenuation that can be overcome by the wireless link.

Nonetheless, in practical systems, an increase in the transmission power will also have a significant impact on the energy consumption of the wireless transceiver. This results from the real power consumption of the transmitter PA, whose efficiency has to be considered. According to Wang and Sodini (2004), it is possible to model the overall power consumption P_{TX} of a wireless transceiver during transmission as

$$P_{TX} = P_{TXO} + P_S \cdot \frac{1}{\eta_{PA}}. \tag{7.15}$$

Within this equation, parameter P_S is the transmission power at the antenna connector, η_{PA} is the efficiency of the PA, and P_{TXO} is an additional offset power representing the remaining parts of the transmitter signal processing chain, whose power consumptions are assumed constant. It is evident that low PA power efficiency will lead to a higher over-all power consumption of the wireless transceiver.

In order to show the relationship between P_S, L_B, and P_{TX}, an example will be shown that uses the energy characteristics of a widespread wireless transceiver named CC1101. The electrical characteristics have been extracted from the datasheet (Texas Instruments 2009). The CC1101 is suitable for the 868 MHz frequency band, and it supports several modulation techniques and data rates. The parameters according to Equation 7.15 have been selected assuming a supply voltage of 3 V and an ambient temperature of 290 K. Furthermore, a frequency shift keying (FSK) modulation at a data rate of 32.768 kb/s has been selected. For these assumptions, the datasheet gives modest values of $\eta_{PA} = 27.68\%$ and $P_{TXO} = 48.58$ mW. The value of η_{PA} indicates that a PA with linear amplitude response is used (Wang and Sodini 2004), which is needed as the CC1101 supports different data rates and several types of modulation.

In order to carry out the calculation of the coverage range, exemplary values according to Konnex-RF, which will be introduced later, have been selected. Therefore, B_{eff} has a value of 200 kHz, and SNR must have a value of 33.75 dB. The calculation of this SNR value will be described in detail within the section covering the system examples. Additionally, a transmitter antenna gain of $G_S = 2.81$ dBi has been assumed, and parameters F, I, and G_R have been set according to their default values that have been introduced during the general link budget calculation.

The resulting building attenuation L_B that can be overcome and the corresponding energy consumption P_{TX} of the wireless transceiver are visualized in Figure 7.3 for a varying transmission power P_S. It can be noted that an increase in transmission power from 5 to 10 mW results in an increase in the maximum coverage range of 3 dB. Besides that, an increase of 5 mW will raise the overall transmission power P_{TXO} by approximately 18 mW according to the PA efficiency of 27.68%. Hence, it must be considered that this higher transmission power results in a shorter battery lifetime equal to 70% of the original value.

In terms of AAL applications, both aspects have to be taken into account if a wireless transceiver has to be designed for a certain application. Since overall power consumption

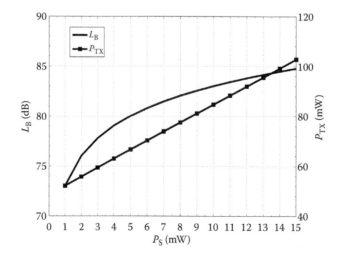

FIGURE 7.3
Relationship between coverage range and overall power consumption.

will increase faster than transmission power due to PA efficiency, electrical characteristics of the selected chipset always have to be considered.

Modulation and Coding

The blocks titled encoder and modulator are generally located within the digital domain of the generic signal processing chain of the transmitter. Here, data are first processed in the channel encoder, which adds redundancy to the information data bits in order to be able to detect and correct errors at the receiver. This procedure is referred to as channel coding. Multiple techniques exist, and further concepts are topics of recent research. Due to the immense number of different channel codes, it is not possible to completely address all aspects within this section. The interested reader should refer to Moon (2005). Nonetheless, the main characteristics and parameters of channel codes are briefly introduced, and their impact on the resulting coverage range and the required energy per packet will be presented. Furthermore, the impacts caused by the applied digital modulation technology are visualized.

In general, a channel code is characterized by its code rate R that is defined as

$$R = \frac{k}{n}. \tag{7.16}$$

Here, k represents the number of information data symbols at the input of the channel encoder. Parameter n describes the number of corresponding coded symbols at the output of the encoder that are forwarded to the digital modulator. The second main parameter, which characterizes a channel code, is its coding gain G_C. The coding gain is a measure that describes how the robustness of a wireless system is increased due to the insertion of the code.

This relationship between modulation and channel coding is visualized in Figure 7.4, which shows the resulting bit error rate (BER) of different digital modulation techniques. This has been carried out for a set of SNR values that have been measured at the input of

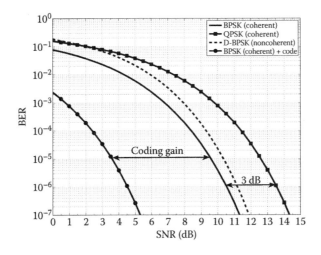

FIGURE 7.4
Impact of modulation and coding on BER and SNR.

the receiver. Furthermore, coherent receivers have been assumed for binary phase shift keying (BPSK) and quadrature phase shift keying (QPSK) modulation. For comparison, a noncoherent receiver has been assumed for a differentially encoded BPSK (D-BPSK) modulation. An additive white Gaussian noise (AWGN) channel has been selected. The applied noncoherent receiver will be investigated in detail in the section presenting the system examples.

Here, the combination of BPSK with an exemplary, quite simple channel code is depicted. The code has a coding gain of about 6 dB. For this example, two orthogonal four-bit-long spreading sequences have been used to encode a single bit of data. It can be clearly seen that the wireless system applying BPSK modulation is able to transmit at a lower SNR due to the insertion of this code. Nonetheless, since more data bits have to be transmitted and if modulation and data rate are kept constant, bandwidth is increased by a factor $(1/R)$ corresponding to the added redundancy. This will result in an increase in the thermal noise according to Equation 7.3, and in the next step, the coverage range L_B will be reduced. This relationship is of great importance, and it will be reinvestigated in the section describing the direct sequence spread spectrum (DSSS) technology. Furthermore, it must be taken into account that the introduction of channel coding can significantly increase the implementation complexity. Hence, the introduction of high-performance channel codes with high implementation complexity is not suitable if a certain AAL application targets simple low-power sensor devices.

Besides these aspects, different digital modulation techniques have varying SNR requirements. In this example, BPSK is able to operate at 3 dB lower SNR than QPSK modulation. This 3 dB difference would lead to additional 3 dB of coverable building attenuation according to Equation 7.12. It is also evident that this additional gain is comparably low among the high attenuations observed in buildings, which have been investigated in the last section. Additionally, if the D-BPSK modulation is further investigated, it can be seen that it needs a higher SNR than the BPSK. Nonetheless, the hardware implementation complexity of a noncoherent D-BPSK receiver is very low. This aspect will be shown in detail in the section describing the system examples.

There is another point regarding the applied digital modulation that has to be considered. Since some modulation technologies have a constant envelope, e.g., minimum shift keying (MSK), it is possible to use a nonlinear PA at the transmitter. This nonlinear PA can have an efficiency η_{PA} of about 70% according to Wang and Sodini (2006), which would result in a significantly lower overall energy consumption. However, since almost all available chipsets support multiple transmission modes with different modulation schemes and data rates, all of these chipsets comprise a linear PA, whose impacts have been described in an earlier section.

Multiplex and Use of Spectrum

In addition to the building attenuation, the impacts of which have been discussed in the prior section, the wireless indoor channel is characterized by additional interference effects caused by multipath propagation. Since radio waves are reflected and scattered on walls or other indoor components, often more than one radio wave will reach the transmitter. These detour paths may interfere at the receiver constructively or destructively. This results in frequency selective fading, which must be regarded in addition to the average attenuation. Several models can be used to describe the frequency selectivity of the wireless indoor channel. Among all available models, the IEEE 802.11 Task Group n (TGn) channel model (Erceg et al. 2004) is widespread and often used for the evaluation of local

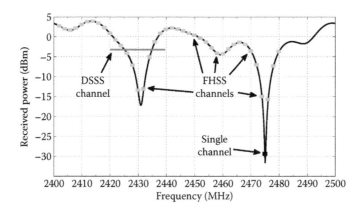

FIGURE 7.5
Different data transmission channels in IEEE 802.11 TGn B channel model.

area wireless systems. This model comprises a set of six scenarios, describing different multipath environments. Regarding the modeling of the wireless indoor channel, the residential environment (scenario B) in non-line-of-sight conditions (NLOS) is applicable, which is characterized by a root mean square delay spread of 15 ns. The delay spread may be interpreted as the difference between the arrival time of the shortest and the longest paths in a multipath environment. Furthermore, the TGn model generates a set of realizations, each representing a static snapshot of a 100 MHz bandwidth indoor channel.

The main challenge regarding wireless indoor communication arises if the impact caused by frequency selectivity is further investigated. Figure 7.5 shows the resulting received power at the receiver for an exemplary realization of the TGn channel model. This realization has been normalized to a mean value of 0 dBm, and it represents a single snapshot of the 2.4 GHz ISM-Band spectrum. It can be seen that the received power strongly depends on the frequency. For instance, at a frequency of 2475 MHz, the received power is more than 30 dB less than at a frequency of 2450 MHz. The main challenge is to cope with this frequency selectivity fading behavior of the wireless indoor channel.

Here, several transmission technologies are applied in current systems for the usage of the spectrum. In order to provide an understanding of them, the following describe the main aspects of certain approaches by summarizing the main advantages and disadvantages.

Single Carrier Data Transmission

The first option is the usage of single carrier (SC) data transmission, which is applied in most available low data rate control networks due to its simple implementation. Furthermore, low data rate control networks tend to have an effective channel bandwidth, which is significantly smaller than the so-called coherence bandwidth of the wireless channel. The coherence bandwidth is a measure for the frequency selectivity of the wireless channel, and it describes the range of frequencies over which the channel can be considered flat. It is reciprocal to the delay spread. The frequency selectivity of the wireless channel will have a significant impact on the performance of a small bandwidth SC PHY. This relationship is depicted in Figure 7.5 that shows a single 2 MHz channel with a center frequency of 2475 MHz. Due to the deep fade, which occurs directly at the center frequency of the channel, the received power is reduced by additional 30 dB. If the curves from Figure 7.4 are taken into account, the selection of this operating channel would lead to a 30 dB increase in the required SNR according to the fading depth.

Furthermore, as all links within the network have an individual propagation characteristic due to the different device locations, it is not predictable where the fades will occur. Besides that, the wireless indoor channel changes, e.g., due to the movement of objects and persons. This temporal behavior can be summarized by the coherence time, which describes how long a channel may be regarded as nearly static in time. During a longer time, the wireless indoor channel can change completely. Due to these facts, low bandwidth wireless systems that operate at a fixed wireless channel must be designed with an additional reserve. This reserve enables them to operate under the presence of deep fades. Additionally, the performance of such systems must be compared under worst case conditions in order to determine the reliable coverage range.

Spread Spectrum Data Transmission (DSSS/FHSS)

Spread spectrum data transmission systems use a larger amount of spectrum compared to small bandwidth SC PHYs. In principle, current spread spectrum systems can be separated into systems applying DSSS and frequency hopping spread spectrum (FHSS). Both technologies try to overcome the fading behavior of the wireless indoor channel by using a larger frequency band. While DSSS uses a single transmission frequency, systems applying FHSS change the transmission channel multiple times during a certain time interval following a predefined hopping sequence. Figure 7.5 depicts a single DSSS channel and 40 single FHSS channels in a realization of the TGn channel model. In this example, the DSSS channel has a bandwidth of 20 MHz, while the FHSS channels have a small bandwidth of 1 MHz.

DSSS

Systems applying DSSS spread their data in the time domain with the help of a spreading sequence. Here, the incoming bit sequence is extended by the spreading factor S_F, which characterizes the DSSS spreading code. For instance, IEEE 802.15.4 at 868 MHz applies a spreading code consisting of 15 elements, which are called chips. In this case, every data bit is multiplied with a 15 chip spreading sequence leading to a sequence that can be characterized by a chip rate. Since the chip rate is S_F times the data rate, the resulting bandwidth will also be S_F times higher than the original bandwidth. At the receiver, the samples are processed in a correlator, which multiplies the received chips with the original chip sequence and finally integrates over the result. This correlation process reverses the spreading, and the original bit sequence with additional noise is available at the output of the correlator. The main advantage of DSSS systems is their immunity against narrow bandwidth interferers, as their interference power can be significantly reduced due to the correlation process according to Proakis and Salehi (2008). Regarding the wireless indoor channel, systems applying DSSS will only have a significant gain compared to SC systems if their effective bandwidth is higher than the coherence bandwidth of the wireless channel. An example has been shown in Figure 7.5, where the DSSS channel bandwidth is higher than the width of the fade at 2430 MHz.

It must be noted that the application of DSSS will not result in an increase in the coverage range in AWGN or general flat fading channels. This relationship can be proven if the spreading sequence is described as a repetition code that has a code rate of

$$R = \frac{1}{S_F}. \tag{7.17}$$

At first, the spreading code will lead to a code gain that equals the spreading factor. In addition to that, the bandwidth will also be enlarged by this factor. Hence, the resulting coverage range according to Equation 7.12 will not change at all for channels that are characterized by a flat spectrum. In addition, it must be considered that an increase in the bandwidth requires faster signal processing. This will result in an increased system clock, and it will thus lead to an increase in the overall power consumption. Furthermore, the multiplications for spreading and de-spreading also lead to higher power consumption. The advantage of using DSSS is the robustness against narrowband fades or interferers.

FHSS

The FHSS spread spectrum technology applies a different approach. In general, the actual data transmission is equal to the SC mode, but the transmission frequency is changed multiple times during a time interval. Therefore, the spectrum is divided into small bandwidth data channels. Figure 7.5 shows an exemplary set of FHSS channels in the TGn channel model. Regarding the channel hopping process, most available systems transmit one or more packets on a channel, and they apply a random hopping sequence that must be synchronous at the transmitter and receiver side. It is also evident that FHSS systems require less energy than DSSS systems, as they do not increase the system bandwidth, and they require less signal processing. For AWGN channels, the system performance of FHSS systems is equal to SC systems. On frequency selective channels, there is always a certain amount of good and bad data channels present in the overall spectrum.

In order to show the performance of FHSS in the TGn channel model, Figure 7.6 depicts simulation results of the Bluetooth LE PHY. Bluetooth LE uses 40 FHSS channels, and it will be introduced and described in detail in the section System Examples for AAL-WHANs. Figure 7.6 shows the resulting PER for a packet length of 32 B and a given SNR at the receiver. The SNR describes the mean SNR of all channel realizations. Here, 100 realizations of the TGn channel model have been used to perform the simulations, and the hopping mechanism changed the center frequency after a packet had been transmitted. In addition, coherent and synchronized receivers have been assumed with perfect channel knowledge.

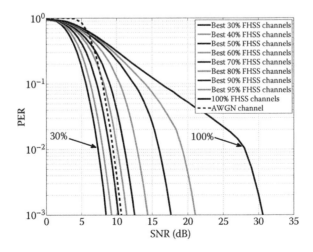

FIGURE 7.6
Performance of FHSS in TGn B channel model.

Figure 7.6 shows the impacts of bad channels on the performance of a FHSS system without automatic repeat request (ARQ). If all FHSS channels are used, the required SNR at the receiver is 18.7 dB higher compared to the AWGN channel at a PER of 10^{-2}. Additionally, the system performance is increased by 9 dB if the worst two channels are removed and only the best 95% of all data channels of each realization are applied. Besides that, the performance can outperform the results of an AWGN channel, if the hopping is only performed on the best 50% of all channels. In this case, the FHSS system would only hop to the parts of the spectrum that benefit from constructive interference.

It can be seen that FHSS has great potential to deal with the challenges of the wireless indoor channel. In addition to that, the implementation complexity of FHSS systems is comparable to SC PHYs, as only the frequency has to be switched according to the hopping scheme. Nonetheless, current systems, like Bluetooth LE, do not fully utilize the high potential of FHSS, as they use all FHSS channels resulting in the 100% curve.

Orthogonal Frequency Division Multiplex

In addition to DSSS and FHSS, there is another transmission technology named orthogonal frequency division multiplex (OFDM), which is applied in almost every new broadband transmission system. Examples for widespread systems applying OFDM are the IEEE 802.11 family of standards and the next generation of mobile communications systems (LTE: long-term evolution). It must be noted that it is very complex to describe all aspects of OFDM. Therefore, only the main points and the impacts regarding the application of OFDM in WHANs are briefly summarized. Further detailed information on the theory and application of OFDM can be found in Prasad (2004).

The main difference between OFDM and the prior described techniques is the fact that more than one data carrier is used for transmission. Hence, the frequency band is divided into subbands each carrying one of the subcarriers, which will be used in the OFDM system. The subbands have a low bandwidth compared to the coherence bandwidth of the wireless channel. Therefore, the channel impact on a SC can be modeled as an additional flat attenuation with a certain phase. This is similar to the effects that occur in low data rate SC transmission systems, which have been presented previously. Here, the information data are allocated on the subcarriers according to a defined allocation scheme. Since the subcarriers are orthogonal to each other, it is possible to separate them at the receiver. Thus, the subcarriers can use different types of linear modulation, and an OFDM system is characterized by a high bandwidth efficiency that is desirable for spectrum-efficient high-speed data transmission.

In order to perform the orthogonal transformation of the subcarriers, the individual constellation points of all subcarriers are processed in an inverse Fourier transformation (IFFT) circuit at the transmitter. The constellation point is the combination of amplitude and phase representing a bit pattern that is transported by a specific subcarrier. Then the so-called cyclic prefix is added to the OFDM symbol, which serves as a guard interval between two successive OFDM symbols. OFDM systems are designed in a way that all multipath components arrive at the receiver during the guard interval. Hence, the guard interval has to be as long as the greatest expected detour path. At the receiver, the information received during the guard interval, which suffers from interference due to multipath propagation, is removed and the channel frequency response is used to equalize the individual attenuation of each subcarrier. Afterward, the remaining OFDM symbol is processed in a FFT block that outputs the received constellation points. All available

OFDM systems use channel coding schemes that are optimized to cope with the frequency selectivity of the channel.

OFDM has some advantages regarding robustness against multipath fading and bandwidth efficiency, but the implementation of an OFDM system is very complex, and it has high power consumption. For instance, OFDM systems require precise synchronization. In addition to that, IFFT and FFT operations require lots of computational power.

Therefore, OFDM data transmission is not feasible for simple and low power devices that are required in WHAN systems. This holds even more because most parts of the energy consuming circuitry of the OFDM receiver must be kept active in order to detect incoming transmissions. Other approaches, e.g., FHSS technology, also have the potential to cope with the challenges of the wireless indoor channel at a much lower implementation complexity making them suitable for simple sensor or control devices.

System Examples for AAL-WHANs

This section gives an overview on current and evolving wireless systems related to the AAL field of application. First, the main characteristics of selected wireless technologies for sensor and control networks are summarized. Then, the resulting transmitter and receiver hardware architectures are presented in order to show the resulting hardware implementation complexity. Finally, the system examples are compared by applying the evaluation methodology that has been derived in the previous sections. Hence, the indoor coverage range and the required transmission energy per packet will be calculated as important parameters for a comparison.

Overview on Available Communication System Concepts and Standards Relevant to AAL

Multiple wireless systems and standards exist that can be used for the interconnection of devices in an AAL wireless home network. They are driven by different industrial consortia that want to place their individual standard as the key technology for low data rate control and automation networks. In addition, wireless local area networks (WLANs) based on the IEEE 802.11 family of standards (IEEE Std. 802.11 2007) are very popular nowadays. In the private environment, they are generally used for transmission of multimedia data and for provision of Internet access. It can be stated that IEEE 802.11 currently is the *de facto* standard for the wireless interconnection of devices in this scenario. In terms of a fully integrated home network, it seems reasonable to reuse the IEEE 802.11 system architecture for the transmission of sensor and control information in an AAL-WHAN. However, since IEEE 802.11 systems apply a convolutional code in combination with OFDM, the resulting hardware complexity and energy consumption will be too high for AAL devices, which require long battery life and simple low-cost hardware architectures. Besides that, IEEE 802.11 systems have not been designed for this additional field of application.

Therefore, it is suitable to use simple and low-power wireless technologies for the interconnection of AAL devices. However, the main challenge arises at this point, as there is no *de facto* communication standard for low data-rate control and sensor networks. Even a trend toward the worldwide usage of a single standard is not noticeable at the moment.

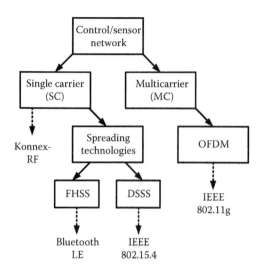

FIGURE 7.7
Classification of WHAN system examples.

Figure 7.7 visualizes a selection of wireless standards, which are currently applied by different projects and researchers for the AAL field of application. They are classified according to their modulation concept and usage of wireless spectrum. Here, Konnex-RF has been selected as an example for a SC PHY. There are a number of proprietary systems that operate in a similar way. Furthermore, Bluetooth LE and IEEE 802.15.4 have been selected as examples for spread spectrum technologies. Many available publications related to AAL-WHANs refer to one of these technologies. The following comprises an overview on the main PHY and MAC characteristics of the selected technologies with respect to AAL requirements.

IEEE 802.15.4 (DSSS)

IEEE 802.15.4 has been specified as a wireless personal area network (WPAN). The first version of the specification was published in 2003. In 2006, this version was revised with an updated specification (IEEE Std. 802.15.4 2006) comprising several enhancements. IEEE 802.15.4 has been designed to transmit messages at a low data rate, while maintaining low energy demand. Its main application target is the transmission of control information for wireless sensor networks. The specification comprises the description of the PHY and MAC layer, which can be used as a basis for higher layer communication protocols and technologies. An example for such a technology is ZigBee®, which adds its own network and application layer on top of IEEE 802.15.4. The current version of the ZigBee specification (ZigBee Alliance 2007) comprises a network layer that is capable of performing meshing between several devices within a ZigBee network. In addition to that, the ZigBee stack has several application-specific profiles (http://zigbee.org). Among these profiles, the so-called *home automation profile* focuses on home automation applications, and the *health care profile* targets the monitoring and management of health care services.

Another protocol that uses the TCP/IP protocol suite on top of IEEE 802.15.4 is named 6LoWPAN (Kushalnagar et al. 2007). Here, IPv6 frames are transmitted via IEEE 802.15.4 with the help of header compression. Hence, simplified web service protocols can run on top of 6LoWPAN. An example of such a protocol that targets on home and building auto-mation is COAP (Shelby et al. 2011).

In general, IEEE 802.15.4 defines several PHY alternatives for usage in different fre-quency bands according to the regulatory requirements. For further evaluations, the two mandatory and applicable PHYs for the European regulatory domain will be considered, the characteristics of which are briefly summarized in the following.

IEEE 802.15.4-2.4 GHz PHY

The first PHY version operates in the 2.4 GHz ISM frequency band and may be used world-wide. This frequency band comprises 16 non-overlapping transmission channels, which are separated by 5 MHz. The majority of the available IEEE 802.15.4 transceivers support this PHY mode. The data are transmitted at a rate of 250 kb/s using DSSS technology.

Figure 7.8 visualizes the corresponding signal processing chain of the transmitter. First, the incoming data bits are mapped into symbols. Here, the incoming data bytes from the PPDU stream are separated into the upper and lower nibble. These groups of nibbles, each corresponding to four bits, are then mapped to the appropriate symbol. In the next step, the spreading mechanism is applied. Therefore, the symbols are mapped to 16 predefined sequences. The sequences have a length of 32 chips and are quasi-orthogonal. Finally, the chips are transmitted using an O-QPSK modulation with half sine pulse shaping at a data rate of 2 Mchips/s. The maximum EIRP is limited to 20 mW in Europe to meet regulatory requirements. Figure 7.9 shows the inphase $i(t)$ and quadrature components $q(t)$ of the com-plex baseband signal. The resulting phase transition diagram at the transmitter output is given in Figure 7.10.

Since half sine pulse shaping is applied, this modulation is sometimes also referred to as minimum shift keying (MSK). As this is a specific form of frequency shift keying, it is possible to use simple noncoherent receiver concepts instead of a coherent receiver.

The receivers differ in implementation complexity, since the coherent receiver depicted in Figure 7.11 demands an equalizer and additional blocks for synchronization and phase

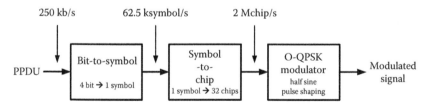

FIGURE 7.8
IEEE 802.15.4-2.4 GHz transmitter signal processing chain.

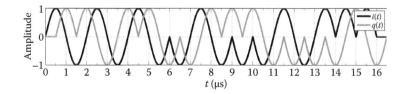

FIGURE 7.9
Complex baseband signal components.

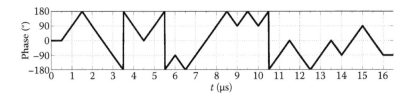

FIGURE 7.10
Resulting phase transition diagram.

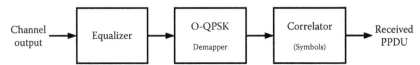

FIGURE 7.11
IEEE 802.15.4-2.4 GHz coherent receiver signal processing chain.

recovery. The main task of the equalizer is to reverse the impact caused by the wireless channel. Since the bandwidth of IEEE 802.15.4 is lower than the coherence bandwidth of the wireless indoor channel, the equalizer only has to turn the received constellation points according to the phase offset at the receiver. After the equalizer, the received samples are forwarded to the demapper, which outputs the received bit stream. This bit stream is then correlated with all possible symbols. Finally, the correlator decides which symbol has most likely been sent and outputs the corresponding PPDU. The PPDU comprises all parts of the frame including protocol overhead, and it will be further explained in the following subsection.

Similarly, different concepts exist for the implementation of a noncoherent IEEE 802.15.4 receiver. Since MSK is used, it is possible to decode the signal with the help of analog frequency demodulation circuits. Furthermore, the receiver depicted in Figure 7.12 can be implemented according to the concepts presented in Notor et al. (2003), where a differential demodulation has been applied in order to decode the received MSK signal.

This differential demodulator outputs the phase difference between two successive symbols, which are then correlated with the prior encoded phase changes of all symbols. This is possible because the phase difference between two successive symbols is always 90°, as depicted in Figure 7.13.

Since the received data bits are restored from the information comprised in the phase changes, no equalizer is needed for this noncoherent receiver. This concept results in a low implementation complexity.

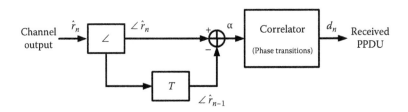

FIGURE 7.12
IEEE 802.15.4-2.4 GHz noncoherent receiver signal processing chain.

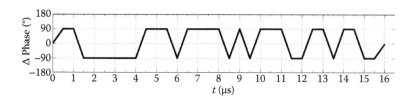

FIGURE 7.13
Phase changes between two successive IEEE 802.15.4 symbols.

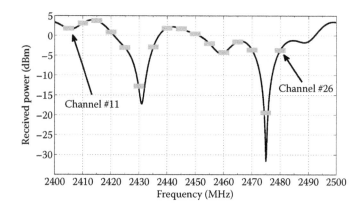

FIGURE 7.14
IEEE 802.15.4 channels in exemplary realization of TGn B channel model.

Due to the small bandwidth of 2 MHz, which is less than the coherence bandwidth of the wireless channel, the characteristics of the wireless indoor channel have a strong impact on the performance of this PHY. The relationship between the data transmission channels and the characteristics of the indoor channel is visualized in Figure 7.14 that shows the IEEE 802.15.4 channels in an exemplary realization of the TGn B channel model. It is evident that the channels differ significantly regarding the received power at the receiver. As every link within the network is characterized by an individual channel profile due to the individual multipath propagation, it is not predictable whether the selected operating channel is a good choice for all wireless links. Besides that, it must be noted that the characteristics of the wireless indoor channel have an additional temporal behavior resulting in a randomly varying channel profile.

IEEE 802.15.4-868 MHz PHY

The second PHY is based on a single transmission frequency in the 868 MHz frequency band. The data rate is set to 20 kb/s and DSSS is applied to spread the data bits. This PHY can only be used in Europe, and the maximum EIRP is limited to 25 mW. The signal processing chain of the transmitter is visualized in Figure 7.15. In the first step, the incoming data bits are differentially encoded and forwarded to the spreading block. Here, the differentially encoded bits are mapped to two predefined bit sequences. The two sequences are orthogonal to each other, and they have a length of 15 chips resulting in a chip rate of 300 kchip/s. The chips are then transmitted with a BPSK modulation, where the baseband chips are represented by a raised cosine pulse shape (roll-off factor of 1).

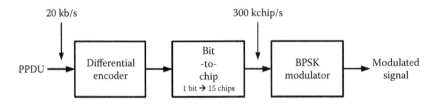

FIGURE 7.15
IEEE 802.15.4-868 MHz transmitter signal processing chain.

Since a differential encoding is applied, two different receiver concepts are applicable for this PHY. The resulting building blocks are visualized in Figures 7.16 and 7.17. Again, both receiver concepts differ in the implementation complexity. The coherent receiver, depicted in Figure 7.16, needs an equalizer in order to correct the phase offset at the receiver. After the correction of the phase offset, the samples are correlated with one of the two spreading sequences. This is possible, since both spreading sequences are orthogonal. The correlated samples are then forwarded to the demapper, which outputs the received differentially encoded bit stream. Finally, the bit stream is differentially decoded in order to get the corresponding PPDU.

The noncoherent receiver, depicted in Figure 7.17, has a significant lower implementation complexity than the coherent receiver. First, there is no need for an equalizer for phase correction, since the noncoherent receiver decodes the data from the phase transitions of the received symbols. In general, the received samples are correlated with the spreading sequence and forwarded to a differential decoder. A noncoherent receiver can be implemented according to the differential decoding concepts presented in Proakis and Salehi (2008). Here, the samples are first processed through a FIR filter that performs the correlation. Therefore, the filter taps correspond to the spreading sequence. The output of the filter is forwarded to a differential decoder that restores the transmitted data by evaluating

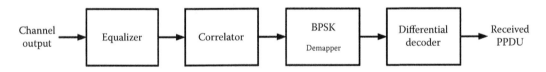

FIGURE 7.16
IEEE 802.15.4-868 MHz coherent receiver signal processing chain.

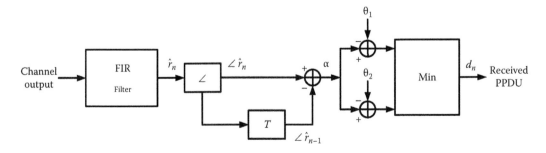

FIGURE 7.17
IEEE 802.15.4-868 MHz noncoherent receiver signal processing chain.

the phase shift between two consecutive symbols. Since BPSK uses an antipodal signaling, the phase difference between two consecutive symbols can be either 0 or π.

IEEE 802.15.4 Frame Formats and MAC Characteristics

Both IEEE 802.15.4 versions use the same frame formats, and they share identical MAC characteristics. The MAC only differs in the temporal behavior due to the different data rates of both versions. Two different schemes exist for channel access. The first option uses a superframe structure that is determined by the coordinator, which is a special device controlling the IEEE 802.15.4 network. Within a superframe, guaranteed throughput slots (GTSs) can be assigned to dedicated devices for guaranteed channel access at a predictable time. The time period comprising the GTS is referred to as the contention free period (CFP). Here, a maximum of 7 GTS is supported. In addition to the CFP, the superframe structure offers another time period, called contention access period (CAP), when the devices can compete for channel access. This competing access is the default channel access mode of IEEE 802.15.4. It is also mandatory, if no superframe structure is employed. Here, a carrier sense multiple access with collision avoidance procedure (CSMA/CA) is used. Hence, devices have to ensure that the channel is free before they access the channel, for instance, by performing energy detection in the assigned frequency band.

IEEE 802.15.4 supports ARQs that can optionally be turned off. The acknowledgements (ACKs) have a fixed MAC frame length of 40 b, and up to three retries are applied as the default value.

The frame formats of the PHY and MAC layer are visualized in Figures 7.18 and 7.19, respectively. The part required for synchronization contains the preamble and the start of frame with a total length of 40 b. The remaining part of the PHY header contains the frame length and an additional reserved bit. Furthermore, the MAC header contains several fields of different length as depicted in Figure 7.19. Since IEEE 802.15.4 supports several types of addressing, the specified addressing fields can vary in length from 0 up to 64 b. Additionally, as data security is optional in IEEE 802.15.4, the field containing information about the applied security also varies from 0 to 122 b. Regarding data security, IEEE 802.15.4 supports an optional AES-128 encryption in order to secure the transmitted data. Finally, the MAC frame comprises a CRC-16 code for detection of transmission errors.

Preamble	SFD Start of frame	Frame length	Reserved	PSDU Payload
32 b	8 b	7 b	1 b	Variable
Sync		PHY		

FIGURE 7.18
IEEE 802.15.4 PHY PDU frame format.

Frame control	Sequence number	Destination PAN	Destination address	Source PAN	Source address	Security (optional)	Frame payload	FCS CRC 16
16 b	8 b	0/16 b	0/16/64 b	0/16 b	0/16/64 b	0/5/6/10/14 B	Variable	16 b
MAC								MAC

FIGURE 7.19
IEEE 802.15.4 MAC PDU frame format.

Konnex-RF (SC)

Due to the historical development of the home automation sector in Europe, several manufacturers prefer to use the wired standard Konnex (KNX) for home and building automation appliances. Konnex is standardized by the KNX Association. Devices must successfully pass a review program in order to get certification. The certification process is only available to members of the KNX Association. The KNX standard emerged from the European Installation Bus (EIB) that has been standardized in the early 1990s. It contains a wireless PHY called KNX-RF (ISO/IEC 14543-3-7:2007). Besides this PHY, several other PHYs exist, for example, PHYs applying wired (via twisted pair cable) or powerline communication. The usage of KNX-RF is restricted to Europe because it operates in the 868 MHz SRD frequency band.

In the following, the main PHY and MAC characteristics of KNX-RF will be summarized.

Konnex-RF PHY

KNX-RF uses a single transmission channel with a center frequency of 868.3 MHz, and the PHY applies a FSK modulation for data transmission. The maximum radiated power is set to 25 mW according to the regulatory requirements.

The transmitter signal processing chain is depicted in Figure 7.20. First the incoming data are processed in a CRC-16 (cyclic redundancy check) encoding block. Here, the data are separated into single 16 b blocks. Each of them is secured with its own CRC-16 sequence. The data rate at the output of the CRC encoder is 16.384 kb/s. Data are transmitted using self-clocking Manchester coding and a FSK applying a frequency deviation of ±50 kHz. Here, the lower frequency represents a logical "0," while a frequency deviation of +50 kHz represents a logical "1." Due to the Manchester coding, the transmitted data rate is 32.768 kb/s.

Since FSK is used, simple noncoherent receivers are applied in practical receiver circuits, the characteristics of which will be briefly summarized. Figure 7.21 visualizes the receiver signal processing chain of an optimum noncoherent FSK receiver, which is also named the correlation detector. A detailed description of the theory regarding optimum noncoherent FSK demodulation can be found in Proakis and Salehi (2008). In general, this optimum noncoherent FSK receiver performs a down conversion of the received signal to the complex baseband. Then it performs a complex correlation with two signals $S_0(t)$ and $S_1(t)$ shifted to frequencies corresponding to the frequency deviation. Finally, the decider selects the frequency that has been sent most likely and outputs the appropriate bit. This process is repeated until the entire PPDU is received.

It must be noted that this optimum noncoherent FSK receiver performs best if the FSK signals are orthogonal. Nonetheless, this will not be reached in practical implementations, as FSK modulators usually comprise simple voltage-controlled oscillators (VCOs). A VCO

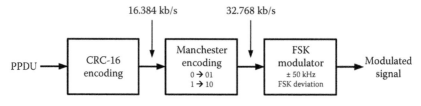

FIGURE 7.20
Konnex-RF transmitter signal processing chain.

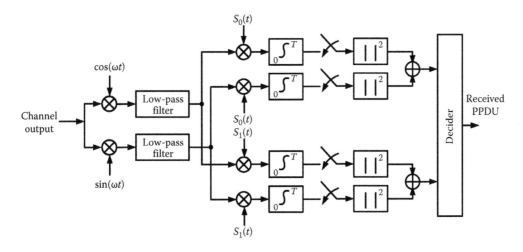

FIGURE 7.21
Optimum noncoherent FSK receiver signal processing chain.

directly converts the bit stream to the corresponding FSK frequency, and VCOs always show a certain inaccuracy. Hence, orthogonality is not reached in practice. For this reason, practical FSK demodulation circuits will always perform worse than the optimum non-coherent FSK receiver. Another aspect regarding the optimum noncoherent FSK receiver is the fact that the performance strongly degrades in the presence of frequency offset between a transmitter and a receiver. Due to the inaccuracies at the transmitter, there will always be a frequency offset. Therefore, practical implementations have to apply automatic frequency offset compensation.

Alternatively, it is also possible to use an analog frequency modulation (FM) demodulator to decode a FSK signal. The corresponding signal processing chain of such a receiver is visualized in Figure 7.22. In principle, the channel output is processed in a prefilter and then demodulated with an analog FM demodulator, which is tuned to the carrier frequency. The output of the FM demodulator is low-pass-filtered and forwarded to the decider that outputs the corresponding PPDU.

It is evident that the description of a noncoherent FSK demodulation would be very complex if all mentioned facts and parameters are taken into account. Therefore, a pragmatic approach has been selected for further evaluation. Here, optimum noncoherent FSK receivers are assumed, and an adequate implementation margin is used to account for all additional effects.

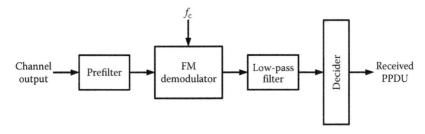

FIGURE 7.22
Noncoherent FSK demodulation with analog FM demodulation circuits.

Konnex-RF Frame Formats and MAC Characteristics

The KNX-RF frame structure is derived from the FT3 data link layer according to IEC 60870-5, and it comprises several data blocks with an appended CRC-16 checksum. In order to perform synchronization, the frame structure comprises additional fields that are sent before and after the data blocks as depicted in Figure 7.23. The preamble has a minimum length of 15 b sequences "01" followed by a *Manchester violation* and the so-called sync word. The Manchester violation is used to detect the end of the preamble, as it is a sequence that cannot occur in a Manchester encoded bit stream. The post-amble finalizes the frame and has a length of 2–8 b.

Among the data blocks, the first block has a length of 10 B, while all the following blocks have a maximum length of 16 B. The first block comprises the length field that is related to the PHY and additional fields from the MAC, as depicted in Figure 7.24. The first field related to the MAC is called the C-Field. The usage of the C-Field is also derived from IEC 60870-5, and it always has a value of 0x44h for KNX-RF, which means "SEND/NO REPLY." It is set to this value, since no ARQ mechanism has been specified for KNX-RF. The second block, which is shown in Figure 7.25, contains the remaining fields of the MAC comprising source and destination address, as well as additional information about KNX-RF application layer services. Furthermore, the second block is able to transmit up to 8 B of application data. Subsequent blocks can each transmit a maximum of 16 B of additional application specific data. The frame format of all the following blocks is shown in Figure 7.26.

Regarding the medium access, KNX-RF applies a simple carrier sense mechanism in combination with random access. In general, the procedure is very simple and can be described as follows. First, a KNX-RF device that wants to start transmitting has to sense the medium for the interframe time and an additional random delay. The interframe time has a length of 15 to 20 ms, and the random time has to be within the time interval of 0 to

Preamble	Manchester violation	Sync word	Block 1-n	Postamble
n × "01" bit	6 b	12 b	Variable	2–8 b
Sync				Sync

FIGURE 7.23
KNX-RF frame format of the synchronization.

L-field Length	C-field Control	ESC	CTRL	Serial number	FCS CRC 16
8 b	8 b	8 b	8 b	48 b	16 b
PHY	MAC				

FIGURE 7.24
KNX-RF frame format of the first block.

CI-Field Control information	Source address	Destination address	L/NPCI	TPCI	APCI	Frame payload	FCS CRC 16
8 b	16 b	16 b	8 b	8 b	8 b	Max. 8 B	16 b
MAC							MAC

FIGURE 7.25
KNX-RF frame format of the second block.

Frame payload	FCS CRC 16
Max. 16 B	16 b
	MAC

FIGURE 7.26
KNX-RF frame format of subsequent blocks.

10 ms. If the device does not detect a preamble or an ongoing transmission during both time intervals, it can start with the transmission of the frame. This procedure is called listen before talk (LBT). In case of an occupied medium, it will start the LBT mechanism again after the medium is detected free. Besides that, KNX-RF assumes a maximum *blind time* of 1 ms for all devices. The blind time represents the time interval that is needed by a transceiver for the transition between receive and transmit state.

Bluetooth LE (FHSS)

The Bluetooth specification is standardized by the Bluetooth Special Interest Group (SIG). Bluetooth targets wireless personal area communications. The standardization of Bluetooth began in 1994, when mobile phone manufacturers started to develop a standard for the interconnection of mobile phones and accessories such as headsets. The work on the initial version of the Bluetooth specification was finished in 1999. This version 1.0 offered a maximum gross data rate of 1 Mb/s while applying FHSS. Furthermore, the standard specifies different application-specific profiles for mobile phone applications. Consecutive versions of the specification introduced higher data rates up to 24 Mb/s based on alternative PHY technologies and extensions to the core protocol.

Bluetooth technology is widespread in the market, as almost every available mobile phone comprises a Bluetooth transceiver. Besides the usage within mobile phones, Bluetooth has also been introduced for the interconnection between sensors and actuators for wireless automation networks. Nonetheless, Bluetooth itself has not been designed for this specific field of application, where sensor devices must have low overall power consumption. Additionally, the basic network topology, which uses a centralized star topology, is not suitable for distributed sensor networks. That has been the reason why the current version 4.0 of the Bluetooth specification (Bluetooth Special Interest Group 2009) introduced Bluetooth low energy (LE) at the end of 2009. Bluetooth LE contains extensions to support the transmission of control information and measurements in sensor and control networks. Besides that, as the name *low energy* indicates, it targets battery-powered applications that require very low power operation. At the moment, Bluetooth LE is not widespread in practice, as the basic PHY technology is not compatible with the prior versions of the specification. Besides that, only few transceiver ICs are available. However, this will most likely change in the near future, since some chip manufacturers have already announced transceiver ICs that support all modes of the Bluetooth specification including the LE physical layer.

Bluetooth LE PHY

Bluetooth LE applies FHSS in the 2.4 GHz ISM-Band and offers a data rate of 1 Mb/s. The frequency band is divided into 40 physical channels that are separated by 2 MHz. The channels numbered 0, 12, and 39 are referred to as advertising channels.

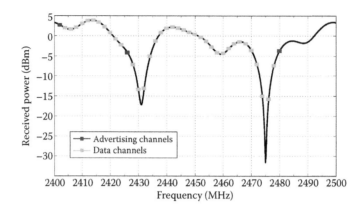

FIGURE 7.27
Bluetooth LE channel in exemplary realization of TGn B channel model.

The remaining channels are called data channels. Figure 7.27 visualizes the Bluetooth LE channels in an exemplary realization of the TGn B channel model. The usage of advertising and data channels is different, as the three advertising channels are applied in order to connect two devices, and data transmission is carried out on the 37 data channels after a successful connection. For Bluetooth LE, these two processes are referred to as events, indicating that they occur in certain time intervals. Figure 7.28 shows a sequence of Bluetooth LE events during an ongoing transmission between two devices. First, the device that wants to initialize a data transmission consecutively scans the advertising channels and listens for so-called advertising packets. The scanning device is called initiator, and the time interval that the initiator spends waiting for advertising packets is named the advertising event.

As soon as the initiator receives a matching advertising packet from the desired peer device, the advertising event is finished and the data transmission is performed in one or multiple connection events. Here, the initiator becomes the master device and the advertising device becomes the slave device. The channel hopping is performed at the beginning of every connection event according to a channel hopping sequence, which is defined by the master. Besides that, the master and the slave alternate in sending data packets within a connection event. The master defines the beginning and the end of each connection event.

Figure 7.29 shows the Bluetooth LE transmitter signal processing chain. The incoming data bits are converted in a low-pass filter to rectangular pulses with a data rate of 1 Mb/s. Then the pulses are forwarded to a Gaussian low-pass filter and afterward transmitted with an FM modulator that is tuned to the current hopping frequency.

This modulation is called Gaussian frequency shift keying (GFSK). The applied modulation index has to be in the interval of 0.45 to 0.55 according to the specification. In principle, GFSK is equal to FSK with an additional filter before the modulator. Due to this additional

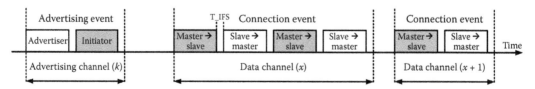

FIGURE 7.28
Bluetooth LE advertising and connection events.

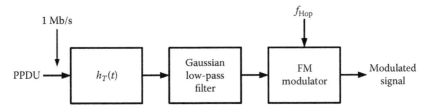

FIGURE 7.29
Bluetooth LE transmitter signal processing chain.

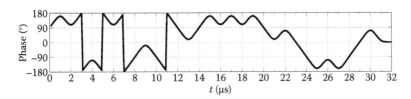

FIGURE 7.30
Bluetooth LE phase transition diagram.

Gaussian low-pass filter, the phase of the transmitted signal has a smooth characteristic. This fact is depicted in Figure 7.30 for clarification.

It must be noted that Bluetooth LE does not apply dedicated forward error control or additional spreading for error correction. Furthermore, the maximum transmission power measured at the antenna connector is limited to 10 mW by the Bluetooth LE specification.

Another interesting aspect arises if the modulation index is further investigated. The minimum value of the modulation index that offers signal orthogonality is 0.5 (Proakis and Salehi 2008). This special case is called MSK for FSK and Gaussian MSK (GMSK) for GFSK. Hence, for this case, the nonlinear FSK modulation can be described as a linear O-QPSK modulation, and coherent demodulation concepts can be applied. Nonetheless, it must be noted that the additional Gaussian filter will result in losses compared to a coherently demodulated O-QPSK.

Bluetooth LE Frame Formats and MAC Characteristics

Bluetooth LE uses the same frame format for advertising packets, which are used during advertising events, and data channel packets that are applied in connection events. The general frame structure for both packet types is depicted in Figure 7.31. After the preamble that is needed for synchronization, the PHY frame contains the access address and the physical layer service data unit (PSDU). The access address is a random 32 b value that is used to identify a Bluetooth LE connection. It is chosen by the initiator during the advertising and connection setup procedure. Furthermore, it is set to a fixed value for advertising packets.

Preamble	Access address	PSDU Payload
8 b	32 b	Variable
Sync	PHY	

FIGURE 7.31
Bluetooth LE PHY PDU frame format.

LLID	NESN Next seq. num.	SN Seq. number	MD More data	RFU Reserved	Length	RFU Reserved	Frame payload	FCS CRC
2 b	1 b	1 b	1 b	3 b	5 b	3 b	Variable	24 b
MAC								MAC

FIGURE 7.32
Bluetooth LE MAC PDU frame format.

Figure 7.32 visualizes the format of the data channel PDU, which contains a 16 b header and a 24 b CRC. The length of the frame payload is variable and limited to a maximum length of 27 B. Among the fields of the header, the fields named next expected sequence number (NESN) and sequence number (SN) are utilized for an ARQ mechanism. Since the master and the slave alternate in sending data packets during a connection event, a packet sent by the master will always be followed by a packet from the slave. Thus, at the beginning of a connection event, the master will set the SN bit to zero and transmit the packet. After the packet is received, the slave will send its own data packet after the interframe space time interval (T_IFS) of 150 μs. Within this data packet, the slave also sets the SN field to zero and increments the NESN field in case the previous packet from the master has been received correctly. After successful reception, the master checks whether the NESN is different from the last sent SN field. If the values are different, then the last sent data packet is acknowledged. Furthermore, identical values indicate a negative acknowledgement (NAK), leading to a retransmission of the last data packet. The master applies the same procedure for the slave. Since this ARQ mechanism requires an alternating transmission of data packets, devices can also send data packets without payload. Furthermore, the connection event is closed if two consecutive erroneous packets are received by either the master or the slave. In addition to that, the connection event will be closed if both devices set the MD field to zero, or one of the devices stops transmitting data packets. Then, the next connection event will be carried out on the next data channel according to the negotiated connection time interval. Since this time interval can be very long, devices can turn to sleep mode in order to save battery power between connection events.

Comparison of Concepts and Performance with Respect to AAL Requirements

All presented system examples are characterized by individual PHY and MAC parameters, whose interrelationship has been presented in the previous sections. Table 7.2 summarizes the PHY and MAC parameters of the evaluated wireless smart home technologies. It can be noticed that all technologies have a small bandwidth compared to the coherence bandwidth of the wireless indoor channel. Thus, the frequency selectivity can significantly influence the system performance if a deep fade occurs at the current transmission frequency. Furthermore, Bluetooth LE and IEEE 802.15.4 both support an ARQ mechanism, while KNX-RF does not have an ARQ mechanism specified in the lower two layers. Regarding the channel access, IEEE 802.15.4 applies a CSMA/CA procedure, whereas KNX-RF uses a simpler LBT function. In contrast to that, Bluetooth LE does not sense the carrier before transmitting. It applies FHSS that results in a generally reduced collision probability. Parameters L_{SYNC}, L_{PHY}, and L_{MAC} describe the protocol overhead caused by synchronization, PHY, and MAC layer, respectively. Among them, parameter $L_{MAC}(ACK)$ represents the MAC frame length of an acknowledgement packet, which is only applicable for systems applying an ARQ mechanism.

TABLE 7.2

Summary of PHY and MAC Parameters

Parameter	Bluetooth LE	IEEE 802.15.4		Konnex-RF
Frequency	2.4 GHz	2.4 GHz	868 MHz	868 MHz
Max. EIRP	10 mW	20 mW	25 mW	25 mW
Data rate	1 Mb/s	250 kb/s	20 kb/s	16.384 kb/s
Use of spectrum	FHSS	DSSS $4 \rightarrow 32$	DSSS $1 \rightarrow 15$	Single carrier Manchester
Channels	40	16	1	1
Modulation	GFSK	O-QPSK	D-BPSK	FSK
B_{eff}	1 MHz	2 MHz	600 kHz	200 kHz
ARQ	Required (1 retry)	Optional (def. 3 retries)		n/a
Channel access	n/a	CSMA/CA		LBT
L_{SYNC}	8 b	40 b		26 b
L_{PHY}	32 b	8 b		8 b
L_{MAC}	40 b	200 b		168 b
L_{MAC}(ACK)	40 b (min)	40 b		n/a

In order to compare the system performance with respect to AAL requirements, two different evaluation parameters have been selected in the following. The first one is the indoor coverage range, which is characterized by the resulting packet loss rate (PLR) for a given building attenuation. The second parameter is the energy demand that is needed in order to transmit a data packet via a specific wireless link. This comparison has been carried out for a real-world AAL scenario that represents a small flat with several AAL sensor devices.

Indoor Coverage Range

The maximum indoor coverage range of all technologies has been calculated by applying Equation 7.12, which has been parameterized for all technologies. The evaluations are based on standard compliant PHY implementations of the technologies in MATLAB®. Regarding the 868 MHz technologies, synchronized optimum noncoherent receivers have been assumed. In addition, all 2.4 GHz technologies used coherent receivers to allow for a fair comparison between them. Hence, a modulation index of 0.5 was assumed for Bluetooth LE. Besides that, the coherent receivers were synchronized and implemented with perfect channel knowledge. Furthermore, an exemplary payload length of 32 B has been assumed, and the simulated packet length contains the PHY and MAC overhead. Additionally, the synchronization part of the frame has been assumed error free. This is feasible, since this part is comparatively short among the remaining parts of the frame.

Since all evaluated systems have a small bandwidth compared to the coherence bandwidth of the wireless channel, deep fades at the transmission frequency strongly degrade the overall system performance. Furthermore, this has a significant impact on the coverage range, which has been shown in the prior sections. Therefore, the evaluations were carried out under worst case conditions in order to compare the reliable communication range, which can be achieved even under the influence of deep fades occurring at the transmission frequency. The IEEE 802.11 Task Group n channel model has been used to model the frequency selectivity by choosing the residential environment in non-line-of-sight conditions. In the next step, 100 realizations were generated and the individual channels of all technologies were filtered out. For all SC and DSSS PHYs, the worst channel of every realization has been selected for the simulation. For Bluetooth LE, which uses FHSS, all wireless data channels were consecutively used, and the implemented hopping mechanism transmitted one data packet per connection event. Regarding the maximum EIRP, a fixed antenna gain of 0 dBi has been selected for all technologies. Besides that, the transmission power of all 868 MHz technologies has been set to 25 mW resulting in an EIRP of 25 mW. This is the maximum value for the European regulatory domain. Since the transmission power of Bluetooth LE is limited to 10 mW measured at the antenna connector, the resulting EIRP of Bluetooth LE equals 10 mW. Finally, the IEEE 802.15.4 PHY operating at 2.4 GHz is limited to 20 mW EIRP by the regulatory requirements.

Figure 7.33 shows a comparison of the resulting PLR for a given attenuation L_B within the building. Two ARQ options have been evaluated for IEEE 802.15.4 and Bluetooth LE. The plots named *no ACK* have been generated by applying a unidirectional transmission, while the plots named *ACK* used the default ARQ mechanisms. Here, Bluetooth LE performed one retransmission, while IEEE 802.15.4 applied three retries.

It is evident that IEEE 802.15.4-868 MHz has the highest coverage range of all technologies at a PLR of 10^{-2}, corresponding to a reliability of 99%. If the 868 MHz systems are compared, it can be noticed that IEEE 802.15.4 (no ACK) can handle a 7 dB higher building attenuation than KNX-RF. Besides that, coverage range is increased by additional 2.2 dB if the ARQ procedure is activated. Among the 2.4 GHz systems, IEEE 802.15.4 (ACK) can operate at a higher building attenuation than Bluetooth LE (ACK). If the ARQ mechanism of Bluetooth LE is enabled, the resulting coverage range is almost equal to IEEE 802.15.4 (no ACK). In addition to that, all Bluetooth LE curves have a less steep characteristic compared to others. This behavior is caused by the frequency hopping technology, which is applied by Bluetooth LE. Since FHSS uses all available channels of the frequency band, there is a certain possibility that a good channel is selected for the next hop.

Another important fact that has to be taken into account is that this figure shows the maximum attenuation within a building that can be overcome by a certain wireless technology. Hence, it must be considered that the building attenuation L_B varies for different transmission frequencies according to Equation 7.14 and Figure 7.2. This relationship will

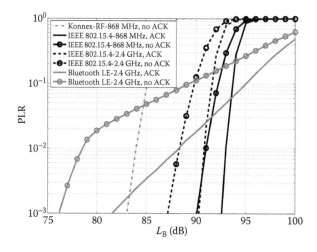

FIGURE 7.33
Comparison of PLR for a given building attenuation L_B.

be examined in the section Evaluation of AAL scenario *Flat*, where the performance of the technologies is compared in a realistic AAL indoor scenario.

Evaluation of AAL Scenario Flat

A realistic AAL indoor scenario named *Flat* has been applied to investigate the individual system performance of the presented technologies. It must be noted that this is only an exemplary analysis using the methods and evaluation parameters described in earlier sections. In principle, this investigation can be carried out for any scenario and for different technologies. The evaluation scenario depicted in Figure 7.34 comprises a small flat with a living space of 62 m², whose dimensions have been taken from an existing German urban multidwelling unit that was constructed in 1962. The flat comprises five rooms including a bathroom and a kitchen. Furthermore, every room contains an AAL sensor device, like a presence or motion detector. The sensors transmit their information to a central unit, named *AAL Home Controller*. This central unit has additional external interfaces, and it can act as a gateway. For instance, it can forward the sensor values to medical services.

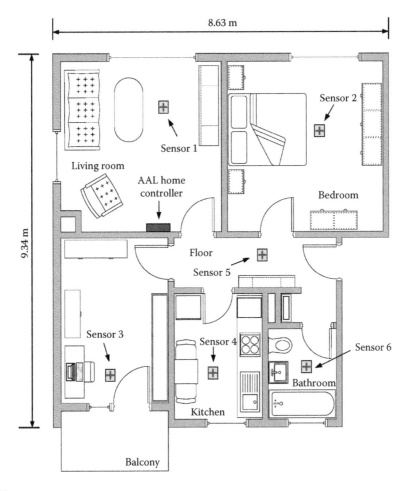

FIGURE 7.34
Scenario *Flat*.

TABLE 7.3

Scenario *Flat* Building Attenuation Parameters

Link	d	n_{walls}	L_B (868 MHz)	L_B (2.4 GHz)
S1	3.02 m	0	40.8 dB	51.3 dB
S2	4.79 m	1	47.8 dB	61.9 dB
S3	3.89 m	1	46.0 dB	59.8 dB
S4	3.89 m	3	52.0 dB	71.8 dB
S5	2.75 m	1	43.0 dB	56.3 dB
S6	5.15 m	4	57.4 dB	80.6 dB

The links between the sensors and the controller are named S1 to S6, where S1 describes the link between sensor no. 1 and the controller. All links are characterized by an individual distance between both devices and the number of walls that intersect the direct path between them. Table 7.3 summarizes all link parameters and the resulting attenuations for transmission frequencies of 868 MHz and 2.4 GHz, which have been determined from Equation 7.14.

In the next step, the required transmission energy per packet E_{Packet} according to Equation 7.7 has been used to compare the systems. Here, a fixed packet length pl of 32 B has been assumed, and the gain of the transmitter antenna has been set to 0 dBi for all technologies. According to the evaluation of the coverage range, the IEEE 802.11 Task Group n channel model has been applied under worst case conditions. Besides that, the ARQ mechanisms have not been used in order to determine the energy that is required to directly transmit a packet of size pl. The simulations have been carried out until a mean SNR value for a PER of 10^{-2} has been reached.

The simulation results for this scenario are depicted in Figure 7.35. This diagram visualizes the required transmission energy per packet (E_{Packet}) in microjoules per link for a certain technology. It can be clearly seen that the technologies that operate in the lower 868 MHz frequency band have significant lower energy demand for links with high attenuation. This results in lower required transmission power, which will lead to longer battery

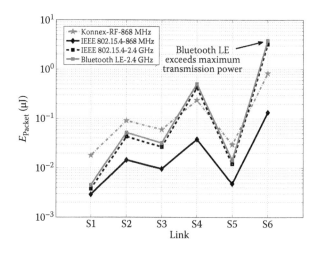

FIGURE 7.35

Evaluation results of scenario *Flat*.

lifetime for battery-powered devices. This is caused by higher attenuation at 2.4 GHz. Besides that, all systems are capable of running the links S1 to S5. In addition to that, the maximum transmission power of Bluetooth LE is exceeded for the S6 link, as the requirements from Equation 7.11 cannot be fulfilled by Bluetooth LE.

In general, the results from this scenario show that the 2.4 GHz technologies can enable a wireless link through three intersecting walls depending on the PHY technology. Beyond this distance, a multihop device, like a wireless repeater, could be added in order to cover the whole flat. Among all systems, IEEE 802.15.4 operating at 868 MHz has the lowest E_{Packet} for all links.

It is evident that the operating frequency of a technology has the greatest impact on the performance, and there are only small differences between the devices that operate in the same frequency band.

Conclusion

This chapter gave an overview on the physical characteristics of wireless data transmission in the field of AAL home automation networks. First, the generic data transmission chain has been introduced, and useful evaluation parameters have been derived from the general link budget calculation. These parameters have been used to compare the performance of different wireless systems and transmission methodologies. Hence, the physical parameters of the generic data transmission chain have been investigated in detail. Among the parameters, the transmission frequency has a large influence on the resulting coverage range, as it is directly related to the attenuation within the building. At this point, a model has been introduced in order to estimate the building attenuation of a wireless link. In addition to that, it has been shown that the overall energy consumption of a wireless transceiver depends on the efficiency of the transmitter PA. Furthermore, the impact caused by modulation and coding has been summarized shortly. Then, different technologies regarding the use of spectrum have been presented. It has been shown that the main challenge is to cope with the frequency selectivity of the wireless indoor channel. Thus, the main characteristics and the performance of SC, FHSS, DSSS, and OFDM data transmission have been evaluated.

The subsequent section presented system examples for WHANs. After a short overview and the classification of the technologies, the main PHY and MAC characteristics of IEEE 802.15.4, Bluetooth LE, and Konnex-RF were presented. Besides the presentation of the transmitter and receiver signal processing chains, the technologies were compared with respect to AAL requirements applying the methods that have been introduced in the earlier sections. Besides a comparison of the maximum building attenuation, the required transmission energy per packet has been evaluated for a realistic indoor scenario taken from an existing living unit.

The evaluations have been carried out in the IEEE 802.11 Task Group n channel model under worst case conditions, and they showed that the transmission frequency and the use of spectrum have the highest impact on the performance of a certain technology. Since the attenuation within the building depends on the transmission frequency, all systems operating in the 868 MHz frequency band required less energy for links between three or more rooms in order to transmit a packet. Besides that, all 2.4 GHz systems have comparable system performance in this scenario. The only difference regarding Bluetooth LE has been caused by the limited transmission power of 10 mW that is required by the specification. Nonetheless, the sole usage of the 868 MHz technologies would cause additional problems. Since they operate on a single channel within a small frequency band, this frequency band would soon be overloaded after a mass rollout of AAL home automation networks, as there is only a single transmission channel available.

Therefore, it seems suitable to use the 2.4 GHz frequency band or to allocate additional sub-gigahertz frequency bands that could be reserved for AAL or general home automation systems. Such a frequency band should have enough bandwidth to be able to overcome the challenges caused by the frequency selectivity of the wireless indoor channel. Especially, FHSS shows potential if bad channels are omitted by an enhanced hopping algorithm, as the effective bandwidth is lower than for DSSS resulting in less thermal noise.

The use of a SC transmission technique is not a promising approach, since deep fades at the transmission frequency would significantly degrade the system performance. Furthermore, OFDM is capable of high bandwidth efficiency, but the implementation complexity and energy consumption caused by the FFT blocks are too high for simple sensor or control devices.

References

Bluetooth Special Interest Group. 2009. Bluetooth Specification Version 4.0.
Erceg, V. et al. 2004. TGn Channel Models. IEEE 802.11 Document 03/940r4.
IEEE Std. 802.11-2007. 2007. IEEE Standard for Information Technology-Telecommunications and Information Exchange between Systems-Local and Metropolitan Area Networks-Specific Requirements—Part 11: Wireless LAN Medium Access Control (MAC) and Physical Layer (PHY) Specifications.
IEEE Std. 802.15.4-2006. 2006. IEEE Standard for Information Technology-Telecommunications and Information Exchange Between Systems-Local and Metropolitan Area Networks-Specific Requirements—Part 15.4: Wireless Medium Access Control (MAC) and Physical Layer (PHY) Specifications for Low-Rate Wireless Personal Area Networks (WPANs).
ISO/IEC 14543-3-7:2007. 2007. Information Technology—Home Electronic System (HES) Architecture—Part 3–7: Media and Media Dependent Layers—Radio Frequency for Network Based Control of HES Class 1.
Kushalnagar, N., Montenegro, G. and Schumacher C. 2007. IPv6 over Low-Power Wireless Personal Area Networks (6LoWPANs): Overview, Assumptions, Problem Statement and Goals (IETF RFC 4919). The Internet Society.
Moon, T. K. 2005. *Error Correction Coding*. John Wiley & Sons, New York.
Notor, J., Caviglia, A. and Levy, G. 2003. CMOS RFIC Architectures for IEEE 802.15.4 Networks. Cadence Design Systems.
Prasad, R. 2004. *OFDM for Wireless Communications Systems*. Artech House, Norwood, MA.
Proakis, J. G. and Salehi, M. 2008. *Digital Communications*, Fifth Edition. McGraw Hill, Boston.
Shelby, Z. et al. 2011. Constrained Application Protocol COAP. IETF Internet-Draft <draft-ietf-core-coap-04.txt>.
Texas Instruments. 2009. CC1101 Datasheet. Document SWRS061F.
Wang, A. Y. and Sodini, C. 2004. A Simple Energy Model for Wireless Microsensor Transceivers. In *Proceedings of IEEE GLOBECOM 2004*.

Wang, A. Y. and Sodini, C. G. 2006. On the Energy Efficiency of Wireless Transceivers. In *Proceedings of IEEE International Conference on Communications 2006*.

Wiesbeck, W. et al. 2006. Minimizing the Exposure of Future Communication Systems—miniWatt II—Final Project Report. miniWatt II. Available at http://www.ihe.kit.edu/download/miniWatt _II_web_version.pdf (accessed August 2, 2011).

ZigBee Alliance. 2007. ZigBee Specification. Document 053474r17. Available at http://zigbee.org (accessed August 11, 2011).

8

Mobility and Multihoming Data Transmission Protocols

João C. Silva, Artur Arsenio, and Nuno M. Garcia

CONTENTS

ABSTRACT This chapter addresses research on context-aware systems for mobility and multihoming, in the scope of ambient assisted living. Always-on connectivity requires efficient management of radio access technologies to enable a terminal device to communicate more effectively. We focus on context-aware systems for mobility management, which are applied to aid the handover process. Based on learning data, users' connectivity can be optimized by deploying entities that have functional intelligence and consistent background knowledge at their disposal. This will enable clever decisions to be made, therefore improving performance. These entities will be able to learn from experience, with special regard to user preferences, user behavior, and recurring situations in the network infrastructure and surrounding scenario.

KEY WORDS: *ambient assisted living, context awareness–based mobility, mobility, multihoming, ontology, wireless health monitoring.*

Introduction

The advent of supplying mobile devices with more processing capabilities, employing reduced power consumption techniques, and incorporating the latest data transmission technologies sets the groundwork for a vast variety of applications.

Information technology has been playing an increasingly stronger role in the health care area of expertise throughout the years, enabling it to be more accurate, faster to respond, and less susceptible to human errors. Wireless access technology has vast applications in health care, including for living assistance at patients' homes, performing such tasks as monitoring patients' health, and taking appropriate actions. The concept of health monitoring conveyed in this work can be extended to sports performance monitoring or job-risk health monitoring (for example, mine workers, track runners), where stationary monitoring is not possible.

Pursuing these mobility requirements, sensor implants became possible, after wireless sensor networks (WSNs) became more advanced and pervasive. To accomplish such goals, communications must exploit the plethora of wireless technologies available to carry patients' information to a health care provider. Sensors must switch between technologies due to constraints on technologies' physical deployment and connectivity challenges.

Radio access technologies integrated with a device, such as the Universal Mobile Telecommunications System (UMTS), IEEE 802.11 [1], IEEE 802.16, global system for mobile communications (GSM), general packet radio service (GPRS), and evolution-data optimized (EVDO), provide the means to transmit the acquired data to a remote point of attachment (PoA; also called point of care for health care applications), where it can be processed and stored for further medical diagnosis. All these technologies combined make Wireless Health Monitoring possible, with a patient being able to have an implant that gathers one or several biosignals and sends them through an internet protocol (IP)-enabled radio interface to a storage entity for further processing.

To support this resiliency and still extend battery life, the monitoring terminal requires efficient management of radio access technologies that enable it to communicate.

Motivation

This chapter will start by reviewing previous literature on mobility and multihoming. But contrary to such approaches, this chapter will then move on to propose an application-level mobility management suite able to seamlessly support the behavior of a patient carrying a body sensor that monitors their biosignals and reports the information to a hospital centralized server. The choice of an application-level mechanism arises from the need to support patient mobility independently of the Internet providers' mechanism for mobility support. As the patient roams between access networks, support must be enforced in order to ensure connection resiliency (due to the crucial aspect of the data to transfer); Internet service provider (ISP), network infrastructure, and access technology independence; and end-to-end operation.

In addition, with such an application-level framework, we can apply more advanced techniques in order to predict users' patterns of connectivity and mobility. This is done by implementing an algorithm that will output the best radio PoA in order to ensure the best transmission performance, taking into account a set of parameters such as available bandwidth, packet loss, received signal strength, power consumption, and cost. We can also make this decision algorithm aware of the sensor's current context by collecting data from the wireless radio interfaces and saving that information in order to make the handover decision based on the state of communications for each location and the past decisions made by the algorithm in an attempt to make the system learn from its experience.

Application to Ambient Assisted Living

The importance of the health care system to the patient's well-being raises many challenges to a health monitoring system. Radio access technology made it possible to improve the effectiveness and nonintrusiveness of such a system by dispensing with the use of wires and allowing it to be always available for reporting the patient's information.

Traditionally, monitoring patient health was done through periodic visits to the doctor in order to undergo on-site tests for blood pressure, pulse, temperature, or sugar level. The alternative is stationary monitoring, upon admission at a health care provider. Currently, patients can take home sensors attached on a belt, for a specific time period (usually 24 h), in order to collect biosignal data for that period. However, the patient still has to move to the health care provider to get the sensor, and afterwards, they have to return to remove the sensor and deliver the data. Nowadays, we are reaching seamless health monitoring by placing a mobile sensor on the patient, executing biosignal collection, and transmitting data through a wireless access technology interface to a storage facility for further medical analysis. The transmission of data must be done on an *always-on* basis, and to use solely one access technology might be very restrictive in terms of the different advantages it can provide with regard to the heterogeneous behavior of the patient. Therefore, it is important to have solutions in which a multiple-network interface sensor is able to adjust itself to patient behavior in order to make monitoring as robust and seamless as possible by changing the network interface when justifiable and being able to learn from the patient's behavior.

Wireless Health Monitoring

Requirements

Ambient assisted living is challenging, imposing severe constraints concerning connectivity, information security, and cost:

1. Monitoring sensors, as well as the monitoring functionality, must be connected permanently.
2. The information that the generated data stream carries is of critical importance and must be given greater priority.
3. At any given moment, the radio resource used for the communication must be the one that bears lowest cost to the user and still guarantees good quality of service (QoS), allowing the former challenges to be addressed.

Adding to the technical challenges of health monitoring, the patient's comfort and the nonintrusiveness of the monitoring system must be taken into account. Health monitoring systems such as the one described in Ref. [2] use GPRS technology to transmit harvested data to a storage server for physician analysis, still relying on the patient (it is user triggered) to enforce the health level measurement. The action of taking a measurement is supervised by a physician using a webcam (that is not wireless), therefore adding another task to be carried out by the patient. This solution is focused very much on the user, developing a friendly user interface for the patient to interact with, in order to perform the measurements. Wireless monitoring, employing radio access technologies for biosignal data transmission, reduces the patient's responsibility in the monitoring action by removing the need to connect wires to the monitoring device. In addition, it provides the patient with the opportunity to perform their daily tasks unaware of their permanent health vigilance. On the other hand, pursuing the stated challenges will allow a monitoring system to capture exceptional episodes or transient abnormalities during real-life physiological states, therefore providing extended information for medical analysis. Indeed, the contextual information can be of high value for further interpretation of biosignal data.

Wireless Technologies for Assisted Living

The wireless technologies that are nowadays widely available are Wi-Fi, Bluetooth (BT), and UMTS. These technologies have certain features and restrictions, which must be taken into account during development of a system that aspires to deliver a fast, intelligent, and robust handover algorithm. This section briefly describes the most important wireless access technologies and their most relevant features for usage in assisted living scenarios.

IEEE 802.11 (Wi-Fi)

Since its entrance into the mainstream of networking technology, Wi-Fi has mostly been used as a replacement and augmentation for wired local area networks. Wi-Fi is well suited for applications requiring high-volume data transfer and distances below 10 m [1].

Wireless local area networks (WLANs) have, through the last decade, been deployed as an extension of other access technologies as a way to expand the reach of Internet broadband access and hence to facilitate the penetration of Voice over IP (VoIP) and other data services. WLANs as complementary networks normally follow an infrastructure mode of operation, where a central controller—the access point (AP)—mixes and controls communication between any two elements.

More recently, there has been a surge of WLANs operating in mesh (ad hoc mode), that is, in a completely decentralized way. This is due to the emergence of soft radio and also of open-distribution operating systems contemplating low-cost APs.

In both situations, the widespread deployment of WLANs is underpinned by the most popular variants of IEEE 802.11 standards, 802.11b/g/n.

IEEE has specified the 802.11 family as the set of standards for WLANs. The IEEE 802.11 specifications define a single medium access control (MAC) layer along with multiple physical layers. Distributed coordination function (DCF) is the fundamental MAC technique that employs a carrier sense multiple access with collision avoidance (CSMA/CA) distributed algorithm and an optional virtual carrier sense using Request to Send (RTS) and Clear to Send (CTS) control frames, originally designed to reduce frame collisions caused by hidden terminals. Any device (other than the sender and intended receiver) receiving the RTS or CTS frames should refrain from sending data by setting its network allocation vector (NAV) for a given time period indicated in the *duration* field of RTS and CTS frames. The other option of extra frames is CTS-to-self frames whose source address and destination address are identical. The 802.11g sender transmits a CTS-to-self frame to inform all the neighboring 802.11g and 802.11b devices to update NAV according to the *duration* field of the CTS-to-self frame. Obviously, extra frames (RTS, CTS, and CTS-to-self) used for ensuring interoperability are viewed as overhead for system performance because they reduce the available medium resource for data delivery.

Universal Mobile Telecommunications System

UMTS is a radio access technology designed for wide coverage of mobile terminals, providing data-oriented high-bandwidth service and operating at a frequency that is different from country to country. This technology is deployed in parallel with GSM technology and therefore limited to locations where UMTS antennas are active. On metropolitan networks, nowadays, UMTS reaches almost full coverage and is now a mature wireless access technology that can provide close to continuous service to mobile terminals. Infrastructure has some important elements, such as the Radio Network Controller (RNC), Node B, and cell, where RNC is responsible for aggregating geographically all Node Bs and Node B is responsible for controlling a group of cells that cover a certain location. Terminals must be handed over between UMTS points of access, and that represents an overhead for the UMTS service.

Bluetooth

The IEEE 802.15.x standard, commonly known as Bluetooth, specifies a short-range radio-frequency technology for low-power wireless communications for portable devices operating at the frequency range of 2.402 to 2.480 GHz. According to the BT specification, BT's range varies between minimum distances of 10 m to 100 m, depending on the BT device class. Yet, there is no range limit for the technology, but it still has a fairly small range compared to UMTS radio access technology. The peak data rate with the Enhanced Data Rate (EDR) feature on BT v2.1 is 3 Mbps. BT's successive releases aim, alongside other features, to reduce power consumption. Wireless personal area networks (WPANs) often employ BT technology, and they are defined on the IEEE 802.15 WPAN standard, which defines a piconet as the most simple association between BT nodes. A piconet can become associated with another piconet using one node present in both networks. BT is characterized as a radio access technology with low bandwidth, close range yet low power consumption, and usually no cost for the *first mile*.

Communication Solutions

Single-Interface Solutions

Nowadays, some deployed systems use one radio access technology, such as GSM [3], to transmit the collected data. Other single-interface solutions have been developed, alongside WSNs, which establish a sensor network on the patient's body and use a single radio access technology as a gateway to report the gathered biosignals. The solution described in Ref. [4] reports an electrocardiogram (ECG) sensor with an integrated BT transceiver monitoring patients in their hospital rooms, enabling them to move freely inside the room, reporting to the doctors' monitors via IEEE 802.11.

The deployment of a WSN for biosignal monitoring, reporting through a PDA device, [5] shows a solution that focuses on the QoS aspect of the data flow. A MAC layer algorithm has been written to provide health care applications with traffic priority over other applications by employing two schemes: preemptive resume priority packet scheduling, in which a health care application packet burst should interrupt all other flows until its transmission is complete, and prioritized channel contention, defining a class for the referred traffic and regular traffic already used on the IEEE 802.11e standard. An exception is that emergency data flow can interrupt any other data flow, and there is no channel contention when emergency data are present.

Dual-Interface Solutions

The existence of a single radio access technology can be a very limiting factor, for instance, in scenarios where radio coverage of the technology is nonexistent, or else it is of limited quality. So the possibility of having a dual radio interface sensor is very empowering for the always-on challenge. However, it raises other questions, related to the efficient handover process between technologies, making the correct handover decision, and making the process transparent to sensor monitoring.

Ref. [6] presents a complete solution for an IEEE 802.16– and IEEE 802.11–enabled biosignal monitoring sensor, although it relies on the service provider to buffer data gathered from the sensor. Such a service has to be bought from the ISP. The solution presents a handover decision algorithm with a strong mathematical basis, focusing on the probability of the patient's transition between a set of locations using a probability matrix and the quantity of connections (ISP service) to be bought to the service provider for each location in the set. In other words, computation is carried on in order to decide how many connections should be brought on top of a previous number. This is decided per location, whenever that number is exceeded by a large number of users on that location. The authors in Ref. [7] propose a monitoring system based on code division multiple access (CDMA) and 802.11 access technologies supporting a 802.15.4 wireless body sensor network (WBSN) that connects a sensor node to ECG collecting devices such as a wrist band or chest band. The data flow generated is aggregated through the 802.15.5 protocol and transmitted through a chosen network interface. Network interface choice is described superficially in this paper by referring to the usage of Java WIPI when developing the solution. Java WIPI is a platform that the Korea Wireless Internet Standardization Forum announced as a standard to enable network applications to be developed regardless of ISPs, mobile carriers, and vendor heterogeneous requirements. This could be a good alternative for a system that aspires to be technology agnostic and easy to implement on any radio access environment.

Mobility and Multihoming

Multihoming

In multihoming, a single computer host makes use of several IP addresses associated with various connected networks. Within this scenario, the multihomed computer host is physically linked to a variety of data connections or ports. These connections or ports may all be associated with the same network or with a variety of different networks. Depending on the exact configuration, multihoming may allow a computer host to function as an IP router.

One possibility for the process of multihoming makes use of what is known as Stream Control Transmission Protocol (SCTP). Essentially, the process involves employing multihoming by making use of a single SCTP end point to support the connectivity to more than one IP address. By establishing connections to multiple addresses, multihoming can help to enhance the overall stability of the connectivity associated with the host [8].

One of the advantages of multihoming is that the computer host is somewhat protected from the occurrence of a network failure. With systems that make use of a single IP address and connection, the failure of the connected network means that the connection shuts down, rendering the end system ineffectual as far as connectivity to the Internet is concerned. With multihoming, the failure of a single network only closes a single open door. All the other doors, or IP addresses associated with the other networks, remain up and functional.

Multihomed networks are often connected to several different ISPs. Routers use the Border Gateway Protocol (BGP), a part of the TCP/IP protocol suite, to route between networks using different protocols [9].

In general, multihoming is helpful for three elements of effective web management. First, multihoming can help to distribute the load balance of data transmissions received and sent by the computer host by lowering the number of computers connecting to the Internet through any single connection. Second, the redundancy that is inherent in multihoming means fewer incidences of downtime due to network failure, which are of special importance for ambient living. Last, multihoming provides an additional tool to keep network connectivity alive and well in the event of natural disasters or other events that would normally render a host inoperative for an extended period of time [8].

Mobility

Mobility has been a topic of concern for many years, bringing many challenges to application developers. Mobility issues vary and are solved differently by the existing technologies.

Mobility support plays a key role in ambient assistance, in order for distributed applications on a service provider to offer living help to remotely ensure users' health, safety, and well-being. Mobility is essential in order to ensure seamless monitoring through quasi permanent connectivity. Building a flexible assisted living platform requires addressing several challenges, such as the following:

1. Fast connection down/up report
2. Robust handover decision
3. Reduced downtime due to handover execution
4. Reduced packet loss
5. Independency of ISP mobility mechanisms

In order to meet these challenges, the aim is to be able to support vertical handover with the workload being done at the application level, which, however, makes the task more difficult because there can be no changes to the TCP stack or other under-layer protocols (as it is usually done on low-level mobility schemes such as Mobile IPv6 [MIPv6] and Host Identity Payload [HIP]). In performing a connection status change report on the application level, performance can be an issue for this kind of mobility solution. Efficient monitoring of transport layers will improve the handover decision and application-level signaling trigger. The next section features some existing solutions on this topic, focusing on the Session Initiation Protocol (SIP; RFC 3261).

Session Initiation Protocol

SIP is able to ensure mobility negotiation on an IP network, providing a high-level dialog to keep two peers connected, despite their whereabouts. SIP architecture standard contains a SIP user agent (UA) and a SIP network server. The UA implements a user agent client (UAC) to initiate SIP calls and a user agent server (UAS) to answer SIP calls.

The most important components of the SIP architecture in terms of mobility support are the redirect server, which accepts a SIP request, maps the address onto zero or more new addresses, and returns these addresses to the client. The redirect server uses the location service to obtain information about a user's possible locations; the register server enables clients to change the address at which they can be reached. A REGISTER request is sent by a SIP client to inform the register server about the change in the client's location and thus the client's address. The register accepts the change and saves the user's new address, maintaining a record of the SIP client's current location. The register server also supports authentication.

Once a SIP transaction is initiated by a SIP-enabled device, the client must register with the register server. These registrations can occur at any time during a session. They are also periodically refreshed so that the most recent information is stored. A register server may be set together with the redirect server to offer location services. After these signaling steps, both application end points have service information about each other as the SIP signaling messages that were sent are written according to the Service Description Protocol (SDP).

This SIP signaling is implemented by SIP methods and SIP responses.

A SIP-enabled mobile node (MN) relies on sending a re-INVITE message to its corresponding node upon link layer address change detection in order to resume a broken transmission due to a location change. In this case, the UA will send another REGISTER request to the home network after receiving a valid IP address from Dynamic Host Configuration Protocol (DHCP) and a re-INVITE request to the corresponding peer. This behavior allows the media session to continue using the new IP address.

SIP is an end-to-end signaling protocol and therefore does not require triangulation such as MIP. Yet this does not solve the underlying handover issues, and it does not comply with Transmission Control Protocol (TCP) (it must be used with the User Datagram Protocol [UDP] protocol only). SIP does not hide each terminal movement, as a third-party entity might eavesdrop and see the plaintext re-INVITE message. SIP has no security practice or standard associated with it, and therefore, this issue must be taken into account by developers. SIP must be complemented by some low-level protocol or any other low-level supporting scheme in order to provide a complete solution for mobility issues.

Many solutions were developed on top of SIP, by extending SIP methods, adding functionality to SIP servers, or developing supporting scheme collaboration, the most important of which are described hereafter.

The solution presented in Ref. [10], describes a framework to support mobility of a multimedia data flow, while roaming between subnets. The framework establishes a SIP core module that implements the SIP stack, a SIP mobility module that manages lower-layer reports and mobility triggering, a call control module that is responsible for SIP message exchange execution, eXosip to manage the socket used for SIP message exchange, and

Windows IP API. The framework uses Windows API to find out when there is an IP address change and to trigger the SIP mobility module, which is in charge of the SIP renegotiation. After retrieving the actual IP address, the SIP mobility module will initiate the SIP negotiation through a UDP socket created for this purpose. After receiving a reply for a re-INVITE, the SIP-enabled MN sends an ACK message to notify the corresponding node that the new agreement is settled. It must be noted that this solution was designed for the transmission of multimedia streams, having a module that implements Real-time Transport Protocol (RTP) support to ensure the stream transport, since SIP is not a transport protocol.

Another framework is described in Ref. [11] that supports application-layer mobility. This particular solution is client-centric, meaning that the workload is on the client side, discarding any network or domain support. This solution implements a connection manager that activates, controls, and monitors failures in the link layers of the radio access technology (RAT)s. This paper defines the concept of cold mobility, which happens when a mobile device changes RAT, changing the IP subnet, yet does not require application-level handover support, because the application session does not need to be kept alive, whereas hot mobility defines a RAT change that does require application handover as well. Applications will still use a connection with an IP address assigned to the interface via DHCP. The difference is that applications monitor connectivity changes and, after any handover, automatically restart their IP connection for the new link.

The solution implements a connection manager that handles low-level mobility tasks and link layer management, allowing mobile-aware applications to be link agnostic. Connection manager features are made available to the application by a mobility API that provides the connect request that triggers the establishment of a path to the infrastructure. The connection manager connects the virtual peer representing the infrastructure, which triggers the selection of a path and its connection. The connection manager reports all route changes through the API as events and requests, described using the XML language. This enables an application to know when a handover has occurred and to trigger the appropriate action.

The lookup request indicates if a specific IP address belongs to one of the locally discovered peers. This enables an application to properly handle local peers that sit on the same network. The paper states that the main integration challenge is to properly handle the restart of IP connections, how this must be done specifically since each application has specific requirements.

Other application-level protocols such as mobile SIP (mSIP) and Scalable Application-Layer Mobility Protocol (SAMP) established improvements to SIP, such as reducing handover time and improving location service, respectively, but both are not exclusively application level.

Low-Level Mobility

Health care service providers often require a mobility workload to be performed at the application level. However, it is still important to review how mobility could be implemented using low-level schemes such as MIPv6, HIP, and IEEE 802.21 Media Independent Handover (MIH) as an alternative.

Whenever a mobile station changes its location to outside the AP's range, thus changing subnets, it may also change its network address, since the old address might have become topologically incorrect. This implies certain modifications to the state of some layers of the Open Systems Interconnection (OSI) model. There are several protocols that operate at one or more of these layers, alone or combined together to create mobility management protocols. There is no protocol that solves all mobility issues efficiently by itself, and while some appear as alternatives, surveys indicate that they represent complementary solutions.

As far as the mobile station is concerned, the mobility scheme should be able to acquire an address from the visiting network's range, while keeping all upper-level connections alive and doing it as seamlessly as possible, such that handover time and packet loss remain low, with minimum effect on the application level. Many protocols have been written to ensure mobility, trying to reduce handover time and packet loss, making the TCP connection resilient, and guaranteeing the safety of the mobility process. Some protocols tend to move the mobility algorithm upwards in the protocol stack, whereas the MN must renegotiate its active connections directly with its peers, such as the mobile Scalable Control Transmission Protocol (mSCTP)—often, they implement security protocols to make sure of both partners' identity. Opposite to this concept, other protocols dislocate the mobility workload to the network, implementing entities that run on network infrastructure and are responsible for executing the mobility functions, working as a mediation platform, thus enabling the MN's mobility process. According to the level of the OSI layer on which they operate, mobility management protocols can be classified as low level, high level, and hybrid, whether they are layer 3, layer 4, or a combination of protocols.

Mobile IPv6

MIPv6 is a mobility management protocol that defines a home agent (HA) that sits in the MN's original network and receives binding updates (BUs) from the MN when it commutes to another network. When the MN realizes that it has changed its location by receiving an IPv6 router advertisement (or sending a router solicitation to receive a router advertisement) from the visited network's access router (AR), it autoconfigures an IPv6 address, which is called a care-of address (CoA), which becomes its secondary address since it still maintains an IPv6 address from its home network. The CoA is sent to the HA on the BU, and it is saved on a table on the HA, who is responsible for forwarding the correspondent node's (CN's) packets to the MN in order to maintain the conversation between them. This builds a triangle between the HA, CN, and MN. When the CN wants to communicate with the MN, it sends packets with the MN's IPv6 address in the destination field, which are delivered on the MN's home network (vertex 1) and are intercepted by the HA, which forwards them to the MN (vertex 2). When the MN wants to communicate with the CN, it simply sends packets with the CN's IPv6 address in the destination field (vertex 3).

IEEE 802.21 Standard

IEEE 802.21, also known as Media Independent Handover, is designed to standardize layer 2 handover operations, providing a normalized framework to upper layers, by defining structures and semantics that are able to aid higher-level protocols. This does not implement a solution to the handover issue and is more of a tool to address the problem. MIH can be considered a new layer to the OSI model, running on top of the link layer and extending its event triggers and commands, establishing a communication model between the MN's layer 2 and the PoA's layer 2 in order for them to correctly decide on handover issues, thus requiring that the MIH suite is deployed at both the MN and the PoA. The standard adds flexibility to the mobility scheme used, enabling it to configure a new connection a priori, by defining link quality thresholds, events that notify the crossing of those thresholds, and commands that trigger configuration actions, therefore reacting faster to location change or link condition variations. This link intelligence and preconfiguration is very important to where mobile devices with strict requirements of power consumption are concerned because all of this prehandover job can be done through the fading media interface, delaying the new media device activation to the time when handover should take place, avoiding time-consuming channel scanning and QoS agreement between the MN and the PoA.

Context Awareness–Based Mobility

Context-aware applications pose a great challenge nowadays as issues of location, device roaming, movement prediction, adaptation to changing scenarios, and location awareness become more important to developers. With respect to mobile connectivity, collecting a wide variety of information that builds the current scenario of the mobile terminal is required as a basis for adaptation of negotiated terms of transmission to the state of the environment. Part of this information may be provided by the mobile network infrastructure, but information from other sources including sensors, information systems, databases, or other mobile devices can be involved as well.

In the context of health care monitoring and in a scenario in which the patient might be constantly moving and must receive a monitoring service that should not restrict their behavior, it is of great relevance that the sensor be able to learn about the environment in which it is currently active. Learning capabilities will allow a monitoring system to adapt promptly to frequently used scenarios or react faster to adverse context conditions, as well as to predict future events. The ability of the sensor to report information about its status regarding battery consumption, signal strength, available bandwidth, and packet loss, alongside other metrics (such as past and current 802.11 Service Set Identifier [SSID], UMTS Cell ID past behavior) that can help to describe a context and set a knowledge base for each patient, is expected to significantly improve the monitoring service.

Existing Solutions

A significant amount of work has been done in the context-awareness field, with some solutions focusing on location capabilities and others on inferring the psychological state of the user, whereas we aim to establish an approach focused on radio access technologies and mobile device status for context collection.

Solutions such as that in Ref. [12] describe a system that can predict certain actions based on context information collection and therefore allow better decisions on commuting radio interfaces. The context collection is done at the transport socket level and at the network interface level and employs the collected data in order to calculate values for the following properties: estimated time until status change, estimated bandwidth available for network interfaces, and estimated lifetime and required bandwidth for transport layer sockets.

Despite the fact that this solution has a strong connection to low layers in terms of monitoring and control, it is considered an application-level approach to a mobility learning system. It sets a shim layer that intersects the system calls and therefore can report the socket's state and radio interface state. When it comes to socket monitoring, expected upstream bandwidth, expected downstream bandwidth, and expected lifetime are calculated using a rolling average. For expected upstream bandwidth and expected downstream bandwidth, calculation is based on the time the socket is open (considering if it is the connection-oriented or connectionless scenario) and the number of bytes that were read and written. Expected lifetime is the average time the socket remained open. Where network interfaces are concerned, an algorithm based on Gaussian process regression (GPR) is used to define X, a random variable that represents the time until a change in the radio interface is expected (up/down), using an N-dimensional vector space defined by N context vectors $x(t)$, whose components were generated by N context collectors. The context collectors are the entities responsible for the collection of the following variables:

1. *Time*: minute of the hour, hour of the day, day of the week
2. *WLAN*: status, current AP, nearby AP, total received data, total sent data
3. *LAN*: status, total received data, total sent data
4. *GSM*: current base station, signal strength
5. *BT*: on/off
6. *System*: memory utilization, running applications
7. *GPS*: on/off, longitude, latitude, altitude, satellites in view
8. *Power*: AC (online/off-line), battery charge

Variables may be of type number, string, or list and therefore must be compared differently. Function $f(x(t))$ is implemented and outputs the time that remains until there is a change in the radio interface. The information describing a context at a certain instant is an N-size vector that is aggregated to other d vectors of context that represent the system past. Function $K(t)$ is implemented, and for each context collector (establishing a proper comparing function k_n for each of them), a relation between the vectors collected consecutively in time is found. Each k_n's output expresses whether there is a strong correlation between the actual parameter and the last one by outputting a number between 0 and 1, that output being weighted according the degree of importance of the context collector it refers to. All k_ns are summed, and an average value is found, where 0 and 1 express the lowest and highest probability of status change in the currently active interface on the next instant, respectively.

The advantages of this solution are that d defines the amount of history that the system uses to estimate the time left until there is a change on an interface; it defines a vast set of parameters that can help to make more precise decisions; it has specific comparison methods that allow the comparison of string values. This system has some negative points as it employs a large data collection process and has poor inference from data, and the general algorithm is purely mathematical, comparing only the actual values and the past, instead of trying to build a consistent scenario based on the past in order to predict more information about the future.

When searching on the subject of context awareness and learning, many solutions were found to address different aspects of this sort of system, some regarding location, motion, and prediction and others based on psychological inference of a user's state or a mobile device's state. The aim of this work is focused on context information that can be extracted from a very narrow scenario, where a mobile device may gather information from its actual state based on the state of the device and radio access technology. Therefore, the solutions presented in the following paragraphs will be restricted to the concepts of context awareness and learning that appear relevant for this work.

Ref. [13] shares a very important and generic overview of the subject, stating that the challenges for context-aware systems are the complexity of capturing, representing, processing, and storing contextual data as well as aggregating it into increasingly more abstract models. In fact, context modeling must be done regarding these challenges to build a solution in which functionality ranges from raw data collection algorithms (e.g., spatial information, network measurement, QoS information) to abstract-based models (decision making, inference engines, task performance, pattern behavior, context reasoning).

The solution in Ref. [14] focuses on context modeling and context reasoning algorithms. Context modeling is done using an ontology, which is a high-level abstract representation of a set of concepts within a domain and the relationships between these concepts, which are domain-specific and can define it. Thus, ontology is a knowledge representation method that can help to denote context. Common items present in an ontology are as follows:

1. *Individuals*: instances, objects
2. *Classes*: sets, collections, concepts, types of object
3. *Attributes*: properties, features, parameters that classes can have
4. *Relations*: ways that classes and objects can be related to each other
5. *Function terms*: complex structures formed from certain relations that can be used in place of an individual term in a statement
6. *Restrictions*: formally stated descriptions of what must be true in order for some assertion to be accepted as input
7. *Rules*: statements in the form of an if–then sentence that describe the logical inferences that can be drawn from an assertion in a particular form
8. *Axioms*: including the theory derived from axiomatic statements
9. *Events*: the changing of attributes or relations

Ontology is a way to describe context by setting a syntactic and semantic definition and arranging it in a hierarchical scheme. The items referred to above are disposed on the hierarchical scheme, establishing the relations between the so-called elements of context. The way the scheme is defined is completely dependent on the domain to be described as well as the depth of information that is to be imposed on the system. Based on the 5W1H (where, when, what, who, why, how) factor, ontology can define class *activity*, whose attributes will be able to describe it (sleeping, awake, walking, running, on emergency) and which sets the *how*; class *user object*, whose attributes will describe the individual (user identification, biological status) and which sets the *what* and the *who*); class *location*, whose attributes will describe all the possible locations where a user might be and which sets the *where*; and class *service object* to characterize any device that is associated with the individual and might contribute with context information. Relations state what the common ground is to relate any set of two classes. For instance, a user behavior is a relation between a user object and an activity.

Context reasoning is achieved using a Bayesian network as a probabilistic inference model, which is useful in expressing uncertain context or situation data. The Bayesian network is a tool for making knowledge representations, reasoning under uncertainty, reasoning with conflicting criteria, and modeling interdependent criteria. A Bayesian network is obtained by using a directed acyclic graph (DAG) in which each node is a relevant variable that poses uncertainty to the system and the arcs that connect them represent the causal or influential relations between them.

However, according to Ref. [15], the Bayesian network approach on its own has an imperfect property: an uncertain result of the context-awareness problem, not covering the fact that reusing and sharing the uncertain knowledge captured by Bayesian networks can make the used ontologies more compact and unique and therefore more precise. Having these limitations in mind, the authors in Ref. [15] propose a fusion scheme between ontology and a Bayesian network, due to their similarities: Both are directed graphs, and there is a direct correspondence between many nodes and relations in the two graphs.

So the Bayesian network will contain the information from the ontology, and defining a conditional probability table (CPT) carries the probability of each item of the DAG. Then, logically connected to the other items as the ontology defines, it is able to make decisions, based on the context parameters of the system. For instance, given a location and user object parameter's probability, infer an activity.

Transposing these concepts to mobility, ontology, and Bayesian networks can be done for context modeling, allowing a good context definition and relationship between entities and parameters as well as context reasoning, inferring a context-aware decision based on conditional probability DAG.

A middleware solution is proposed in Ref. [16], where an architecture for context management is proposed in order to make the appropriate services available to users in dynamically changing environments. The architecture consists of five modules and three databases (DB). A context integrator module is the first entity to interact with the raw data that come from sensors and perform context normalization, i.e., it aggregates data in terms of the MN or user that produced it and the location from which they were gathered. It will perform some data conversion as well. The rules to this procedure and data aggregation can be modified, enabling the system to be more or less tuned according to how accurate the system needs to be. This filtered information is stored on the current context database. A learning engine module will apply appropriate learning methods to the data in history DB, such as a neural network or a decision tree, among other algorithms. The output of this module will be stored on a knowledge database. A context prediction engine is used to make predictions upon data, such as predicting user movements over user position. It supports the creation of a future context database and decision making over its data. This module can be used to reduce monitoring cost. The methodology used for the prediction is based on the naive Bayes classifier seen as an equivalent Bayesian network. Using the naive Bayes classifier, a user's next location can be predicted from historical data. The same methodology can be applied to any knowledge predicate for which historical data is available. The knowledge base database and history database will feed context prediction to predict a context that, together with current context, will supply information to the reasoning module that will reason about context information, using predefined rules and trigger actions or set inferences that will be sent to the learning engine module. The solution has a clearly separated context-aware functionality yet does not specify the data module nor the storage model in detail.

Aiming to specify the way that the context parameters are measured in order to adapt the measuring method to the type of parameter, the following concepts have been proposed:

1. *Acquisition type*: explicit, where context parameters are directly acquired by context collection entities; implicit, where context parameters are inferred from other stored context parameters

2. *Acquisition mode*: instantaneous, where context parameter is acquired only once at the beginning of a certain interaction; continuous, where context parameter is acquired continuously during a certain interaction

3. *Relevance*: active, where context parameter is relevant to the current interaction; passive, where the context parameter is not relevant to the current interaction yet can be stored for future usage or inference

4. *Evolution*: dynamic, where context parameter changes during the interaction; static, where context parameter does not change during interaction

5. *Adaptation*: adaptable parameter during interaction; nonadaptable parameter during session

In this list, the concept of interaction refers to a certain connection established by the MN to a certain PoA within a certain time interval that has specific parameters for each time it occurs, varying with the radio access technology used for the connection as well as the status of the mobile device.

The solution in Ref. [17] is, in fact, a middleware for context-aware applications and establishes a model for context awareness with its workload on several entities. One of these entities enforced the concept of context updating: the notion that the context parameters must be updated with different frequency rates in order to ensure freshness, yet not adding unnecessary overhead to the system. For instance, some context parameters may require updating every month or year, whereas sensed contextual elements may need to be updated more frequently due to the dynamic nature of the sensed data. It is worth noticing that the applications that will run on top of this middleware have a completely different purpose than the methodology that we propose, but the classification of the context parameters contains important information.

Focusing on the handover process between RATs, the solution in Ref. [18] presents a very complete handover support platform, covering the subjects of context awareness, learning, and handover decisions (where the latter is left to be discussed in the next section of this chapter). The solution proposed by Ref. [18] uses a multiple-criteria decision-making (MCDM) method based on the concept of Bayesian networks, specifically the Bayesian belief network. The algorithm defines three types of nodes: chance nodes, which represent both criteria and subcriteria; the utility node, which represents the set of objectives; and decision nodes, which represent the set of possible decisions or actions.

The MCDM method utilizes a Bayesian network with states, relationships, preferences, and relations between them. The nodes present on the DAG must aid the handover process by establishing relations between criteria, available networks, constraints and possible actions. A set of variables is defined (cost, interface power consumption, bandwidth, data rate, application tolerable delay, jitter, data loss) as well as a set of constraints (properties of the criteria). No mention is made concerning the method used to collect this information.

Chance nodes have a level of indirectness by building synthetic variables that can be characterized similarly to simple variables, yet aggregating their information in a single output per set of variables. Every chance node has a CPT that sets the probabilities for a certain configuration. For instance, a CPT for cost defines the probabilities of (high/low) cost for the different RATs. Synthetic variable chance nodes establish the same CPT but set the probabilities relating the simple variables they refer to. User preference (high or low) output will depend on the high/low state of the simple variables. Synthetic variables will feed into the utility node, which, in turn, outputs a utility value for each target network in order to compare the utility of each candidate network given the actual conditions of the system. The fact that the nodes are connected by conditional probability allows any change made to any point of the graph (i.e., system) to propagate through all the nodes it affects and alter the utility output.

The handover decision algorithm is delegated to the decision nodes, set in a chain. The algorithm is used solely for the target network decision node, which requires a decision over multiple criteria as all the other decision nodes use rule-based policies.

The authors in Ref. [18] present a complete algorithm for decisions and context-aware reasoning for vertical handover foreseeing the GPRS and Wi-Fi technologies. Application requirement oriented, this solution fully describes a methodology to make context-aware decisions based on user preferences, QoS parameters, and algorithms to prioritize and score these parameters.

The context model for the algorithm contemplates static parameters: service types, QoS requirements for service, and user preferences for the terminal side and provider's profile for the network side (for charging models). It also contemplates dynamic parameters: running application type and reachable APs for the terminal side and current QoS parameters of APs for the network side. The five service types have specific QoS parameters set a priori. For any of the service types, the available radio interfaces, service type requirements, and system objectives are prioritized from one to nine, where one is high priority. Six nonfunctional requirements, after being prioritized, tune the system towards which of them are more important to the system's execution. The six that are defined in the document are interface priority, minimizing cost, maximizing mean throughput, minimizing delay, minimizing jitter, and minimizing bit error rate (BER). Then it sets boundaries to QoS parameters to discretize all the values that the parameters can take and make further comparison and setting up maximum values such as maximum jitter easier. It then compares the values that are collected from the network interfaces with the QoS boundaries and user preferences (which represent the values that are associated which a certain service type) and ranks the candidate networks using an algorithm called Analytical Hierarchical Process (AHP). AHP is designed to make complex decisions by separating system elements into hierarchies and making choices based on their weighted properties. The model consists of a goal (ideal network to be handed over to); a set of criteria (all the parameters at stake, such as user preferences, QoS parameters); and a set of alternatives (candidate networks alongside their QoS properties). The criteria are compared one by one, producing relative scores. Using these values, a pair decision matrix is set. The size of the matrix is (number of interfaces) (objectives). The rank given to a candidate network is the sum of the products of the weight of each parameter and its relative score for each candidate network. Light network capability discovery (LNCD) sweeps the radio interfaces, acquiring their current network parameters, and simultaneously, the Adaptation of Application module (AfA) acquires the application requirements and sends them to the light session transfer management (LSTM) module where the main algorithm is implemented. The handover process is triggered, and the LSTM notifies the AfA module of which applications should connect to what interfaces.

The aforementioned solution does not show many learning capabilities but shows strong context-awareness features being highly customizable, admitting user preferences to great extent, defining priorities for them as well as six different service types for application requirements. It does not mention the periodicity of the interface sweep to read the required network parameters, making it unclear about the battery consumption of this algorithm. It does not use MIP; instead, it implements a custom scheme to perform handover. AfA is responsible for application mobility management. The whole handover process, including interface sweeping, decision making, and session transfer, takes 60 ms in the case of GPRS to Wi-Fi handover and 20 ms in a Wi-Fi to GPRS handover. The fact that the second is faster than the first is explained as follows: "[T]he time taken for inter-face detection is much higher for Wi-Fi than for GPRS because the former is in influenced by the technology-specific detection mechanism, whereas the interface is always active in the latter case [18]." This fact can be much criticized as the battery consumption is, among others, a strong requirement in this work.

Bayesian networks deal well with incomplete data. For instance, implementing a clas-sification algorithm that requires a set of variables that are correlated in some manner poses no inconvenience if all the required parameters are present. If they are not, which, in terms of this work, might represent an incorrect or incomplete network parameter read-ing, Bayesian networks can, for example, be employed to deal with dependencies.

A New Approach Based on Machine Learning

Hereafter are presented the system architecture entities, together with the description of the relationships between them, which constitutes a new approach based on machine learning for context-aware mobility in assisted ambient living scenarios (among other applications as well).

System Ontology

The ontology contains a formal and high-level description of the entities and relation-ships among these entities that constitute the system. The synthetic parameters have no semantic value to the system other than the one that is given by the elementary parameters that constitute them. The synthetic parameter's relevance is that it aggregates elementary parameters logically, simplifying the update operations and providing a system that can be tuned to provide different relevance to different sets of parameters at different points in time (Figure 8.1).

Ontology Element Description

The *BT successful handover* element represents a learning parameter that infers if the past handovers to BT have been successful. The purpose of this parameter is to introduce learn-ing functionality towards successful handover for each technology.

It should be given a low weight on the overall system as it may be inaccurate, but it can still be important if UMTS or BT conditions are not good for a given terminal localization.

The *moving* element infers the terminal state by assuming TRUE or FALSE based on handover frequency. If a terminal is being handed over very frequently on BT, it may be due to BT conditions for a certain AP that may not be acceptable. But in the UMTS case, it may represent movement since UMTS range is much larger than BT's.

The *UMTS successful handover* element represents the learning parameter that infers if the past handovers to UMTS have been successful. The purpose of this parameter is to introduce learning functionality towards successful handover for each technology.

The *cost* element will be used to influence BT or UMTS in terms of what the cheapest technology is. BT is free, and therefore, this element will be more important to UMTS. Concerning BT, it may be just a measure of preferred technology.

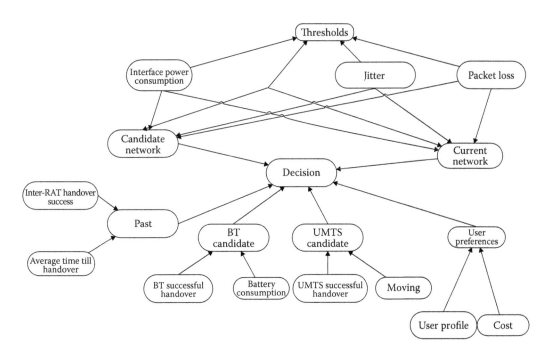

FIGURE 8.1
The system's description of ontology.

Battery consumption reports the evolution of battery state by updating battery depletion every handover. This allows the general algorithm to take into account the battery state of the terminal when deciding which network it should change to.

The purpose of the *user consumption profile* element is to introduce information about the user state in terms of user behavior configuration. Adding this to the algorithm will allow the user to tune the system whether they plan to take a big hike through the countryside or stay within BT range (home, hospital) for a while. A profile element set to *high* represents high movement. An element profile element set to *low* represents low movement. This is done to prevent unnecessary handover to vestigial BT networks along the user's path.

The *average time until handover* element should provide the system with an average measure of how frequently handover happens with the passage of time. Having this element updated every handover can provide a raw estimate of when the next handover should take place.

Inter-RAT handover success is used to build past knowledge about the intertechnology handover. Since the decision element has information about one BT and one UMTS target network as well as the original RAT, it may provide some information that shows whether inter-RAT handover has proved worth it through time.

The *decision* element combines the four synthetic elements from the ontology. The decision element's purpose is to choose a target RAT from a BT candidate and a UMTS candidate. Both should be chosen based on the highest received signal strength indicator (RSSI). A decision is to be made based on knowledge acquired from execution. Therefore, the parameters described in this section, which contain information about context, and past history, will influence it. A decision is ultimately a Bayesian CPT carrying all combinations of past, BT candidate, UMTS candidate, and user preferences.

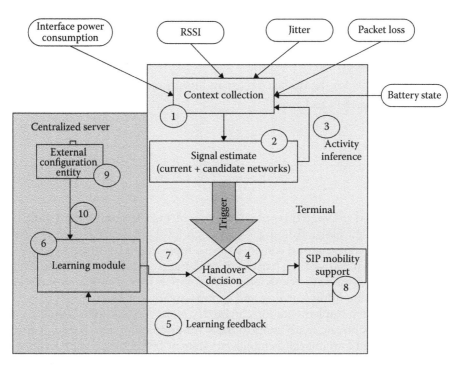

FIGURE 8.2
The system's architecture.

The ontology elements will then be translated to another learning structure, based on the Bayesian network algorithm, which combines probabilities and dependencies for every entity (Figure 8.2). Whenever one element is updated, the changes will be reflected on every other element of the structure.

Architectural Design

The system will be deployed on both the client and server sides. The client side will be responsible for the collection of network parameters, handover detection, and application of the probabilistic model that will output the new RAT system for receiving the call. The server side will be a serving point for mobile terminals and will apply an update algorithm to each terminal's probabilistic model according to a prior handover information report, which is received every time a terminal handovers to a different RAT. The report will contain information on success/failure, new RAT information, a handover timestamp, and battery level. After these parameters are received, the central server will update the element value probabilities to reflect the values received.

1. Context collection from interfaces/terminal gathering parameters with period P
2. Data uniformization; threshold testing; handover triggering; interface probing
3. Activity feedback to control periodicity P
4. Decision algorithm with Bayesian network
5. Feedback to learning module: SIP information: success/failure, new address; new RAT; handover time stamp; battery level

6. Update of learning module

7. Sending of updated model to terminal

8. SIP mobility support

9. Entity responsible for the update of cost and user profile (ISP UMTS cost update)

10. Update of user profile and cost

Conclusions

This chapter presented research on context-aware systems for mobility and multihoming, in the scope of ambient assisted living. Many high-level solutions regard the handover issue without energy concerns and consider the multiple interfaces always connected. It is of relevance that an exhaustive search of the prior literature revealed that there is not much information available for a network-independent solution with a single centralized server to report to and implementing learning and context-awareness elements.

Context-aware system implementation can be driven to very complex scenarios as some algorithms had a very strong mathematical basis yet oriented on a narrower feature, such as monitoring time until an interface changes its state or predicting what transition from a set of possible states the user will make. Other systems turned to the radio access technology parameters in order to make handover more precise and efficient. Parameters such as the received signal strength indicator, packet loss, or mean packet delay were taken into account by these systems.

But still, context information must be addressed in a generic and focused way. Bayesian networks are used to address these questions probabilistically and provide a tool that can establish a model that relates the chosen parameters in terms of their dependencies. Finding these dependencies by evaluating the system key requirements and aiming at setting some inferences upon data based on these dependencies can be an excellent starting point to build a Bayesian network. In order to present a formal system definition regarding these dependencies, an ontology must be designed (where all the system entities are present), while a Bayesian network will determine the probabilistic relations between entities. This system's objective is to implement a cost function that outputs the best radio access technology at a given handover point. Not forsaking this objective, the Bayesian network's ultimate purpose is to decide the output. The learning functionality of this system comes from the possibility of updating it in order to reflect the passage of time and subsequent execution of the algorithm.

To make use of a centralized server can constitute a bottleneck and may not scale, but it relieves the mobile terminal of heavy probability computations (taking into consideration their reduced processing power). The centralized server update can provide the adjustment capabilities to the probabilistic model externally to the mobile device without requiring the user's presence. In prior context-aware-oriented solutions, the parameters specified to define context are very much left to each implementation's concern.

Context-aware information can thus be of high value in order to predict handover, aiding the handover process. Based on learning data, users' connectivity can be optimized. Deploying entities that have functional intelligence and consistent background knowledge at their disposal, it will enable clever decisions to be made, therefore improving its performance. Ideally, these entities will be able to learn from experience, with special regard to user preferences, user behavior, and recurring situations in the network infrastructure and surrounding scenario.

References

1. Ferrari, P., Flammini, A., Marioli, D., and Taroni, A. IEEE 802.11 Sensor Networking Dept. of Electronics for Automation and INFM (Istituto Nazionale Fisica della Materia), University of Brescia, Italy.
2. Marko, H., and Maija, M. K. Wireless System for Patient Home Monitoring. In *2nd International Symposium on Wireless Pervasive Computing, (ISWPC '07)*. San Juan, February 2007.
3. Kumar, A., and Rahman, F. System for Wireless Health Monitoring Sensors for Industry. In *Proceedings the ISA/IEEE Conference, 2004*, 2004, pp. 207–210.
4. Niyato, D., Hossain, E., and Camorlinga, S. Remote Patient Monitoring Service using Heterogeneous Wireless Access Networks: Architecture and Optimization. In *IEEE Journal on Selected Areas in Communications*, Vol. 27, Issue 4, pp. 412–423, 2009.
5. Benhaddou, D., Balakrishnan, M., and Yuan, X. Remote Healthcare Monitoring System Architecture using Sensor Networks. In *2008 IEEE Region 5 Conference*. Kansas City, April 2008.
6. Sung-Nien, Y., and Jen-Chieh, C. A Wireless Physiological Signal Monitoring System with Integrated Bluetooth and WiFi Technologies. In *27th Annual International Conference of the Engineering in Medicine and Biology Society, 2005. IEEE-EMBS 2005*. Shanghai, January 2006, pp. 2203–2206.
7. Chiew-Lian, Y., and Wan-Young, C. IEEE 802.15.4 Wireless Mobile Application for Healthcare System. In *Proceedings of the 2007 International Conference on Convergence Information Technology*. Washington, DC, 2007.
8. Charoenpanyasak, S., and Paillassa, B. SCTP Multihoming with Cross Layer Interface in Ad-hoc Multihomed Networks. In *Third IEEE International Conference on Wireless and Mobile Computing, Networking and Communications*. France, 2007.
9. Choi, Y., Kim, B., Kim, S., In, M., and Lee, S. A Multihoming Mechanism to Support Network Mobility in Next Generation Networks. In *IEEE Asia-Pacific Conference on Communications*, 2006.
10. Yeh, C. H., Wu, Q., and Lin, Y. B. *SIP Terminal Mobility for both IPv4 and IPv6*. 26th IEEE International Conference on Distributed Computing Systems Workshops. Portugal, 2006.
11. Tourrilhes, J. *L7-MOBILITY: A Framework for Handling Mobility at the Application Level*. Hewlett Packard Laboratories, Palo Alto, CA.
12. Herborn, S., Petander, H., and Ott, M. Predictive Context Aware Mobility Handling. In *IEEE International Conference on Telecommunications*, 2008, pp. 1–6.
13. Khedo, K. Context-Aware Systems for Mobile and Ubiquitous Networks. In *International Conference on Systems and Networking*, 2006.
14. Kwang-Eun, K., and Kwee-Bo, S. Development of Context Aware System Based on Bayesian Network Driven Context Reasoning Method and Ontology Context Modeling. In *International Conference on Control, Automation and Systems*. Seoul, October 2008, pp. 2309–2313.
15. Mokhesi, L., and Bagula, A. Context-Aware Handoff Decision for Wireless Access Networks using Bayesian Networks. In *Proceedings of the 2009 Annual Research Conference of the South African Institute of Computer Scientists and Information Technologists*. ACM New York, 2009.
16. Chun-dong, W., Xiao-qin, L., and Huai-bin, W. A Framework of Intelligent Agent Based Middleware for Context Aware Computing. In *Fifth International Conference on Natural Computation*. Tianjin, August 2009, pp. 107–110.

17. Malek, J., Derycke, A., and Laroussi, M. A Middleware for Adapting Context to Mobile and Collaborative Learning. In *Fourth IEEE International Conference on Pervasive Computing and Communications Workshops (PERCOMW'06)*. Pisa, Italy, March 2006.

18. Ahmed, T., Kyamakya, K., and Ludwig, M. Architecture of a Context-Aware Vertical Handover Decision Model and Its Performance Analysis for GPRS—WiFi Handover. In *Proceedings of the 11th IEEE Symposium on Computers and Communications*. Washington, DC, 2006.

9

Power-Aware Communication in Body Area Networks

Hassan Ghasemzadeh and Roozbeh Jafari

CONTENTS

ABSTRACT Monitoring human movements using wireless sensory devices promises to revolutionize the delivery of health care services. Such platforms use inertial information of their subjects for motion analysis. Potentially, each action or disease can be discovered by collaborative processing of sensor data from multiple locations on the body. This functionality is provided by a body area network (BAN), which consists of several wireless sensor nodes positioned on different parts of the body. In spite of the revolutionary potential of this platform, power requirements and wearability have limited the commercialization of these systems. This chapter presents energy-efficient communication models for BAN applications using buffers to limit communication to higher-rate short bursts, decreasing power usage and simplifying the communication. Transmission at higher rates and in short bursts will create opportunities to reduce the energy per bit for communication, hence decreasing the overall energy consumption. This energy minimization is achieved via proper buffer allocation in this chapter. The buffer allocation problem is formulated as an optimization problem that reduces transmissions among sensor nodes. Both an integer linear programming (ILP) solution and a fast greedy heuristic algorithm are discussed to solve this power optimization problem. It is shown that despite the decreased transmission efficiency, the greedy algorithm can be adopted for fast allocation of buffers in real time. Performance of both the near-optimal and greedy solutions is compared against an unbuffered system using experimental analysis. It is demonstrated that ILP and greedy solutions can reduce the amount of transmissions by an average factor of 70% and 41%, respectively.

KEY WORDS: *buffer allocation, collaborative signal processing, power optimization.*

Introduction

Technological advances in wireless communication, sensor design, and embedded processors have led to the development of pervasive body area networks (BANs) that enable wearable and mobile health care monitoring systems. Such platforms consist of a set of miniaturized sensor nodes that sense physiological and environmental data, initiate actions, and trigger alarms during an emergency [1]. BANs can be used for remote patient monitoring and testing, which enables a shift of health care from a traditional clinical setting to the home. This shift will reduce costs, allow collection of information previously unavailable, and give patients more control over their care. Despite the variety of potential applications, proliferation of continuous health monitoring is still limited due to application-dependent platform constraints in terms of computation, communication, battery lifetime, and storage. Often, the problem is overconstrained, so the designer must relax some constraints to produce a solution. Consequently, techniques improving the efficiency of resource usage can greatly expand the efficiency of the platform.

In BANs, energy is constrained to a small battery for each sensor node. One of the biggest consumers of energy is communication [2]. In traditional wireless sensor networks, a significant amount of energy can be saved by improving the routing protocol. However, on a BAN, sensor nodes are quite proximate, which results in a single-hop network. From the application perspective, communication cost depends only on the amount of data to be sent. Because of this, energy saving techniques frequently focus on decreasing the amount of data that needs to be communicated through greater local processing [3]. There is still an advantage to be gained by application-aware, data-agnostic communication optimizations. In many applications, channel usage is fragmented—that is, communication is frequent but sparse.

This chapter presents a method for using buffers to transmit in bursts. Burst transmission can reduce energy per bit [4] and can simplify communication by lowering packet scheduling overhead [5]. The buffer allocation technique assigns each signal processing module a large buffer, which is sized to minimize communication. Since many medical monitoring applications require only periodic reports, real-time results are unnecessary [6]. Removing immediate data-processing deadlines permits an interesting optimization based on burst transmissions. Signal processing is modeled as a directed acyclic dependency graph in which processing modules use results from other nodes for data fusion. The dependency graphs are used to introduce an integer programming (IP) of the optimization problem with a separable convex function. A polynomial-time greedy algorithm is then introduced to compensate for the computational complexity of the integer linear programming (ILP)–based solution for dynamic allocation of buffers in real time.

Burst transmission requires buffers to accumulate results between transmissions [7]. The concept of buffers has been utilized in several domains in order to optimize communication systems. It has been traditionally used in asynchronous transfer mode (ATM) networks to improve system throughput by allowing communication parties to dynamically allocate their buffers to multiple nodes [8]. In networks on chip (NoCs), efficient distribution of buffers among input channels of on-chip routers can significantly increase overall performance of the system [9]. Buffers have been used in embedded software to minimize memory requirements of runtime software components [10]. In real-time distributed systems, buffers have been employed to avoid communication delay among synchronous processes and to preserve data semantics [11].

Besides buffer allocation, power-aware signal processing techniques have been proposed to reduce power consumption of the system by minimizing the number of active nodes in the network. For instance, Ref. [12] poses optimization problems for minimizing the number of active nodes and for maximizing system lifetime while maintaining high classification accuracy for action recognition. Similarly, a task graph can be constructed using timing constraints and data dependencies [13]. Using the task dependency graph, the system can determine the critical paths, which can be used in the development of a scheduling mechanism to distribute the unused time (slacks) among tasks such that the overall energy cost is minimized. The decision tree model in Ref. [14] is used for incremental movement classification, where only informative nodes are involved in each classification decision. The node activation policy in Ref. [15] activates sensor nodes dynamically according to the local observations made by individual nodes.

Preliminaries

Before formulating the problem of buffer allocation in BANs, several concepts must be discussed, including a more thorough description of the platform, signal processing model, and definition of dependency graphs in the context of this problem.

Communication Power Efficiency in BANs

Recent studies [1,16–19] have revealed various power limitation and challenges in realizing BSN applications. Optimization approaches that address the power-constraint issue span a wide range of research fields from hardware design to communications and signal processing. One strategy of addressing energy constraint relies on modifications of standard communication protocols. Ref. [17] shows that, based on the specifications of popular BAN communication protocols, such as 802.15.1 (Bluetooth®) and 802.15.4 (ZigBee®), and specific needs of the considered application, it is possible to modify the set of protocol commands to enhance the power performance of the sensor nodes. The concept of a power-aware sensor node proposed in Ref. [18] is another mechanism to address the energy constraint problem. It can be effective if sensor nodes are capable of estimating the required level of transmission power to maintain network connectivity. This idea is further utilized by the authors in Ref. [19], where, based on power awareness, nodes can gracefully trade off performance for energy efficiency.

System Architecture and Signal Processing

A BAN system consists of several sensor nodes, each equipped with a processing module, a set of sensors, a battery, and a radio module for communications. In physical movement monitoring applications, each node has several motion sensors, such as accelerometers and gyroscopes. For action recognition applications, the system aims to detect physical movements of the subject wearing the system. A number of sensor nodes are placed on different joints of the human body. Inertial data obtained by each sensor node are subject to physical action recognition and further processing.

A typical system of physical activity recognition intends to classify a set of movements of interest. Pattern classification techniques are mostly employed to distinguish each action from the rest. Per-node signal processing involves several modules, including *preprocessing, segmentation, feature extraction,* and *classification* [12]. In the preprocessing phase, the data are collected from each sensor node and are passed through a filter to reduce high-frequency noise. During segmentation, the signal is divided into parts, each representing a complete action. This is done by annotating the start and end of each movement. A feature extraction block calculates a set of statistical and morphological features from each signal segment. Each sensor node makes a local classification decision on the movement being performed by the subject. A final decision based on the all local results is made by a central node.

Collaborative Model

The signal processing model described in the previous section is usually implemented in a distributed manner over a BAN. Information flow across the network is represented with a dependency graph model. In a system of n sensor nodes, a dependency graph is composed of n subgraphs connected through internode links. Each subgraph represents static information dependencies within a node, as shown in Figure 9.1, where u_i^R, u_i^S, u_i^F, and u_i^C denote *sensor reading* and *preprocessing, segmentation, feature extraction,* and *classification* blocks, respectively. As mentioned previously, features are extracted by locating the annotation points in the filtered signal and calculating a set of statistical and morphological features from the resulting segment.

Definition 1

Given a set of n sensor nodes $s_1,...,s_n$, the intranode dependency subgraph for node s_i is defined by $G_i = (V_i, E_i)$ where V_i is the set of four vertices and E_i is the set of four edges. Each vertex, denoted by u_i^μ, corresponds to a processing unit, and each edge is denoted by $e_{ii}^{\mu\eta}$ (μ, $\eta \in \{R, S, F, C\}$) representing intranode dependencies. ∎

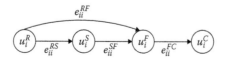

FIGURE 9.1
Intranode dependency subgraph.

Internode links that represent dependencies across sensor nodes are used to connect subgraphs and form a dependency graph. An internode link is determined according to dependencies induced by the application of interest.

Definition 2

Given a set of n sensor nodes $s_1,...,s_n$ and internode dependencies, dependency graph $G = (V, E)$ is formed by connecting n intranode dependency subgraphs $G_1,...,G_n$ through dependency links E_b defined by the application criteria. The set of edges E is given by ■

$$E = E_w \cup E_b \tag{9.1}$$

where the set of intranode edges E_w is given by

$$E_w = \bigcup_{i=1}^{n} E_i \quad i = 1,...,n \tag{9.2}$$

and the set of vertices V is defined by

$$V = \bigcup_{i=1}^{n} V_i \quad i = 1,...,n \tag{9.3}$$

where each V_i is the set of vertices within subgraph G_i.

As an abstract example, Figure 9.2 shows a dependency graph for a network of three sensor nodes where processing units are connected through 10 internode dependency links. Intranode subgraphs are highlighted by the dashed boxes.

In the example of an activity monitoring system, practical internode links $e_{ij}^{\mu\eta}$ connecting the processing block μ at node s_i to the processing block η at s_j are presented as follows. A link e_{ij}^{SS} shows that the segmentation block at sensor s_j requires segmentation results from sensor s_i. A lack of prominent patterns prevents s_j from properly determining the start and

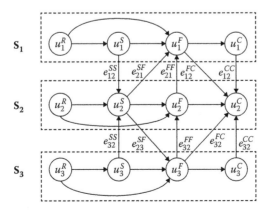

FIGURE 9.2
An example of a dependency graph for a three-node network.

end of actions. When a subject is walking, a node placed on the leg observes a high-quality pattern, but a head node observes irrelevant patterns. A link e_{ij}^{SF} is required when node s_i becomes a master node for segmentation and provides node s_j with the annotation points (fragment of sensor data stream signifying a certain activity of predefined class type) for feature extraction. When s_j requires information on features calculated by s_i to extract features, a link e_{ij}^{FF} is added. If classification at node s_j is contingent on certain features from s_i, a link e_{ij}^{FC} is required. A segmentation unit may need information on current movement detected by another node. In this case, a link e_{ij}^{CS} is added to the dependency graph. A link e_{ij}^{CF} is required if the feature extraction depends on classification results provided by other nodes. When sensor node s_j is considered as a classifier aggregator, links of the form e_{ij}^{CC} are considered, allowing other nodes to transmit local classification to a central node.

Problem Definition

The idea behind using buffers is to transmit the maximum amount of data in short time intervals. The large number of data blocks produced by each processing unit are stored locally and are transmitted using available bandwidth. This would conform to real situations of health care systems where physicians are interested in receiving reports on daily activities rather than immediate reports. By assuming no immediate deadlines in the system, individual buffers on each link are maintained, and the data blocks are transmitted separately for each internode link.

Problem 1

Given dependency graph G, each internode link $e_{ij}^{\mu n}$ is associated with a number $x_{ij}^{\mu n}$ denoting the number of actions for which data blocks produced by the source unit u_i^μ are buffered prior to every transmission. The objective is to find values $x_{ij}^{\mu n}$ that minimize the number of transmissions subject to memory constraints on nodes. ∎

Buffer Assignment

The buffer allocation rechnique is discussed through an illustrative example (Figure 9.3) in this section.

The amount of data that can be stored within buffers is constrained by the available memory of the nodes. Different processing units, including reading (raw sampled sensor data), segmentation, feature extraction, and classification, produce data blocks of different sizes.

Definition 3

The amount of data produced by unit u_i^μ per action is called a data unit and denoted by b_i^μ. In the example shown in Figure 9.3, reading, segmentation, feature extraction, and classification generate data blocks of size 200, 2, 10, and 1 byte, respectively. ∎

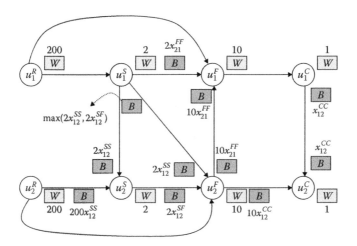

FIGURE 9.3
Example of the buffer assignment method.

The communication model maintains two types of buffers for each sensor node as follows. A buffer of size b_i^μ associated with processing unit u_i^μ is called an *intranode buffer* in order to enable in-node processing. The data stored in this buffer will be consumed by the next processing unit within the same node. In this example, shown in Figure 9.3, the total amount of intrabode buffers, labeled W, maintained for nodes s_1 and s_2 is $W_1 = W_2 = 200 + 10 + 2 + 1 = 213$. Furthermore, a buffer allocated to a processing unit u_i^μ due to internode dependencies is called an *internode buffer*. These buffers provide data for consequent dependent units.

Internode buffers are sized according to the number of actions each link would store. An internode link with $x_{ij}^{\mu\eta}$ number of actions allocates a buffer to the source unit and another buffer to the destination unit. When a source unit has more than one outgoing edge, only one buffer is enough to store data for both links. The size of such a buffer is determined based on the maximum amount of data required to be transmitted among the links. In Figure 9.3, the processing unit u_1^S has two outgoing edges. The internode buffer (labeled B) is then sized according to the values of x_{12}^{SS} and x_{12}^{SF}. However, only a single buffer with the maximum required size would be sufficient to accommodate the data generated by this unit. That is, a buffer of size $\max(2x_{12}^{SS}, 2x_{12}^{SF})$ is allocated where the coefficients are determined as the absolute number of data units that are required per processing block per action (e.g., segmentation block generates two data units for each action). Destination units, however, require $2x_{12}^{SS}$ and $2x_{12}^{SF}$. Moreover, an internode dependency prevents the destination unit from performing any processing until it receives data from the source. That is, for link $e_{ij}^{\mu\eta}$, the data produced by the predecessor of the destination unit ($b_j^{\eta-1}$) must be buffered as well. In Figure 9.3, link e_{12}^{SS} enforces a buffer of size $200x_{12}^{SS}$ on the incoming link e_{11}^{RS} because sensor reading produces 200 bytes. For the same reason, the $2x_{21}^{FF}$ bytes buffer on e_{11}^{SF} and $10x_{12}^{CC}$ bytes buffer on e_{22}^{FC} are allocated and sized.

To formulate the problem, certain assumptions are made about the frequency of occurrence of the actions. The number of movements occurring in a given time period T is assumed to follow a Poisson distribution [20]. The probability of observing x number of actions in a given time interval is represented by

$$p(x) = \frac{\lambda^x e^{-\lambda}}{x!} \tag{9.4}$$

where λ is the expected number of movements that occurred in the given interval. With a confidence level of $1 - \alpha$, the Poisson model provides an upper bound k on the number of actions that occurred during the interval:

$$p(x \leq k) = \sum_{x=0}^{k} p(x) = 1 - \alpha \tag{9.5}$$

Definition 4

The upper bound on the number of actions that occurred during a given time interval is known as action rate, k, which is obtained according to a Poisson distribution model. ∎

Problem Formulation

Given the dependency graph G as described earlier, let $d_{ij}^{\mu\eta}$ be a binary that represents the existence of internode links, given by

$$d_{ij}^{\mu\eta} = \begin{cases} 1, & \text{if } s_i \text{ and } s_j \text{ are dependent through } u_i^{\mu} \text{ and } u_j^{\eta} \\ 0, & \text{otherwise} \end{cases} \tag{9.6}$$

The number of actions A that occurred at action rate k during time period T is given as $A = k \times T$, and the number of transmissions can be calculated by

$$Z = \sum_{i \neq j} \sum_{\mu,\eta} A \frac{d_{ij}^{\mu\eta}}{x_{ij}^{\mu\eta}} \tag{9.7}$$

The total size of the intranode buffers W_i for node s_i is given by

$$W_i = \sum_{\mu} b_i^{\mu}, \tag{9.8}$$

and the total size of the internode buffers for node s_i is determined by

$$B_i = \sum_{\mu} \left(\max_{j,\eta} \left(d_{ij}^{\mu\eta} b_i^{\mu} x_{ij}^{\mu\eta} \right) + \max_{j,\eta} \left(d_{ji}^{\eta\mu} b_j^{\eta} x_{ji}^{\eta\mu} \right) + \max_{j,\eta} \left(d_{ji}^{\eta\mu} b_j^{\mu-1} x_{ji}^{\eta\mu} \right) \right) \tag{9.9}$$

Let M_i be the size of the memory on node s_i. The problem of minimizing the number of transmissions can be formulated as a convex optimization problem as follows:

$$\min Z \tag{9.10}$$

subject to

$$W_i + B_i \le M_i \qquad \forall i \in \{1,\dots,n\} \tag{9.11}$$

$$x_{ij}^{\mu\eta} \in Z^+ \qquad \forall i, j, \mu, \eta \tag{9.12}$$

Problem Complexity

Both A and d_{ij} in Equation 9.7 are known a priori. Thus, the objective function in Equation 9.10 is to minimize $\sum_{j=1}^{m} \dfrac{1}{x_j}$. Furthermore, the nonlinear constraints in Equation 9.11 can be written as linear constraints by expanding the *max* functions in Equation 9.9 over all possible values of j and η. With these modifications, the optimization problem in Equations 9.10 through 9.12 can be represented as the following problem **P**:

$$\min \; w(x) = \sum_{j=1}^{m} \frac{1}{x_j} \tag{9.13}$$

subject to set of feasible solusions *F*:

$$a_{i1}x_1 + a_{i2}x_2 + \dots + a_{im}x_m + W_i \le M_i \qquad \forall i \in \{1,\dots,n\} \tag{9.14}$$

$$x_j \in Z^+ \qquad \forall j \in \{1,\dots,m\} \tag{9.15}$$

In Equations 9.13 through 9.15, each x_j is associated with one of the existing internode links in the graph. The coefficients a_{ij} in Equation 9.14 are calculated according to the transformation of nonlinear constraints in Equation 9.9 into linear equations by expanding every *max* function over all values taken by the function. Therefore, the set of feasible solutions can be represented by vectors of the form $x = \{x_1, x_2, x_m\}$. The new formulation in Equations 9.13 through 9.15 will simplify subsequent discussions.

The objective function $w(x)$ is a summation over several convex functions, turning the objective function into a convex separable function. According to the literature, no polynomial solution exists that solves this problem in its full generality. However, polynomial solutions exist for several special cases. In particular, a greedy algorithm is presented in Ref. [21] when the set of feasible solutions forms a jump system. Another study [22] shows that if the integer linear version of an integer convex separable minimization problem over linear constraints is polynomial, it can be solved in polynomial time with the number of variables m, the number of constraints, and the absolute value of the largest subdeterminant of the constraints matrix.

Since the IP problem is hard to solve in general, two methods are discussed in this chapter for approximating the solution. First, the integrality condition Equation 9.15 can be relaxed as in Equation 9.16 to solve the problem using common convex programming tools.

$$x_j > 0 \qquad \forall j \in \{1,\dots,m\} \tag{9.16}$$

The solution obtained due to integrality relaxation will not carry the optimality condition but helps in finding a lower bound on the size of memory for which the result is optimal.

Theorem 1

For each sensor node s_i, the convex optimization problem **P** with integer relaxed constraints finds optimal solutions for memories of size ∎

$$M_i - \sum_{j=1}^{m} (1-\varepsilon)a_{ij} \tag{9.17}$$

Relaxation of a variable x_j will round the variable down to closest integer. Thus, the size of optimal buffer associated with x_j would increase by factor $1 - \varepsilon$ of the coefficients a_{ij} represented in Equation 9.14. Therefore, memory usage on each node is optimized as shown in Equation 9.17.

In investigating polynomial time solutions for the buffer assignment, a greedy algorithm is discussed in the next section, which has less computational complexity than the IP technique.

Greedy Algorithm

A greedy solution is discussed in this section for solving the buffer assignment problem. The algorithm starts with an initial feasible solution and reiterates an augmentation process that moves greedily toward the final solution. Since the algorithm is motivated by several basic concepts mostly used in combinatorial optimization over jump systems, these basic terms are defined first.

Definition 5

For any two lattice points [23] x and y in Z^m, the box spanned by x and y is denoted by $[x, y]$ and defined as the set ∎

$$\{z \in Z^m \mid \min(x_j, y_j) \le z_j \le \max(x_j, y_j)\} \qquad \forall j \in \{1,\dots,m\} \tag{9.18}$$

The spanned box $[x, y]$ contains all the points z such that

$$d(x, z) + d(z, y) = d(x, y) \tag{9.19}$$

where $d(x, y)$ denotes the Manhattan distance between two vectors x and y and is given by

$$d(x,y) = \|x - y\|_1 = \sum_{j=1}^{m} |x_j - y_j| \tag{9.20}$$

Definition 6

For any two points x and y in Z^m, a step s from x to y is a point $x' \in Z^m$ such that $x' \in [x, y]$ and $d(x, x') = 1$. ▪

The definition of a step implies that in any step from x to y, only one of the components x_j should change. This component is denoted by s (i.e., $x' = x + s$) and refers to such a step $St(x + s)$ as used in Ref. [21].

Algorithm 1: Greedy Solution for Buffer Allocation Problem

Input: Optimization problem P:(w, F) and initial solution $x^0 \in F$
Output: Solution x for P
$x \leftarrow x^0$
while $\exists St(x + s)$ s.t. $x + s \in F$ and $w(x + s) < w(x)$
$\qquad \hat{s} \leftarrow \arg\min_s w(x + s)$
$\qquad x \leftarrow x + \hat{s}$
endwhile
return x

The greedy approach is shown in Algorithm 1. It takes the convex optimization problem **P**: (w, F) and an initial feasible solution x^0 as input and generates a final solution x. A comparison of the results obtaned from this algorithm and those of IP will be discussed later in the section "Performance of Buffer Allocation Algorithms." The algorithm iterates through subsequent steps as follows. At each time, it checks all components x_j within vector x and finds the step $St(x + s)$ that minimizes the objective function w. It then updates the current vector x and chooses the next step by setting $x \leftarrow x + \hat{s}$. The algorithm terminates when no other feasible solution exists that improves the objective function. This happens when either all following steps would violate the constraints F or every feasible step increases the value of $w(x)$.

Lemma 2

Any step s from a current feasible solution x^{curr} to the final solution x^{final} updates the objective function w only by increasing one variable x_j. ▪

Assume that step s takes the algorithm for x^{curr} to a next step x^{next}, updating the objective function $w(x^{curr})$ to $w(x^{next})$. This means $w(x^{next}) < w(x^{curr})$. By definition of the step, $d(x^{curr}, x^{next}) = 1$. To keep the distance between the two vectors at 1, one component x_j should be either increased or decreased by 1. However, decreasing x_j would result in increasing the value of the objective function ($w(x^{next}) > w(x^{curr})$), which contradicts greedily minimizing the objective function w. Therefore, any step s increments one component of the vector x.

Definition 7

Within each step s of the greedy algorithm, an augmented link is defined as the internode edge e_j whose corresponding variable x_j is incremented.   ∎

Static Buffer Allocation

The greedy algorithm can be used offline to determine initial buffers associated with different links. This is required at the system startup, where dependencies are fixed and defined by the application. In addition to the objective function w and feasible solutions F defined by Equations 9.13 through 9.15, the algorithm needs an initial feasible solution x^0 as input. An obvious value for x^0 is (1,1,1), which is obtained by initializing every variable x_j to the smallest possible value introduced by Equation 9.15. As a result, we initialize all x_j to 1 at the beginning of the program. At each iteration, the algorithm will increment the variable (see Lemma 2) that maintains a locally optimum solution. Each link augmentation allocates some buffer to both processing blocks connected by the link, as discussed in the section on "Static Buffer Allocation".

Lemma 3

Unless memory constraints in Equation 9.14 are violated, in each round of the greedy algorithm, all dependency links are augmented.   ∎

Proof for Lemma 3 is by induction on value of variables x_j. At the beginning of the algorithm, $x_j = 1$ for all the links x_1, x_2, x_m. Let w_1 be the value of the objective function by augmenting all the links, through one round of the algorithm (e.g., m steps). Further, let w_1' be the objective function by augmenting all the links but x_l, which remains unchanged ($x_l = 1$), and x_p, which is increased by 2, through m iterations. Therefore,

$$w_1 = \sum_{j=1}^{m} \frac{1}{x_j + 1} = \frac{m}{2}$$

$$w_1' = \frac{1}{x_l} + \frac{1}{x_p} + \sum_{j=1, j \neq l, p}^{m} \frac{1}{x_j + 1} = \frac{m}{2} + \frac{5}{6}$$

(9.21)

Obviously, $w_1 < w_1'$, which means that the algorithm will evenly augment the links. Now assume, in the kth round of the algorithm, that all variables $x_1 = x_2 = = x_m = k$ increased by 1. We need to prove that in the $(k + 1)$th round, all the links will be augmented. Let w_{k+1} be the result of augmenting all the links ($x_j = k + 1$), and w_{k+1}' the value of the objective function by augmenting all the links except x_l, which remains $k + 1$, and x_p, which is augmented twice ($x_p = k + 3$). Thus,

$$w_{k+1} = \sum_{j=1}^{m} \frac{1}{x_j + 1} = \frac{m}{k + 2}$$

(9.22)

$$w'_{k+1} = \frac{1}{x_l} + \frac{1}{x_p} + \sum_{j=1, j \neq l, p}^{m} \frac{1}{x_j + 1} \tag{9.23}$$

$$= \frac{m}{k+2} + \frac{2}{(k+1)(k+2)(k+3)}$$

Since $w_{k+1} < w'_{k+1}$ the algorithm will augment all internode links evenly in any round of the algorithm.

Theorem 4

The greedy algorithm for a given buffer allocation problem **P** as in Equations 9.13 through 9.15 is polynomial in the number of dependency links m and the size of memory M. ∎

Without loss of generality, assume that all the sensor nodes have equal memory sizes M and within-node buffers of size W. Also, assume that the algorithm starts with an initial solution x^0, which holds inequality constraints as described previously. The algorithm takes steps that minimize the objective function in Equation 9.13. This convex separable function forces the algorithm to choose the next step such that variables x_j get close to each other. Based on Lemma 3, the greedy approach would make all x_j equal unless incrementing a variable violates some constraints. This procedure can be interpreted as follows. The algorithm takes m steps to augment each of the m internode links. For each node s_i, the amount of memory assigned by this round of the algorithm is given by

$$\theta_i = \sum_{j=1}^{m} a_{ij} \tag{9.24}$$

where a_{ij} are given by the constraints in Equation 9.14. The remaining memory $(M - W - \theta_i)$ will be further assigned to different buffers in following steps. When increasing a variable x_j violates constraints, the algorithm excludes that variable from further buffer allocation. The number of such rounds that eliminate variables from future augmentation differs from one variable to another. However, in the worst case, a link may require $\dfrac{M-W}{\theta_i}$ rounds before running out of memory. Because each round of the algorithm takes, at most, m steps, the number of iterations is bounded by $m \times \dfrac{M-W}{\theta_i}$. Assuming fixed W and θ_i for a given problem, the total number of steps $St(x + s)$ required for the algorithm to converge has a complexity of $O(m \times M)$.

Dynamic Buffer Allocations

The goal of dynamic buffer allocation is to reassign buffers based on changes in the dependency graph. At each point in time, one or more internode links may be removed from the graph, and several edges can be added. Since the system is expected to operate in real time, it is extremely important to quickly decide what the size of each buffer should be. In this section, a simple and effective approach for dynamic assignment of the buffers based on the greedy algorithm is presented. Deletion of an internode link makes some memory available on the nodes. The new memory space can be used to assign buffers to the existing or newly inserted links. However, the optimality of the solution is not guaranteed if only memory of the deleted links is taken into consideration when reassigning buffers. To overcome this problem, certain properties of the greedy algorithm are explored that allow for drastic reduction in the number of steps for real-time buffer allocation. The key idea is that, by means of information obtained from the static case, the algorithm can restart with a significantly large initial feasible solution and yet achieve the same solution as the static buffer allocation approach.

Definition 8

Given probelm **P** with objective function w as in Equation 9.13, feasible solutions F as in Equation 9.14 through 9.15, and initial solution $x^0 = (1,1,1)$, a saturation point is a point x^{sat} within spanned box $[x^0, x]$ ($x \in F$) such that all components of x^{sat} have the same value v^{sat}, and v^{sat} is maximized.   ■

$$x^{sat} = (v^{sat},\dots,v^{sat}) \tag{9.25}$$

$$v^{sat} = \arg\max_{v}(v_1,\dots,v_m) \in F \qquad \forall j \; v_j = v \tag{9.26}$$

When the greedy algorithm iterates through steps, different links will be saturated one after another. Once a link is saturated, it is ignored in the subsequent iterations. The saturation point, in fact, refers to the first link that is eliminated from further augmentation. Figure 9.4 shows the evolution of the algorithm for three variables x_1, x_2, and x_3. The algorithm starts with the initial solution (1,1,1) and reiterates by evenly incrementing the variables. The point (4,4,4) is the saturation point because all variables have the same value

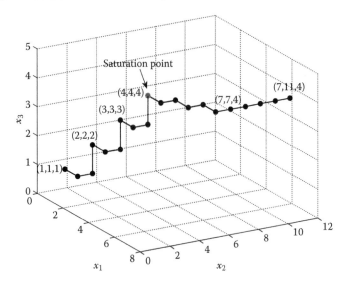

FIGURE 9.4
Illustration of saturation point.

and one of the links (x_3) is saturated. This link cannot be further augmented in following steps due to memory constraints. The algorithm continues by augmenting other links than x_3 until x_1 becomes saturated at (7,7,4). However, it keeps increasing x_2 until the algorithm converges at (7,11,4).

Lemma 5

Given the final solution $x = (v_1,\ldots,v_m)$ obtained from the greedy algorithm, the saturation point $x^{\text{sat}} = (v^{\text{sat}},\ldots,v^{\text{sat}})$ is calculated by ∎

$$v^{\text{sat}} = \min(v_1,\ldots,v_m) \tag{9.27}$$

The proof follows from the definition of the saturation point. The saturation point is identified by the first link that is saturated. Since such a link will not be augmented in the future, its value remains fixed throughout subsequent steps. Therefore, at the end of the algorithm, the value of such a link is the same as its last augmentation, but other links have been augmented in subsequent iterations (see proof for Theorem 4).

Link Deletion

Removing an existing link will create free space for other links to be augmented. On deletion of a link, the greedy algorithm is executed with the initial feasible solution given by the saturated point. This guarantees the same final solution as the static algorithm and reduces the number of steps required for the algorithm to converge.

Lemma 6

Given a buffer allocation problem **P**, any point in the box spanned by two feasible solutions x and x' remains a feasible solution if any memory size M_i increases. ∎

Let **P** be the problem that allocates buffers to sensor nodes s_1, s_n with memories of size M_1, M_n. The set of feasible solutions F for problem **P** is defined by the box spanned by the smallest initial solution x^0 and the optimal solution x^{opt}. Increasing M_i by δ will expand this box according to the constraints in Equation 9.14. Therefore, the new expanded box contains all previous feasible solutions. In particular, it contains all the points within the box $[x, x']$.

Theorem 7

By removing a link from dependency graph, the greedy algorithm with initial solution x^{sat} produces the same result as that with the initial solution x^0 used for the static approach. ∎

Let v^{sat} refer to the saturation point for the original problem with m links. Without loss of generality, assume that link e_m has been removed from the dependency graph. The problem turns into finding final solution for $x = (x_1,\ldots,x_{m-1})$. Let w and w' be the values of the objective function using initial solutions $x^0 = (1,1,1)$ and $x^{sat} = (v^{sat},\ldots,v^{sat})$, respectively. Because link deletion makes some memory available, any point within the box $[x^0, x^{sat}]$ is a feasible solution (see Lemma 6). Thus, x^{sat} could be an initial point for the greedy algorithm. Based on Lemma 3, this point is on the path from x^0 to the final solution. Therefore, both static and dynamic approaches will take the same steps after reaching x^{sat} and output the same solutions.

Link Insertion

When a new link is added to the network, the saturation point is still used to restart the algorithm. However, this point would not necessarily be a feasible solution for the new problem with extra link. The reason for this is that the new variable added to the constraints in Equation 9.14 may shrink the feasible solution space. Yet, we are interested in finding an initial point whose components all have the same value. This point would necessarily lie within the box $[x^0, x^{sat}]$. To find this initial point, a quick binary search is performed. This gives a feasible point in $[x^0, x^{sat}]$, which has largest components. Once this point is found, it is fed to the greedy algorithm. The algorithm will then go through different steps by evenly augmenting existing links. When incrementing a variable results in violating memory constraints, the algorithm skips that link and excludes it from further augmentation and iterates through the rest of the edges in the dependency graph as accomplished for the static case.

Performance of Buffer Allocation Algorithms

The effectiveness of the discussed buffer assignment techniques is presented in this section through several networks with varying internode dependencies.

Setup

Suppose a set of experiments are conducted on several networks, each composed of homogenous sensor nodes. The nodes are assumed to be a typical mote (e.g., TelosB) and have memories of size 10 KB. The results are discussed for two different networks with respect to typical dependencies required in BAN applications. Here, x_j denotes the number of actions for which data is buffered before transmission over the given link.

Assume that the movements occur at a rate of 1 action per minute and each movement spans 200 samples. These assumptions ensure a high confidence level (95%) with the Poisson model. In fact, processing blocks will have sufficient computational throughput to process incoming actions. Further, assume that the size of the intranode buffer is 2 bytes for segmentation, 10 bytes for feature extraction, and 1 byte for classification.

Experiment 1

The first arrangment is a network of two sensor nodes with emphasis on information dependencies for segmentation and classification, as shown in Figure 9.5. A brief description of this configuration is as follows. The second node is the master node for segmentation and classification. It performs segmentation based on its local knowledge and the information received from node 1. In order to provide the first node with a more confident segmentation,

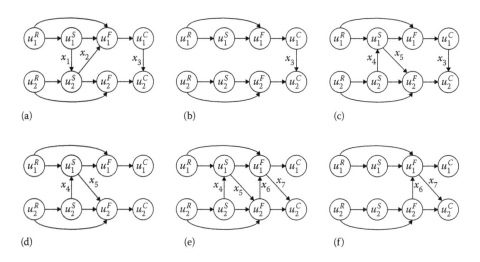

FIGURE 9.5
Evolution of dependency graph for a body sensor network with two sensor nodes (used for Experiment 1). (a) Initial network with 3 dependency links x_1, x_2, and x_3. (b) The network after removal of x_1 and x_2. (c) The network with two new dependency links x_4 and x_5. (d) The network after removing x_3. (e) Two new dependency links x_6 and x_7 are added. (f) The final network after x_4 and x_5 are removed.

node 2 transmits the results to node 1 for feature extraction. Furthermore, the classifier at node 2 is assumed to be dependent on the results of classification provided by node 1.

The network is initially constructed to satisfy the three information dependencies labeled as x_1, x_2, and x_3. Figure 9.5b shows the situation where x_1 and x_2 are removed from the network. The network model is then updated as shown in Figure 9.5c due to the addition of two new edges, x_4 and x_5. The network changes afterward, as shown in Figure 9.5d through f.

The buffer allocation problem is solved using both integer relaxation and a greedy algorithm. A standard IP solver (e.g., Ref. [24]) can be used to specify and solve the convex optimization problem. To evaluate the effectiveness of the combinatorial algorithm, a developer further needs to develop the greedy algorithm using a high-level programming language such as MATLAB. In the absence of buffers, each node is required to transmit its local data to the other node on the occurrence of every action. This results in 1440 transmissions per node during 24 h of system operation. Table 9.1 shows the difference between the relaxed ILP and greedy buffer allocations for each of the six configurations in Figure 9.5. When the network model changes from one configuration to another (e.g., from

TABLE 9.1

Number of Transmissions for Experiment 1 for 24 h of System Operation

Conf.	# Packets (w/o Buffer)	ILP		Greedy	
		# Packets	% Saving	# Packets	% Saving
a	2880	52	98.19%	89	96.91%
b	2880	2	99.93%	2	99.93%
c	2880	41	98.58%	88	96.94%
d	2880	36	98.75%	58	97.99%
e	2880	73	97.47%	128	95.56%
f	2880	9	99.69%	9	99.69%
Avg	2880	35.50	98.77%	62.33	97.84%

TABLE 9.2

Time Complexity Comparison for Experiment 1

| Conf. | ILP Time (s) | Greedy Static | | | | Greedy Dynamic | | | |
		Time (µs)	# Steps	Speedup	Time (µs)	# Steps	Speedup (ILP)	Speedup (Static)
a	1.453	188	144	7728	–	–	–	–
b	1.234	3172	911	389	2750	863	448	1.15
c	1.625	206	145	7888	15.6	1	104,166	13
d	1.518	196	98	7744	27	2	56,222	7.2
e	2.030	294	176	6904	20	4	101,500	14.7
f	1.478	1978	668	747	1740	1160	849	1.1

a to b), both static and dynamic algorithms achieve the same results. For this particular experiment, the ILP and the greedy algorithm reduced the number of transmissions by an average factor of 81 and 46, respectively. The results of the greedy algorithm and convex solver (ILP based) are shown in Table 9.2, which verifies the effectiveness of the buffer allocation algorithm in terms of convergence time. Number of steps in this table corresponds to Definition 6. For each of the networks b through f, the last two columns in Table 9.2 show the speedup of the dynamic algorithm compared with that of the ILP and static buffer allocation schemes.

Experiment 2

The second experimental network is illustrated in Figure 9.6. The initial configuration shown in Figure 9.6a has six internode dependency links (labeled as x_1 to x_6) for segmentation, feature extraction, and classification. Figure 9.6b through f illustrates dynamic changes in the network due to potential requirements of the application. First, the network loses its all internode dependencies for feature extraction and classification (x_2, x_3, x_5, and x_6) but not for segmentation. Network configuration is then updated as in Figure 9.6c to enable classification at the second node. In this configuration, the second classifier is assumed to combine features from all the sensors for highly accurate movement classification. In Figure 9.6d, the network has only dependencies for classification at node 2, as a result of deleting links x_1 and x_4 from the previous network. The model is further updated, as shown in Figure 9.6e, by adding four new dependencies (x_9, x_{10}, x_{11}, and x_{12}), which makes the second node the master for segmentation. Node 2 receives segmentation data from the two other nodes and provides them with final annotations. Figure 9.6f shows a situation where node 2 is not a classifier combiner as it was in c, d, and e. This is done by deleting x_7 and x_8 from the network. However, node 2 is still the master for segmentation.

Note that when no buffering scheme is employed, a transmission is initiated after occurrence of each movement. This yields a large number of transmissions, as shown in Table 9.3. This table also shows the number of transmissions reported by both ILP and greedy solutions. For this experiment, the number of transmissions is reduced by a factor of 60 and 37 using the ILP-based and greedy solutions, respectively. An interesting observation is that for Figure 9.6b, the ILP solver outputs a larger number of packets than the greedy algorithm. This is, in fact, due to integer relaxation of the variables x_j when using a convex solver (see Theorem 1).

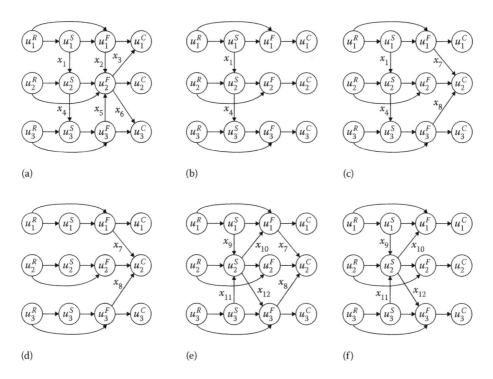

FIGURE 9.6
Example of dependency graph for three sensor nodes with dynamic reconstruction of internode links (used for Experiment 2). (a) The network with 6 information dependency links x_1–x_6. (b) The network after removal of all links except x_1 and x_4. (c) The network after addition x_7 and x_8. (d) x_1 and x_4 are removed from the network. (e) Four new dependencies are added including x_9 to x_{12}. (f) Dependency links x_7 and x_8 are eliminated from the network.

In Table 9.4, timing complexity of different solutions, including ILP and static and dynamic greedy solutions, are compared. As demonstrated, the greedy algorithm can drastically reduce CPU time while maintaining higher savings in terms of packet transmissions. Moreover, real-time allocation of buffers using a dynamic greedy solution serves a considerable time reduction compared to both ILP and a static greedy solution. This verifies the importance of employing saturation point as the initial solution of the greedy algorithm for dynamic reconfiguration.

TABLE 9.3
Number of Transmissions for Experiment 2 for 24 h of System Operation

Conf.	# Packets (w/o Buffer)	ILP		Greedy	
		# Packets	% Saving	# Packets	% Saving
a	4320	81	98.13%	194	86.5%
b	4320	59	98.63%	58	95.9%
c	4320	95	97.80%	128	91.1%
d	4320	6	99.86%	6	99.5%
e	4320	117	97.29%	191	86.7%
f	4320	71	98.36%	116	91.9%
Avg	4320	71.50	98.34%	115.5	97.33%

TABLE 9.4

Time Complexity Comparison for Experiment 2

		Greedy Static			Greedy Dynamic			
Conf.	ILP Time (s)	Time (µs)	# Steps	Speedup	Time (µs)	# Steps	Speedup (ILP)	Speedup (Static)
a	2.532	6266	261	404	–	–	–	–
b	1.484	2343	98	633	297	12	4996	7.8
c	2.078	4031	176	515	109	4	19,064	36
d	1.612	8563	1002	188	8175	914	1763	1.09
e	2.555	3520	266	725	150	2	17,033	23
f	2.152	2872	196	749	109	20	19,743	26

Concluding Remarks

A communication model was outlined in this chapter in order to reduce the number of transmissions over the BAN networks. An efficient buffer assignment technique was presented for distributed lightweight sensory systems with limited storage. The approach maps the communication minimization model into a convex optimization problem and provides an IP as well as a greedy algorithm to calculate buffer sizes associated with each processing module. The dynamic resource allocation technique is based on the basic greedy approach, which reduces the time required for buffer assignment in real time. This model can be used to realize different BAN applications with relaxed processing deadlines.

The buffer allocation approach presented in this chapter provides a unique way to achieve energy conservation, context awareness, and collaborative communication in BANs. The proposed techniques have several advantages in addition to the main objective of transmission reduction. They can simplify the communication, reduce the overhead of communication coordination, and enhance the system lifetime.

The simple communication model presented in this chapter can be suitably extended to incorporate needs for real-time deadlines. Immediate reactions can be initiated when certain actions (e.g., falling) are observed. For each such action, one master node can detect the movement locally and initiate the communication [25].

The choice of the number of packets as a performance metric makes the evaluation independent of the communication protocol. Moreover, the larger packet sizes provided by the presented model can potentially enhance the communication system by reducing energy consumption and supporting self-configuration [26].

References

1. Lo, B. and Yang, G.-Z. Body sensor networks—Research challenges and opportunities. pp. 26–32, April 2007.
2. Raghunathan, V., Schurgers, C., Park, S. and Srivastava, MB. Energy-aware wireless microsensor networks. *IEEE Signal Processing Magazine*, 19(2):40–50, 2002.

3. Luprano, J., Sola, J., Dasen, S., Koller, J. M. and Chetelat, O. Combination of body sensor networks and on-body signal processing algorithms: The practical case of MyHeart project. *BSN '06: Proceedings of the International Workshop on Wearable and Implantable Body Sensor Networks*, pp. 76–79, 2006.

4. Kahn, J. M., Katz, R. H. and Pister, K. S. J. Next century challenges: Mobile networking for *Smart Dust. MobiCom '99: Proceedings of the 5th Annual ACM/IEEE International Conference on Mobile Computing and Networking*, pp. 271–278, 1999.

5. Liu, R.-S., Fan, K.-W. and Sinha, P. Locally scheduled packet bursting for data collection in wireless sensor networks. *Ad Hoc Networks*, 7(5):904–917, 2009.

6. Chigan, C. and Oberoi, V. Providing QoS in ubiquitous telemedicine networks. *PERCOMW '06: Proceedings of the 4th Annual IEEE International Conference on Pervasive Computing and Communications Workshops*, p. 496, 2006.

7. Chandrakasan, A., Amirtharajah, R., Cho, S., Goodman, J., Konduri, G., Kulik, J., Rabiner, W. and Wang, A. Design considerations for distributed microsensor systems. *IEEE Custom Integrated Circuits Conference (CICC)*. pp. 279–286, 1999.

8. Kung, H. T. and Chang, K. Receiver-oriented adaptive buffer allocation in credit-based flow control for ATM networks. *INFOCOM '95: Proceedings of the Fourteenth Annual Joint Conference of the IEEE Computer and Communication Societies*, Vol. 1, p. 239, 1995.

9. Jingcao, H., Ogras, U. Y. and Marculescu, R. System-level buffer allocation for application-specific networks-on-chip router design. *IEEE Transactions on Computer-Aided Design of Integrated Circuits and Systems*, 25(12):2919–2933, 2006.

10. Hahn, J. and Chou, P. H. Buffer optimization and dispatching scheme for embedded systems with behavioral transparency. *EMSOFT '07: Proceedings of the 7th ACM & IEEE International Conference on Embedded Software*, ACM, New York, pp. 94–103, 2007.

11. Benveniste, A., Caspi, P., di Natale, M., Pinello, C., Sangiovanni-Vincentelli, A. and Tripakis, S. Loosely time-triggered architectures based on communication-by-sampling. *EMSOFT '07: Proceedings of the 7th ACM & IEEE International Conference on Embedded Software*, ACM, New York, pp. 231–239, 2007.

12. Ghasemzadeh, H., Guenterberg, E., Gilani, K. and Jafari, R. Action coverage formulation for power optimization in body sensor networks. *Design Automation Conference, 2008. ASPDAC 2008. Asia and South Pacific*, pp. 446–451, 2008.

13. Liu, Y., Veeravalli, B. and Viswanathan, S. Critical-path based low-energy scheduling algorithms for body area network systems. *The 13th IEEE International Conference on Embedded and Real-Time Computing Systems and Applications (RTCSA 2007)*. pp. 301–308, 2007.

14. Ghasemzadeh, H., Barnes, J., Guenterberg, E. and Jafari, R. A phonological expression for physical movement monitoring in body sensor networks. *Mobile Ad Hoc and Sensor Systems, 2008. MASS 2008. 5th IEEE International Conference on*, pp. 58–68, 2008.

15. Ghasemzadeh, H., Loseu, V. and Jafari, R. Structural action recognition in body sensor networks: Distributed classification based on string matching. *IEEE Transactions on Information Technology in Biomedicine*, 14(2), 2010.

16. Quwaider, M., Rao, J. and Biswas, S. Transmission power assignment with postural position inference for on-body wireless communication links. *ACM Transactions on Embedded Computing Systems (TECS)*, 10(1): Article 14, 2010. doi: 10.1145/1814539.1814553.

17. Yan, L., Zhong, L. and Jha, N. K. Energy comparison and optimization of wireless body-area network technologies. *BodyNets '07: Proceedings of the ICST 2nd International Conference on Body Area Networks*, ICST (Institute for Computer Sciences, Social-Informatics and Telecommunications Engineering), Brussels, Belgium, Belgium, pp. 1–8, 2007.

18. Min, R., Bhardwaj, M., Cho, S.-H., Ickes, N., Shih, E., Sinha, A., Wang, A. and Chandrakasan, A. Energy-centric enabling tecumologies for wireless sensor networks. *Wireless Communications, IEEE*, 9(4):28–39, 2002.

19. Xiao, S., Dhamdhere, A., Sivaraman, V. and Burdett, A. Transmission power control in body area sensor networks for healthcare monitoring. *IEEE Journal on Selected Areas in Communications*, 27(1):37–48, 2009.

20. Panangadan, A., Mataric, M. and Sukhatme, G. Detecting anomalous human interactions using laser range-finders. *Intelligent Robots and Systems, 2004. (IROS). Proceedings. 2004 IEEE/RSJ International Conference on*, 3:2136–2141, 2004.
21. Ando, K., Fujishige, S. and Naitoh, T. A greedy algorithm for minimizing a separable convex function over a finite jump system. *Journal of Operations Research*, 38(3):352–375, 1995.
22. Hochbaum, D. S. and Shanthikumar, J. G. Convex separable optimization is not much harder than linear optimization. *Journal of the ACM*, 37(4):843–862, 1990.
23. Krätzel, E. *Lattice Points*. Springer, New York, 1988.
24. Grant, M. and Boyd, S. Graph implementations for nonsmooth convex programs. In *Recent Advances in Learning and Control* (a tribute to M. Vidyasagar), V. Blondel, S. Boyd and H. Kimura, editors. Lecture Notes in Control and Information Sciences, Springer, London, pp. 95–110, 2008.
25. Ghasemzadeh, H., Jain, N., Sgroi, M. and Jafari, R. Communication minimization for in-network processing in body sensor networks: A buffer assignment technique. *IEEE/ACM. Design, Automation & Test in Europe Conference & Exhibition, 2009. DATE '09*. Nice, France, pp. 358–363, 2009.
26. Ye, W., Heidemann, J. and Estrin, D. An energy-efficient MAC protocol for wireless sensor networks. *The Twenty-First Annual Joint Conference of the IEEE Computer and Communications Societies (INFOCOM 2002)*. vol. 3, pp. 1567–1576, 2002.

10

Wireless Systems Applied to e-Health: Radio-Planning, Energy Efficiency, and System Integration

Francisco Falcone, Antonio López-Martín, Carlos Fernández-Valdivielso, Luis Serrano, Santiago Led, and Miguel Martínez Espronceda

CONTENTS

ABSTRACT   In this chapter, the impact of radio-planning strategies, transceiver electronic design, and overall wireless system planning will be discussed. By following a complete approach, from physical layer limitations derived from radiopropagation losses to transceiver requirements and the functional elements of the overall wireless system, performance of such wireless systems applied in e-health environments is increased. The

225

fundamental loss mechanisms for radiopropagation will be described, as well as the models employed to analyze them. The elements of transceiver architecture and the challenges in order to reduce power consumption will be described. The practical example of a functional wireless HOLTIN system is described, as well as the main trends in building automation technologies, giving a complete overview of the elements within wireless systems applied to e-health scenarios.

KEY WORDS: *wireless systems, wireless body area networks, radioplanning, energy efficient electronics.*

Introduction

The use of wireless systems holds clear benefits, such as ease of installation, noninvasive behavior, and interconnectivity, among others. The progress in microelectronic circuit design and in the adoption of converging wireless standards has led in recent years to their widespread adoption in diverse areas, such as communication networks, intelligent buildings, and telemetering in utilities or logistics, to name just a few. One of the key issues to take into account in the near future is the way in which these wireless sensor networks are deployed, in order to enhance their performance in terms of capacity while reducing the required energy consumption. Consideration of the radio wave channel characteristics has a direct impact not only on the topology of the wireless system but also on the design of the transceiver.

One of the main characteristics is the use of a wireless carrier to convey the information of the system. Radioelectric channels allow for almost immediate deployment within a determined service area. However, due to the complexity of the environment (given not only by surrounding elements such as buildings or trees but also by variable elements such as vehicles or persons), radio wave channels suffer strong degradations, which are time dependent. This variability has a strong impact in the overall performance of a wireless system, in which the following considerations must be taken into account:

- As the distance increases, propagation losses are higher in line-of-sight conditions. If non-line-of-sight conditions hold, losses will be increased due to absorption, diffraction, and scattering mechanisms.
- The use of higher frequency bands allows higher channel capacity, as stated by Shannon's limit, but leads to higher propagation losses.
- Scenarios with structural complexity, such as dense urban and indoor, exhibit strong multipath components.
- Wireless sensor networks tend to use a large amount of elements. It is therefore desirable to work with transceivers with low power consumption, increasing the overall energy efficiency.
- The proliferation of wireless systems implies the possibility of nondesired signals, which can interfere with the system deployed for ambient assisted living (AAL) purposes. This is aggravated when nonlicensed spectral bands are used, which is the normal case when using WLAN/WPAN/WBAN standards.

The use of wireless systems applied to AAL is usually focused on the following applications:

- Wireless sensor networks within the household of the user. In this case, radioelectric propagation is mainly driven by strong multipath due to the complexity of the topology as well as the morphology of the indoor scenario.
- Wireless public land mobile networks and wireless LAN/MAN, in order to establish connectivity with the user out of the household. In this case, radio wave propagation will be determined by terrain profile and the possibility of indoor/outdoor operation. In this case, other factors such as network load and its impact on network availability have to be considered.

In this chapter, the considerations for optimal rollout of wireless sensor networks will be described in terms of coverage/capacity relations. The coexistence with other existing wireless networks will be analyzed in order to optimize system performance. Energy-efficient transceivers will be described in this wireless ecosystem, with examples of operation of real telemonitoring devices and the impact that radio wave propagation considerations have on the overall performance. Finally, integration with building automation systems (BASs) will be covered in order to have a full system view of the wireless solution applied to AAL.

Characterization of Radio Wave Propagation

Analysis of a wireless channel can be performed in order to estimate time-dependent as well as frequency-dependent variables. The usual parameters under consideration are received power level (mean level and instantaneous level), power delay profiles, and Doppler spectrum, among others. In the case of broadband communications in mobile systems with large channel variability, all of the previous parameters must be analyzed in detail. In the case of confined areas, with moderate bandwidth and quasi-static behavior of the transceivers, the estimation of the received power level is the main parameter for initial deployment.

In order to analyze the mean value of received power of a wireless system, it is necessary to consider if the received signals are within the thresholds of sensitivity of the receiver for a given quality of service. To this extent, a link balance calculation is performed, given by

$$P_{RX} = P_{TX} - L_{feed\ TX} + G_{ANT\ TX} - L_{prop} + G_{ANT\ RX} - L_{feed\ RX} \tag{10.1}$$

where
P_{RX} and P_{TX} are the values of received and transmitted power, respectively.
$L_{feed\ TX}$ and $L_{feed\ RX}$ are the losses due to feeding and coupling elements to transmit and receive antennas, respectively.
$G_{ANT\ TX}$ and $G_{ANT\ RX}$ are the gains of the transmitter and receiver antennas, respectively.
L_{prop} is the propagation loss in the path within the transmitter and the receiver.

When the given value of received power P_{RX} is greater than the receiver sensitivity threshold, the communication link can be established. In the case of wireless systems placed within an indoor scenario, such as a household, the transceivers exhibit low transmission power and the values of the antenna gain are moderate. This is due to the fact that the wireless standards usually applied for this type of communication are within the scope of 802.15, mainly ZigBee® and Bluetooth®, which are inherently parameterized for low transmit power. As for the performance of the antennas, usually low profile antennas, such as planar antennas in microstrip or coplanar waveguide technology, or chip antennas are used. The overall size of the devices tends to be minimized, which leads to lower values in antenna gain, usually in the vicinity of 0 to 3 dBi. Therefore, the initial consideration in evaluation of performance in terms of a wireless channel is the influence of the indoor scenario in radio wave propagation losses.

The term L_{prop} that accounts for the losses in the wireless channel can be further expanded as

$$L_{\text{prop}} = L_{\text{basic losses}} + L_{\text{diffraction losses}} + L_{\text{body losses}} \qquad (10.2)$$

where

$L_{\text{basic losses}}$ is the term that accounts for propagation losses due to field decay with distance, considering the influence of the surrounding environment.

$L_{\text{diffraction losses}}$ is the term that accounts for the interaction of the impinging wave with the elements within the scenario, leading to diffraction from one or more sources.

$L_{\text{body losses}}$ is the term that accounts for absorption losses due to the presence of the user body.

Figure 10.1 depicts the radio wave propagation components received by a wireless terminal in a conventional urban environment, in which penetration losses, diffraction losses, and multipath propagation are the main contributions to the overall received power. Each one of the contributions is identified in the previous figure, schematically represented by the corresponding arrow and legend.

Calculation of the propagation losses can be performed either by analytical or by numerical calculation [1–5]. In the case of analytical calculation, there are several models that have been defined by consideration of ideal conditions (i.e., point sources in free space) where subsequently the influence of other elements such as terrain or climate has been introduced. The complexity and variability of the radio wave propagation scenario have led to empirically based models, extracted by nonlinear regression. Some of these models are the following:

- *Okumura-Hata*, based on field measurements for different effective heights and a reference receiver height of 1.5 m. The estimation of propagation losses, which is influenced by the type of environment (urban, suburban, and rural), is given by

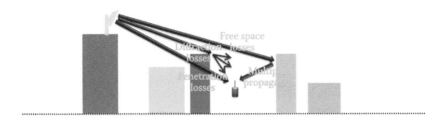

FIGURE 10.1
Propagation mechanisms within a conventional urban environment. Penetration losses (mainly due to buildings and vegetation), diffraction losses, and multipath propagation are the main causes for signal loss in wireless systems. Each one of the components is represented by the corresponding arrow in the figure.

$$L_{\text{prop Okumura-Hata}} = 69.55 + 26.16 \log f - 13.82 \log h_b - a(h_m) + (44.9 - 6.55 \log h_b)\log d \quad (10.3)$$

where

f is the operation frequency in megahertz (valid for a frequency range between 150 and 1500 MHz).

h_t is the effective height of the transmitter antenna in meters (valid in the range between 30 and 200 m).

h_m is the effective height of the receiver antenna in meters (valid in the range between 1 and 10 m).

d is the distance between the transmitter and the receiver in kilometers (valid in the range between 1 and 20 km).

$a(h_m)$ is a height correction factor; the value of this coefficient depends on the type of environment that is considered (urban, suburban, or rural).

- *Cost 231*, obtained by intensive measurements within the framework of COST action 231, to characterize propagation conditions in typical urban scenarios in Europe. The estimation of propagation losses in this case, which takes into account basic propagation losses, multiscreen diffraction, and the last term of roof to street diffraction, is given by

$$L_{\text{prop COST 231}} = 32.45 + 20 \log(f) + 20 \log(d) - 8.2\text{–}10 \log(w) + 10 \log(f) + 20 \log(\Delta h_R)$$
$$+ L_{\text{street axis}} - 18 \log(1 + \Delta h_B) + k_a + k_d\log(f) - 9 \log(b) \quad (10.4)$$

The values of the coefficients in the last expression are given by

$L_{\text{street axis}} = -10 + 0.354\varphi$	for $0 < \varphi < 35°$
$L_{\text{street axis}} = 2.5 + 0.075(\varphi - 35°)$	for $35° < \varphi < 55°$
$L_{\text{street axis}} = 4 - 0.114(\varphi - 55°)$	for $55° < \varphi < 90°$
$k_a = 54$	for $\Delta h_B \geq 0$
$k_a = 54 - 0.8\Delta h_B$	for $\Delta h_B < 0$ and $d \geq 0$
$k_a = 54 - (0.8\Delta h_B)(2d)$	for $\Delta h_B < 0$ and $d < 0.5$
$k_d = 18$	for $\Delta h_B \geq 0$
$k_d = 18 - 15(\Delta h_B/h_R)$	for $\Delta h_B < 0$
$k_f = -4 + 0.75(f/925 - 1)$	for medium-size urban areas
$k_f = -4 + 1.5(f/925 - 1)$	large dense urban areas

where

f is the frequency of operation in megahertz.

d is the distance between the transmitter and the receiver in kilometers.

w is the width of the street where the receiver is located.

h_m is the mean value of the height of the receiver relative to the ground.

h_R is the mean value of the height of buildings.

h_B is the height of the transmitter relative to the ground.

b is the distance between the center points of the buildings.

- *Cost 231 multiwall* is an enhanced model in order to take into account the effect of indoor elements, such as walls and floors. These elements are considered by loss coefficients, which are given by the type of walls (thin, thick) and floors, leading to different values of propagation losses.
- *Ikegami* is based on geometric optics, in which rays are divided into primary and secondary rays, where primary rays are the main contribution (with only one interaction due to diffraction and one reflection), since secondary rays will suffer higher losses. This model is useful for outdoor urban environments, where a uniform building scenario is considered and parameters such as base station and mobile terminal height, street orientation, operation frequency, and distance are considered.
- *Walfish-Bertoni* is a model that can be considered an evolution from the previous Ikegami model. In this case, based on geometric optics, the overall effect of the profile of the surrounding buildings is taken into account. Diffraction losses are taken into account by considering the final roof to street diffraction component and the previous diffraction losses by the rest of the buildings in the profile, which is modeled as a multiscreen diffraction component. Parameters such as the mean height of surrounding buildings, the distance between the transmitter and the receiver, the height of the mobile terminal, or the distance between buildings are taken into account in the model.

The previous empirical methods need additional calculation in order to take into account diffraction losses due to interaction of radio waves (i.e., buildings, vehicles, surrounding vegetation, people, etc.) in the propagation path between wireless transceivers. The calculation of diffraction losses is mainly performed by simplification of Fresnel diffraction integrals to the following types of objects:

- *Knife profile*: the objects are modeled with a sharp profile as compared to the wavelength of the impinging wave.
- *Round profile*: the objects are modeled with a smooth profile, with large contact surface as compared to the wavelength.
- *Grouped objects*: the objects are a collection of closely spaced elements, each one of them with a knife profile.

Empirical methods are strongly dependent on the environment in which the regression was performed to obtain the analytical expressions for path loss, requiring frequent calibration measurements. In order to gain precision in the estimation of path losses, as well as obtaining time-dependent parameters (e.g., power delay profiles), deterministic methods can be used [6–9]. In this latter case, propagation of the electric field in magnitude and phase are calculated within the simulation scenario. Several methods can be applied, such as

- Approximations based on geometrical optics, such as ray tracing or ray launching techniques. Power emitted from the sources is modeled as a set of rays launched from a solid angle, which represent the equivalent wave vectors of the propagating wavefronts.
- Full wave electromagnetic methods, such as finite element, method of moments, finite difference time domain, or finite integration time domain. In this case, Maxwell equations are solved for the entire calculation domain.

An adequate balance between computation time and accuracy is essential to perform valid wireless system planning analysis. Figure 10.2 depicts the trade-off between computational complexity and accuracy from empirical to deterministic and full wave methods.

To illustrate the benefit of applying deterministic methods to analyze wireless system performance, the power distribution of a Bluetooth-based sensor network named HOLTIN (which will be described in detail in the section "Examples of Wireless Systems Applied to AAL") is shown for different network topologies in Figure 10.3.

As can be seen from the power density plots depicted in Figure 10.3, there is a significant change in the values of received power for different positions within the scenario. The topology of the network as well as the position of the user play a key role in the overall performance of the wireless systems. The previous calculations give valuable information in order to determine the regions where connectivity with the Bluetooth host device is available, and therefore, monitoring of vital constants will be achieved successfully.

Once the values of propagation losses have been obtained, the influence of traffic can be taken into account, giving rise to coverage–capacity relations. In the case of a digital system with multiple users, the sensitivity of the receiver can be modeled by the following expression:

$$S\,(\text{dBm}) = -174 + 10\log R\,(\text{bits/s}) + \left(\frac{E_b}{N_o}\right)_{\text{dB}} + F_r\,(\text{dB}) + 10\log\left(\frac{K_{\text{max}} - 1}{K_{\text{max}} - K}\right) \qquad (10.5)$$

where
S is the receiver sensitivity.
R is the binary rate of the transmitter.
E_b/N_o is the energy per bit to interference ratio (considering internal interference, external interference, and noise).
F_r is the noise factor of the receiver.
K_{max} is the maximum number of users allowed in the system in terms of interference condition (also known as pole capacity).
K is the actual number of users in the system.

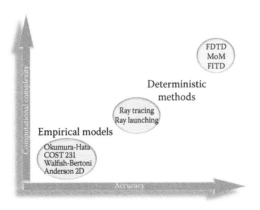

FIGURE 10.2
Trade-off between accuracy and computational complexity from empirical to full wave electromagnetic analysis. Deterministic methods based on ray tracing/ray launching provide an adequate balance between computational complexity and accuracy for medium-sized scenarios.

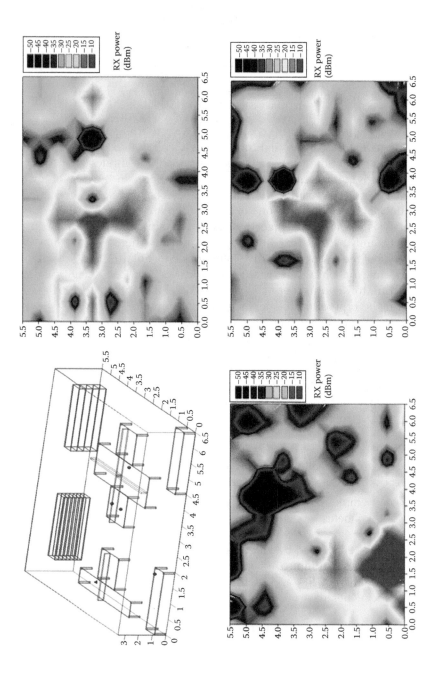

FIGURE 10.3

Power distribution for a Bluetooth sensor network (scale reference in dBm, at an operating frequency of 2.45 GHz) for the transmission of vital constants within an indoor scenario, for different transmitter positions at a vertical cut plane of 1.25 m. As can be seen, power distribution varies as a function of the topology as well as the morphology of the sensor network.

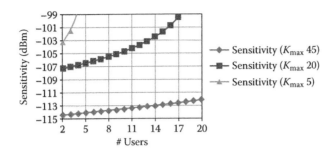

FIGURE 10.4
Coverage–capacity relation for services operating at different bit rates (K_{max} 45 = 100 Kbps, K_{max} 20 = 500 Kbps, and K_{max} 5 = 1 Mbps) as a function of the number of users.

Depending on the bit rate R of the transmitted service, different values of maximum allowed users due to interference (i.e., pole capacity of the system for that particular user) will be possible (the number being lower as the bit rate per user increases). Therefore, the sensitivity of the receiver will vary as a function of the total interference of the system, leading to dynamic values of coverage, which is termed as coverage–capacity relations. The influence on sensitivity for different values of pole capacity (which correspond to bit rates of K_{max} 45 = 100 Kbps, K_{max} 20 = 500 Kbps, and K_{max} 5 = 1 Mbps) as a function of the amount of users is shown in Figure 10.4.

The combination of morphological/topological properties of the radio wave signals with the indoor scenario as well as the coverage–capacity relations determine the overall performance of the resulting heterogeneous wireless systems. This knowledge in combination with careful transceiver design and integrated BASs leads to energy-efficient and performance-oriented systems, as will be seen next.

Wireless Systems Design for Health Monitoring

The analysis of the wireless channel reveals that both topology and morphology modify the received power levels and signal-to-noise ratios. The performance in terms of power consumption is clear, since sensitivity values will differ. Moreover, power consumption is a key parameter in the design and operation of wireless systems. Portable and wearable electronics for wireless health monitoring require extreme miniaturization, and this restricts the available battery size and power drawn. In some applications, even the minute energy harvested from the environment is employed to power these devices. This scenario represents a challenge to the development of the required electronics, in terms of signal acquisition, processing, and transmission. New techniques both at the system and circuit level are needed to achieve the required degree of integration and power consumption. Discrete, lightweight, and comfortable devices are essential for user acceptance in applications demanding long monitoring periods, such as Holter monitors, epilepsy diagnosis, or brain–computer interfaces [10]. In the following, some techniques aimed to face these demands are described.

System Architecture

Figure 10.5 shows a typical wireless sensor node architecture for health monitoring. The different elements that form the system are described below.

- *Sensor*: a device in charge of sensing the required parameter. Depending on the parameter, it can be an electrode, a temperature, etc.
- *Analog front-end*: an analog interface circuit that processes the sensor signal. Typical tasks performed by this block are amplification, filtering, offset cancellation, temperature compensation, etc.
- *Analog-to-digital converter (ADC)*: this block converts the analog signal delivered by the preceding front-end to digital form. In wearable wireless health monitoring systems, the critical ADC requirement is often low power consumption, while the required speed and resolution are usually modest.
- *Processor*: it performs the required signal processing in the digital domain and controls the overall system. In particular, it may run the communication protocols required by the transceiver unit.
- *Transceiver*: this block includes the wireless transmitter and receiver to communicate with other wireless devices. Typically the transmitter and the receiver share some circuits such as frequency synthesizers and oscillators.
- *Memory*: it allows storage of signal, control, and configuration data. Usually an EEPROM memory is employed, allowing simple rewriting operations. The memory size is strongly determined by the communication standard employed, as well as the sampling rate and resolution of the ADC.
- *Power unit*: this block includes the power source and energy management circuits to properly supply the different modules of the system. The power source is typically a battery, although in energy harvesting transceivers, this battery may be supplemented (or even replaced) by an energy harvester. This harvester is a transducer that acquires energy from the environment (for instance, a solar cell to acquire light energy, a piezoelectric transducer to get energy from movement or vibrations, a thermoelectric generator to get thermal energy, an antenna to acquire energy from RF signals, etc.). The energy management circuits are mainly based on DC/DC or AC/DC regulators, depending on the energy source.

The analog front-end, the ADC, and the receiver in the transceiver are critical elements in terms of achieving a low-energy, minimum size device. In the next paragraphs, design techniques proposed by some of the authors to build these modules will be described.

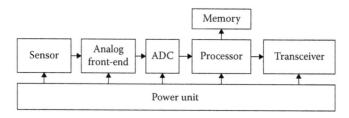

FIGURE 10.5
Diagram of a typical wireless monitoring system.

Analog Front-End

Figure 10.6 shows a typical analog front-end employed in monitoring of biological signals [11], such as the electrocardiogram (ECG), electroencephalogram (EEG), electromyogram (EMG), or evoked potentials (EPs). The differential signal coming from the two electrodes is applied to a preamplifier with high input resistance. The preamplifier also requires low noise and removal of the baseline drift of the input signal. This drift can originate from electrode changes due to perspiration, respiration, or movement, and can be more relevant in tests recorded during exercise. Particularly, in ECG recording, measures of the ST segment (used, for example, for diagnostic ischemia) can be strongly influenced by this drift. To avoid degradation of the biosignal record by baseline drift, it needs to be properly removed. Hence, a high-pass filtering is typically applied to minimize the baseline drift generated by the electrode. This high-pass filter is usually external and is the main limitation for achieving a fully integrated front-end.

Then a second amplification stage is applied where most of the gain is provided. Next, low-pass filtering is required to filter out all the frequency components beyond the maximum frequency of interest (which is around 150–200 Hz for ECG signals and in any case less than around 10 kHz for other biosignals). This filter removes out-of-band noise and interference and serves as an antialiasing filter for the subsequent ADC. Finally, a buffer is employed to drive the ADC.

A compact implementation for the shaded elements of Figure 10.6 (the preamplifier and the high-pass filter) based on quasi-floating gate (QFG) techniques [12] is shown in Figure 10.7. Using QFG input transistors in the amplifier, the DC input voltage is set to the negative rail thanks to the large leakage resistance of the pull-down n-channel MOSFET (metal–oxide–semiconductor field-effect transistor) (NMOS) transistors of Figure 10.7a, without altering AC operation. The circuit can provide N voltage gain values $A_1, A_2,\ldots,$ A_N selectable by properly activating switches SW_i. Two $N + 1$ input QFG transistors form the input differential pair of the amplifier. N input branches with capacitances of values $A_1C, A_2C,\ldots, A_NC$ are connected to the selection switches, whereas the input branch with capacitance C is connected to the output. The resulting capacitive feedback leads to an input resistance considerably larger than in conventional inverting amplifiers with resistive feedback, which are also subject to gain errors if the impedance of the source is not very low. This is a key performance issue to interface ECG and EEG electrodes.

Due to the amplifier feedback, a variation Δv_{din} in the differential input voltage leads to a net charge transfer to the feedback capacitors of $A_iC\Delta v_{din}$ ($i = 1, 2,\ldots, N$ depending on the gain selected), and therefore to a variation Δv_{dout} in the differential output voltage of $v_{dout} = A_i\Delta v_{din}$, yielding a voltage gain A_i.

To reduce noise, a PMOS input amplifier has been designed. The required amplifier was implemented using a modified version of a differential two-stage Miller topology, as shown in Figure 10.7. Note that feedback is only in AC, so the DC offset of the amplifier needs to be compensated in order not to appear amplified by the same gain as the signal at the

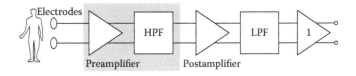

FIGURE 10.6
Analog front-end for biosignals.

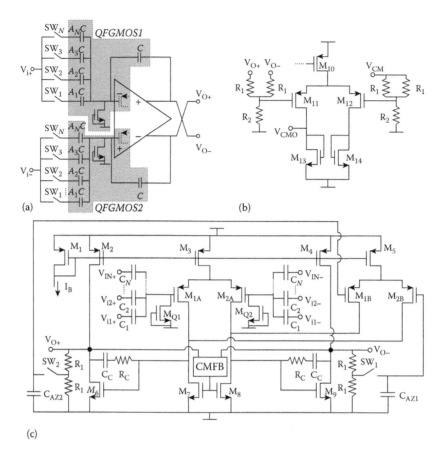

FIGURE 10.7
Programmable preamplifier. (a) Diagram, (b) CMFB circuit, and (c) schematic.

output. To this purpose, an autozeroing technique has been implemented in the circuit of Figure 10.7c. It consists of the differential pair M_{1B}–M_{2B}, switches SW_1 and SW_2, capacitors C_{AZ1} and C_{AZ2}, and two resistive dividers. The dividers are used to shift the output voltages close to the negative rail. This minimizes the supply requirements of the autozeroing amplifier. The offset cancellation, based on a technique described in Ref. [13], is as follows: during an initial phase, the input is shorted, so that the differential input voltage corresponds to the amplifier offset. Switches SW_1 and SW_2 are closed, and the output, once attenuated and level-shifted by the resistor dividers, is applied to capacitances C_{AZ1} and C_{AZ2}. The resulting feedback sets the voltages at these capacitances so that the differential DC in the autozeroing pair M_{1B}–M_{2B} exactly compensates the differential DC of the amplifier pair M_{1A}–M_{2A} caused by the input DC offset. Then, switches SW_1 and SW_2 are opened and capacitors C_{AZ1} and C_{AZ2} keep the charge required for compensating the offset. The input short ceases and normal operation then starts. The refreshing time required for this autozeroing can be very large (several seconds as verified experimentally) since the circuit operates in ac. Hence, a small DC drift of the output caused by a slight discharge of C_{AZ1}–C_{AZ2} is unimportant.

The common-mode feedback (CMFB) circuit is a simple PMOS differential pair with resistive input dividers. These are also used to shift the output voltages close to the negative rail and to minimize supply requirements of the CMFB circuit as shown in Figure 10.7b. The gate of transistor M_{10} is connected to those of M_1–M_5 in the amplifier.

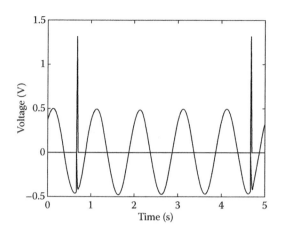

FIGURE 10.8
Output voltage at 1 Hz and autozeroing clock signal.

The circuit of Figure 10.7 was fabricated in a 0.5 μm complementary metal–oxide–semi-conductor (CMOS) n-well process. The voltage gains implemented were 1, 2, 4, and 8, respectively. Note that with gain equal to 1, the circuit just eliminates the baseline drift and buffers the electrodes without providing any gain. A single 1.5 V supply voltage was employed, and the common-mode output voltage was set to 0.75 V. The unit capacitance C was 0.25 pF. Bias current I_B was set to 20 μA. Figure 10.8 shows the measured differential output voltage for a 1 Hz, 0.25 V_{pp} input sinusoid and the amplifier gain set to 4, as well as the pulses of the autozeroing phase (which takes place when these pulses occur). The same output is obtained for different DC input levels; thus, the circuit properly cancels the DC input. Note that autozeroing intervals as long as 4 s can be employed without significant degradation in the output voltage. Note also how the circuit can operate even for these very low frequencies as required for biosignal analog front-ends, due to the extremely large pull-down QFG resistance values.

Analog-to-Digital Conversion

The ADC required is a critical module in terms of power consumption. Specific designs are required to maximize the efficiency in the use of the energy available, exploiting the features of biological signals. These signals are typically very slow (tens of hertz). In this context, Sigma-Delta architectures are advantageous.

As an example of ADC suited to this scenario, Figure 10.9 shows an extremely low-power (160 nW), low-voltage (1.2 V), 50 Hz Nyquist frequency Sigma-Delta modulator with 10 b resolution aimed to ECG signals [14]. The converter has been implemented using a second-order switched capacitor (SC) Sigma-Delta modulator topology. This architecture has been shown to be very power efficient to deal with biomedical signals [15,16]. The architecture is composed of two correlated double sampling integrators: a comparator and a 1 b digital-to-analog converter.

To achieve low energy consumption, a simple and efficient low-voltage two-stage operational amplifier with class AB output stage presented in Ref. [17] has been used. On the other hand, to allow rail-to-rail operation in switches that require it (those highlighted in Figure 10.9) with supply voltage near to one transistor threshold, the QFG technique is also employed [18].

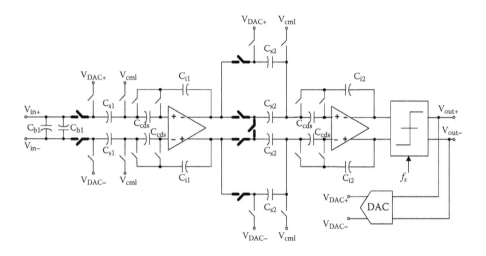

FIGURE 10.9
Sigma-Delta modulator (critical switches highlighted).

The Sigma-Delta modulator was implemented in the same 0.5 μm CMOS technology as the circuit of Figure 10.3. Figure 10.10 shows the chip microphotograph. A sinusoidal input of 5 Hz and 362 mV$_{pp}$ has been used to characterize the dynamic performance. Figure 10.11 shows the output spectrum of the modulator, where an signal-to-noise-and-distortion ratio (SNDR) of 60.82 dB is measured. Under these conditions, the power consumption is only of 160 nW (110 nW of static power consumption).

Low-Power Receivers

There are several choices available for the architecture of the receiver. Besides certain solutions suited to particular applications (like super-regenerative receivers [19]), they can be grouped into two main categories: heterodyne and homodyne (also named direct conversion or zero-IF) receivers. The most employed heterodyne architectures are superheterodyne receivers with a fixed, relatively high intermediate frequency (IF) or two different IF sections. A variant suited to highly integrated receivers is the low-IF architecture.

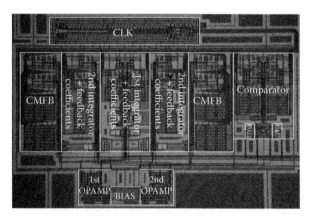

FIGURE 10.10
Microphotograph of the Sigma-Delta modulator.

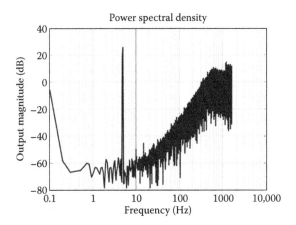

FIGURE 10.11
Output spectrum with an input signal of 362 mV$_{pp}$ and 5 Hz.

The conventional superheterodyne receiver achieves high sensitivity and its design is well known. However, this is not the best solution in terms of power consumption, and it requires highly selective filters for image rejection and channel selection, which cannot be implemented on a chip. Typically external surface acoustic wave (SAW) resonators are used. Therefore, this topology is not suited to energy-efficient wearable devices. The two basic architectures that allow achieving high integration density and low power consumption at the same time are the low-IF and zero-IF topologies. Each one has inherent advantages and shortcomings.

Low-IF Receiver

Figure 10.12a shows a typical architecture of a low-IF receiver. The signal is down-converted to a low-IF frequency (typically in the order of the channel spacing) by a quadrature mixer, and then amplified, filtered, digitized, and demodulated. The main advantage of this

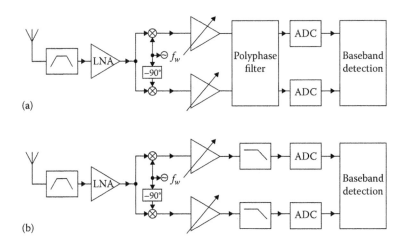

FIGURE 10.12
(a) Low-IF receiver. (b) Zero-IF receiver.

solution is that it keeps the signal spectrum out of baseband, thus overcoming two important signal degradations typical at baseband frequencies:

1. *DC offsets*. These offsets may arise from the inherent DC offset of baseband signal processing circuits, but their main (and most important) contribution in wireless receivers is due to the self-mixing at the mixer. Due to the imperfect isolation, in practice, from the local oscillator (LO) output to the input of the mixer, the LO signal is coupled to the mixer input, and as a result of the mixer action, a DC component appears. The level of this offset may be orders of magnitude larger than the desired signal, so if it is not removed, it leads to strong signal degradation or even saturation of the baseband circuits. This offset tends to be slowly time-varying, which reduces the effectiveness of conventional offset cancellation solutions (e.g., autozero techniques). In low-IF receivers, by processing the signal at a nonzero IF, the inherent band-pass response of the baseband circuits efficiently removes this offset.

2. *Flicker noise*. The flicker or $1/f$ noise of CMOS circuits may be the dominant noise source up to moderately high frequencies. The corner frequency (boundary between dominance of flicker and thermal noise) in modern submicron CMOS technologies may be as high as hundreds of kilohertz. Hence, as in low-IF topologies, the signal spectrum is far enough from DC; signal processing in the IF chain can remove most of the flicker noise power. In order to reduce power consumption, the IF is typically chosen large enough to avoid limitation by flicker noise, but not too much to decrease power consumption. A typical choice in Bluetooth is IF = 2 MHz.

Despite these advantages, the low-IF solution has some shortcomings:

1. *Need for image rejection*. Since the IF is nonzero, rejection of the image spectrum must be considered. In the low-IF receiver, the image spectrum is rejected thanks to the independent processing of the I and Q signal components. However, a complex polyphase band-pass filter as shown in Figure 10.12a is usually needed for channel filtering, which requires good linearity and good gain and phase matching between I and Q components.

2. *Increased power consumption*. At least in principle, processing at a nonzero IF requires more power than processing at the baseband (which corresponds to the lowest possible frequencies). However, for this to be true, the extra complexity required when processing at baseband frequencies to compensate for the degradation due to noise and offset must be small.

3. *More sensitivity to I and Q gain/phase mismatch*. Mismatch in the gain of the I and Q channels, as well as in the orthogonality of the quadrature LO signals for down-mixing, is more severe in low-IF architecture since it has a direct impact on the rejection of the image band. Considering typical mismatch in conventional CMOS processes, image rejection may be in the order of 35 dB.

Zero-IF Receiver

Figure 10.12b shows a typical zero-IF receiver. It is based on the direct conversion of the RF signal to baseband, allowing the use of simple low-pass filters for channel selection. This is the simplest receiver and features important advantages.

1. *No image rejection required.* In the zero-IF architecture, there are no image frequencies since the signal is directly converted to baseband, i.e., there is no intermediate frequency. Stated otherwise, the signal itself is its own image.
2. *Simpler channel filtering.* Moreover, the channel filters are simpler low-pass filters operating at lower frequencies. Band-pass channel filtering requires more power than a low-pass filter of the same bandwidth and order.

This simplicity makes zero-IF receivers the most promising choice in terms of cost, integration density, and power consumption. However, in this receiver, the signal is at baseband so it suffers from the degradations just mentioned (mainly DC offset and flicker noise). Thus, these problems must be properly solved.

The simplest way to get rid of DC offset is to use a simple RC high-pass filter after the mixer. This has typically been done for modulations with negligible DC components (like FSK signals with a high modulation index) used in paging receivers [20]. There are other solutions, typically based on feedback loops. However, they are more complex and usually do not remove completely time-varying offset.

Depending on the bandwidth and resolution required, the ADCs in Figure 10.11 can consume a large percentage of the total power. In ultralow-power applications, alternative demodulation schemes not requiring multibit A/D conversion may be advantageous. Among other techniques, those based on detection of zero crossing of linear combinations of the I and Q signal components are widely used due to their simplicity and performance.

Examples of Wireless Systems Applied to AAL

Once the impact of the wireless channel and the design strategies for optimizing transceiver design have been analyzed, examples of real systems and the standardization bodies will be discussed. It is compulsory to state that advances in information and communication technologies are bringing new opportunities to health care applications. Improvements in medical devices, standard-based designs, and ubiquitous solutions focused to patient oriented services, the so-called patient empowerment [21], can increase the users' quality of life and the efficiency of the health system. These evolutions are making possible new scenarios and applications like AAL, home monitoring, chronic disease management, or health and fitness, characterized by the user's ability to get around and perform their daily activities while being followed up.

Ubiquitous health (uHealth) services are based on the well-known ambient intelligence (AmI) [22] concept; furthermore, they rely on wearable monitoring systems that acquire the user's biomedical and environmental information (blood pressure, weight, ECG, temperature, and fall detection, among others) and transmit it to be analyzed later by health care staff [23]. In these systems, the availability of wearable devices [24–26] with features such as low form factor (reduced dimensions and low weight), ergonomic design, wireless communication, and enough intelligence is essential in order to perform nonintrusive data acquisition, help users to self-manage their monitoring process, and therefore improve their quality of life [27].

Within uHealth services, indoor and outdoor management of chronic cardiovascular disease is the most widespread health care application due to its high prevalence in society

[28], and especially those ambulatory ECG monitoring applications aimed at following up patients that suffer from no-risk sporadic arrhythmias and syncopes. Since these symptoms may occur occasionally, the ambulatory services require long-term monitoring periods in order to acquire the outstanding data and diagnose the patient's cardiovascular disease. In this regard, two main ECG remote monitoring systems with clinical utility are used by health care staff: the conventional Holter device and insertable cardiac monitors like the so-called Reveal® system from Medtronic [29]. A large number of research and innovation proposals that are focused on ECG monitoring have been developed over recent years: CardioNet, Biotronik, CardioSmart, V-Patch system, Alive cardiac monitor, and the CorBELT device are some of the most important commercial solutions [30–35]. These systems provide functionalities (real-time monitoring, cardiac event detection, portable/wearable design, wireless communication, etc.) that are required in any innovative uHealth service, but suffer from not being clinically evaluated enough. Next, a new ambulatory ECG monitoring system developed to fulfill the entire health care staff's functional requirements, and evaluated from clinical, economical, and user satisfaction points of view, is described, for example, wireless systems applied to AAL scenarios.

HOLTIN Service

HOLTIN (acronym for Intelligent Holter) [36,37] is a uHealth service for ambulatory ECG monitoring of patients that suffer from cardiovascular diseases whose symptomatic signs are paroxysmal arrhythmias (supraventricular tachycardia, bradycardia, atrial fibrillation, etc.) and sporadic faints. The service has been designed to fulfill the health care staff's requirements and improve key issues of conventional ECG systems like diagnostic performance, operation autonomy, outstanding data availability, and wearable and user-friendly design, among others (see Table 10.1).

As with any new uHealth application, the HOLTIN service has been clinically compared with conventional Holter device in a pilot project, which has also included cost-effectiveness analysis and questionnaires for patient/cardiologist satisfaction [38,39]. With more than 100 patients evaluated, the main conclusions obtained are as follows:

- The HOLTIN service provides greater diagnostic performance thanks to long-term monitoring and improved detection of arrhythmias. This new service led to implant one implantable cardioverter defibrillator (ICD) and five pacemakers in patients that were not previously diagnosed with the Holter device.

TABLE 10.1

Comparative Table of Ambulatory ECG Monitoring Systems

	Insertable Monitors	HOLTIN	Conventional Holter
Invasive	Yes	No	No
Limited Memory	Yes	No	Yes
Portability	+++	++	+
Operation Autonomy	Until battery end (12 months)	Variable (7–30 days) Rechargeable battery	24–48 h
Price	+++	+	+
Configurability	+++	+++	+
Data Access	+	+++	+

- The HOLTIN service provides high comfort and satisfaction levels in most patients. However, its usability should be improved to allow elderly people to self-manage the service.

Technological Platform

The HOLTIN service is based on a wearable system for long-term and continuous cardiac activity monitoring. The system architecture is shown in Figure 10.13 and consists of three elements: wearable front-end, gateway device, and management center.

The wearable front-end is a smart device placed on the patient's chest and it performs the acquisition and processing of standard ECG lead II. The device is designed with a low form factor, very low power consumption, and ergonomic design. These features together with using disposable electrodes provide a high device wearability and patient comfort level. Figure 10.14 shows a real view of the front-end device. The device is able to detect specific cardiac events suffered by the patient, store the outstanding information, and transmit it later to a near gateway device through Bluetooth technology.

Since the front-end device is battery powered, low voltage–low power (LV–LP) hardware design has been accomplished in order to obtain long-term operation autonomy. The core of the device is an ultralow-power microcontroller that performs all the required processing tasks: signal A/D conversion, heart rhythm and cardiac event detection, information storage, etc. The technical features of the microcontroller together with optimized software development allow the front-end device to have very low power consumption. Moreover, several volatile and nonvolatile memories with low-power consumption and

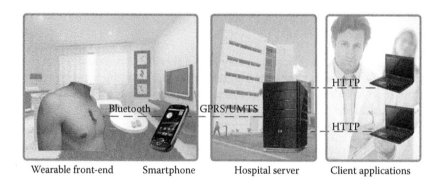

| Wearable front-end | Smartphone | Hospital server | Client applications |

FIGURE 10.13
HOLTIN service architecture.

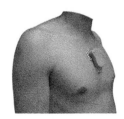 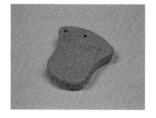

FIGURE 10.14
Real view of wearable front-end device.

high data access rate are included in the front-end device; volatile memory is used for temporary storage of the ECG signal while it is processed, and nonvolatile memory is used for permanent storage of cardiac event information for later transmission. Wireless communication of the front-end device is performed through Bluetooth technology implemented in a single-chip solution. The wireless component includes all the hardware and software resources required to use Bluetooth technology: radio frequency block, low firmware layers (baseband, link manager), and internal microcontroller with high software layers (logical link control, serial port emulation, application). This single-chip solution is highly optimized in order to reduce the power consumption of the front-end device.

The gateway device is implemented in a commercial smartphone with customized service software, and performs data transmission from a wearable front-end device to a management center through Bluetooth technology and 3G/4G mobile phone network. This bridge device manages all the communications, wireless connections, storage of patient's information, and visual/in voice alarm messages. With this aim, a customized software application based on Android OS is implemented in the smartphone device. In this way, minimal intervention of the patient is required thanks to the whole device functionality achieved in an autonomous way; that is, wireless communications are established without requiring patient confirmation. A smartphone device provides high usability and user-friendly interfaces to the patient and HOLTIN service.

The management center is located at a hospital and is based on a client–server paradigm. This element receives and stores the patient's acquired information. These data can be analyzed later by a health care specialist in order to diagnose the patient's disease. Moreover, this reception center stores all information required by service operation: patient's demographic information, a wearable front-end device assigned to each patient, time of data reception, etc.

Functional Description

The HOLTIN service consists of an extremely elaborate functional model that includes the whole requirements of health care staff and takes into account the technological solutions that make possible to fulfill them. Next, the main functional aspects of the HOLTIN service are briefly described.

Cardiac Event Detection and Storage

A front-end device is able to detect and store a patient's outstanding cardiac information in two different operation modes:

- *Automatic detection*: the device performs continuous ECG signal processing and detects automatically specific types of cardiac arrhythmic events based on the patient's heart rhythm and several diagnostic settings established by the health care specialist. The front-end device is able to acquire the outstanding data associated with three cardiac events: tachycardia, bradycardia, and asystolia.
- *Patient notification*: the device receives storage notifications through a gateway device when some outstanding symptomatic event (syncope, dizziness, or even arrhythmia) occurs. These notifications are achieved by means of pushing a specific key in the smartphone device. This action triggers the establishment of Bluetooth communication with the front-end device and the exchange of service data.

In any operating mode, the device always stores a time period of the patient's ECG signal around the cardiac event, allowing the health care specialist to have the outstanding diagnostic information. The diagnostic criteria and storage times are the front-end device's configurable operational parameters, which provide a high versatility level to the HOLTIN service.

Data Communication

The detected cardiac events are temporarily stored in a front-end device. When storage capacity reaches a specific and configurable level, the device establishes Bluetooth communication with a smartphone device in order to transmit all the ECG information. In case wireless connection fails because devices can be out of range, the front-end device is able to continue the storage of new cardiac events until communication is available. In this way, a permanent Bluetooth communication with high power requirements is avoided, and no patient's outstanding information is lost. In a similar way, the smartphone device establishes 3G/4G communication with the management center in order to transmit the cardiac event information. If connection has not been established because the patient is at an out-of-coverage location or the reception server is down, the smartphone device is able to store the information for later communication attempts. These functional features of front-end and smartphone devices ensure the health care specialist has all the patient information as soon as the environment and communication technologies make it possible.

Once the patient's information is received at the management center, the health care specialist can access to it through a specific client application. This application provides all the required functionalities in order to diagnose patient cardiac disease: visualization, amplitude and time measurement, medical reports, operational front-end device parameters, etc. Figure 10.15 shows a screenshot of the HOLTIN service client application.

Alarm Notifications and Messages

The HOLTIN service includes several alarms related to functional operation. On the one hand, a low battery alarm indicates that the battery in the front-end device should be

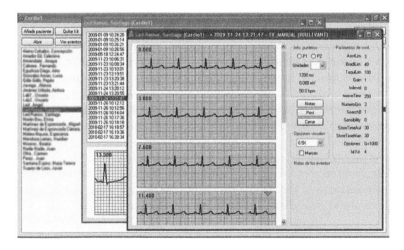

FIGURE 10.15
Screenshot of HOLTIN client application.

changed and recharged. For this aim, the device has been designed with an easy mechanism allowing the patient to remove the battery with minimal effort. The use of rechargeable and removable batteries makes it possible to have a long-term and quasi-continuous monitoring service. On the other hand, a low-quality signal alarm indicates that the ECG signal acquisition is being performed without correct quality, usually due to poor electrode contact or front-end device movements. The patient must correctly replace the device and switch on again. All these alarm notifications are shown to the patient through visual and voice messages in the smartphone device.

The smartphone device also shows specific messages when an outstanding symptomatic event is notified by the patient. These messages make it possible to know whether the notification has been correctly processed or, on the other hand, it has failed. This method of operation improves the usability and user-friendly features of the HOLTIN service.

Standardization in uHealth Services

Solutions based on electronic health care record (EHR) storage, standardized communication within the components of a monitoring system, and intersystem coordination are essential features in any uHealth application in order to exploit clinically all the information gathered [40–42]. At present, several norms for medical information interoperability are being developed by the main organizations of standardization: DICOM [43] for medical imaging and communication, HL7 [44] focused on medical message exchange, EN13606 [45] for interoperable data exchange with EHR, and ISO/IEEE 11073 [46] oriented to medical device communication. The integration in the use of so many standards and their huge-scale implementation is a complex method that requires external associations to play an important role. In this integration effort, two initiatives stand out: integrating the Healthcare Enterprise (IHE) [47], which is an organization that aims to adopt the most suitable standards for each health care service, and Continua Health Alliance [48], which is a nonprofit alliance of technology and health companies to establish interoperable personal health systems.

Actually each manufacturer provides its own medical devices and communication protocols making it possible to build only proprietary health care solutions. Thus, a standardized end-to-end communication framework is required in order to solve the interoperability problem that now exists. With patient surroundings in mind, there is a need for developing open sensors that allow transparent integration and plug-and-play interoperability of monitoring devices and systems. To this aim, several protocols have been proposed, but the ISO/IEEE 11073 standard has reached the highest development and adoption level.

Originally focused on covering medical device communication at the Point of Care (ISO/IEEE 11073 PoC) of the patient [49], the emergence of new uHealth scenarios has made essential its evolution toward a more lightweight version focused on personal health devices: the so-called ISO/IEEE 11073 PHD version [50]. The standard is developed by the PHD Working Group, and the results obtained are adopted by Continua Health Alliance for medical device certification. Figure 10.16 shows the standard method for medical device interoperability.

Next, the main features of the ISO/IEEE 11073 PHD standard and its implementation in wearable devices with processing and memory constraints are described.

ISO/IEEE 11073 Standard for Personal Medical Devices

The ISO/IEEE 11073 family of standards has undergone an evolutionary process from the beginning of its development to the present. The development of new wearable medical

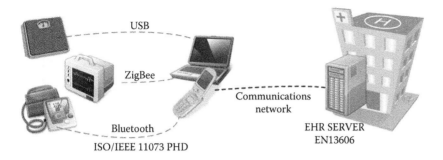

FIGURE 10.16
Standardized monitoring system.

devices and wireless low power technologies such as Bluetooth or ZigBee and the increase in broadband accesses to multimedia networks have made the standard evolve toward an optimized version adapted to ubiquitous scenarios and personal health devices: the so-called ISO/IEEE 11073 PHD version. The standard has thoroughly simplified the architecture of the protocol into three different models (see Figure 10.17):

- A *domain information model* (DIM) represents the medical device and its functionality through a set of objects and attributes. Attributes describe the device's measurement data that are sent to the manager, and elements that control the behavior of the agent. The ASN.1 notation is used for describing the information related to the model.

- A *service model* provides methods to access DIM's data exchanged between an agent and a manager.

- A *communication model* describes the network architecture in which several agents communicate with a single manager via point-to-point connections. This model describes a finite state machine that controls the system behavior.

ISO/IEEE 11073 PHD defines a protocol stack that makes possible the connection between agents and managers. This stack is divided into three levels (see Figure 10.17):

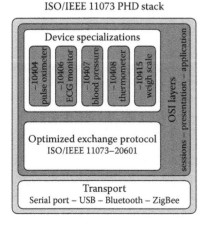
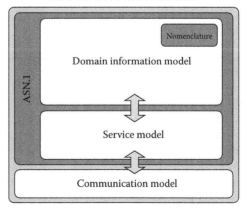

FIGURE 10.17
ISO/IEEE 11073 PHD architecture.

- *Device specializations*: each type of a medical device is specified in a specialization as a set of model descriptions that include all the objects and attributes related to the device's characteristics and functionalities. At this time, the standard has adopted the most basic device specializations (blood pressure, thermometer, ECG basic monitor, and weigh scale, among others), but new medical devices are being continuously added.

- *Optimized exchange protocol*: this core layer defines the architecture of the standard (DIM, service model, and communication model) and consists of several components: medical and technical terminology framework, messages and instructions to retrieve data from agents, modeling objects, communication's state management, etc.

- *Transport layer*: data transmission is held over wired/wireless transport technologies of which specifications are out of the standard scope. This layer only specifies the basic requirements (type and characteristics of communication channels) that the transport technology must support. Thus, special interest groups have developed specific application profiles for technologies like USB, Bluetooth, and ZigBee, which refer to the ISO/IEEE 11073 PHD standard for being used in health applications.

The development of the ISO/IEEE 11073 PHD standard requires to define a set of closed conditions where it should be used. These are called use cases (UCs) and claim to collect both the standard's potential application and user's requirements. Advances in information and communication technologies together with the appearance of uHealth applications have forced the development of new UCs: healthy living, fitness, AAL, and home monitoring, among others. All these UCs have been arranged in three main groups: *disease management, health and wellness,* and *elderly monitoring*.

The ISO/IEEE 11073 PHD architecture, and especially the object-oriented paradigm used in DIM, is one of the main features and advantages of the standard. As it combines basic classes with extending/adding attributes when needed, new medical devices can be brought into the specialization list. With this in mind, a wearable front-end device of the HOLTIN service allows it to be used not only as a proof of the concept of adopted basic ECG specialization but also to propose a new advanced ECG device specialization with diagnostic functionalities added.

Implementation in Wearable Medical Devices

Due to new uHealth services, a double aim must be overcome in the implementation of the ISO/IEEE 11073 PHD standard: (1) the incorporation of new wired/wireless technologies such as USB, Bluetooth, and ZigBee; and (2) the reduction of standard complexity in order for it to be used in low voltage–low power devices with processing and memory constraints. Thus, the RAM available in most common ZigBee devices based on system-on-chip solutions is a few kilobytes, and it must be shared between application and communication protocol stack. Depending on the ISO/IEEE 11073 PHD device specialization to be implemented, the size of incoming and outgoing protocol messages could require as much memory as 64 and 8 kB, respectively. In these situations, it is really difficult to implement the standard into embedded and wearable devices [51,52].

In order to optimize resources and reduce power consumption in agents, a pattern methodology to implement the ISO/IEEE 11073 PHD standard has been proposed [53]. Several

TABLE 10.2

Comparative Table between Different Approaches

	Memory Needs	Processor Needs	Power Consumption
One process	++++	+	+
OS-based	+++	++	++
Multithread	++	+	+
Pseudocode	+	++	++

software implementation approaches can be used depending on factors such as memory space, microcontroller resources, real-time operating system (RTOS) type, wireless communication stack, etc. The main approaches are as follows [54]:

- *One process with nonblocking functions*: all the application protocol units are managed in one piece, and the system uses nonblocking functions in order to process write/read operations.

- *Multiprocess within an operating system*: each transmission channel has two processes: the writer one focused on formatting and transmission of protocol data units, and the reader one for reception and matching of data according to pattern methodology. Thus, data units are processed part by part reducing the needs of the RAM.

- *Multithread implementation*: it consists of a threaded application where the threading algorithm is optimized for implementing the ISO/IEEE 11073 PHD standard.

- *Pseudocode-based implementation*: this approach improves the footprint and memory resources by means of using a set of high-level instructions (pseudocode) that represent blocking operations. The tasks are executed by a pseudocode *ad hoc* virtual machine.

A qualitative comparison between the different approaches is given in Table 10.2. As is shown, there are compromises among memory needs, processor usage, and power consumption, which indicates that the suitability of each one for a specific low voltage–low power device depends on its own features.

Integration of AAL in the Home Environment

In order to control and optimize the use of wireless systems in AAL, with a large number of services and nodes, BASs are introduced for overall control purposes. Moreover, the concept of assisted living systems fits perfectly well into the new research field of AmI. The ambition of ambient intelligent systems is to enhance the quality of human life when living, working, in leisure time, and so on. AmI systems are characterized by distributed sensing, actuating, and computing components and the use of an intelligent and unobtrusive human system interface.

Applications of AmI technology can be conceived in many areas, for example, intelligent working environments, home automation, hotels, hospitals, etc. It is clear that there is huge potential in the area of living assistance for handicapped and elderly people suffering from all kinds of disabilities.

In this context, AmI systems represent a new generation of systems that show the following characteristics [55]:

- Invisible, i.e., embedded in clothes, watches, glasses, etc.
- Mobile, i.e., being carried around.
- Spontaneous (*ad hoc*) communication among the nodes.
- Heterogeneous and hierarchical, i.e., they comprise different kinds of system nodes regarding their computational power and rendered functionality.
- Context-aware, i.e., they are aware of their local environment and spontaneously exchange information with similar nodes in their neighborhood, taking into account different privacy policies.
- Anticipatory, i.e., acting on their own behalf without explicit extrinsic requests.
- Natural communication with users by voice and gestures instead of keyboard, mouse, or text on screens.
- Natural interaction with users by means of devices they are used to, e.g., clothing, watches, TV, smartphones, household appliances.
- Adaptive, i.e., capable of reacting to all abnormal and exceptional situations in a flexible way.

In order to achieve all these characteristics, AmI systems and all the involved devices must be equipped with some kind of intelligence. On the other hand, with the aforementioned characteristics, AmI systems apparently bear some interesting potential for building energy management systems (BEMSs) and home care systems (HCSs). These two concepts of systems are described next.

Building Energy Management Systems

BEMSs have a considerable impact on the control of building services. This concept was developed 20 years ago, but it came into focus only after the introduction of electronic devices that are capable of retaining data for the purpose of managing services such as power, access control, security, lighting, and heating. There are many terms used for BEMSs, such as building management systems (BMSs), energy management systems (EMSs), and BASs. All these refer to the same equipment—BEMSs.

In order to establish a definition, BEMS is a computer-aided program installed in a building in order to control the mechanical and electrical equipment and installations such as ventilation, lighting, power systems, fire systems, access systems, and security systems. Thus, BEMSs have a great impact on the control of the building service plant and energy efficiency.

The ancestors of BEMSs were electromechanical systems, but the microelectronic and computing revolution in recent years has changed the outlook of BEMSs.

One of the benefits of BEMSs is constant monitoring of the building and the ability to recall the monitored data at a later time. This enables technicians and the engineers to develop a better understanding of the buildings. As a result, it leads to improvement of the building and energy saving.

Home Care Systems

Living assistance systems that are focused on the support of people with special needs (elderly, disabled, etc.) in their own homes are called HCSs [56].

The aim of an HCS is to allow assisted people to live better and for longer in their preferred environment at home, while retaining their independence, even when they have handicaps or medical diseases. As illustrated in Figure 10.18, the HCS domain can roughly be structured into emergency assistance services, autonomy enhancement services, and comfort services.

First, an AmI approach for HCSs is discussed. The system is composed of three subsystems: the body area network (BAN), the home network (HAN), and the central processing node, which also acts as a gateway to the Internet and other external telecommunication services like the telephone network [55].

The BAN is composed of special sensors that monitor body vital functions such as blood pressure, temperature, and pulse frequency, and transmit their results to the body gateway via wireless connection. The body gateway collects the measurements from the different sensors and periodically transmits them to the central station for further processing. The body network is invisibly embedded in clothes such as shirts, in watches, and in glasses so that the handicapped and elderly persons do not have to put on those sensors explicitly; in fact, they should not even be aware that sensors exist.

The HAN consists of a different kind of electronic devices (sensors, actuators, displays, etc.) attached to walls in rooms for collecting and exchanging data about the behavior of the person under observation. Part of the HAN might also include loudspeakers, microphones, and video cameras for communicating with the person. It is assumed that video cameras are usually switched off; they will be activated only after detection of an emergency or under an explicit order of the patient. This option is only available in order to provide external medical personnel the opportunity to look at the patient. This constraint is very important and will guarantee the privacy of patients under observation. Nowadays, manufacturers are working in miniaturizing all these devices decreasing their size in order to define such an *invisible network*.

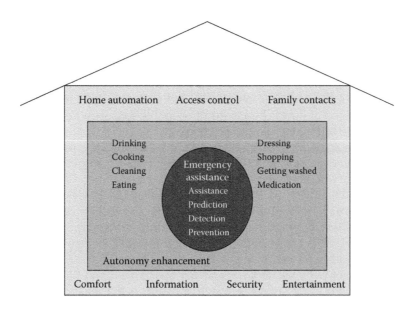

FIGURE 10.18
HCS domain.

Sensor Network

Because of its transparency, AmI technology enables novel ways of unobtrusive sensing. First, monitor and assistance devices will be embedded invisibly in objects of daily life, reducing the stigmatization of these devices and increasing their acceptance. Second, a considerable amount of sensors that can also be used to detect specific situations from an external perspective will be integrated in the living environment. With this, the availability of the sensing functionality does not depend on the actual usage of devices, e.g., the wearing of special devices, which is a serious problem these days. By fusing and drawing conclusions from different measured variables, the system can compensate for the low accuracy and uncertainty of single sensor values, especially of environmental sensor values. On the one hand, an accurate automated system has a clear benefit compared to existing methods such as surveys in providing a continuous monitoring activity at home or in a building, i.e., a log along with times and durations for a wide range of activities. On the other hand, it also enables the system to recognize some mid-term or long-term trends and short-term deviations from the usual daily routine. Through enhanced self-awareness and context awareness, the systems are able to adapt themselves to changing situations (e.g., changing capabilities of the users). Thus, they can render their services at a new level of experience and enhance the quality of service.

Fortunately, advances in sensing, object localization, event monitoring, and wireless communication technologies make possible the unobtrusive supervision of the basic needs of frail elderly and thereby replicate services of on-site health care providers. It is postulated that implementation of a cost-effective, reliable, secure, and open personal system that provides real-time interaction between elderly people and remote care providers can delay their transfer to skilled nursing facilities (SNFs) and improve the quality of their lives (by preserving independence). It is further postulated that the money saved by delaying transfer to SNFs will significantly offset the deployment cost of personal assistant systems (PASs).

With this architecture, several applications can be provided [57]. These include PASs for helping residents to perform daily activities through active wireless-enabled devices (PDAs, digital frames, cell phones) and reminder messages; measurement of physiological functions (blood glucose, daily body weights, O_2 saturation) by means of Bluetooth- or ZigBee-enabled medical meters and their transmission to a hospital in order to be evaluated by health care providers; real-time tracking of objects through ultrasonic/RFID tags attached to eyeglasses, hearing aids, key chains, and purses/wallets; and detection of falls and early warning signs of illness by means of wearable sensors equipped with an accelerometer converted to bracelets/watches or pendants.

Some of the health applications for sensor networks in hospitals provide interfaces for the disabled, integrated patient monitoring, diagnostics, drug administration, and tracking and monitoring of doctors and patients inside a hospital.

The design of the sensor network that is part of an assisted living system is influenced by many factors, which include fault tolerance, scalability, production costs, operating environment, sensor network topology, hardware constraints, transmission media, and power consumption. These factors are important because they serve as a guideline to designing a protocol or an algorithm for sensor networks.

Many existing sensor network deployments use specialized and highly optimized protocols that require the presence of a gateway that connects the sensor network to the outside world. The gateway must be tailored to the specific protocols used inside the sensor network. To be able to avoid the use of a specialized gateway, several recent systems use the IP inside the sensor network. Running the IP inside the sensor network has the benefit of interoperability at the network layer. The IP does not, however, automatically enable integration at a higher layer [58].

To integrate sensor networks with existing living assistance systems, the use of web services can be a good solution. Web services are a mechanism that is widely used in general-purpose information technology (IT) systems, such as business logic systems, intelligent building management, and databases. Web services provide a structured and interoperable mechanism for data acquisition, data storage, and data replication both within and outside of the sensor network. A web service-based sensor network can be integrated into building automation or home EMSs that are built on standard IT system components. Unlike specialized gateway-based approaches, web services provide an architecture that is able to evolve as the field grows.

Impact of BEMSs and HCSs in Assisted Living

With the considerable system functionality of BEMSs and ambient HCSs (AHCSs), the combination of nonfunctional properties becomes especially important. They have a major impact on the overall acceptance of the system and the chance to let elderly people learn to get used to the assistance provided. BEMSs and AHCSs have to fulfill the following interface-related requirements [55]:

- *Robustness*: as the system is watching the health of the patient, it must be extremely robust against all kinds of misuse and errors. Wrong inputs must not lead to a system malfunction or crash.
- *Availability*: the system must do its job even in the presence of hardware component crashes, shortage of hardware resources such as storage or communication bandwidth, and other exceptional conditions.
- *Extensibility*: the system must support its extension by new components at runtime, e.g., sensors to measure specific vital functions or actuators for active assistance, in order to adapt the system to changing disabilities.
- *Safety*: the system should do exactly the job it was designed for. This requires precise system specifications and a guided design process including verification and validation steps, which assures that the specifications are met. Faulty system components and exceptions must never result in system misbehavior.
- *Security*: a living assistance system, although continuously monitoring persons, must guarantee a well-defined degree of privacy for the persons under observation. The privacy rules must be precisely formulated and verified.
- *Timeliness*: although living assistance systems are not considered hard real-time systems, some of their services, such as the emergency treatment, have to be carried out in time. Long propagation delays after the detection of an emergency are not tolerable.
- *Resource efficiency*: the available resources, i.e., processing power, memory, communication bandwidth, and energy, have to be utilized as efficiently as possible in order to allow
  - An affordable price of the systems.
  - The realization of highly integrated, autonomous sensor nodes with high endurance, which is of particular interest if the sensor nodes have to be mobile.

- *Natural, anticipatory human–computer interaction (HCI)*: living assistance systems have to provide human interfaces for three groups of people: the assisted persons, the medical personnel, and the maintenance personnel. Each of these groups has different requirements for interacting with the system. The human interface for the handicapped and elderly persons must be based on voice, gesture, and visual animation, and must avoid any kind of particular skills. Multimodal interaction paradigms that combine several modes are a powerful approach to enhance usability. Anticipatory interfaces, which proactively contact persons in certain situations, are considered mandatory.
- The service interface for medical personnel should allow input/output of medical data such as critical situation indicators and behavioral patterns of the persons under observation in a domain-specific notation, avoiding any specific IT knowledge.
- *Adaptability*: the systems are able to adapt themselves at runtime. Adaptability on different levels and scales is considered one outstanding characteristic of living assistance systems. To support this, the systems must monitor themselves, i.e., continuously check critical system conditions such as resource bottlenecks, exceptions raised by components indicating upcoming crashes, low battery status, etc., before they lead to a disruption of operation. Based on the identified situations, the system can perform
  - *Self-optimization*, which denotes the ability of the system to adapt its algorithmic behavior to the changing needs of the application. An example of self-optimization is the dynamic increase in the volume of loudspeakers for persons with increasing deafness.
  - *Self-configuration*, which denotes the ability of the system to integrate dynamically new software components and remove existing ones not needed anymore. Self-configuration is a form of self-adaptation at the architectural level of a system. Self-reconfiguration may be triggered by changes in the hardware configuration aiming at better use of resources or a higher degree of fault tolerance.
  - *Self-maintenance*, which denotes the ability of the system to perform standard maintenance tasks such as downloading new updates and releases automatically from a remote service center.

At the same time, ethical, social, medical, and technological constraints must be considered [56–61].

- *Formalization of domain knowledge*: developing BEMSs and AHCSs requires domain knowledge to be transformed for machine processing. In many cases, this knowledge is difficult to formalize, e.g., the diagnosis of a disease pattern; decisions depend mostly on the expertise of the medical staff and cannot be translated easily into information models and algorithms.
- *Elderly people as the most important stakeholders*: some of the currently available solutions put a strong focus on the technological solution and neglect usability issues. Any HCS, which requires special skills from the elderly people to handle it, will fail. In addition, requirements are usually elaborated together with the end users. This is a difficult task since elderly people often have insufficient knowledge of the

possible technical solutions available and are usually unaware of their increasing disabilities.

- *Late learning*: still many of today's elderly people (especially in Europe) are not used to modern IT systems, and even worse, they are afraid of using them. Here, big cultural differences become apparent. To meet this challenge, BEMSs and HCSs must either rely on the interaction paradigms they are used to or there must be special training programs offered to teach the users.

- *Low acceptance of health assistance solutions*: assistance solutions that solely tackle health problems are hard to sell due to the negative associations raised by them and the social stigma identifying the assisted person's disabilities.

- *Integration of available technologies*: many different electronic devices are available on the market. However, most of them do not provide standardized interfaces or integration specification. Many of these technologies have been developed for other purposes or are not intended to be integrated in larger solutions with other components. Good usability of applications is essential.

- *Immaturity*: driven by upcoming problems due to the diverse changes, it is common sense that the assisted living domain will be a huge market. However, there is only limited knowledge on how products will look, how they can be introduced to the market, who will pay for them, and how they will be accepted. To meet this challenge, the products must provide some kind of flexibility that will also affect the HCI.

In summary, the potential of integrating all aspects of assisted living systems in home automation systems and intelligent buildings is very important. Two different scenarios can be distinguished: the integration of applications for assisted living systems at the patient's home and the integration of these applications in a hospital environment.

Nowadays, as noted above, the installation of such applications is increasing in order to improve the environment and the quality of life of patients in their homes. With this kind of solution, the main goal is to enhance the economic savings in health costs, decreasing the number of visits to different health centers and hospital days. In this scenario, integration between assisted living systems and home automation systems is not only immediate but also necessary. The benefits are as follows: it is economical (optimization of control and sensor networks, using the captured data by the sensors for different actions such as turning on or off lights, turning on heating, showing a special message on TV or in a touch panel, or controlling the patient's presence in his or her bed) and it is able to bring technology to the patient (by the aforementioned *invisible network*).

Moreover, today, the integration of assisted living systems in hospitals seems an indispensable alternative. Designing new hospital environments includes the installation of intelligent control systems with the integration of different technical systems of the building (lighting, HVAC, access control, fire alarms, surveillance, security, etc.). With such infrastructure deployed throughout the building, the integration of assisted living systems is immediately obtaining obvious benefits from the beginning of use of the building. Again, saving on installation and sharing optimized networks also facilitate their maintenance, and more importantly, they allow the direct communication between all systems sharing information and giving the building greater intelligence for making decisions in the activation and deactivation of facilities (lighting, air conditioning, etc.), monitoring of patients, the location of doctors, sending notices and reports, etc.

For all these reasons, the integration of assisted living system services in control networks (KNX, LON BACNET, or any other communication protocol) of a building proves to be ambitious and also emerges as an opportunity to obtain all the benefits described above providing the use of new technologies in these environments and improving the quality of life of patients.

Conclusions

Wireless systems have become key elements in order to provide services to enable AAL scenarios. In order for these systems to operate adequately, coverage capacity relations have to be optimized, overall interference has to be reduced, and energy consumption should be kept at the minimum level possible. In order to achieve the best performance in terms of quality of the wireless links as well as operating distance, the topology and the morphology of the working environment of the system should be considered. In this way, losses due to material absorption as well as multipath propagation can be considered prior to wireless network deployment, with the capability of selecting the optimal network configuration. Moreover, interference sources can be detected and taken into consideration, minimizing overall system degradation. The use of such radio-planning techniques can also optimize the necessary transmission power by locating wireless transceivers in positions with lower losses and hence longer transmission ranges.

Radio-planning techniques can be combined with the implementation of ultralow-power transceivers. By carefully choosing the transceiver topology as well as the power supply mechanisms, overall power consumption can be greatly reduced. This leads to increased freedom of use of the wireless sensors, especially in the case of on-body wireless sensors. A particular case of the u-Health service has also been described as an example of an implemented system that is functional thanks to the use of multiple wireless access technologies. These technologies can all coexist and collaborate with more complex systems, such as those applicable to building automation solutions. The combination of wireless sensor networks with BASs and global communication networks leads to a true u-Health ecosystem, which can increase the quality of life of assisted individuals and optimize overall cost.

References

1. Iskander, M.F., Yun, Z. "Propagation Prediction Models for Wireless Communication Systems," *IEEE Transaction on Microwave Theory and Techniques*, Vol. 50, No. 3, pp. 662–673, 2002.
2. Katuiski, R.J., Kiedrowski, A. "Calculation of the Propagation Loss in Urban Radio-Access Systems," *Antennas and Propagation Magazine, IEEE*, Vol. 50, No. 6, pp. 65–70, 2008.
3. de Adana, F.S., Gutierrez Blanco, O., Diego, I.G., Pérez Arriaga, J., Cátedra, M. "Propagation Model based on Ray Tracing for the Design of Personal Communication Systems in Indoor Environments," *IEEE Transactions on Vehicular Technology*, Vol. 49, No. 6, pp. 2105–2112, 2000.
4. Erricolo, D., Uslenghi, P.L.E. "Propagation Path Loss—A Comparison Between Ray-Tracing Approach and Empirical Models," *IEEE Transaction on Antennas and Propagation*, Vol. 50, No. 5, pp. 766–768, 2002.

5. Rossi, J., Gabillet, Y. "A Mixed Ray Launching/Tracing Method for Full 3-D UHF Propagation Modeling and Comparison with Wide-Band Measurements," *IEEE Transaction on Antennas and Propagation*, Vol. 50, No. 4, pp. 517–523, 2002.

6. Gorce, J., Jaffrès-Runser, K., de la Roche, G. "Deterministic Approach for Fast Simulations of Indoor Radio Wave Propagation," *IEEE Transaction on Antennas and Propagation*, Vol. 55, No. 3, pp. 938–948, 2007.

7. Jiang, L., Tan, S.Y. "Geometrically Based Statistical Channel Models for Outdoor and Indoor Propagation Environments," *IEEE Transactions on Vehicular Technology*, Vol. 56, No. 6, pp. 3587–3593, 2007.

8. Fuschini, F., El-Sallabi, H., Degli-Esposti, V., Vuokko, L., Guiducci, D., Vainikainen, P. "Analysis of Multipath Propagation in Urban Environment through Multidimensional Measurements and Advanced Ray Tracing Simulation," *IEEE Transaction on Antennas and Propagation*, Vol. 56, No. 3, pp. 848–857, 2008.

9. Thiel, M., Sarabandi, K. "3D-Wave Propagation Analysis of Indoor Wireless Channels Utilizing Hybrid Methods," *IEEE Transaction on Antennas and Propagation*, Vol. 57, No. 5, pp. 1539–1546, 2009.

10. Casson, A.J., Yates, D.C., Smith, S.J., Duncan, J.S., Rodriguez-Villegas, E. "Wearable Electroencephalography," *IEEE Engineering in Medicine and Biology Magazine*, Vol. 29, No. 3, pp. 44–56, 2010.

11. Bronskowski, C., Schroeder, D. "A Programmable Analog Front End for the Acquisition of Biomedical Signals," *Proc. of the 15th ProRISC Workshop*, pp. 474–477, 2004.

12. Ramirez-Angulo, J., Lopez-Martin, A.J., Carvajal, R.G., Chavero, F.M. "Very Low-Voltage Analog Signal Processing Based on Quasi-Floating Gate Transistors," *IEEE Journal of Solid-State Circuits*, Vol. 39, No. 3, pp. 434–442, 2004.

13. Enz, C.C., Temes, G.C. "Circuit Techniques for Reducing the Effects of Op-Amp Imperfections: Autozeroing, Correlated Double Sampling, and Chopper Stabilization," *Proceedings of IEEE*, Vol. 84, No. 11, pp. 1584–1614, 1996.

14. Lopez-Morillo, E., Carvajal, R.G., Muñoz, F., El Gmili, H., López Martín, A.J., Ramírez-Angulo, J., Rodriguez-Villegas, E. "A Low-Voltage and Low-Power QFG-Based Sigma-Delta Modulator for Electroencephalogram Applications," *IEEE Transactions on Biomedical Circuits and Systems*, Vol. 2, No. 3, pp. 223–230, 2008.

15. Goes, J., Paulino, N., Pinto, H., Monteiro, R., Vaz, B., Garção, A.S. "Low-Power Low-Voltage CMOS A/D Sigma-Delta Modulator for Bio-Potential Signals Driven by a Single-Phase Scheme," *IEEE Transactions on Circuits and Systems—I: Regular Papers*, Vol. 52, No. 12, pp. 2595–2604, 2005.

16. Lee, H.-Y., Hsu, C.-M., Huang, S.-C., Shih, Y.-W., Luo, C.-H. "Designing Low Power of Sigma Delta Modulator for Biomedical Application," *Biomedical Engineering Applications, Basis & Communications*, Vol. 17, No. 18, pp. 181–185, 2005.

17. Ramirez-Angulo, J., Carvajal, R.G., Galan, J.A., Lopez-Martin, A. "A Free but Efficient Low-Voltage Class-AB Two-Stage Operational Amplifier," *IEEE Transactions on Circuits and Systems II: Express Briefs*, Vol. 53, No. 7, pp. 568–571, 2006.

18. Munoz, F., Ramirez-Angulo, J., Lopez-Martin, A., Carvajal, R.G., Torralba, A., Palomo, B., Kachare, M. "Analogue Switch for Very Low-Voltage Applications," *Electronics Letters*, Vol. 39, No. 9, pp. 701–702, 2003.

19. Otis, B., Chee, Y.H., Rabaey, J. "A 400uW-RX, 1.6mW-TX Super-Regenerative Transceiver for Wireless Sensor Networks," *Proc. ISSCC 2005*, pp. 396–397.

20. Wilson, J., Youell, R., Richards, T., Luff, G., Pilaski, R. "A Single-Chip VHF and UHF Receiver for Radio Paging," *IEEE Journal of Solid-State Circuits*, Vol. 26, pp. 1944–1950, 1991.

21. Monteagudo, J., Moreno, O. "eHealth for Patient Empowerment in Europe," 2009, available at http://www.ehealthnews.eu/images/stories/pdf/eh_era-patient-empower.pdf (accessed April 4, 2015).

22. Ducatel, K., Bogdanowicz, M., Scapolo, F., Leijten, J., Burgelman, J-C. "Scenarios for Ambient Intelligent in Europe," Institute for Prospective Technological Studies, IPTS. 2001.

23. Bonato, P. "Wearable Sensors and Systems," *IEEE Engineering in Medicine and Biology Magazine*, Vol. 29, pp. 25–36, 2010, doi: 10.1109/MEMB.2010.936554.

24. Binkley, P.F. "Predicting the Potential of Wearable Technology," *IEEE Engineering in Medicine and Biology Magazine*, Vol. 22, pp. 23–27, 2003, doi: 10.1109/MEMB.2003.1213623.

25. Korhonen, I., Parkka, J., Van Gils, M. "Health Monitoring in the Home of the Future," *IEEE Engineering in Medicine and Biology Magazine*, Vol. 22, pp. 66–73, 2003, doi: 10.1109/MEMB.2003.1213628.

26. Pentland, A. "Healthwear: Medical Technology Becomes Wearable," *Computer*, Vol. 37, pp. 42–49, 2004, doi: 10.1109/MC.2004.1297238.

27. Sungmee, P., Jayaraman, S. "Enhancing the Quality of Life through Wearable Technology," *IEEE Engineering in Medicine and Biology Magazine*, Vol. 22, pp. 41–48, 2003, doi: 10.1109/MEMB.2003.1213625.

28. World Heart Federation, available at http://www.world-heart-federation.org/about-cvd/global-facts-maps/global-facts (accessed April 4, 2015).

29. Medtronic, available at http://www.medtronicdiagnostics.com/us/cardiac-monitors/Reveal-XT-ICM-Device/index.htm (accessed April 4, 2015).

30. CardioNet, available at https://www.cardionet.com/medical_06.htm (accessed April 4, 2015).

31. Biotronik, available at http://www.biotronik.com/wps/wcm/connect/en_de_web/biotronik/sub_top/healthcareprofessionals/Products+and+Therapies/Arrhythmia+Monitoring/#jump (accessed April 4, 2015).

32. Cardiplus, available at http://www.cardiplus.com/cardiplus.html (accessed April 4, 2015).

33. V Patch Medical Systems, available at http://vpatchmedical.com/pages/vpms-components.php (accessed April 4, 2015).

34. Alive Technologies, available at http://www.alivetec.com/alive-bluetooth-heart-activity-monitor (accessed April 4, 2015).

35. Corscience, available at http://www.corscience.de/en/medical-engineering/products/ecg/bluetooth-ecg-device.html (accessed April 4, 2015).

36. Led, S., Serrano, L., Galarraga, M. "Intelligent Holter: A New Wearable Device for ECG Monitoring using Bluetooth Technology," *Proc. of International Federation for Medical and Biological Engineering*, 2005.

37. HOLTIN, available at http://www.lqtai.com/product/index (accessed April 4, 2015).

38. Quintana, A., García, L., Mendoza, H. et al. "Rendimiento diagnóstico de un sistema de telemonitorización ECG ambulatoria por eventos (HOLTIN) y Holter convencional en pacientes con síncope o palpitaciones," *Proc. of Congreso de la Sociedad Española de Cardiología*, 2010.

39. Maldonado, E., García, L., Quintanilla, J. et al. "Evaluación de la satisfacción de un servicio de telemonitorización ECG ambulatoria por eventos (HOLTIN) frente a Holter convencional gestionado por enfermería," *Proc. of Congreso de la Sociedad Española de Cardiología*, 2010.

40. Stead, W., Miller, R., Musen, M., Hersh, W. "Integration and Beyond: Linking Information from Disparate Sources and into Workflow," *Journal of the American Medical Informatics Association*, Vol. 7, pp. 135–146, 2000.

41. Pedersen, S., Hasselbring, W. "Interoperability for Information Systems among the Health Service Providers Based on Medical Standards," *Informatik-Forschung Und Entwicklung*, Vol. 18, pp. 174–188, 2004.

42. Kennelly, R.J. "Improving Acute Care through Use of Medical Device Data," *International Journal of Medical Informatics*, Vol. 48, pp. 145–149, 1998.

43. NEMA National Electrical Manufacturers Association, DICOM Digital Imaging and Communications in Medicine, available at http://medical.nema.org/standard.html (accessed April 4, 2015).

44. HL7 Health Level Seven, available at http://www.hl7.org/implement/standards/index.cfm (accessed April 4, 2015).

45. CEN European Committee for Standardization, ENV13606CEN/TC251 Electronic Healthcare Record Communication, available at http://www.en13606.org/the-ceniso-en13606-standard (accessed April 4, 2015).

46. ISO International Organization for Standardization, ISO/IEEE11073, available at http://standards .ieee.org/findstds/standard/11073-20601-2014.html (accessed April 4, 2015).

47. Integrating the Healthcare Enterprise (IHE), available at http://www.ihe.net (accessed April 4, 2015).

48. Continua Health Alliance, available at http://www.continuaalliance.org (accessed April 4, 2015).

49. ISO International Organization for Standardization, ISO/IEEE11073 Point-of-Care, Medical Device Communication Standard, Health Informatics, available at http://standards.ieee.org /develop/project/11073-20101.html (accessed April 4, 2015).

50. ISO International Organization for Standardization, ISO/IEEE11073 Personal Health Devices Standard, Health Informatics, available at http://standards.ieee.org/develop/project/11073 -20601.html (accessed April 4, 2015).

51. Warren, S., Lebak, J., Yao, J. "Lessons Learned from Applying Interoperability and Information Exchange Standards to a Wearable Point-of-Care System," *Proc. of Transdisciplinary Conference on Distributed Diagnosis and Home Healthcare*, pp. 101–104, 2006.

52. Martínez de Espronceda, M., Serrano, L., Martínez, I. et al. "Implementing ISO/IEEE 11073: Proposal of Two Different Strategic Approaches," *Proc. of IEEE International Conference Engineering in Medicine and Biology*, pp. 1805–1808, 2008.

53. Martínez de Espronceda, M., Martínez, I., Serrano, L. et al. "Implementation Methodology for Interoperable Personal Health Devices with Low-Voltage Low-Power Constrains," *IEEE Transactions on Information Technology in Biomedicine*, Vol. 15, p. 398, 2011, doi: 10.1109/TITB .2011.2134861.

54. Martínez de Espronceda, M., Martínez, I., Serrano, L. et al. "Lessons Learned Implementing the ISO/IEEE11073 Standard into Wearable Personal Devices," *Proc. on IEEE International Conference on Information Technology and Applications in Biomedicine*, pp. 1–4, 2010.

55. Nehmer, J., Karshmer, A., Becker, M., Lamm, R. "Living Assistance Systems—An Ambient Intelligence Approach," *Proceedings of the 28th International Conference on Software Engineering*, 2006.

56. Kleinberger, T., Becker, M., Ras, E., Holzinger, A., Müller, P. "Ambient Intelligence in Assisted Living: Enable Elderly People to Handle Future Interfaces," C. Stephanidis (Ed.), *Universal Access in HCI, Part II, HCII 2007*, LNCS 4555, pp. 103–112, 2007.

57. Hou, J.C., Wang, Q., AlShebli, B.K. et al. "PAS: A Wireless-Enabled, Sensor-Integrated Personal Assistance System for Independent and Assisted Living," *High Confidence Medical Device Software and Systems*, Boston MA, June, 2007.

58. Yazara, D., Dunkels, A. "Efficient Application Integration in IP-Based Sensor Networks," *Proceedings of the First ACM Workshop on Embedded Sensing Systems for Energy-Efficiency in Buildings*, November 2009.

59. Virone, G., Wood, A., Selavo, L., Cao, Q., Fang, L., Doan, T., He, Z., Stoleru, R., Lin, S., Stankovic, J.A. "An Assisted Living Oriented Information System Based on a Residential Wireless Sensor Network," *Proceedings of the 1st Distributed Diagnosis and Home Healthcare Conference*, Arlington, VA, April, 2006.

60. Andrushevich, A., Staub, M., Kistler, R., Klapproth, A. "Towards Semantic Buildings: Goal-Driven Approach for Building Automation Service Allocation and Control," *Emerging Technologies and Factory Automation (ETFA), 2010 IEEE Conference on*, 2010.

61. Eklund, J.M., Hansen, T.R., Sprinkle, J., Sastry, S. "Information Technology for Assisted Living at Home: Building a Wireless Infrastructure for Assisted Living," *Proceedings of the 2005 IEEE Engineering in Medicine and Biology 27th Annual Conference*, Shanghai, China, September 1–4, 2005.

Section III

AAL Applications to Specific Areas

11

Video Care Services: AAL Solution for Dementia Support—State of the Art of Research and Intervention

Jorge Nunes Monteiro, Liliana Dias, and Susana Espadaneira

CONTENTS

ABSTRACT Isolation, depression, and cognitive impairment are major factors that impact health, well-being, and care costs of elderly people. Information systems and in particular those supported by video (e.g., video call, video-conferencing, video immersion) can help in connecting elderly, care providers, health personnel, and family and friends to address dementia challenges. According to the World Health Organization, dementia is one of the major problems of public health in Europe. The United States forecasts for 2040 that 7.3 million of citizens will have a dementia problem compared to 3 million in 2000. Maintaining elderly with some kind of cognitive impairment (e.g., dementia, Parkinson's, and Alzheimer's) at home, supervised and with a cost-effective level of care, is a major challenge for families and for health and social organizations. Psychological and social support, particularly companionship, can produce a major outcome in biopsychosocial indicators for this population. Online counseling has been considered by many authors as a service that not only overcomes physical, economic, and psychological barriers but also has a pertinent and large scope of intervention nowadays. Providing counseling, support, and companionship using up-to-date information and communication technologies can be an important cost-effective solution to address the increasing and widespread demand for support.

KEY WORDS: *telecare, video care, counseling, social support, elderly, dementia, ambient assisted living.*

Introduction

In this chapter, the integrative literature review presents the state of the art in terms of e-companionship and e-counseling solutions, particularly for elderly cognitive challenged people, and the major lessons learnt from previous projects using video technologies in health and social contexts. The aim is to identify the major benefits obtained, the success factors considered in project implementation, the pitfalls to avoid, and the business and operations models used.

Considering the structure of this chapter, we will begin to conceptualize the problems that the elderly population face nowadays, particularly when challenged with dementia, the specific needs and costs of all the stakeholders involved, and the barriers to technology utilization in services delivery.

The technological layer is then presented, and the concept of *video care* is defined.

Within the ambient assisted living (AAL) approach, the development focus will be distributed in revealing the state of the art of solutions that use video technology as a means of home-based provision of professional services.

After considering the benefits, success factors, and pitfalls of these solutions, we will end by considering cost-effective argumentation and actual limitations and trends-related business models to address the increasing demand for dementia support and treatment.

Aging and Dementia

Population aging is one of the greatest challenges of the twenty-first century in terms of global economic and social demands.

In *Active Ageing: A Policy Framework* from the World Health Organization (WHO 2002), it is established that the proportion of people of age 60 and above is growing faster than any other age groups. By 2025, there will be about 1.2 billion people of age over 60 years, and about 2 billion by 2050 are expected, with 80% of them living in developing countries. Although people with the age of 80 make up just 1% of the world's population and represent 3% of the population in developed countries, this age group is the fastest growing segment of the older population.

The demographic trends like the increase in the number of women without children, the smaller number of children, rates in divorces, and different patterns of marriages contribute to the reduction of family support. On the other hand, the health needs of the elderly population will lead to incremental costs on the industry of health care and social services; one of the major challenges in the health policy will be achieving the economical balance between informal support and formal care (health and social services) for the constantly growing elderly population.

As the population in our society is aging, the number of people with chronic diseases is growing. One of the conditions with a rising concern is the increasing number of people with dementia (Lauricks et al. 2010). The prevalence of dementia rises with age, doubling every 5 years after the age of 65, from 3% at the age of 70 to 20% at the age of 85. Across the world, 4.6 million new cases of dementia will emerge every year, and the number of people living with dementia will almost double every 20 years from 42.3 million in 2020 to 81.1 million in 2040 (Cahil 2007).

Dementia is a syndrome characterized by disturbance of multiple higher cortical functions, including memory, thinking, and orientation, and comprehension, calculation, learning capacity, language, and judgment. Impairments of cognitive function are commonly accompanied by deterioration in emotional control, social behavior, and motivation. Besides this, there are neuropsychiatric changes that are nearly universal: psychological symptoms include delusions, hallucinations, depression, anxiety, and misidentifications; behavioral symptoms may include aggression, wandering, sleep disturbances, and inappropriate behavior (Luxenberg 2000).

The most common type of dementia is Alzheimer's disease (65% of all cases), followed by vascular dementia (25%); rarer dementia disorders include dementia with Lewy bodies and front-temporal dementia. Different types and stages of dementia manifest different symptoms in psychological, behavioral, and motoric functioning (Cahil 2007).

The challenge is that dementia needs to be understood in terms of world demographic trends, increased life expectancy, and difficulties that low-income countries will experience in the future given the high number of people likely to experience dementia there.

Most persons with dementia live at home and are supported by family and friends, as well as formal caregivers; it is fundamental to find services that could help families and caregivers in maintaining these people at home, with quality of life for both the elderly and the caregiver.

Providing care services at home is a major trend to address the needs and wishes of the aging population. Home care prevents unnecessary institutionalization, and maintains individuals in their home and community for as long as possible and guarantees their well-being at home (family, friends, memories, artifacts, etc.; World Health Organization 2008).

The Telemedicine Systems for Home Care can be used for (1) prevention, (2) health surveillance, (3) health management, (4) health monitoring, and (5) health treatment. All those services must address major requirements: increase individual biopsychosocial indicators and support reducing health costs strategies (Warner 1997).

The societal cost of dementia is huge, and it is already significantly affecting every health and social care system in the world. *World Alzheimer Report 2010* (Wimo and Prince 2010) demonstrated that the total estimated worldwide cost of dementia was 418 billion euros in 2010, and about 70% of the cost occur in Western Europe and North America. "If dementia care were a country, it would be the world's 18th largest economy, ranking between Turkey and Indonesia," as stated in *World Alzheimer Report 2010* (Wimo and Prince 2010).

The costs associated with dementia are recognized in three social and health areas:

1. Informal care (usually family or relatives and friends)
2. Social care (community care professionals and residential homes)
3. Medical care

There is an imperative need to develop cost-effective packages of medical and social care that meet the needs of people with dementia and their caregivers throughout the development of the illness. Governments and health and social care systems need to be adequately prepared for the future and must seek ways now to improve the lives of people with dementia and their caregivers.

The accelerating adoption of microprocessor-based technology might lead to beneficial outcomes on the aging population. Technology holds a promise for reorganizing care, playing an important role in work and leisure and in health care provision, like the prevention of age-associated impairments, the amplification of its effects, or substitution of some physical impairment (Charness and Boot 2009), helping and facilitating the lives (Wimo and Prince 2010) of people with dementia and their families or caregivers (Cahil 2007).

A literature review of Brownsell et al. (2007) to identify the trigger factors associated with a need for increased levels of care and support for elderly people demonstrated that telecare could be used to assist, prevent, and minimize the impact of about 66% of the identified factors and 75% of the top 12 factors. This identification suggests that telecare has a significant role in the support of elderly people.

The trigger factors associated with the increased level of care are

- Fear of failing
- Major health event
- Perceived decline and concern of own health
- Person feeling lonely
- Abuse (physical and mental)
- Bereavement of a family member or friend
- Cognition impairment
- Consequences of admission to hospital
- Depression, mental breakdown, or deterioration
- Deterioration of physical functioning
- Difficulty cooking for themselves
- Difficulty in managing stairs and steps

The elderly with dementia have similar needs with regular elderly, but some of the needs of persons with dementia are insufficiently met by regular care. People with dementia have different needs during the progression of the disease, varying from memory support in the early stages to support in every areas of functioning in severe dementia (Lauricks et al. 2010).

The common needs can be categorized in four areas (Nugent 2007; Lauricks et al. 2010):

1. Need for general and personalized information
2. Need for support regarding symptoms of dementia

3. Need for social contact and company

4. Need for health monitoring and perceived safety

The use of technology can contribute to meet the most frequently unmet needs of people with dementia and their informal caregivers. Several studies in the area of information and communication technologies (ICTs) revealed that persons with dementia are capable of handling this equipment and benefit in terms of confidence and enhanced positive effect; and, as a side effect, informal caregivers receive a reduction in the perceived burden (Lauricks et al. 2010).

It has been widely supported that elderly people can use technology, especially if they are provided with adequate training (Rogers et al. 1996). Careful attention has to be given to elderly people with dementia in the development of technology to support their needs.

Factors like individual and caregiver needs, the design of the product, including its familiarity, and the fact that no new learning should be required on the part of the person with dementia are essential factors to develop technology applied to ease the quality of life of the elderly people with dementia, promoting the aging in place and additional reduction in health and social care costs (Mynatt and Rogers 2001; Nugent 2007; Orpwood 2007).

Video Care

Introduction

Information systems and in particular those supported by video (video call, video-conferencing, video immersion) can help in connecting elderly, caring providers, health personnel, family, and friends to address dementia challenges.

The utilization of videophones and video-conferencing to provide health, psychological support, social support, and educational services is referred to in several studies. All these services use interactive video technology in conjunction with services provided by caregivers and other health personnel. In some cases, video technologies can be integrated with other AAL technologies.

In this study, the concept of video care applies to an application system that can provide video calls (one to one, or many to many) in order to deliver health, social support, and psychological and educational services from a distance.

Video Care System Defined

The video care system can rely on different video technologies and can provide different types of services to address specific user or organizational needs.

Conceptually, a video care system is the result of the integration of the following components: digital encounter, services, applications, hardware and operating systems software, and service delivery operations model (Figure 11.1).

According to Monteiro (2001), the capabilities necessary to address digital markets are (1) business strategy and (2) technological capacity and a business model. The video care system integrates the technological capacity and must support the business strategy and business model of the organization that provides the video care services.

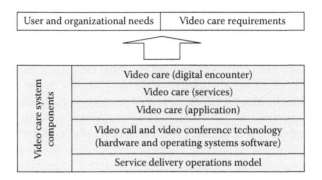

FIGURE 11.1
Video care system components.

Video Call Adoption

Video technology remains an emerging technology, but the first experience was made early in the twentieth century. The first video call took place in 1927. The first commercial system, the picturephone, became available in 1964 (Kraut and Fish 1995).

Several studies have reported problems in video call adoption by the users (Egido 1988; Webster 1998; O'Hara et al. 2006). The industry has concerns about the penetration of video call technology in the market (O'Hara et al. 2006), but at the same time, the market and technology analysts report that now is the moment for video technology adoption:

> After years of false starts and unfulfilled promises, conferencing and collaboration solutions have reached reliability, ease-of-use, and utility levels whereby the technologies are finally being integrated into the enterprise core and are helping to reinvent business processes. New software, new services, and increasingly powerful hardware are making enterprise investments in collaboration solutions not only more useful, but also easier-to-use and far more cost-effective. (Davis and Weinstein 2005)

On the other hand, several studies reported significant success in using video technology for health care services, an enthusiastic adoption of the videophone by the elderly, and evidence that it improves the quality of life (Nakamura et al. 1999, p. 127; Harrington and Harrington 2000; Arnaert and Delesie 2007; Jönsson and Willman 2009). However, evidence of the adoption of home telehealth is limited to pilot projects most of the time.

It seems that the one who has made a video call likes the experience, but the experience is limited to pilot projects and does not seem to have success yet in mass markets (Hebert et al. 2004). This leads this study to identify the factors behind this (what influences elderly and their families in adoption of video calls for video care purposes?).

Besides the video experience, there are other factors that need to be considered to understand what influences the elderly and their families in the usage of video call technology. There are several information systems studies and theories that can help to understand the phenomenon of new technology adoption; in this work, we highlight the studies developed by Venkatesh and Brown (2001), Webster (1998), Venkatesh et al. (2003), and van der Heijden (2004) that contribute to the following questions:

- What influence the adopters and non-adopters about the use of new technology at home? An investigation of the adoption determinants of personal computers in homes reports the following: "…adopters were influenced by different outcomes (utilitarian, hedonic and social), non-adopters were influenced strongly by the fear of obsolesce," (Venkatesh and Brown 2001, p. 94).

- What are the explanations for the underutilization of information technology? In an investigation of the introduction of video-conferencing technology, Webster (1998) reports several reasons behind the underutilization: insufficient training, lack of awareness by users of the technology's functionality, its widespread implementation and its potential value, and users' concerns regarding privacy.

- What are the determinants behind the user acceptance of a new information technology? According to the Unified Theory of Acceptance and Use of Technology (UTAUT; Venkatesh et al. 2003, p. 425), there are four determinants of intention and usage (performance expectancy, effort expectancy, social influence, and facilitating conditions) and up to four moderators of key relationships (gender, age, experience, and voluntariness of usage). Perceived enjoyment is a stronger determinant also for hedonic information systems (van der Heijden 2004, p. 695).

Video Call Technology Background

The image definition, image size, and interaction reliability is related to the technology used to support the video conversation. The three main technologies used over copper telephones lines are (1) plain old telephone service (POTS), (2) integrated services digital network (ISDN), and (3) asymmetric digital subscriber line (ADSL).

The POTS is the traditional analog telephone service for personal and business utilization. The ISDN permits digital transmission of voice, video, and data. The ADSL is a data communications technology that permits faster data transmission. Nowadays it is very popular because it permits high-speed Internet access at an affordable price.

There are other technologies for voice and data transmission that permit permanent connection, that are more reliable, and that permit very high transmission rates, but they are more expensive.

The costs, bandwidth, availability, video experience, and reliability of the technology are important factors to consider in the decision of what technology to adopt. Table 11.1 presents a comparison between the different options to consider in an implementation of video care services.

Nowadays, the ADSL and IP video are the solutions that offer better relation quality/ price (Wakefield et al. 2004; Weinstein 2006).

State of the Art and Trends

We forecast that the video care market can grow very fast and be leveraged by the fact that the major technology global players are pushing for the voice-over-IP and video-over-IP. *The New York Times* (2011) reported that in the last year or two, video use has surged, now accounting for 40% of Skype's traffic. There are also other global IT companies like Apple, Cisco, and Microsoft that have video on their growth strategies.

TABLE 11.1

Telecommunications Technology Options

Technology Options	Price	Availability and Access	Video Experience	Reliability
POTS/PSTN	Low	High	Low	High
ISDN/IP video	Medium	Medium	Medium	High
ADSL/IP video	Medium	Medium	High	Medium
Dedicated line/IP video	High	Medium	High	High

- *Apple has launched Face Time*: a video call system that permits Macs to make a video call for 19 million iPhone 4 and iPod touch users (Apple 2010) and 15 million of iPad users (Apple 2011) and much more.

- *Microsoft buy Skype*: have entered into a definitive agreement under which Microsoft will acquire Skype. With 170 million connected users and over 207 billion minutes of voice and video conversations in 2010, Skype has been a pioneer in creating rich, meaningful connections among friends, families, and business colleagues globally (Microsoft 2011).

- *Cisco buy Tandberg*: "Cisco and TANDBERG have remarkably similar cultures and a shared vision to change the way the world works through video communications technologies," said Cisco Chairman and Chief Executive Officer John Chambers. "Collaboration is a $34 billion market and is growing rapidly—enabled by networked Web 2.0 technologies. This acquisition showcases Cisco's financial strength and ability to quickly capture key market transitions for growth," (Cisco 2009).

At the same time, we assist in major technological transformations of the TV industry. Those transformations can provide more interaction with the user, improved accessibility (terrestrial digital television [TDT], fourth generation [4G], and internet protocol television [IPTV]), customized content, and fusion with the Internet.

Those transformations have impact on three major industries: TV, computers, and data and voice telecommunications. Companies like Apple (Apple TV), Google (Google TV), and Microsoft (Microsoft Mediaroom) are designing the future of the merging of TV and the Internet. This merging is going to have a major impact in the technological accessibility to make video calls from different devices that we use every day (TV, computer, mobile phone, game console, etc.).

Lessons Learned from Video Care Projects

Benefits from the success and failure of previous video care projects are valuable knowledge (Kasvi et al. 2003) that must be integrated into future projects.

The first use of technology to support the practice of medical, psychological, and social support dates back to the invention of the telegraph and telephone. Physicians were among the first to adopt it. The current telemedicine systems originated from the pioneering developments of the National Aeronautics and Space Administration (Zundel 1996).

Professional organizations such as the American Telemedicine Association (ATA), the American Psychiatric Association (APA), and the National Association of Social Workers have issued standards and guidelines that shall be considered in telecare. For instance, Practice Guidelines for Videoconferencing-based Telemental Health issued by the American Telemedicine Association (2008) state several specifications that must be incorporated in telemental health services: standard operating procedures/protocols, clinical specifications, technical specifications, administrative issues, etc.

There is considerable knowledge and experience that must be integrated in future video care projects. The major benefits, major success factors, and pitfalls considered in the projects analyzed are given as follows:

- *Major benefits*: (1) convenience and improved health access; (2) earlier interventions; (3) clients *love the video phone*; (4) quality of health encounter and trust in telecare; (5) reduced travel; (6) more efficiency; (7) extended support (advice and emotional support for patients and for families); and (8) improving health

- *Major success factors*: (1) other equipment to change information; (2) awareness about computer-mediated communication and digital encounter; (3) IT implementation project management best practices; (4) video and audio quality; (5) usability; (6) support; (7) training; and (8) technical reliability
- *Major pitfalls*: (1) integration with other IT systems; (2) privacy; (3) physician expectations; and (4) elderly expectations regarding independence

E-Companionship and E-Support

Belonging to a group and to be connected is major need of human beings. After satisfying humans basic needs—food, drink and other physiologic needs, feeling secure—it is very important for seniors' wellbeing and quality of life to be connected to others (society, family, friends, health professionals and formal and informal caregivers, etc.).

To be connected to others can be conceptualized as "social network." The social network as frail elderly persons can be defined as following: "is a description of their social identity in their network of significant others who can assist and interact in caring and other important aspects of life" (Sävenstedt 2004). The interactions of the elderly can be seen in Figure 11.2.

There are several factors, such as the loss of significant others, social and geographic isolation, and difficulties in relating to or developing relations with others, that can turn the elderly network much smaller.

The lack of social relationships and support may have severe consequences. Weyerer et al. (1995) demonstrated that the lack of social support via relatives and friends was a significant predictor of depression after admissions of seniors in nursing homes.

Some families are elderly and have some difficulties in engaging in visits because of physical disabilities or because they live in geographically distant locations. Video applications have enormous potential in this population to facilitate communication and relations with all the persons included in the identified network areas.

Given the decrease in social networks in the elderly, enhancing the quality of the remaining relationships has extreme importance. Our focus in this chapter is to present the state of the art in terms of e-companionship, particularly for elderly with dementia.

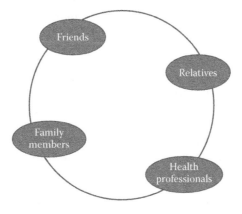

FIGURE 11.2
Social network of an elderly person.

TABLE 11.2

Supportive Functions of Social Support

Emotional support	Confidant support, esteem support, reassurance of worth, attachment, intimacy
Instrumental support	Tangible support, practical support, behavioral assistance, material aid
Informational support	Advice/guidance, appraisal support, cognitive guidance, problem solving
Companion support	Belonging, socialization, integration
Validation	Feedback, social comparison

We define *e-companionship* as a concept of telecare, which involves social support (and its supportive functions) given by families, friends, professionals, and other informal caregivers to the elderly population, provided at a distance via the use of interactive communication.

Social support includes not only the structural characteristics of the social networks but also the functional aspects of the interaction between the members (Portero and Oliva 2007). The supportive functions of social support include emotional, instrumental, informational, and companion support and validation (see Table 11.2; Wills and Shinar 2000).

The aim of e-companionship is to enhance the quality of relations of the elderly, amplifying the kind and nature of support that they receive from these relations. In this section, we will focus on three areas of e-companionship: *televisits, telenursing,* and *support groups.* In all areas, we justify how video support technology can facilitate remote conversations between elderly adults and their care providers.

Televisits

Televisits are the definition of contact (audio and video support) between elderly people, usually living in a nursing home, and their family or friends (Mickus and Luz 2002).

Televisits are a way of enhancing the quality and frequency of communication and relationships between elderly and their families or friends that are geographically distant or have physical limitations, which precludes physical encounters. In this type of e-companionship, the most frequent support function is emotional, but it is possible to facilitate all kinds of support functions.

Elderly people with dementia have difficulties in the reception and expression of language, and this complicates the communication and care process (Sävenstedt 2004). The interaction by videophones can accommodate visual nonverbal cues like face expression, gestures, posture, movements, and physical appearance, making possible a better *social presence* that enables personal interaction, and sending and receiving affective information (Hensel et al. 2007).

Videophone can be used successfully to enhance social interactions regardless of the distance, and can be used by individuals with mild dementia and physical limitations. Evidence was found in the study by Mickus and Luz (2002) that showed that the contact between elderly and family via videophone promotes social contact. A similar study showed that videophone conversations between patients with dementia and their family reduced the feelings of guilt in the latter (Sävenstedt et al. 2003). This study also showed that with televisits, the number of visits between the family and the elderly increased, and the family felt that they could actively participate in elderly care because they could see the physical and emotional state of the patient. In a case study of televisits by Hensel et al. (2007), visual images on the videophone allowed the participants to feel part of the other's environment, which was not possible without video communication. Participants reported psychological benefits using videophones to check on each other and share each other's life.

Another benefit found in this study area of elderly people with dementia is the tightening effect of the relations between the family and the staff members. Sävenstedt et al.

(2003) showed that the relations have improved as a side effect of the help given by the staff during the utilization of the videophone.

A curious fact in this same study was the finding that, in some cases, the conversations between the elderly and families were more focused and had better quality, showing that videophone conversations could help ameliorate the cognitive state of people with dementia. Sävenstedt et al. (2003) demonstrated that the videophone helped subjects to focus to a greater extent with personal communication, because these situations induce the orientation response and maintain individual focus on the monitor, preventing distractions and enabling patients with dementia to focus on the videophone.

The same effect was reported by Mochizuki-Kawai et al. (2008). In their study, there were elderly residential participants with and without dementia, who had televisits from a group of persons (nonfamily). The study reported that even the demented participants were able to maintain focus on the videophone conversations and improve their verbal ability.

These facts could be explained because motion pictures and real-time voices from a videophone might prevent distraction and help participants to focus on the present task. Videophone communication may be beneficial in cognitive rehabilitation for elderly adults including people with dementia.

All these studies show that it is possible to have communication of good quality via video-conferencing with frail elderly persons, enhancing their relations with the participants, even those that have mild or midlevel dementia, if the conditions provided are right (Sävenstedt 2004).

The studies have demonstrated that there are also benefits for family members. Videophone conversations allowed relatives of people in nursing homes to be involved in the caring process, and communicating with these demented patients was different.

- These patients needed the assistance of the nursing home staff to use videophone; but this permitted those family members to have a much closer relationship with the staff.
- Being involved in the caring process minimized the feelings of guilt.
- Families can see the day-to-day well-being of their elderly.
- Videophone interactions compensate for the lack of semantic responses from the elderly with dementia because it was possible to see visual cues.
- Videophone conversations were more focused and demanding than face-to-face conversations, and so they contributed to a better quality of interaction.

The most common limitations found in this literature that interfere with videophone use are

- Physical impairments (vision and hearing)
- Low tolerance to deal with the problem related to the operation of videophones
- Impaired cognitive ability to operate with the equipment
- Technical problems like screen size and lack of synchronization between what was said and what was viewed
- Frustration in using the equipment
- Value placed on video

People with severity of vision loss or low tolerance to frustration may not benefit from the use of videophones.

Telenursing

Nursing care is usually associated with instrumental procedures (giving injections, treatment wounds, etc.), but it is a broad concept that includes more interventions (quoted by Arnaert and Delesie 2001):

1. Advising
2. Giving physical support
3. Giving psychological support
4. Creating an environment to promote personal growth
5. Providing instruction or education

These aspects of communication and support are as important as instrumental interventions.

Care applications using video-conferencing have been very successful in consultations and support by health professionals (Arnaert and Delesie 2001). This type of nursing intervention stimulates communication and encourages the maintenance of social contact with care staff, increasing the communication abilities and reducing social isolation for people with dementia as well as their caregivers at home.

Telenursing is a type of e-companionship, because it permits the elderly to receive emotional support from people besides the family, who most of the time are absent or do not exist, informational support about physical and health-related problems, and instrumental support related to the common activities of nursing.

One of the first projects in this area was The ACTION project—Assisting Careers Using Telematics Interventions to Meet Older Persons' Needs—a multicenter European gerontechnology project (Magnusson et al. 1998).

The aim of the project was to explore to what extent the autonomy, independence, and quality of life of frail, older, and disabled people and their family caregivers could be maintained or enhanced with the combined use of new and familiar technology.

This project used a videophone, a TV, and a remote control connected to a video-conferencing system and a network computer. The videophone enabled the elderly and family to communicate with other families, elderly, and health professionals, and the system provided access to various multimedia programs with information about diseases and caregiving.

Early findings showed that many of the families involved in the study did not have experience in using a personal computer, but used other electronic devices like microwaves or remote controls. The utilization of the TV set (the most familiar technology) as an interface was the best way of enhancing participation (Magnusson et al. 1998). Similar findings of facility and familiarity in using TV as an interface could be seen in the review of assistive technology by Orpwood (2007), even in elderly people with dementia.

The major findings in the study showed that families that access the system on a regular basis were more likely to benefit from ACTION than those who access the system once in a while. And the sooner the families have access to information, the greater the benefits were to the elderly's health and the psychosocial well-being of the caregiver (Tetley et al. 2001).

A version of the ACTION project was later established only in Sweden (Magnusson et al. 2005). The Swedish ACTION Project was used to explore the role of user-friendly ICT to inform and enable families to care more effectively and work in partnership with professionals.

The major findings in the study were as follows:

- ACTION services facilitated videophone contact with formal and informal sources of support at a distance, facilitated group support, and enhanced the social contacts of the families. In some cases, this reduced social isolation for the elderly and their families.
- With appropriate education and support, older people can fully engage with technology.
- Services were most appropriate for those who experienced the desire to care for an older relative at home.
- ACTION also facilitated a deep understanding of caregiver needs and promoted a more inclusive and empowering way of working with the professionals.
- The scheme was most effective when delivered at the earliest opportunity because it enables the caregiver early access to information, education, and support services, and to be actively involved in developing new services.

In both projects, the major difficulty encountered to fully develop this support was the cost. The main costs in ACTION are the equipment, installation, making reproduction of videos, and programming and updating programs. It was difficult to find local partners to invest in new technologies when there were already cost pressures in maintaining the existing levels of services. The cost of new technology is decreasing permanently and it is possible to offer a system like ACTION in digital television, making it available to a greater number of people (Tetley et al. 2001; Magnusson and Hanson 2005).

A study by Jönsson and Willman (2009) has demonstrated that virtual encounters did not have negative impacts in elderly and quality of care; in fact, virtual encounters offer the opportunity for more information about the patient's clinical status than did the physical encounter. Their study on patients with leg wounds in which they were submitted to distant care with videophones at home demonstrated that patients felt secure and positive about the video encounter, enhancing the relation and support with the nurses. And nurses felt that the videophone provides the possibility for a direct and quick connection to the patients' home for assistance in everyday caregiving.

Similar findings were expressed by Demiris et al. (2003). Telenursing permits the care provider to assess the patient medical condition, educate the patient and promote compliance, as well as discuss personal matters, which are essential for the emotional support of the elderly. The study demonstrated that the nurses participated in conversations about topics unrelated to health but seemed important to the patients (like family matters); in some visits, nurses spent more time on these conversations than on medical topics.

Other studies in the area of video care that do not have the direct interventions of nurses but other professionals in the health area showed the positive effects of this technology on the communication, socialization, and health of the elderly.

Smith et al. (2007) showed that televideo monitoring can improve auto-administration of medication and improve the mood of elderly with mild dementia who live alone; the family were reassured by the monitoring and felt that it could improve the elderly's compliance to medication and could prevent patient relocation. The study by Constantinescu et al. (2010) demonstrated the validity and feasibility of video-conferencing of a treatment to speech disorder with Parkinson's disease. In their study, the treatment provides the patient with high satisfaction and motivation because the patient did not need to travel several miles to go to speech treatment; this type of treatment can reduce the effects of physical disability and transport and travel difficulties.

Besides the advantages of saving travel time and costs, making nursing care more readily available, improving compliance with therapy, and preventing, delaying, or limiting admissions to nursing homes, unscheduled visits to the doctor, and hospital admissions (Whitten et al. 1997; Jönsson and Willman 2009), telenursing has demonstrated social benefits for the elderly and their families. Telenursing enhances the social relation with formal caregivers and facilitates easy informational support as well.

Telenursing must be seen as complementary and not as a replacement for necessary face-to-face encounters, because it does not permit real care in real time (like wounds, injections, etc.) but is a supplement to routine home care to observe and monitor the patient condition (Demiris et al. 2003; Magnusson et al. 2005; Jönsson and Willman 2009).

E-Counseling and Online Therapy

Counseling and the Elderly

Older adults, particularly people over 65 years of age, constitute a unique population that has been underserved in the area of counseling services (Myers and Schwiebert 1996), although an estimated one-third of individuals in this population have mental problems that require professional intervention, such as anxiety, depression, and other diagnosable mental disorders (Smyer and Qualls 1999). This estimate does not incorporate normative development issues such as the transition to retirement, grandparenthood, and second careers, which once included will increase considerably the incidence of mental health needs (Smyer and Qualls 1999).

There is a growing literature that documents the effectiveness of psychotherapy with older adults, despite the difficulties this population faces to get access to mental health services through the traditional primary care context and gateway (Haley 1999).

The first barrier for seniors to get access to counseling services seems to be the lack of training of physicians to assess and treat mental disorders; also due to time pressures to treat clients quickly, highly prevalent psychological problems are rarely treated effectively in medical settings (Higgins 1994).

Other barriers to the use of these services by this population include bias against older persons among service providers, a lack of adequate training and supervised clinical practice with this population, and a reluctance of older people to seek counseling (Nordhus and VandenBos 1998).

Counseling presents itself as an efficacious service for older people, particularly in the treatment of anxiety and depression and in improving well-being (Hill and Brettle 2006).

This study revealed that individual, as opposed to group, counseling is the psychological treatment of choice among the community-dwelling elderly and that home-based individual counseling may be the most feasible and effective modality with this population.

There is an urgent need for counselors to take a proactive approach to the identification of psychological problems in older people to ensure that they receive effective and high-quality treatments (Hill and Brettle 2006).

Several challenges need to be addressed by counselors with this population; for instance, typically counselors are younger than their older clients and need to consider the impact of differences in age and life experience on the counseling relationship; building rapport may take longer because of the reluctance to seek counseling, or the lack of familiarity with counseling processes, and the lack of experience in discussing or dealing with feelings (Myers and Schwiebert 1996).

Considering the several barriers common to older adults, remote provision of counseling, through telephone for instance, may be an efficient and effective mental health resource for this population, and online counseling via video-conferencing may become a more practical option in the near future (Mozer et al. 2008).

Online Counseling

Online counseling is now a current and growing medium for providing mental health and psychotherapy services particularly in Anglo-Saxon countries like the United States and the United Kingdom, and has its onset in the 1980s as an evolution of previous computerized therapy developed in the 1960s and 1970s (Fletcher-Tomenius and Vossler 2009).

In some other contexts and markets in the world, the implementation of online counseling is still in its infancy and mainly restricted to a younger, more *digital native* population (Hanley 2006; Bambling et al. 2008).

The exact definitions of e-counseling or online therapy are still a source of debate in the literature, and some authors tend to view the concept as being completely defined by the specific means of provision of the service or by the therapeutic approach used by the counselor.

Abbott and Ciechomski (2008), for example, consider online counseling as the provision of advice and support via textual communications relayed back and forth between a therapist and a consumer, usually in real time, and it rarely includes a structured *treatment* program. On the other hand, the same authors consider e-therapy as a more Internet-based program for the treatment of specific disorders, deeply embedded in cognitive-behavior therapy principles, structured and with an evidence base.

These authors present in their article a proposal of distinction for the different types of mental health services provided on the Internet that we present partially in Table 11.3.

The approach that we strongly advocate is that e-counseling and online therapy are interchangeable concepts and refer to any kind of professional therapeutic interaction that makes use of the Internet (i.e., asynchronous e-mail, synchronous chat, and video-conferencing) to connect qualified mental health professionals and their clients (Roclen et al. 2004).

Notwithstanding, online counseling sessions may differ considerably because a significant time may elapse between responses, and the sessions may occur via synchronous or asynchronous channels. Synchronous communication is a distance-based conversation that occurs in real time and may be facilitated via chat rooms, real-time video, or telephone. Asynchronous conversations are accomplished through e-mails, message board postings, or video e-mails, where there may be a significant amount of time between responses (Trepal et al. 2007).

Chester and Glass (2006) found in their study that online counselors are primarily Western-based, relatively experienced, cognitive-behavioral therapy or eclectic practitioners, who combine online work with face-to-face practice.

Online clients according to the same authors are mainly female, presenting with a range of problems commonly seen in face-to-face practice, and receive services for a relatively short period, typically by e-mail.

Although the majority of online therapy takes place via e-mail (Stofle 1999), it is easy to foresee as Internet technology evolves that the use of text-based online counseling may become obsolete, giving way to video- and audio-based interventions (Haberstroh et al. 2008).

TABLE 11.3

Types of Mental Health Services Provided on the Internet

Type of Internet Mental Health Service	Definition
e-Therapy	Communication between a therapist and a consumer with directive treatment-oriented communications and the addition of an Internet-based treatment program for the treatment of specific disorders.
e-Counseling	Provision of advice and support in real time (most commonly by chat-based communication) and rarely including a structured *treatment* program.
Mental health information websites	Websites that provide information (usually text-based) such as self-help suggestions, resources for further help, and referrals. They do not involve treatment or therapist interaction (quoted by Abbott and Ciechomski 2008).
Self-guided treatment program websites	Internet-based treatment programs without consumer and therapist interaction (quoted by Abbott and Ciechomski 2008).
Online support groups	A means for persons with a mental issue to communicate with one another (either in real time or time-delayed, e.g., by discussion forums, e-mail, or chat-rooms) without the aid of a therapist (quoted by Abbott and Ciechomski 2008).
Online mental health screening and assessments	Online websites where consumers can fill in screening questionnaires to obtain an indication of their physical or mental health status (quoted by Abbott and Ciechomski 2008).

Technology advancements have the potential to profoundly impact the field, broadening its scope, practice, and range of creativity. With appropriate conditions in place, online counseling may show promise for providing a practical, therapeutic alternative or adjunctive resource to face-to-face counseling for some populations (Haberstroh et al. 2007).

There seems to be a general support in the literature for the use of video-conferencing to deliver psychological services, considering that the video-conferencing process is both clinically reliable and positively accepted by consumers (Capner 2000).

Psychotherapy experts predicted that computerized therapies, use of virtual reality, self-help resources, and self-help techniques will substantially increase in the next 10 years (Norcross et al. 2002).

Thus, the proliferation of e-counseling as a business opportunity to deliver psychological support using Internet and video technology is becoming real; also, including technology into the equation proves to be only an additional consideration when developing a service rather than a factor, which means we have to start afresh with counseling and therapy framework (Hanley 2006).

Challenges of Online Counseling

Some of the factors that can impede online counseling are clinical, personal, and environmental processes (Haberstroh et al. 2008).

In this study, technical problems seem to have the potential to not only frustrate the counselor but also create a serious barrier when the client's concerns are serious and in need of immediate attention.

The clinical limitations are specifically linked to the fact that not having access to nonverbal cues (particularly in using chat or IM means of communication) limits the participants' ability to make comprehensive assessment of the dynamics in the session in addition to assessing the severity of client's concerns, and also the slow pace of online counseling breadth, if not the depth, of the session's content (Haberstroh et al. 2008).

Other challenges in online therapeutic settings are the difficulties of developing a therapeutic relationship, but the literature seems to point out that the main obstacle is the absence of face-to-face interaction that could easily be addressed through video technology (Bloom 1998). In fact, by video-conferencing, we can actually see and hear the other person, and thus it is more similar to face-to-face than other forms of computer-mediated communication in counseling (Mallen et al. 2005).

A productive strategy to address these clinical challenges is to develop methods of maximizing the focus and impact of the online therapeutic sessions, such as making use of precounseling questions to enable interactive information gathering and identify client problems, goals, contextual factors, and resources without requiring the immediate presence of a counselor (Bambling et al. 2008).

Other issues present in online therapeutic context are security, legal, and ethical concerns associated with the delivery of mental health services via the Internet.

Technology has the potential to guarantee confidentiality of communications and client records more securely than conventional systems, but without awareness of Internet protocols and utilization of encryption solutions, online therapists may inadvertently increase the risk of divulging sensitive information (Grohol 2000).

Considering legal and ethical issues, opponents worry about licensure issues related to doing therapy across jurisdictional boundaries, legal responsibility in the event of a crisis, and the appropriateness of client anonymity, among other concerns. Many of these issues (especially pertaining to licensing) are culture- or nation-specific (Bloom 1998).

Online counseling has several challenges and clinical limitations, but one way to mitigate them is to carefully identify the target of the solution. Stofle (1999) argues that it is ideal for clients in outpatient settings and possibly even in intensive outpatient settings. However, it is not appropriate for patients who are hospitalized or who have severe psychiatric disorders, and also for those who have suicidal ideation, thought disorders, borderline personality, or unmonitored medical issues.

Other authors consider that online counseling is potentially suitable for client concerns that are not especially complex or serious or do not require face-to-face assessment (Haberstroh et al. 2008).

The authors of this study clearly anticipate that future technologies would assist counselors to assess nonverbal dynamics during online counseling sessions and also help them to visually identify their clients.

Actually most counselors provide information to clients about the possible limitations of online counseling and referred clients to face-to-face counseling where they considered it appropriate as a means to address the fact that some problems seem to be unsuitable for online counseling (Chester and Glass 2006).

Perhaps the technology of today may already answer some of the technological, clinical, and environmental challenges, as we have seen throughout the previous sections in particularly in "Aging and Dementia," "Video Care," "E-Companionship and E-Support," and "E-Counseling and Online Therapy."

Benefits of Online Counseling

Online counseling has several benefits; one of the most frequently cited is convenience and increased access for both clients and therapists (Mitchell and Murphy 1998). Plus, it also has the ability to link clients to limitless multimedia resources (Grohol 2000).

Other advantages perceived by counselors are the ability to provide services to those in remote areas (92% of respondents), decreased client defensiveness due to perceived anonymity (74% of respondents), increased flexibility of services (69% of respondents), low cost (58% of respondents), and electronic records of practitioner–client correspondence (25% of respondents) (Chester and Glass 2006).

Another advantage of online therapy is the ability to use the power of the Internet to feed relevant supplementary material to clients quickly and easily, such as links to informational websites, video clips, documents, and assessment tools that are readily supplied via all online therapy modalities. The online therapeutic context is characterized by limitless resources (Grohol 2000).

It clearly has the potential to serve people with limited mobility, time restrictions, and limited access to mental health services, or that would ordinarily not seek traditional counseling (Alleman 2002).

People who are physically disabled, such as those with dementia, or their caretakers represent another group with significant barriers to visiting a psychotherapist (Mitchell and Murphy 1998).

Despite the fact that the literature is still in need of efficacy studies of online counseling services (Bloom 1998) that will clearly establish online counseling as a truly effective mode of service, some recent studies revealed interesting results.

Considering the effectiveness of online counseling, some studies reveal significant improvements in symptom relief after participating in different online therapy interventions, reported by participants experiencing a range of clinical concerns including panic disorders (Klein and Richards 2001), eating disorders (quoted by Roclen et al. 2004), and posttraumatic stress and grief (quoted by Roclen et al. 2004).

One study that evaluates the effectiveness of Internet-based psychotherapeutic interventions, based on a comprehensive summary of 92 studies involving 9764 clients, concludes that online work is moderately effective, with an average effect size quite similar to the average effect size of traditional, face-to-face therapy (Barak et al. 2008).

Jedlicka and Jennings (2001) also concluded that online-only therapy was effective in a similar manner to that which has been described for face-to-face therapy couples. These findings were particularly evident according to the authors for couples who seemed actively engaged in problem solving, the cognitive focus of therapy.

An additional study addressing an important area within the process of online therapy found comparable, and relatively high, evaluations of the working alliance for the online sample using the frequently applied working alliance inventory (quoted by Cook and Doyle 2002). More specifically, significantly higher scores were observed on the client's ratings of the therapeutic bond and tasks involved in therapy between the online therapy and face-to-face normative data (Cook and Doyle 2002).

Day and Schneider (2002) concluded in their study that "the similarities among the three modes of therapy—face-to-face, video teleconference, and audio conference—came through more strongly than any differences" (p. 501).

Also, in a series of studies, Glueckauf et al. (2002) compared video-conferencing to face-to-face counseling for families with epileptic children, and concluded across all treatment types that participants reported significant reduction in both severity and frequency of family problems.

Implementation Success Factors

Since the e-counselor and consumer are more removed from one another than they would be if working face-to-face, they may require greater motivation and self-management ability to successfully engage in and complete treatment, particularly considering the elderly population or their caregivers (Abbott and Ciechomski 2008).

One possible way to reinforce consumer self-management and motivation is with the incorporation of videos, audio files, pictures, and graphics into the treatment material and by setting exercises and homework activities (Manhal-Baugus 2001).

It has been noted that synchronous communications may produce more immediate, direct responses, whereas asynchronous communications allow for more reflection and purposeful responses (quoted by Trepal et al. 2007). Other authors have suggested that synchronous discussions lend themselves to social interactions, whereas asynchronous discussions may be more task-oriented (quoted by Trepal et al. 2007), suggesting that different forms of communication may serve different purposes.

Guidelines for online practice have also begun to proliferate. For example, in 1997, the American Psychological Association (APA) published a statement on Internet services (American Psychological Association 1997), and two years later, the American Counseling Association (ACA) produced a document entitled Ethical Standards for Internet Online Counseling (ACA 1999, 2005). Shaw and Shaw (2006) compiled a checklist composed of 16 items to assess the current practices of online counseling services from the ACA (1999), because they found that ACA standards are viewed as the most exhaustive, and most stringent, guidelines written for Internet counseling.

In 2001, comprehensive guidelines were developed in the United Kingdom by the British Association for Counseling and Psychotherapy (Goss et al. 2001), and these were revised in 2005. Similar guidelines exist in a range of countries including Canada and Australia.

Barak et al. (2008) in their meta-analysis study concluded that most approaches to online therapy are technical (e.g., cognitive behavioral therapy), rather than those that place more emphasis upon the curative nature of the relationship (e.g., person-centered therapy). In online therapeutic settings, the three main psychotherapeutic approaches are cognitive behavioral therapy, psychoeducational interventions, and behavioral interventions.

In addition, e-therapy treatment programs are generally well structured, and guidelines are provided so the consumer is aware of what should be done (e.g., week by week); and they should incorporate a variety of multimedia modalities and specify homework exercises as a means to increase participant engagement and treatment adherence (Abbott and Ciechomski 2008). The authors referred as examples audio files that can be downloaded to practice relaxation techniques, and self-monitoring forms can also be downloaded.

Some authors find that there may be differences among telephone, synchronous chat, asynchronous e-mail, and video-conferencing in terms of quality of care. Yet, at this point, the literature still neglects these questions. For instances Mallen et al. (2005) argue that perhaps counseling by telephone and video-conferencing is superior to synchronous chat and asynchronous e-mail because nonverbal cues are transmitted instead of text.

Online Counseling and Dementia

The older adult experiencing dementia seems to have been traditionally seen as a recipient of respite care rather than as a client for mental health practice; however, Woods (2001) argued that the impaired older adult should be represented in research as well as interventions in order to address the myriad of cognitive, behavioral, and emotional concomitants of dementia.

The success of psychological interventions with dementia patients depends largely on the stage of dementia. Roth and Fonagy (1996) provided in their book a brief synopsis of different kinds of interventions with dementia patients: special design of the care environment, reality orientation, reminiscence, validation therapy, psychotherapy, cognitive-behavioral therapy, and behavior modification.

Reality orientation is the most extensively evaluated psychological approach to treating dementia, but it is only researched so far in inpatients settings, and the literature is lacking in studies of interventions for older people with dementia that are living in the community (Roth and Fonagy 1996).

Another aspect for the success of psychological intervention with this population is the important role of family members and caregivers, and the need to involve members of family systems in treatment (Myers and Schwiebert 1996).

Video-conferencing technology has also been used to conduct neuropsychological assessment interviews, particularly in dementia illnesses (Ball and McLaren 1997).

According to these authors, assessment by video-conferencing is at an early stage of development, but it clearly shows promise for the future because it allows for a much wider range of assessment than the telephone.

More recent studies, such as that of Schopp et al. (2000), have randomly assigned 98 participants with a wide range of neuropsychological problems to two modes of evaluation: video-conferencing or face-to-face interaction. In Schopp et al.'s study, no significant differences were found between the conditions on measures of client satisfaction, ease of communication, and the level of relaxation during the interview.

In fact, clients seemed to report a greater willingness to repeat the experience in the video-conferencing condition than in the face-to-face condition. However, interviewers (i.e., neuropsychologists) expressed significantly lower satisfaction with the video-conferencing condition.

Video Care Services—From Laboratory to Market

The scientific literature acknowledges a lack of projects that have reached an ongoing phase (Broens et al. 2007), and one of the major problems reported is the lack of integration of telemedicine services with traditional health systems (Botsis et al. 2008). There are also several barriers to telemedicine that make the expansion of telemedicine services difficult, like cost, legal, culture, infrastructure, policy, priorities, standards, expertise, and knowledge (World Health Organization 2009).

But according to the market analyst BCC Research (2011), we are going to contribute to a considerable market growth in the next few years. "The global telemedicine market is expected to grow from $9.8 billion in 2010 to $23 billion in 2015, at a compound annual growth rate (CAGR) of 18.6% over the next 5 years...the telephone market, which represented 28.5% of the market in 2009, is expected to capture nearly 35% by 2015. This sector is valued at nearly $2.9 billion in 2010 and is expected to increase at a 22.5% compound annual growth rate (CAGR) to reach $7.9 billion in 2015."

The private health sector is going to have a increasing role in providing telecare services and telemedicine services to their clients. This expected growth can generate new and innovative business models, similar to the one assisted with B2B and B2C markets (Timmers 2000).

Video Care: A Cost-Effective Solution

Providing health services to the elderly covers several resources and infrastructures and affects the daily lives of the elderly and their families, friends, and others.

TABLE 11.4

Cost Savings Using Video Care

Care Actors	Cost Perspective[a]		
	Cost of Care Provision	Impact of Preventing Institutionalization	Impact on Disease Progression
	7.9 € per day	Nursing home: 121 € per day Respite care: 137 € per day Day care: 72.7 €	
Elderly	+ Savings: improved access to social and health services by family and friends without travel needs.		
Family and friends	+ Savings: family and friends can interact without travel needs.	+ Savings: family and friends can be part of the symptom-based surveillance (Johansen et al. 2010). + Savings: reduce the burden placed on caregivers and provide them with more personal freedom.	
Employers	+ Savings: the employees can be more engaged with their job and can better manage the family demands and reduce absenteeism.		
Society	+ Savings: more efficiency (number of patients visited per day).	+ Savings: reduce unnecessary hospital admissions. + Savings: support hospital discharge and intermediate care. + Savings: reduce the need for residential/nursing care.	

[a] Costs used in the study by Magnusson and Hanson (2005).

The economic analysis of telehealth is one of the key research areas considered by the ATA. Economic analysis is one of the biggest issues we have in the telehealth and health-care in general today, and there is very little sophistication in the economic analyses of telehealth to date. A lot of the research is in an exploratory phase at this point. For example, the economic perspective that one wishes to study should be stated (i.e., societal, healthcare system, etc.). According to Krupinski et al. (2006) "we need methodologies and statistics that are designed for the type of multi-site, longitudinal, complex, dynamic system that we know telehealth is." We propose to analyze the problem of costs in three perspectives (Bayer 2007): (1) the cost of care provision, (2) the impact of preventing institutionalization, and (3) the impact on disease progression. The costs are also analyzed using perspectives from different actors that participate in the care process (World Health Organization 1998): (1) elderly, (2) family and friends, (3) employers, and (4) society.

In Table 11.4, the cost savings are summarized according to the perspectives mentioned.

The major predictors of institutionalization (Luppa et al. 2010) in the elderly are the following:

- *Strong evidence*: self-rated health status, low; cognitive impairment, dementia; prior institutionalization; number of prescriptions
- *Moderate evidence*: employment status, employed; social network, low contacts; activity level, low; diabetes

Those predictors can be addressed by video care services as presented in the previous sections. Video care services can improve health indicators* (World Health Organization 1998), improving the quality of life and at the same time obtaining cost savings and improving access to social, health services, and family and friends support.

---

* Mortality and morbidity, impact of disease and impairment on daily activities and behavior, perceived health, disability/functional status measures.

This study advocates that the video care services can mitigate the risks associated with major predictors of institutionalization, contributing to minimizing the probability or retarding the institutionalization. In the study by Magnusson and Hanson (2005), the cost presented for supporting frail people and their family caregivers at home using information and communications technology was 7.9 € per day. The average savings per day was 26.8 €, which represents a benefit of 239.7% (ROI).

Video Care Services Development in Portugal

In Portugal, the authors are engaged in an AAL4ALL Project. The main objective of the AAL4ALL project is the development of an ecosystem of products and services for AAL associated to a business model and validated through a large-scale trial. The authors are engaged in developing a video care system to provide services for seniors and their relatives. The catalog of services includes companionship and general information and assistance, geriatric case management, nursing support, and psychological counseling.

In the process of developing the services, the major requirements considered are the following:

1. The services utilization must have a positive contribution for improving quality of life of the future users (Monteiro 2012).
2. The services must provide a high quality of user experience and address the paradigm of ubiquitous computing.

The scientific body of knowledge used in the new service process development are the following: information systems artifact design, information technology acceptance, psychology, service design, and design thinking.

Conclusion

We are assisting nowadays two important sociocultural trends. The first is the outstanding increase in longevity that began in the twentieth century especially in the developed countries. The second is the accelerating development of technology. The confluence of these two trends might lead to positive outcomes on the aging population, with cost reduction and efficacy benefits in the health and social care industry.

However, a larger number of older people are living in developed countries, and therefore it is essential to look carefully to the developing world, in which the estimates suggest that in the future, the number of people with dementia in the developing world will vastly exceed those in the developed world.

The increased number of people with dementia will have an impact on the economy and health care and social protection systems, and developing countries particularly are not prepared for this impact.

The demand for qualified health care professionals has never been greater.

E-companionship is an area that is of great advantage to enhance the communication and network relations of elderly people. This area of interactive video prevents social isolation and can help the elderly with dementia and their families.

Studies show that the use of video facilitates communication and in some cases enhances the quality of communication over face-to-face, because dementia patients are more focused. In addition, families that are far from their elderly relatives can have a direct channel for talking, watching, and participating during the caregiving. Health and social care professionals also benefit from this approach, since it makes possible direct contact for instrumental support and emotional support, saving travel and time expenses.

The limitation of these studies is partly related to the attitude of health care professionals (Arnaert and Delesie 2001; Sävenstedt 2004; Jönsson and Willman 2009; Lauricks et al. 2010). Health care practitioners, besides nurses, need to be open to this new current practice and be in favor of new technologies, like communication via video telephony with the elderly about their needs, expectations, and feelings. Usually, the formal health care caregivers are enhancers for families in order for them to learn and use the new technologies.

Another barrier for these kinds of studies is that several ICT applications and services were developed for the elderly but not tested for people with dementia (Lauricks et al. 2010). People with dementia have specific needs and requirements for equipment that are different from the specific requirements of an elderly person, and so cautious analysis, evaluation, and testing are required.

People with early and mild dementia can express themselves and are capable of identifying their needs; special attention has to be given to their needs and not only from the perspective of informal caregivers, because it could be different. A need for user-centered design (Mynatt and Rogers 2001) is the best approach in developing video technology that best fits the needs of people with dementia.

We can conclude that older adults have been clearly underserved in the area of counseling services, despite the considerably high incidence of mental health needs, and the proven effectiveness of counseling and psychotherapy interventions with this population.

Traditionally, older adults experiencing dementia have been seen as recipients of respite care rather than as clients for mental health practice, but the success of psychological interventions with dementia patients depends largely on the stage of the dementia and the important role of family members and caregivers in the treatment process.

The provision of these services via online and video technology presents a unique opportunity to overcome physical, psychological, and community professional offering, and also guarantees an efficient and effective mental health resource for this population.

The online counseling field is to be profoundly impacted by technology advancements by broadening the scope, practice, and range of creativity, but the inclusion of technology reveals itself only as an additional consideration when developing these services.

Some challenges of online counseling need to be addressed in order for these services to succeed, such as clinical limitations, technical problems, and security, legal, and ethical concerns.

Considering the clinical aspects, in the provision of online counseling, the target of intervention should be well defined, and treatment design should be more structured and concise. Professionals also need to strongly focus on the development of the therapeutic relationship and client motivation and self-engagement in the process.

Although through video-conferencing counselors will have access to nonverbal cues, such as in face-to-face interventions, there is still some advice in the literature to maximize the focus and impact by precounseling questions to enable interactive information gathering, and also by enriching the therapeutic context with a variety of multimedia resources and specifying homework exercises.

Technology problems need to be addressed in order to prevent frustration and lack of immediacy in the provision of services.

Confidentiality of communications and client records should be secure and abide by Internet protocols and utilization of encryption solutions.

When implementing online counseling services, developers need to consider legal and ethical issues, such as licensure issues and legal responsibility, which are culture- and nation-specific.

The major advantages reported seem to be convenience and increased access; decreased client defensiveness; increased flexibility of services; the power of the Internet to easily feed relevant supplementary material to clients in different multimedia supports; and the possibility to conduct neuropsychological assessment interviews.

Several studies show no significant differences in outcomes when comparing face-to-face, video teleconference, and audio conference, reporting significant problems and symptom reductions, and relatively high evaluations of the working alliance. Thus, the use of video-conferencing to deliver psychological services to dementia patients seems to be both clinically reliable and positively accepted by consumers.

References

Abbott, J.-A. M., and Ciechomski, L. "Best practices in online therapy." *Best Pratices in Online Therapy* 26 (2008): 2–4.

Alleman, J. R. "Online counseling: The internet and mental health treatment." *Psychotherapy: Theory: Research, Practice, Training* 39 (2002): 199–209.

American Counseling Association (ACA). "ACA history: 1999." Alexandria, VA: ACA, 1999.

American Counseling Association (ACA). "Code of Ethics." Alexandria, VA: ACA, 2005.

American Psychological Association (APA). "Statement on services by telephone, teleconferencing and internet." 1997.

American Telemedicine Association. "Practice guidelines for videoconferencing-based elemental health." 2008.

Apple. "Apple brings FaceTime to the Mac." *Apple website*. October 20, 2010. http://www.apple.com/pr/library/2010/10/20facetime.html (accessed June 5, 2011).

Apple. "Apple launches iPad 2." *Apple website*. March 2, 2011. http://www.apple.com/pr/library/2011/03/02ipad.html (accessed June 6, 2011).

Arnaert, A., and Delesie, L. "Telenursing for the elderly. The case for care via video-telephony." *Journal of Telemedicine and Telecare* 7 (2001): 311–316.

Arnaert, A., and Delesie, L. "Effectiveness of video-telephone nursing care for the homebound elderly." *Canadian Journal of Nursing Research* 39(1) (2007): 20–36.

Ball, C., and McLaren, P. "The tele-assessment of cognitive state: A review." *Journal of Telemedicine and Telecare* 3 (1997): 126–131.

Bambling, M., King, R., Reid, W., and Wegner, K. "Online counselling: The experience of counsellors providing synchronous single-session counselling to young people." *Counselling and Psychotherapy Research* 8(2) (2008): 110–116.

Barak, A. H., Boniel-Nissin, M., and Shapira, N. "A comprehensive review and meta-analysis of the effectiveness of internet-based psychotherapeutic interventions." *Journal of Technology in Human Services* 26 (2008): 109–160.

Bayer, S. "Assessing the impact of a care innovation telecare." *System Dynamics Review* 23(1) (Spring 2007): 61–80.

BCC Research. "Research report telemedicine: Opportunities for medical and electronic providers." 2011. http://www.bccresearch.com/report/HLC014D.html (accessed June 6, 2011).

Bloom, J. W. "The ethical practice of Web counseling." *British Journal of Guidance* 26 (1998): 53–59.

Botsis, T., Demiris, G., Pedersen, S., and Hartvigsen, G. "Home telecare technologies for the elderly." *Journal of Telemedicine and Telecare* 14 (2008): 333–337.

Broens, T. H. F., Huis in't Veld, R. M. H. A., Vollenbroek-Hutten, M. M. R., Hermens, H. J., van Halteren A. T., and Nieuwenhuis, L. J. "Determinants of successful telemedicine implementations: A literature study." *Journal of Telemedicine and Telecare* 13 (2007): 303–309.

Brownsell, S., Aldred, H., and Hawley, M. "The role of telecare in supporting the needs of elderly people." *Journal of Telemedicine and Telecare* 13(6) (2007): 293–297.

Cahil, S. M. "Technology in dementia care." *Technology and Disability* 19 (2007): 55–60.

Capner, M. "Videoconferencing in the provision of psychological services at a distance." *Journal of Telemedicine and Telecare* 6 (2000): 311–319.

Charness, N., and Boot, W. R. "Aging and information technology use potential and barriers." *Current Directions in Psychological Science* 18(5) (2009): 253–258.

Chester, A., and Glass, C. A. "Online counselling: A descriptive analysis of therapy services on the internet." *British Journal of Guidance and Counselling* 34 (2006): 145–160.

Cisco. "Cisco makes recommended offer to acquire TANDBERG. Acquisition of TANDBERG to expand Cisco's collaboration offering to transform how they do business globally." *Cisco*. Edited by CISCO. October 1, 2009. http://newsroom.cisco.com/dlls/2009/corp_093009.html?print=true (accessed June 6, 2011).

Constantinescu, G., Theodoros, D., Russell, T., Ward, E., Wilson, S., and Wootton, R. "Home-based speech treatment for Parkinson's disease delivered remotely: A case report." *Journal of Telemedicine and Telecare* 16 (2010): 100–104.

Cook, J. E., and Doyle, C. "Working alliance in online therapy as compared to face-to-face therapy: Preliminary results." *Cyberpsychology and Behavior* 5 (2002): 95–105.

Davis, A. W., and Weinstein, I. M. "The business case for videoconferencing—Achieving a competitive edge." 2005. http://www.wainhouse.com/files/papers/wr-bizcase4vc-v2.pdf (accessed February 29, 2012).

Day, S. X., and Schneider, P. L. "Psychotherapy using distance technology: A comparison of face-to-face, video, and audio treatment." *Journal of Counseling Psychology* 49 (2002): 499–503.

Demiris, G., Speedie, S., Finkelstein, S., and Harris, I. "Communication patterns and technical quality of virtual visits in home care." *Journal of Telemedicine and Telecare* 9 (2003): 210–215.

Egido, C. "Videoconferencing as a technology to support group work: A review of its failure." *Proceeding CSCW '88 Proceedings of the 1988 ACM Conference on Computer-supported, Cooperative Work*. New York: ACM, 1988.

Fletcher-Tomenius, L. J., and Vossler, A. "Trust in online therapeutic relationships: The therapist's experience." *Counselling Psychology Review* 24 (2009): 24–33.

Glueckauf, R. L., Fritz, S. P., Ecklund-Jonhson, E. P., Liss, E. P., Dages, H. J., and Carney, P. "Videoconferencing-based family counseling for rural teenagers with epilepsy: Phase 1 findings." *Rehabilitation Psychology* 47 (2002): 49–72.

Glueckauf, R. L., Ketterson, T. U., Loomis, J. S., and Dages, P. "Online support and education for dementia caregivers: Overview, utilization, and initial program evaluation." *Telemedicine Journal and E-Health* 10 (2004): 223–232.

Goss, S., Anthony, K., Jamieson, A., and Palmer, S. *Guidelines for Online Counseling and Psychotherapy*. Rugby: BACP Publishing, 2001.

Grohol, J. M. *The Insider's Guide to Mental Health Resources Online*. New York: Guilford Press, 2000.

Haberstroh, S., Duffey, T., Evans, M., Gee, R., and Trepal, H. "The experience of online counseling." *Journal of Mental Health Counseling* 29–23 (2007): 269–282.

Haberstroh, S., Parr, G., Bradley, L., Morgan-Fleming, B., and Gee, R. "Facilitating online counseling." *Journal of Counseling and Development* 86 (2008): 460–470.

Haley, W. E. "Psychotherapy with older adults in primary care medical settings." *Journal of Clinical Psychology* 55(8) (1999): 991–1004.

Hanley, T. "Developing youth-friendly online counselling services in the United Kingdom: A small scale investigation into the views of practitioners." *Counselling and Psychotherapy Research* 6(3) (2006): 182–185.

Harrington, T., and Harrington, M. *Gerontechnology Why and How.* Maastricht: Shaker, 2000.

Hebert, M. A., Jansen, J. J., Brant, R., Hailey, D., and van der Pol, M. "Successes and challenges in a field-based, multi-method study of home telehealth." *Journal of Telemedicine and Telecare* 10(Suppl. 1) (2004): 41–44.

Hensel, B., Parker-Oliver, D., and Demiris, G. "Videophone communication between residents and family: A case study." *Journal of American Medical Directors Association* 8 (2007): 123.

Higgins, E. "A review of unrecognized mental illness in primary care." *Archives of Family Medicine* 3 (1994): 908–917.

Hill, A., and Brettle, A. "Counselling older people: What can we learn from research evidence?" *Journal of Social Work Practice* 20–23 (2006): 281–297.

Jedlicka, D., and Jennings, G. "Marital therapy on the Internet." *Journal of Technology in Counseling* 2 (2001): 1–15.

Johansen, M. A., Johnsen, J.-A. K., Shrestha, N., and Bellika, J. G. "Symptoms from patients as the primary information source for real-time surveillance." In *MEDINFO 2010—Proceedings of the 13th World Congress on Medical Informatics*, Series: Studies Health Technology Informatics, volume 160, pp. 427–431, edited by S. Reti, H. F. Marin, and C. Safran. Cape Town, South Africa: IOS Press, 2010.

Jönsson, A.-M., and Willman, A. "Telenursing in home care services experiences of registered nurses." *Electronic Journal of Health Informatics* 4(1) (2009): 1–7, e9.

Kasvi, J. J. J., Vartiainen, M., and Hailikari, M. "Managing knowledge and knowledge competences in projects and project organisations." *International Journal of Project Management* 21 (2003): 571–582.

Klein, B., and Richards, J. C. "A brief internet-based treatment for panic disorder." *Behavioral and Cognitive Psychotherapy* 29 (2001): 113–117.

Kraut, R., and Fish, R. "Prospects for video telephony." *Telecommunications Policy* 19 (1995): 699–719.

Krupinski, E., Dimmick, S., Grigsby, J., Mogel, G., Puskin, D., Speedie, S. et al. "Research recommendations for the American Telemedicine Association." *Telemedicine Journal and e-Health* 12(5) (2006): 579–589.

Lauricks, S., Reinersmann, A., Roest, H., Meiland, F., Davies, R., Moelaert, F. et al. "Review of ICT-based services for identified unmet user needs in people with dementia." In *Supporting People with Dementia Using Pervasive Health Technologies*, Mulvenna, M. D. and Nugent, C. D. (editors), pp. 37–61. London: Springer-Verlag, 2010.

Luppa, M., Luck, T., Weyerer, S., König, H.-H., Brähler, E., and Riedel Heller, S. G. "Prediction of institutionalization in the elderly. A systematic review." *Age and Ageing* 39(1) (2010): 31–38.

Luxenberg, J. "Clinical issues in the behavioural and psychological symptoms of dementia." *International Journal of Geriatric Psychiatry* 15 (2000): 52–54.

Magnusson, L., and Hanson, E. "Supporting frail older people and their family carers at home using information and communication technology: Cost analysis." *Nursing and Health Care Management and Policy* 51 (2005): 645–657.

Magnusson, L., Berthold, H., Chambers, M., Brito, L., Emery, D., and Daly, T. "Using telematics with older people: The ACTION project." *Nursing Standard* 13 (1998): 36–40.

Magnusson, L., Hanson, E., and Nolan, M. "The impact of information and communication technology and family careers of older people and professionals in Sweden." *Aging and Society* 25 (2005): 693–713.

Mallen, M. J., Vogel, D. L., Rochlen, A. B., and Day, S. X. "Online counseling: Reviewing the literature from a counseling psychology framework." *The Counseling Psychologist* 6 (2005): 819–871.

Manhal-Baugus, M. "Etherapy: Practical, ethical and legal issues." *Cyberpsychology and Behavior* 4 (2001): 551–563.

Mickus, M., and Luz, C. "Televisits: Sustaining long distance family relationships among institutionalized elders trough technology." *Aging and Mental Health* 6(4) (2002): 387–396.

Microsoft. "Microsoft to acquire Skype-combined companies will benefit consumers, businesses and increase market opportunity." *Microsoft News website*. October 5, 2011. http://www.microsoft .com/presspass/press/2011/may11/05-10corpnewspr.mspx (accessed June 6, 2011).

Mitchell, D. L., and Murphy, L. M. "Confronting the challenges of therapy online: A pilot project." *Proceedings of the Seventh National and Fifth International Conference on Information Technology and Community Health*. Victoria, British Columbia, Canada, 1998.

Mochizuki-Kawai, H., Tanaka, M., Suzuki, T., Yamakawa, Y., Mochizuki, S., Arai, M. et al. "Elderly adults improve verbal fluency by videophone conversations: A pilot study." *Journal of Telemedicine and Telecare* 14 (2008): 215–218.

Monteiro, J. *Estratégias de Negócio e Capacidade Tecnológica em Mercados Digitais: As Lojas Virtuais Portuguesas*. Lisboa: ISEG/UTL, 2001.

Monteiro, J. "Improve quality of life—Additional criteria for health and social care information technology acceptance in an ageing world." *pHealth 2012 Proceedings of the 9th International Conference on Wearable Micro and Nano Technologies for Personalized Health*. Netherlands: IOS Press, 2012, 59–64.

Mozer, E., Franklin, B., and Rose, J. "Psychotherapeutic intervention by telephone." *Clinical Interventions in Aging* 3(2) (2008): 391–396.

Myers, J. E., and Schwiebert, V. *Competencies for Gerontological Counselors*. Alexandria: American Counseling Association, 1996.

Mynatt, E., and Rogers, W. "Developing technology to support the functional independence of older adults." *Ageing International* 27 (2001): 24–41.

Nakamura, K., Takano, T., and Akao, C. "The effectiveness of videophones in home healthcare for the elderly." *Medical Care* (Lippincott Williams and Wilkins, Inc.) 37(2) (1999): 117–125.

Norcross, J. C., Hedges, M., and Prochaska, J. O. "The face of 2010: A Delphi poll on the future of psychotherapy." *Professional Psychology* 33 (2002): 316–322.

Nordhus, I. H., and VandenBos, G. R. *Clinical Gero-Psychology*. Washington, DC: American Psychological Association, 1998.

Nugent, C. D. "ICT in the elderly and dementia." *Aging and Mental Health* 11(5) (2007): 473–476.

O'Hara, K., Black, A., and Lipson, M. "Everyday practices with mobile video telephony." *CHI '06 Proceedings of the SIGCHI Conference on Human Factors in Computing Systems*. New York: ACM, 2006.

Orpwood, R. S. "Designing technology to support quality of life of people with dementia." *Technology and Disability* 19 (2007): 103–112.

Portero, C., and Oliva, A. "Social support, psychological well-being, and health among elderly." *Educational Gerontology* 33 (2007): 1053–1068.

Roclen, A. B., Zack, J. S., and Speyer, C. (2004). "Online therapy: Review of relevant definitions, debates, and current empirical support." *Journal of Clinical Psychology* 60(3) (2004): 269–283.

Rogers, W., Cabrera, E., Walker, N., Gilbert, D., and Fisk, A. "A survey of automatic teller machine usage across the adult lifespan." *Human Factors* 38 (1996): 156–166.

Roth, A., and Fonagy, P. *What Works for Whom? A Critical Review of Psychotherapy Research*. New York: Guilford Press, 1996.

Sävenstedt, S. *Telecare of Frail Elderly—Reflections and Experiences among Health Personnel and Family Members*. Umeå: Umeå University, 2004.

Sävenstedt, S., Brulin, C., and Sandman, P.-O. "Family members' narrated experiences of communicating via video-phone with patients with dementia staying at a nursing home." *Journal of Telemedicine and Telecare* 9 (2003): 216–220.

Schopp, L. H., Johnstone, B., and Merveille, O. C. "Multidimensional telehealth care for rural residents with brain injury." *Journal of Telemedicine and Telecare* 6(Suppl. 1) (2000): 146–149.

Shaw, H. E., and Shaw, S. F. "Critical issues in online counselling: Assessing current practices with an ethical intent checklist." *Journal of Counseling and Development*, 84 (2006): 41–53.

Smith, G., Lunde, A., Hathaway, J., and Vickers, K. "Telehealth home monitoring of solitary persons with mild dementia." *American Journal of Alzheimer's Disease and Other Dementias* 22(1) (2007): 20–26.

Smyer, M. A., and Qualls, S. H. *Aging and Mental Health*. Malden, MA: Blackwell, 1999.

Stofle, G. S. *Choosing an Online Therapist*. Harrisburg, PA: White Hat Communications, 1999.

Tetley, J., Hanson, E., and Clark, A. "Older people, telematics and care." In *Care Services for Later Life: Transformations and Critiques*, pp. 243–258, edited by L. Warren, and M. N. T. Warnes. London: Jessica Kinglsey, 2001, 243–258.

The New York Times. "For Microsoft, Skype opens vast new market in telecom." *The New York Times website*. May 10, 2011. http://www.nytimes.com/2011/05/11/technology/11skype.html (accessed June 6, 2011).

Timmers, P. *Strategies and Models for Business-to-Business Trading Electronic Commerce*. West Sussex: John Wiley and Sons, Ltd., 2000.

Trepal, H., Haberstroh, S., Duffey, T., and Evans, M. "Considerations and strategies for teaching online counseling skills: Establishing relationships in cyberspace." *Counselor Education and Supervision* 46(4) (2007): 266–279.

van der Heijden, H. "User acceptance of hedonic information systems." *MIS Quarterly* 28(4) (2004): 695–704.

Venkatesh, V., and Brown, S. "A longitudinal investigation of personal computers in homes: Adaptation determinants and emerging challenges." *MIS Quarterly* 25 (2001): 71–102.

Venkatesh, V., Morris, M. G., and Davis, F. D. "User acceptance of information technology: Toward a unified view." *MIS Quarterly* 27(3) (2003): 425–478.

Wakefield, B. J., Holman, J. E., Ray, A., Morse, J., and Kienzle, M. "Nurse and patient communication via low-and high-bandwidth home telecare systems." *Journal of Telemedicine and Telecare* 10 (2004): 156–159.

Warner, I. "Telemedicine applications for home health care." *Journal of Telemedicine* 3(1) (1997): 65–66.

Webster, J. "Desktop videoconferencing: Experiences of complete users, wary users, and non-users." *MIS Quarterly* 22 (1998): 257–286.

Weinstein, I. M. *The ISDN to IP Migration for Videoconferencing*. Duxbury, MA: Wainhouse Research, 2006.

Weyerer, S., Hafner, H., Mann, A., Ames, D., and Graham, N. "Prevalence and course of depression among elderly residential home admissions in Manheim and Camden." *London International Psychogeriatrics* 7(4) (1995): 479–493.

Whitten, P., Mair, F., and Collins, B. "Home telenursing in Kansas: Patients' perceptions of uses and benefits." *Journal of Telemedicine and Telecare* 3(Suppl. 1) (1997): 67–69.

Wills, A., and Shinar, O. "Measuring perceived and received social support." In *Social Support Measurement and Intervention. A Guide for Health and Social Scientists*, pp. 86–135, edited by L. Underwood, B. Gottlieb, and S. Cohen. New York: Oxford University Press, 2000.

Wimo, A., and Prince, M. *World Alzheimer Report 2010—The Global Economic Impact of Dementia*. London: Alzheimer's Disease International, 2010.

Woods, R. T. "Discovering the person with Alzheimer's disease: Cognitive, emotional, and behavioral aspects." *Aging and Mental Health* 5 (2001): S7–S16.

World Health Organization. "WHOQOL- user manual—Programme on mental health." 1998.

World Health Organization. *Active Ageing: A Policy Framework.* Madrid: Noncommunicable Disease Prevention and Health Promotion Department; Ageing in Life Course, 2002.

World Health Organization. *The Solid Facts—Home Care in Europe.* Copenhagen: WHO Regional Office for Europe, 2008.

World Health Organization. *Telemedicine—Opportunities and Developments in Member States.* Geneva: WHO Press, 2009.

Zundel, K. M. "Telemedicine: History, applications, and impact on librarianship." *Bull Med Libr Assoc* 84(1) (1996): 71–79.

12

Telemedicine Scenario for Elderly People with Comorbidity

César P. Gálvez-Barrón, Maged N. Kamel Boulos, Sandra Prescher, Carlos Abellán Cano, Emilio Suárez Ortega, Ada Font Tió, Jordi Morales Gras, Karol O'Donovan, Marta Díaz Boladeras, Friedrich Köhler, and Alejandro Rodríguez-Molinero

CONTENTS

ABSTRACT   Progressive population aging is associated with negative social and economic impacts mainly due to its associated comorbidity rather than to aging *per se*. In this regard, information and communication technology resources may provide useful tools to assist the population with comorbidities through the use of telemedicine systems. However, despite their potential, such systems have not yet been effectively implemented due to a number of different reasons: absence of a clear business plan, poor acknowledgment of their clinical usefulness, and ethical and legal issues, among others. An analysis of the current scenario from the point of view of the different actors (patients, health care providers, and health care systems) aimed at identifying the needs to be covered by telemedicine systems that could contribute to overcoming such problems. This chapter is intended to offer such an analysis.

KEY WORDS: *telemedicine, telehealth, telecare, telemonitoring, remote patient management, older people, comorbidity, health systems, social services.*

Introduction

Progressive population aging and increasing chronic diseases (WHO 2011) have promoted interest in the development of solutions for the health-related, economic, and social adverse effects of this phenomenon, which are precipitated by aging-related comorbidity rather than by aging *per se*. An important development sector dedicated to researching these solutions focuses on the application of information and communication technologies (ICTs) to providing assistance and medical care to older people, including telemedicine, telehealth, and telecare. However, despite the large potential for ICT applications in this field, such solutions have not yet been effectively implemented due to a number of factors: absence of a clear business plan, poor acknowledgment of their clinical usefulness (evidence-based medicine), ethical and legal issues, usability problems with the required devices, failure to meet the actual needs of the target population, and a need for organizational changes in current health systems, among others.

A major step toward overcoming such obstacles is consideration of the scenario where these technological resources could potentially be introduced. Unfortunately, there is not a single scenario for the use of ICT due to high variability among both the technological applications and the users.

The goal of this chapter is to provide a description and analysis of the specific scenario for a telemedicine application to monitor and provide health care to older people with comorbidity. To that end, the main actors in this scenario have to be identified along with the set of technologies included in the telemedicine solution.

As far as the identification of scenario actors is concerned, the Ambient Assisted Living Innovation Alliance (AALIANCE) platform, in the published Ambient Assisted Living Roadmap (AALIANCE 2009), identifies the following actors for the global ambient assisted living (AAL) scenario:

- *Primary stakeholders*: users and caregivers
- *Secondary stakeholders*: organizations offering services
- *Tertiary stakeholders*: organizations supplying goods and services
- *Quaternary stakeholders*: organizations analyzing the economic and legal context of AAL

In this chapter, we use a modified classification adapted to the telemedicine services for older people:

- *Older patients*: potential end users
- *Health care professionals*: all medical (clinical) and nonmedical professionals involved in providing assistance to older people
- *Health systems*: health organizations who are potential contractors of telemedicine systems

Furthermore, due to the high heterogeneity of ICT resources, those to be included in a particular telemedicine solution should be clearly specified. A definition of telemedicine by the World Health Organization (WHO) states (WHO 1998a, p. 10), "Telemedicine is the delivery of healthcare services, where distance is a critical factor, by all healthcare professionals using information and communication technologies for the exchange of valid information for diagnosis, treatment and prevention of disease and injuries, research and evaluation, and for the continuing education of healthcare providers, all in the interests of enhancing the health of individuals and their communities."

The scenario described in this chapter is intended for telemedicine systems aimed at domiciliary remote patient monitoring and assistance (consultation/diagnosis, monitoring/management/surveillance) for older patients with comorbidity by the health care providers involved in their care.

The contents of this chapter are organized into three sections:

1. "Aging, Comorbidity, and Target Diseases" reviews the impact of comorbidity and its consequences, as well as those conditions that should be covered by telemedicine systems.
2. "Scenario for Each Stakeholder of Telemedicine Systems" analyzes and describes the scenario for each stakeholder—patients, health professionals, and health systems (organizations).
3. "Potential Scenarios for Telemedicine Systems" describes potential situations, scenarios, and use cases for the use of the telemedicine systems covered in this chapter.

Aging, Comorbidity, and Target Diseases

Aging and Comorbidity

Progressive population aging is a well-known phenomenon, especially in developed countries, including most of the European countries. Data published in the EUROSTAT 2008 report (Giannakouris 2008) illustrate this demographic phenomenon and its possible socioeconomic consequences in the coming years:

- Population aged 65 years or over will grow from 17.1% in year 2008 to 30% of total Europeans (151.5 million, including Switzerland and Norway) in 2060.

- The current 4:1 ratio of persons of working age (15–64 years) to persons aged 65 or over is expected to decrease to 2:1 by 2060.

Several studies have demonstrated that aging is associated with (different than *being the cause of*) an increase in the prevalence* of different chronic diseases (Guralnik 1996). However, aging is associated not only with an increasing number of persons who suffer from a chronic disease but also with an increasing number of diseases that affect them: 1.88 associated chronic diseases for persons aged 65–69 years and 2.71 associated diseases for persons over 85 years (Wolff et al. 2002). In 1999, 24% of patients over 65, who were managed by the Medicare (United States), had more than four chronic diseases (Wolff et al. 2002). Unlike what used to be the case in past decades, managing patients with coexisting chronic diseases is nowadays the norm rather than the exception (Starfield 2006).

Comorbidity is a term with more than one definition. We take the following as a reference: "comorbidity is the concurrent presence of two or more medically diagnosed diseases in the same individual, with the diagnosis of each contributing disease based on established, widely recognized criteria" (Fried et al. 2004, p. 258).

However, the consequences of comorbidity go beyond the *coexistence* of diseases (Fried et al. 2004; Gijsen et al. 2001; Karlamangla et al. 2007; Valderas et al. 2009). A study by Ettinger et al. (1994) conducted on 4059 patients with either knee arthropathy, cardiac disease, or pulmonary disease revealed that the risk for motor disability was 4.4 (odds ratio) in patients with arthritis, 2.3 in patients with cardiac disease, and as high as 13.6 in patients with both conditions. This is due to the *interaction* between different conditions—often apparently unrelated (e.g., arthritis and heart disease)—so that the consequences (in this example, evaluated as motor disability) are not always simply summational (Fried et al. 2004; Gijsen et al. 2001; Karlamangla et al. 2007; Valderas et al. 2009).

A foreseeable consequence of the increasing number of chronic diseases associated with population aging is an increase in health-related costs. Wolff et al. (2002) performed a study on health care costs for 1.2 million persons aged 65 or over, randomly selected from Medicare, for the year 1999. Several observations can be drawn from their study:

- Health care costs increase with an increase in the age and number of coexisting diseases; however, the increase is very much higher in persons with chronic conditions compared to persons without chronic conditions. Costs increase from $195 for a person aged 65 to 69 without chronic conditions to $999 for a person of the same age with one chronic condition.

---

* The proportion of persons that suffer from a certain disease in relation to the total population at a certain moment.

- The number of conditions coexisting in a person influences the health care costs more than their age; thus, health care costs for a person aged 65–69 with two associated chronic conditions are higher ($2055) than those for a person over 85 years with one associated chronic condition ($1579). In other words, health care costs for a person aged 65–69 with one associated chronic condition ($999) rise more if the person develops a second associated chronic condition than when the person simply gets older.

Thus, the comorbidity affecting a certain person is more relevant than their aging *per se.*

Target Diseases for Telemedicine Systems

It is essential that telemedicine systems are aimed at providing assistance for conditions that are most relevant to older people. In order to evaluate the clinical relevance of diseases, the following main parameters can be used: disease prevalence or frequency, diseases that lead to hospitalization, associated mortality, and associated functional impairment.

The Health Survey for England (HSE) consists of a group of annual studies, each year with special emphasis on a different topic concerning the English Health System. In 2005, these studies were especially focused on older people (The Information Centre 2007). In this study, the most frequently reported diseases (physician-diagnosed chronic conditions reported by the person taking the questionnaire) were cardiovascular diseases (CVDs) for men (37%) and joint diseases (mainly arthritis) for women (47%). Since women outlive men (a finding habitually observed for this age group worldwide), osteoarticular disorders are commonly reported as the one most frequent chronic disease. However, the mortality caused by CVD (stroke, acute myocardial infarction, heart failure, etc.) is usually higher than that caused by osteoarticular disorders (WHO 1998b). In turn, disability produced by osteoarticular disorders is rather important. A study conducted by Boult et al. (1996) on the US population with projections for years 2001 and 2049 predicted that 1% biannual reductions in the prevalence of arthritis would reduce the number of functionally limited older persons more than equivalent reductions in the prevalence of other conditions such as coronary artery disease, stroke, diabetes, cancer, or delirium.

As a reference for conditions most often causing hospitalization, we include information from the Minimum Basic Data Set (MBDS) from the Spanish National Surveillance System for Hospital Data* (Ministerio de Sanidad y Consumo 2006). Major causes of admission to hospital of persons aged 65 or over, reported by the MBDS in 2005 (Table 12.1), include the following five most frequent main diagnoses: heart failure, chronic bronchitis, osteoarthritis and related disorders, pneumonia, and hip fracture.

Notice that cardiovascular, respiratory, and osteoarticular diseases are the most frequent causes of admission to hospital within this age group. Together they account for 18% of total hospitalizations; although apparently low, this proportion is not meaningful without taking into account the long list of different diagnoses (total number 571) and the considerable overlapping of related diagnoses. Grouping diseases into affected organs and systems shows that cardiovascular diseases (including stroke), respiratory diseases, and osteoarticular disorders (including fractures) account for 37% of total admissions to hospital. Hip fracture, being the fifth cause of hospitalization, deserves special attention because of the massive changes in quality of life and functional situation that it usually brings about in

---

* Database including 99% of the hospitals belonging to the National Health System (more than 95% of the hospitals in Spain).

TABLE 12.1

Hospitalization Causes (Aged 65 and Over, 2005)

Disease	#(%)
Heart failure	68,363 (16.37%)
Chronic bronchitis	63,964 (15.32%)
Osteoarthritis and other osteoarticular diseases	43,647 (10.45%)
Pneumonia	41,075 (9.84%)
Hip fracture	40,934 (9.80%)
Colelithiasis	35,864 (8.59%)
Acute myocardial infarct	35,033 (8.39%)
Stroke	34,290 (8.21%)
Cardiac arrhythmia	28,766 (6.89%)
Other lung diseases	25,650 (6.14%)
Total	417,586 (100%)

Source: Ministerio de Sanidad y Consumo, Conjunto Mínimo Básico de Datos 2005. Spain, 2006. Available at http://www.msc.es (accessed October 17, 2012).

a rather short period of time (one out of five patients dies within a year after the fracture; Cooper et al. 1993; Koike et al. 1999; Walker et al. 1999), and only 40% of patients recover their previous functional situation (Koot et al. 2000). Many of these fractures are the consequence of falls, which are not managed until several hours afterward, due to the fact that 20%–40% of older people are unable to stand up without help after the fall and cannot call for help (Nevitt et al. 1989, 1991; Vellas et al. 1998).

We can conclude that cardiovascular, respiratory (especially chronic bronchitis or chronic obstruction pulmonary disease), and osteoarticular diseases should be particularly regarded, because of the high total burden of morbidity they produce. Other important diseases include stroke and cardiovascular risk factors (mainly diabetes mellitus and hypertension).

Medical Trends in Telemedicine Research

We conducted a nonsystematic review of studies published in the medical literature (PubMed Database [only *free* access articles were considered]) and two additional journals (*Journal of Telemedicine and Telecare* and *Telemedicine and e-Health*) from 2005 to 2010 on the use of telemedicine systems and services.* The *keywords* were (*Telemedicine* OR *Telehealth*) AND (*Heart* OR *Diabetes* OR *respiratory* OR *COPD* OR *Asthma* OR *Psychiatry* OR *Dementia* OR *Neurology* OR *Stroke* OR *Parkinson*).

The following findings are derived from our literature search and review (144 studies) for noninvasive remote patient monitoring systems:

Concerning the conditions addressed by this research (Table 12.2), cardiovascular diseases (especially heart failure) and risk factors (hypertension and diabetes) formed the largest group. Respiratory diseases were the second largest group in Europe. A further distinct group of conditions identified in our surveyed studies were psychiatric and neurological diseases (mainly diagnosis and treatment of the acute phase of stroke).

Few studies about telemedicine systems are aimed at treating more than one group of diseases. We found just 20 research articles with such a multidisciplinary assistance

---

* Survey performed for enhanced Complete Ambient Assisted Living Experiment (eCAALYX) EU Project Consortium (http://ecaalyx.org); Ambient Assisted Living Joint Programme.

TABLE 12.2

Frequency of Telemedicine Studies per Type of Health Disorder

Type of Health Disorder	Frequency	Percentage
Cardiac disorders	50	34.7
Respiratory disorders	24	16.7
Psychiatric disorders	27	18.8
Neurological disorders	23	16.0
Diverse health conditions	20	13.9
Total	144	100.0

approach, and most of them (7 studies) were focused on combined care for cardiovascular and respiratory disorders involving different diseases. This observation is important because older people usually present more than one of these diseases. Designing individual telemedicine systems for each of these diseases is not practical.

The technologies predominantly used in the reviewed studies were telemonitoring devices such as electrocardiogram (ECG) equipment, blood pressure monitors, weighing scales, and video-conferencing equipment. Furthermore, a number of combinations of these technologies with telephone/mobile phone and the Internet were used.

The typical telemonitoring system generally consisted of a computer or mobile phone equipped with peripheral medical devices for measuring health parameters and submitting the results to a health care or telemedicine center. In most of the reviewed studies, telemonitoring was combined with other technologies, especially with communication technologies: web-based applications (14.6%), standard or mobile telephone (9%), both telephone and web applications (2.1%), or both telephone and web applications plus video-conferencing (4.9%). A clear trend emerged toward the integration of all of the technologies for remote health assistance into a unique system.

Video-conferencing was often used for consultations between a patient and a specialist clinician or between a patient and a nurse. Systems were usually installed at the patient's home or in primary care centers lacking a specialized service. As the search was based on remote patient monitoring systems, video-conference systems used for consultation between physicians (*doc2doc*) were not included in this review. In general, the use of different technological solutions appeared to be based on the specific needs associated with different interventions. Thus, interventions aimed at treatment and in-depth follow-up promote the use of telemonitoring; interventions focused on follow-up and keeping contact with the patient promote the use of telephone; and interventions focused on remote consultation promote the use of video-conferencing.

Scenario for Each Stakeholder of Telemedicine Systems

Patient Scenario

Multimorbidity

Due to increasing life expectancy and improvements in medicine and medical technologies, multimorbidities—two or more diseases—are present in a growing proportion of older people. The cardiovascular, respiratory, musculoskeletal, and metabolic systems are most frequently affected. However, there are insufficient data and less well designed longitudinal studies on the impact of multimorbidity on the social system as well as the medical (e.g., guideline-based therapy for family physicians, poly-pharmacies) and nursery systems (Schäfer et al. 2009).

The Health Survey for England 2005 (The Information Centre 2007) showed that the proportions of persons in England older than 65 years with two or more diseases were 37% for men and 40% for women; these proportions were larger in the subgroup of persons older than 85 years with 46% of men and 45% of women in that age group having two or more diseases. The average number of diseases per person did not increase significantly with age: 1.8 diseases per person in the group of 65–69 years and 2 diseases per person in the group of older than 85 years.

A telephone-based (GEDA) survey in 2009 in Germany showed similar findings: while only 54.3% of people aged 50–64 years have two or more diseases, nearly 80% of the 75 age group have two or more diseases (30.3% have 5 and more diseases; Figure 12.1; Fuchs et al. 2012).

The "Randomized Controlled Trial of Telemonitoring in Older Adults with Multiple Health Issues to Prevent Hospitalizations and Emergency Department Visits" (Takahashi et al. 2012) focused on these patient groups (older than 60 years with high risk of hospitalization). The vital signs of the weighing scales, blood pressure cuff, glucometer, pulse oximeter, and peak flow meter were overseen by a registered nurse who contacted the patients in case of alerts and assessed the symptoms with the family physicians of the patients. In case of an emergency, the patients were advised to call the emergency department by themselves because the telemonitoring system had no emergency components (e.g., emergency button). Even though the results for the telemonitoring group showed no benefit for the primary nor secondary end points, the trial revealed a research demand for telemonitoring-supported medical care systems within this target group: the direct inclusion of medical and nursing competence for symptom assessments is necessary, and for multimorbidity patients, disease-related experts are also needed for effective clinical intervention, at least with doc2doc communication.

From these results, it can be concluded that telemedicine systems aimed at the older population should be capable of monitoring several diseases rather than one specific disease, but with the inclusion of medical and nursing disease-related specialists. Standard

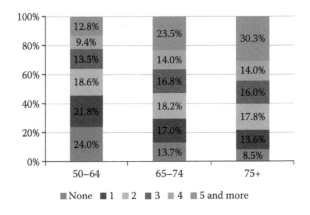

FIGURE 12.1
Number of conditions/diseases by age group. (From Fuchs J et al., 2010, *Bundesgesundheitsblatt, Gesundheitsforschung, Gesundheitsschutz* 55 (4): 576–586.)

operating procedures in medical services are necessary to perform effective telemedical care as well as to assess the medical benefits.

Furthermore, telemedicine systems could be useful to support physicians in different disease interventions particularly in the case of multimorbidity whereby medical interventions for one disease have to consider the impact for other diseases and the interactions of different medications.

Sensory Capabilities and Impairments: Vision and Audition

All domains of a patient's personal life are affected by the deleterious effect of comorbidity associated with aging and result in important barriers, e.g., functional and mental limitations, and social needs. Many older users have limited short memory, poor coordination ability, poor sensory capability, and slower ability to react (Dong et al. 2002). Moreover, they often also have visual and hearing impairments, reduced tactile senses, impaired balance, and higher susceptibility to falls (Gaßner and Conrad 2010). Additional physical and psychological health barriers are pain, fall-related injuries, loneliness, cognitive impairment, and adverse drug reactions.

Even considering the use of visual and hearing aids, 12% of older people (65–74 years) and 24% of people over 75 years in Germany have visual impairment, and 12.5% of older people (65–74 years) and 22.3% of people over 75 years have hearing-related impairments (Table 12.3; Robert Koch Institute 2009).

These characteristics of the population should be taken into account when developing telemedicine systems for older people.

Need of Care and Age Target for Telemedicine Systems

As sensory and mental abilities decline and the possibility of developing one or more chronic diseases increases, the need for aid for activities of daily living (ADL) and care for older people increases.

The predominant model of support for older people is family or ambulatory nursing services (Robert Koch Institute 2009). While persons (aged 65–69 years) who need care in most cases get cared for at home by family members, with further aging, the majority of care is provided by nursing homes. Home care by ambulatory nursing services is relatively constant across all ages. With the growing trend to have fewer children and single generation/households, family support is entering a state of crisis. Additionally, the demographic change will lead to a lack of formal support in the future. The gap between the desire to

TABLE 12.3

Exemplary Limitations (Visual, Auditive, Cognitive)

Visual limitation	Aging is associated with a decline in the ability to discriminate color as well as contrast sensitivity and limitations in motion perception and peripheral vision.
Auditive limitations	Aging can affect hearing function as well as the ability to concentrate on audio and text at the same time. Most likely there could be impairments in absolute sensitivity, sound localization, and speech recognition.
Cognitive impairments	Aging can affect information-processing capacity (speed, longer thinking time, loss of memory) and reduces the ability to perform information selection and extraction from a display leading to a decline of spatial and working memory, which in turn leads to difficulty with learning.

Source: Robert Koch Institute (RKI), 2009, *Gesundheit und Krankheit im Alter*. Berlin: Gesundheitsberichterstattung des Bundes.

live at home and the lack of family and ambulatory support might be compensated for by home care solutions and assistive technology. AAL technologies and services may help older people live independently and autonomously in their domestic environment and postpone placing older people into the unfamiliar and anonymous environment of nursing homes.

In contrast to telemedicine-based care for secondary and tertiary prevention, primary prevention of illness when the person is healthy or telemonitoring for lifestyle, fitness, and wellness is not very well accepted. The fear of surveillance (*big brother*) is higher than the potential of support. Also primary prevention is difficult to justify because the disease may never occur (Rogers 2003). For this reason, the monitoring of older patients with important comorbidity looks most promising.

Attitude toward the ICTs

According to the German SENTHA Study (Mollenkopf 2006), ICT devices are perceived as a support for independence by 67% of older German people. Fears of ICT were expressed by 15% of the respondents; nearly 50% said they liked to use ICT while 45% prefer to use it as little as possible. These findings support the European study MOBILATE (enhancing mobility in later life; Mollenkopf et al. 2005), which showed that access to modern technologies in general depends on age, income, education, gender, experience, and attitudes. Negative acceptance factors can be described as fear of the new, lack of motivation for use, unwillingness to try out ICT and its specific functions, ease or complexity of use, and lack of advice, training, and encouragement.

Actual Situation

An important aspect for the acceptance of telemedicine systems in general is the acceptance/use of the Internet; however, currently the use of the Internet in the target group of AAL (65 years and older) in Germany is under 40%. The proportion of persons of age 70 years and older using the Internet was only 28.2% (INITIATIVED21 2012), and the average age of *offliners* (persons who do not use the Internet) was 62.5 years (INITIATIVED21 2011).

While the older people of tomorrow will have more experience in technologies than today's older people, the actual technical developments have to take into account the user-specific requirements of older people today to achieve accessibility, usability, and acceptance in usage; as shown in the section "Sensory Capabilities and Impairments: Vision and Audition," this is especially important for older people with impairments, e.g., in sight, hearing, or ability to control ICT equipment.

The potential and interest for telemonitoring devices for persons aged 65 years or older are high. But individual adaptation or tailoring of the systems is necessary (e.g., volume of signals) to prevent feelings of stigmatization. Older people also ask for TV programs on health-related issues and news (e.g., healthy nutrition, diseases, function of medical examination devices, etc.), because interest in health and disease is very high in this age group.

Design Requirements for Telemedicine Systems for Older People

The "success of AAL solutions greatly depends on an effective design" (Leonardi et al. 2009). All home devices have to be selected and designed for use by patients above the age of 65 with little or no previous technical background and with poor health (sensory/perceptual and psychomotor abilities) and mental/cognitive conditions.

Along with impairments to older people, trust (access just for persons with appropriate reason) and security (prevention of unauthorized access) are other major concerns that affect ICT acceptance, especially in sensitive areas such as banking and health information/ provision of medical care.

The needs and desires of older people are the focus of accessible design, which is well defined in the specialized literature and addresses requirements for system interface (including web-based text and graphics design), support and training of users, content, and security.

Table 12.4 shows examples for the correlation between healthy needs, desires, and design outcomes (Bernard et al. 2001; Dong et al. 2002; Edwards and Englehardt 1989; Hartley 1994; Hawthorn 2010).

These physical and cognitive impairments are often combined with inexperience in computer use as described previously. The aim of a web-based information system is to increase functional accessibility in order to maximize the number of potential users who can easily use the system (Demiris et al. 2001).

Because of the desire for mobility, the mobile phone is a central element in telemedicine systems. A study on older people and their requirements regarding mobile phones showed very different results depending on physical abilities (Glende et al. 2008). Active older people asked for the Global Positioning System (GPS) for hiking tours and an integrated flashlight. Older people with vision impairments asked for an integrated electronic magnifier and a reading function or the possibility to expand the mobile phone should such functions become necessary. Also an easy-to-use reminder for medication or an emergency button to call for help or put off an attacker was requested. Besides these requirements, the desire for getting a nonstigmatizing handset for seniors was emphasized. The mobile phone should be easy to use and fault-tolerant.

Research showed that the user model of older people, e.g., in browsing the web, differs from that of other regular users. The user model is based on prior experience and expectations, limitations, and capabilities. But consideration of usability only for older people—barrier free, accessible design, assistive technology—often yields stigmatizing and separate (noninclusive) solutions. For this reason, the concept of *design for all* has been developed, which is related to the political concept of an information society. This concept consists of three strategic requirements (Malanowski et al. 2008):

- Usable services and products regardless of physical and mental abilities, age, and context of use
- Easy adaption to a different user
- Standardized interfaces that also cater for special users

It is a balancing act to consider the specific requirements of older people and not develop a stigmatizing product. Usability tests during the development stage with the target groups will help to understand their requirements.

Other System Requirements from Older People for Telemedicine Systems

Users' awareness and purpose of technology affect user acceptance (Mackie and Wylie 1988), and the perception of an ICT system as a useful tool depends on the ability to perform tasks without errors in a reasonable time (*fault-tolerant*).

TABLE 12.4

Requirements Relating to Impairments

Physical Limitations (Visual, Auditory, Tactile)	Cognitive Limitations	Safety Needs	Desires for Functionality
• High-contrast colors • Font size of at least 14 points • Antiglare displays • Avoidance of sound effects and background noise • Provide text equivalent to auditory and visual content lower frequencies • Large buttons and enough space between them • Buttons labeled according to functionality	• Clear, comprehensible, readable language • Simple menu/low hierarchy • Show only necessary information, highlighting important information • Show error messages with explanation of its cause and offering possible solution • Context sensitive • User manual with images and examples • Intuitive use	• High reliability (functional safety) • Robust system • Fast and secure error diagnosis and removal • Guarantee of data protection and transparency of the data use • Emergency call button	• Comfortable to wear • Individualized and targeted for specific groups • Record of medication compliance • Require little space/small devices and fewer sockets

Source: Bernard M et al., 2001, The Effects of Font Type and Size on the Legibility and Reading Time of Online Text by Older Adults. Available at http://psychology .wichita.edu/hci/projects/elderly.pdf (accessed October 17, 2012); Dong H et al., 2002, Accommodating older users' functional capabilities. In *A New Research Agenda for Older Adults, Proceedings of BCS HCI*, eds. Brewster, S and Zajicek, M. London: HCI BCS, pp. 10–11; Edwards R and Englehardt KG, 1989, *International Journal of Technology and Aging* 2: 56–76; Hartley J, 1994, *British Journal of Educational Technology* 25 (3): 172–188; Hawthorn D, 2010, *Interacting Computers* 12 (5): 507–528.

Despite the mobile applications of technology, the main area of use remains the patient's home. A home is much more than a building to live in with furniture; a home has personal meanings such as familiarity and long-established neighbors (Kellaher 2001; McCreadie and Tinker 2005). The interdependence of pleasures, esthetics, and emotions with utilitarian and functional dimensions leads to a desire to live at home for as long as possible. Home becomes the "emotional centre of older peoples' life" (Leonardi et al. 2009), which also means stability and safety. The issue of safety is complex because some places feel more comfortable, safer, and emotionally important than others. While bedrooms and leisure rooms are places associated with safety, intimacy, and closeness, the bathroom is related to accidents (more than the kitchen). For this reason, the acceptance of safety-related technologies depends on the patient's own characterization of the home as well as the role of telemedicine technology. Acceptance may increase in non-emotional places such as kitchen or bathroom and when the technology is not defined as embarrassing, disrupting, complex, or intrusive (Leonardi et al. 2009).

While technology use in general declines with age, it is necessary to design more established and easier-to-use technology and to create a positive attitude toward technology as useful and useable. If older people have a positive attitude toward technology in general, they will be more likely to use a specific device. Therefore, communication on the usefulness and the advantages of telemedical technologies is very important. A study on digital pens for pain assessment showed that when the technology is accepted, patients can take a greater role in managing their own health care, develop better contact with their caregivers, and feel an increased sense of security (Lind et al. 2008).

In the case of telemedicine system acceptance, this can be stimulated by user-friendliness of the sensors, user-friendliness of the mobile device (phone), user-friendliness of the user interface, and alleviation of the personal fears of data abuse as shown before.

Self-Empowerment

Besides the successful use of telemedicine devices, a further aim of telemedicine is to empower patients by helping them understand their disease and participate in decision-making processes, as well as encouraging them to influence their health status ("self-empowerment"; Bruegel 1998). Education has a major role to play in the process of providing help for self-care (prevention and treatment). The importance of health literacy for patients with heart failure was proven in a retrospective cohort study of 1494 patients (Peterson et al. 2011). Low health literacy was associated with a significant increase in risk of overall mortality (low vs. adequate health literacy: 17.6% vs. 6.3%; HR, 1.97 [95% CI, 1.3–2.97]). An influence on hospitalization could not be shown.

Telemedical technology could involve patients in their own medical care and improve their health literacy as the first step for improving their self-empowerment.

Health Professional Scenario

Trigger Factors Causing Care Demand for Older People

A study by Brownsell et al. (2007) presents a literature review aimed at identifying trigger factors associated with an increase in older patients' need for support and care. Identified trigger factors were then classified into a priority ranking by a group of experts, mainly composed of workers in the social services, housing, health, and voluntary services. Older persons also participated in the ranking by responding to postal questionnaires; 107 trigger factors were initially identified, and 36 of them were selected for a second evaluation and ranking by the group of experts with the participation of older persons through the postal questionnaires. At the end, 12 factors were selected and ranked as follows:

- A major health event—such as support following a stroke or hip replacement
- Cognition impairment (e.g., dementia)
- Deteriorating physical functioning
- Inability to care for self at home
- Mobility problems
- Needing assistance with personal care, hygiene, bathing, washing, dressing
- Occurrence of falls
- Presence of chronic diseases
- Difficulty in toileting/continence management
- Consequences of admission to hospital
- Depression, mental breakdown, or deterioration
- Inability to cope with independent ADL

Notice that these factors are heterogeneous in nature and involve medical, cognitive-emotional, functional, and social situations.

Medical and Nonmedical Health Professionals for Older People Care

Following from the section "Trigger Factors Causing Care Demand for Older People," it can be concluded that health care services for older people require the involvement of not only physicians and nurses but also other groups of clinicians such as physiotherapists, occupational therapists, and social workers. Usually, these geriatric service groups work in an interdisciplinary manner and have regular meetings to discuss various aspects related to the patient's health: clinical problems, functional and cognitive status, destination upon discharge, etc. Telemedicine systems could provide an important platform to allow home use not only for strictly clinical objectives (such as monitoring vital signs) but also to meet the needs of other health care groups involved (Figure 12.2).

Older People Information That Should Be Monitored

Independent of patients' diagnosis, health professionals dedicated to older people care need to know information that includes not only physiological parameters (heart rate, respiratory rate, temperature, etc.) but also knowledge about functional status, ability to perform basic activities of life, cognitive status, and other details. This information is collected from geriatrics through *comprehensive geriatric assessment* (CGA) and includes mainly the evaluation of clinical, functional, cognitive, and social aspects of the older person. The CGA has been demonstrated to improve the diagnosis and treatment of older people with comorbidity in different settings (e.g., urgency services and hospitalization units). More importantly, it is more useful when the patient's case is more complex from a medical point of view. Not using formal CGA may result in mistakes in diagnosis or prescription of inappropriate treatments to older patients (Ellis et al. 2011a,b; Stuck et al. 1993; van Craen et al. 2010).

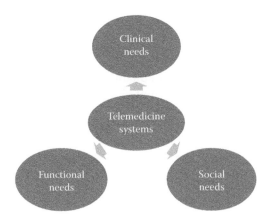

FIGURE 12.2
Needs to be covered by telemedicine systems for older people with comorbidity.

Often, information for CGA is obtained by applying medical scales to patients (for example, the Barthel index for functional status evaluation), and these scales are specifically validated for older people. These may also be applied by a telemedicine system, and its use may improve patient monitoring. Thus, according to the monitored clinical parameter, a telemedicine system's *sensors* might include (Figure 12.3)

- A technological/electronic medical device: an ECG monitor, a blood-pressure meter, a weighing scale, etc.
- A medically validated questionnaire: pain-intensity scale, Barthel's scale of functional performance, Yesavage's scale of depression, etc.

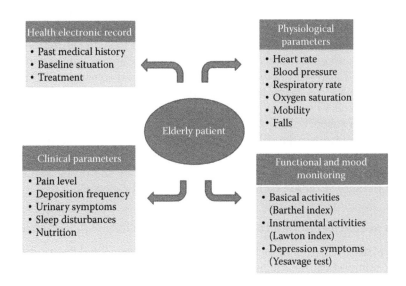

FIGURE 12.3
Patient's information that should be monitored by telemedicine systems for older people with comorbidity.

Potential Uses for Telemedicine Systems during Treatment and Follow-Up

Target situations where telemedicine systems could be implemented correspond either to short time periods—during which the health provider considers them to be important to evaluate certain health parameters for suitable follow-up—or to longer periods for the same purposes, where home stay is promoted and visits to the emergency department, justified or not, are prevented.

One of the most clearly suitable situations for home monitoring with telemedicine systems corresponds to the so-called postdischarge period, when a patient leaves the hospital after a short or a long intervention. Currently, the postdischarge situation is managed through postdischarge visits or telephone follow-up. Through telemedicine system, health professionals from primary care services could have access to certain health parameters of patients at home, and then visits to the hospital would be reduced, thus saving usually dramatic and complicated journeys.

Structure and Flexibility of Telemedicine Systems for Older People

As described in the section "Multimorbidity," a large proportion of older patients have two or more diseases, so that a telemedicine system specifically focused on one disease would probably not be suitable. Telemedicine systems for this population should be able to monitor at a minimum the most significant group of conditions, such as cardiovascular (including stroke and cardiovascular risk factors such as diabetes mellitus and hypertension), chronic respiratory, and osteoarticular diseases. For this reason, telemedicine systems should have extensive interfaces to include/exclude monitoring devices independent of the patient's condition.

A telemedicine system that monitors more than one disease is feasible, since the control or monitoring of several conditions usually requires information from some common clinical parameters. Thus, a patient with heart failure would probably need to have their weight, blood pressure, ECG, heart rate, oxygen saturation level, exercise tolerance level, and other data monitored; while a patient with a chronic respiratory disease (e.g., chronic obstructive pulmonary disease) would need their oxygen saturation level, blood pressure, heart rate, and exercise tolerance level monitored, as well as their respiratory symptoms and statistics tracked. Notice that certain identical clinical parameters are monitored in the control of both conditions: blood pressure, heart rate, and oxygen saturation and exercise tolerance levels. Alternatively, the same technological resources could obtain information on more than one clinical parameter: the patient's functional capacity could be monitored, or a check of sleep patterns or urinary symptoms could be carried out by remote usage of clinical questionnaires or scales administered through a computer and the Internet.

Another important aspect of telemedicine systems is the flexibility needed with regard to choosing and programming the different clinical parameters to be monitored. Physicians should be able to choose the most relevant clinical parameters according to the pathologies they wish to monitor in their patients (Figure 12.4), and they should be able to modify the alert levels of the sensors or algorithms implemented in the system.

Other System Requirements from Health Professionals for Telemedicine Systems

As a part of a research project of the AAL program,* we organized two focus groups (medical and nonmedical health professionals) with the aim of analyzing the opinions

---

* Enhanced Complete Ambient Assisted Living Experiment (eCAALYX) EU Project Consortium (http:// ecaalyx.org); Ambient Assisted Living Joint Programme.

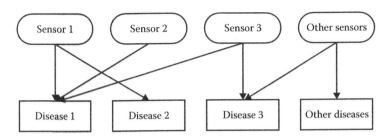

FIGURE 12.4
Required flexibility by telemedicine systems for older people with comorbidity. Doctors should be able to choose the most relevant clinical parameters according to the pathologies they wish to monitor in their patients.

of health care providers on the requirements that telemedicine systems should meet in order to be accepted and used in monitoring older patients with comorbidity. These focus groups provided the following relevant information on telemedicine systems:

- The telemedicine system has to work 24 h, 7 days a week: "there should always be someone (a person) at the other end of the system."
- The system must be able to send automatic alerts (without false positives).
- The system should be easily incorporated into the patient's daily life. It should not significantly change the patient's routines or home environment.
- The system should complement and not replace the health care that patients routinely receive.
- Access to the patient's medical record through the system is considered very useful.
- There was conflict on the question of whether patients should or should not have access to their measured vital sign values. Some physicians thought this property may cause undesirable alarm to the patients. The system has to show vital sign data without causing unneeded and undesirable alarm to the patients.
- System configuration (choice of sensors, etc.) should be performed by medical physicians according to the clinical profile of their patients.
- For nonmedical health professionals, the issues that they considered important to monitor are medication compliance, monitoring nutrition, fall detection, and GPS tracking of patients with cognitive impairment.
- The system should allow nonmedical health professionals more freedom of action, when they detect certain risk situations, e.g., poor medication adherence, neglecting nutrition, etc. The possibility of using the telemedicine system as a means of direct communication between this group and the group of medical professionals is very important.

Health System Scenario

The most significant and vital aspects of health care systems that are required to successfully implement telemedicine systems aimed at the comorbid older population are analyzed next.

Before describing the determining factors, it is important to define telecare and tele-health services and their scope. Therefore, in this chapter, we use the following definitions (Kamel Boulos 2009):

- Telecare involves monitoring patients' daily activity and the safety of their home environment with mechanisms such as panic buttons, fall sensors, furniture occupancy sensors, movement detectors, fire/smoke and flood detectors, dangerous gas sensors, room temperature sensors, property exit detectors, intruder alarms, etc., which are connected to a 24/7 emergency call and response service. Additionally, these services may be classified as follows:
    - First-generation telecare refers to user-activated—e.g., push button, pendant, wristbands—telealarm calls to a control center, where a call handler can organize a response, usually via a neighbor, a relative, or a care service provider.
    - Second-generation telecare evolved on the basis of telealarms, though incorporating other components, such as smoke alarms, fall sensors, and others.
    - Third-generation telecare is focused on identifying risk situations in order to anticipate adverse situations, usually by evaluating behavior patterns (e.g., low water intake, reduced mobility detected by door sensors, etc.).
- Telehealth is the remote monitoring of vital signs and other clinical indicators, such as body temperature, heart rate/ECG, respiratory rate, blood pressure, pulse oximetry, blood glucose, body weight, etc., by remote clinicians who can then send instructions to the patient on medication, diet, or lifestyle, or call them in for consultation.

Also the remote patient monitoring systems can be defined in several generations by the type of data transfer, the sensor platform, and the integration level in primary care (Anker et al. 2011):

- In the first generation, only a few measurements (e.g., ECG event recorders) were asynchronously transmitted to the primary care physicians or nurses who can only react within consultation hours.
- The second-generation systems are using synchronous data transfer to a tele-medicine center with medical staff assessing the measurements. But also this care model is dependent on office hours of the telemedicine center.
- The third generation uses remote patient management systems with constant medical assessment by specialized nurses (e.g., heart failure nurses) and physicians 24/7.
- The fourth-generation systems are an extension of the third-generation systems and are providing fully integrated remote management systems using data from invasive (e.g., defibrillator or point-of-care for biomarkers) and noninvasive tele-medical devices.

Important in this regard is the research report on the state of the art of ICTs, entitled *ICT & Ageing. European Study on Users, Markets and Technologies. Final Report* (Kubitschke et al. 2010). This review analyzes the current situation of telecare and telehealth resource implementation and the main factors (drivers and barriers) involved in this. With regard to the more advanced telecare and telehealth services, this review describes the issues that are shown in Table 12.5.

TABLE 12.5

Drivers and Barriers for More Advanced Telecare and Telehealth Services

	Drivers	**Barriers**
More advanced telecare services	There is a lack of a common pattern discernable across countries as regards market drivers. Many countries have the infrastructural potential in place. Combination of product innovation and social care service receptivity is the key to market takeoff. Public provision and/or reimbursement seem to be a key facilitator of market development.	Significant variability across countries on infrastructural readiness. Fragmentation of the provision/reimbursement situation and uncertainty about who should be responsible and who should pay for installation. The lack of a demonstrated *business* and/or *quality* case. Nature of the response delivery system seems to be a critical issue from the market point of view (reliance on family caregivers or formal care staff to provide the response). Concern on distribution of payments and benefits between community care and institutional care providers. If the main benefit of telecare services were to be in delaying a move to institutional care, then the main costs might accrue to community social care services, and the main savings would be in terms of reduced institutional care costs. The challenge of transitioning from pilots to mainstream. Organizational changes that are needed to get a successful implementation of telecare services (and social/professional resistance in some cases). Concerns about privacy, data access, sharing, and ethical/regulatory issues.
More advanced telehealth services	The extent of mainstreaming is very limited to date. In the forerunner countries, somewhat different specific drivers have been apparent: 1. United States: transparent and accepted cost–benefit rationale (savings in health care costs). 2. Germany: home telehealth has emerged in the context of a new approach to provision of integrated care and emerging reimbursement of this by insurers (this makes the German *market* one of the most likely for more widespread mainstreaming in the near future).	Lack of a recognized *business case* in Europe (in contrast to the United States). Lack of a generally accepted *clinical case* for home telehealth. Perceived lack of awareness at the policy/funding level. The generally poorly developed *continuity of care* structures and processes in many health care systems, as well as the typically episodic-based payment models in many systems. The administrative fragmentation on delivery of health services (regional and even local level) makes it difficult to implement coordinated national policy in this field. Medicolegal uncertainties in relation to home telehealth (in some countries). The difficulties of scaling up/moving beyond the local level. Current technology limitations can also be a barrier, and the lack of interoperability between the many different devices and systems emerging on the marketplace.

Source: Kubitschke L et al., 2010, ICT & Ageing. European Study on Users, Markets and Technologies. Final Report. Available at http://ec.europa.eu/information_society/activities/einclusion/library/studies /docs/ict_ageing_final_report.pdf (accessed October 17, 2012).

Another important review on this topic was carried out for the European Commission: European Countries on Their Journey towards National eHealth Infrastructures— Evidence on Progress and Recommendations for Cooperative Actions—Final European Progress Report (Stroetmann et al. 2011). In this report, telehealth services are emphasized as one of the key fields of eHealth (together with computerized records and electronic prescriptions) in Europe.

In the following, some of these factors are analyzed individually, and the analysis is adapted to the scenario of older people with comorbidity.

Perception of Usefulness

Developing the necessary technological infrastructure for implementation of advanced telecare (second and third generations) and telehealth is not enough to ensure successful take-up of these services. Major barriers for the implementation of these services by the practitioners are the poor perception of their usefulness and the suspicion of trends toward high-tech medicine with less human support and substitution of the current outpatient care; physicians are also afraid that telemedicine-based care is negatively influencing their daily work and patient contact by substitution of their medical care and treatment authority (this is opposite to what occurred with first-generation telecare services; Percival and Hanson 2006).

Technologies of second- and third-generation telecare and telehealth are perceived by potential payers as expensive and with a poor cost/benefit ratio. This perception is most probably influenced by the general view that technological innovations are expensive while in-depth health economic analysis is lacking and depends on country-specific conditions of the health system. Information exchange between countries in the European area and large-scale studies were proposed as tools to overcome cost–benefit and usefulness-related barriers.

The usefulness of these services, as managed by health providers (physicians, nurses, etc.), is also not clear, despite the abundant related literature, including specific journals (e.g., *Journal of Telemedicine and Telecare, Telemedicine Journal and e-Health*, etc.) indexed in main databases (MEDLINE, etc.). This finding leads to the conclusion that these communication media are not sufficient or adequate, since most people in the medical community probably ignore the current state of technological developments or even their existence. Habitual resistance to adopt technological innovations is a relevant factor that needs to be taken into account.

Options for self-managed health care, offered by some telehealth solutions, are not always perceived as adequate by health providers.

As an example of medical benefit through telemedical treatment, heart failure is one of the conditions most frequently studied. In total, 33 randomized controlled trials (RCTs) with telemedical interventions for heart failure have been published since 1999. Two meta-analyses of remote patient monitoring (telemonitoring or telephone support; Inglis et al. 2010; Klersy et al. 2009) showed significant reduction in mortality and/or hospitalizations. At present, a definition of the relevant parameter of the used devices is not presented.

The Telemonitoring to Improve Heart Failure Outcomes (Tele-HF) Study (Chaudhry et al. 2010) examined the influence of telemonitoring systems in 1653 patients with heart failure. The intervention was described as daily telephone calls from the patient to an automated interactive voice response system to answer standard questions about the health status, symptoms of the disease, and weight. Every 30 days, a screening on depression was performed. The study centers evaluated the answers every weekday for patient-related changes and missing data transfer. The trial results showed no significant difference for the overall mortality between the control and intervention groups.

Telemedical Interventional Monitoring in Heart Failure (TIM-HF) trial (Koehler et al. 2011) involved 710 patients with chronic heart failure and New York Heart Association class II-III. The follow-up of this RCT was at least 12 months (median 26 months). The intervention consisted of daily monitoring of ECG, weight, blood pressure, self-assessments, and a weekly 6 min walk test. After 12 and 24 months, the Patient Health Questionnaire (PHQ-9) and the questionnaire for physical life quality (SF36) were used. The results showed no reduction in all-cause mortality but an increase in life quality. Furthermore, a patient subgroup (LVEF ≤ 25%, depression score about ≤10) showed significant reductions in loss due to death or heart failure hospitalization.

Although no significant benefit for all heart failure patients has been shown in these trials, a specific group of patients has been identified who have benefited from telemedical intervention. These results need further investigation. While the compliance in TIM-HF was, at 81%, very high (Koehler et al. 2011), one reason for the results of TELE-HF could be the decreasing compliance rate to 55.1% at the end of the 6 month follow-up (Everett et al. 2011).

The *Whole System Demonstrator (WSD)* program (funded by the Department of Health [2011]) was launched by the United Kingdom's Department of Health in May 2008 with 3230 people with diabetes, chronic obstructive pulmonary disease, or heart failure, recruited from 179 general practices in three areas in the United Kingdom. The trial has already finished, and the first results show reductions in mortality, the need for admissions to a hospital, the number of bed days spent in the hospital, and the time spent in urgency services (Department of Health 2011; Steventon et al. 2012).

At the European level, the RENEWING HEALTH (Regions of Europe Working Together for Health; http://www.renewinghealth.eu/) project, which is partially supported by the European Commission (Competitiveness and Innovation Framework Programme), is finished and has implemented large-scale real-life test beds for the validation and subsequent evaluation of innovative telemedical services using a patient-centered approach and a common rigorous assessment methodology. In nine of the most advanced regions in the implementation of health-related ICT services, service solutions are already operational at the local level for telemonitoring and the treatment of chronic patients suffering from diabetes, COPD, or CVD diseases.

Technological Infrastructure

Most countries have the necessary technological infrastructure for the application of first-generation telecare services (social alarms) to a considerable level of implementation. This has often been considered as a platform for the implementation of more developed services. However, implementation of the additional infrastructure necessary for these more advanced services varies greatly across European countries and even across different regions of certain countries. Overcoming such difficulties requires considerable effort by both public and private actors, an effort that is subordinated to the perceived value of the new services. Public–private joint initiative has been proposed, where the public sector would offer the service to potential clients and the private sector would provide the technological resources. Promoting investment in basic infrastructures (where these are not developed at a country-wide level) by the EU Structural Funds has also been proposed.

The Current Marketplace

First-generation telecare services can be considered as implemented in most countries of the European Union, since they are regularly provided (with some exceptions) in all of these countries. Regarding second- and third-generation services, none of these countries provides them on a regular basis, with the United Kingdom being the closest to this goal. In terms of telehealth implementation, northern countries are the most advanced (Stroetmann et al. 2011). For instance, Scotland has already started to offer eHealth services to its population. The Scottish Government of Health Department started a strategy in 2009 (Scottish Centre for Telehealth and Telecare 2009) to introduce these kinds of technologies gradually, and now they are offering services such as video-conference and remote patient monitoring (http://www.sctt.scot.nhs.uk/stories.html). After WSD's trial results, there is a plan to extend these services to 3 million people in the 2012–2017 period (Department of Health 2011). At the same time, in the region of Lombardy, Italy, after the success of the pilot Telemaco (Bernocchi et al. 2012), a Chronic Disease Management platform is under deployment. Spain has a lot of pilots going on around the country, but real implementation has not been documented (Kubitschke et al. 2010).

In Germany, some health insurance companies signed integrated health care contracts with hospitals and medical caretakers for providing telemedical services for heart failure patients (e.g., AOK Nordost 2011 for the South-Brandenburg; IKK Südwest 2012).

The poor implementation of these services does not imply poor market potential. The profile of users who may benefit most from these services is described in the above sections ("Scenario for Each Stakeholder of Telemedicine Systems," "Patient Scenario"). Telehealth systems have been mainly developed for monitoring patients with chronic diseases, especially heart diseases, respiratory diseases, and diabetes mellitus. Estimates suggest a potential use of these services by 25%–60% of these patients (Empirica and Work Research Center [WRC] 2005). On this basis, a potential of 3.3 million to 10.9 million users can be estimated in the European Union (Kubitschke et al. 2008).

Ethical and Regulatory Issues

Ethical and regulatory issues must also be considered in order to prevent barriers to implementation of these technologies.

No major problems are expected in relation to second- and third-generation telecare. However, some concern has been expressed in certain countries in relation to privacy protection and the role of sensor monitoring. Greater difficulties are expected in this regard as third-generation products and continuous monitoring systems become more affordable and also with the increasing importance of cloud computing. A forum for information exchange among European member countries has been proposed. Taking telephone and e-mail medical consultations as an example, noticeable differences across countries can be expected in terms of regulation and practice.

The legal validity of *remote* (not *face-to-face*) consultation between a patient and a physician is a further topic to be taken into account (especially in some countries such as Austria and Poland; Stroetmann et al. 2011). In Germany, some trends indicate a willingness among the medical fraternity as well as the legislative organs to face these challenges; for example, in Germany on the 113th German Medical Assembly, a catalog about inner medical and legal requirements (liability, data protection, professional law) for the tele-medical patient care was decided (Deutscher Ärztetag 2010). In the 114th German Medical Assembly, the amendment of the professional law was carried out. Although this amend-ment enables physicians for remote care via print and communication media, a direct care (via face-to-face) communication of the patients has to be ensured ("ban on remote treat-ment"; Deutscher Ärztetag 2011). Remote patient management must only be considered as an addition to normal medical services but not as a substitution.

Incentives for Technology Development

Availability of financial incentives (for hospitals, physicians, social services, primary care teams, etc.) as well as the quality of such incentives is important. Evidence indicates that incentives are not adequate enough for health care providers working in the health and social services of several EU member countries. Furthermore, currently available incentives might discourage rather than encourage implementation of advanced telecare and telehealth.

Although current development of systems' technology and components is rather advanced, some aspects still need to be reinforced:

- Mobile devices and monitoring services.
- End-user devices for telecare and telehealth.
- Monitoring and processing systems for telecare and telehealth centers.
- Clinical support systems to give relevant information and guidance to health and social care providers. Data are unlikely to be useful without a filtered presentation that allows providers to extract value from huge amounts of monitoring data.
- Improved interoperability between the various system components and the differ-ent products and services in the European marketplace.

Organization

Implementing services such as telemedicine services has important organizational impli-cations. Providing innovative systems for simultaneous health and social care requires high-level coordination between health services and social services, which might be dif-ficult to achieve in some European countries. These services are usually managed by dif-ferent, not always collaborating organizations. Implementing collaborative work may need restructuring of the involved organizations, as well as training staff in the use of the new systems—technical and also on the different kind of care (e.g., communication training), all of which may be received reluctantly. Fortunately, initiatives for integration of health services and social services are being undertaken in some European countries (e.g., in England, through the Care Trusts).

Heterogeneity of the social and health care providers (public, private, mixed) is a further factor to be taken into account. Implementation also requires agreement between involved organizations in terms of funding.

Responding to a system alarm requires coordinated action, since different causes may need different agents to respond: caretakers, relatives, health care providers (ambulance, emergency practitioners, etc.), social services, or external service providers.

Potential Scenarios for Telemedicine Systems

The potential scenarios or situations where telemedicine systems can be used with the comorbid older population arise from interaction with the key players involved, the health care actions required, and the locations where these could be carried out. This section describes examples of possible use of these systems.

Potential scenarios for a telemedicine system are described below. For all of them, the following features and/or components are assumed to be present:

- The patient's physician (usually the family general practitioner [GP] or medical specialist), who has access to the system.
- A qualified teleoperator (nurse or physician) in a telemedical center, who is available 24 h, 7 days a week for patients being monitored. The teleoperator has access to the data gathered from the patients by the sensors and receives any alarm signals sent by the system. The teleoperator can send notes to the patient's physician and notify the patient as well as emergency services with regard to patient transfer, etc.
- The patient has a telemedicine system at home that includes
  - Vital signs sensors for blood pressure, heart rate, breathing rate, temperature, blood glucose, etc.
  - A mobile phone for mobile relaying (uploading) of measured vital signs and GPS localization.
  - A computer or other similar device, which allows video-conferencing and where the patient receives instructions sent by the teleoperator or GP. This would include changes to treatments, completion of medical scales or questionnaires, appointments for medical checkups, etc.

Telemedical Care by Telemedical Centers in Hospitals

1. If a GP or a specialist decides that a patient needs a telemedicine system, he or she speaks with his or her patient about this option. When the patient agrees, the GP contacts the telemedical center that is responsible for telemedical treatment in this region/for this disease.

2. The patient gets the necessary devices/sensors for his/her home by post for installing alone or with the help of a technician. The patient also gets a manual for using the sensors and devices (plug-and-play). If the patient needs (re-)training in using the device, a nurse visits him/her. This nurse can also take other information about the patient (relatives, environment, need for help, etc.), as well as help in building the patient's confidence and trust with regard to the new technique and to telemedicine in general.

3. Besides the sensors, the patient gets the contact number of the telemedical center where the patient can call 24 h per day for emergency, questions, or any other problems. If the patient needs help, he/she shall at first contact the caretaker in the telemedical center.

4. Every day in the morning, the patient measures his/her vital parameters (determined by the family physician and/or caretakers), and the measured values are

then sent to the electronic patient record. In the telemedical center, the measured values will be assessed by a caretaker. If the sensors detect a change, the caretaker calls the patient and speaks about the cause of this change. The caretaker (a physician or a suitable person with direct access to a physician) can decide to change the treatment or the medication, or give an appointment for visiting the family physician/specialist.

5. In case of an emergency, the caretaker calls the emergency service. If there is deterioration in the course of the patient's disease, the family physician will be advised about the situation and sent all information. The family physician can inquire at any time for information at the telemedical center and can get it by phone, fax, e-mail, or post. When the patient visits his/her family physician, he/she can get a list of the measured values by the telemedical center. With telemedicine systems, it should be possible to log in on a webpage to see the electronic patient record when the patient has agreed for this access.

6. When necessary, the caretaker may suggest that the patient makes a video-conference call to speak about his/her actual state/problems (perhaps once a month). If the patient asks for a video-conference, the caretaker arranges an appointment depending on the urgency of the situation, within the same or the next day.

Monitoring of Patients with Chronic Heart Failure and Respiratory Disease

Scenario: A patient with a history of previous hospitalizations for heart failure and/or chronic respiratory disease exacerbation, who is at a high risk of decompensation and has been recently discharged.

1. The family physician decided that the patient needs a telemedicine system. He/she contacts the telemedical center and speaks with the caretakers about the needed sensors and the following treatment. The medical personnel in the telemedical center monitor the course of the disease of the patient and advise the family physician in case of deterioration. The physician gets all information about any emergency. When the patient visits his/her family physician, he/she can get a list of the measured values from the telemedical center.

2. The system allows the patient's family physician to select the sensors that will be used to monitor the patient, to exclude sensors considered unnecessary, or to reintroduce initially excluded sensors. Furthermore, the physician may modify the alert threshold or the monitoring frequency of each sensor (the system notifies the patient of such changes, so that the physician does not need to contact the patient).

3. The physician may request evaluation of the functional performance by completion of the Barthel's scale every 4 weeks. The system will notify the patient of such a request.

4. The physician may request a video-conference at any time. The system will notify the patient of such a request. Alternatively, the physician may fix a date and time for a visit. The system will notify the patient of the appointment details.

5. Treatment changes scheduled by the physician—on the basis of the evolution of the system-measured patient's vital sign values—are introduced into the system, which will in turn notify the patient of such changes.

Patient with Decompensated Cardiac/Respiratory Disease, Who Visits the Emergency Department

Scenario: The emergency physicians consider that further hospitalization is unnecessary if the patient is monitored at home. They prescribe outpatient treatment and discharge the patient during the night. Thus, the family physician/telemedicine physician is in charge of controlling and monitoring the patient.

1. The emergency physicians notify the caretaker of the patient's discharge from the emergency department. The caretaker notifies the family physician if the physician has not already been notified (e.g., patient discharged during the night).

2. The family physician contacts the patient through video-conference and requests a scanned copy of the emergency report and prescribed treatment.

3. The family physician reviews the report and accordingly selects the most suitable monitoring sensors, alarm thresholds, and monitoring frequencies.

4. The patient progresses favorably, and thus the physician changes the sensors' monitoring frequency and modifies the treatment through the system. The system communicates such changes to the patient and the caretaker provides assistance if necessary.

5. The physician arranges a visit for examining the patient, if necessary. The system notifies the patient of the date and time.

Patients with Osteoarticular Disease and Poor Control of Pain

Scenario: Patient with gonarthrosis and moderate associated pain that impairs the gait. The patient decides to consult the caretaker.

1. The caretaker notifies the family physician of the patient's poor control of pain. The family physician contacts the patient through video-conference and evaluates the intensity of pain through the Face Pain Scale and the impact on functional performance through the Barthel's scale.

2. The physician adjusts the analgesic treatment and advises the patient that the system will periodically (e.g., every 48 h) request completion of both scales or of other scales without the need to contact the patient again. The patient completes the requested scales without the need to contact the physician (although a caretaker may provide help if necessary).

3. The physician may access the pain measurement results and adjust the corresponding analgesic treatment without contacting the patient. Treatment changes are recorded and communicated to the patient by the system. To solve possible queries about the submitted treatment schedule, the patient may contact a caretaker (who would in turn contact the physician if necessary).

4. The physician may change the frequency of pain evaluations according to the progression of pain. The system will notify the patient of such changes.

5. The physician may request an evaluation of the patient's functional performance (by using the Barthel's scale, gait speed, etc.) together with the pain evaluation;

otherwise, the physician may request both evaluations some time after a certain change in the analgesic treatment has been introduced.

6. Patient's queries or comments intended for the physician will be first screened by the caretaker.

7. The physician may resume direct communication with the patient at any time through video-conference (the system will notify the patient of the physician's request to communicate with him/her). Alternatively, the physician may schedule a video-conference at a certain time or make an appointment for the patient to visit (the system will notify the patient of the appointment details).

Patients with Diabetes Mellitus

Scenario: Patient with diabetes mellitus and poor control of glycemia despite prescribed treatment.

1. After an initial physician–patient interview, the physician sets a glycemia-control schedule with measurements on Tuesdays and Saturdays, before and after breakfast, lunch, and dinner. The system notifies the patient of this schedule and delivers reminders of the controls. The glucometer automatically enters the measured results into the system, where the physician may access them at any time.

2. The physician reviews the measured glycemia values in the following days and modifies the antidiabetic treatment accordingly. Such changes are recorded and notified to the patient by the system. To solve possible queries about the submitted treatment schedule, the patient may contact a caretaker, who would in turn contact the physician if necessary.

3. According to the progression of glycemia, the physician modifies the days and/or daily frequency of controls (e.g., only before breakfast, 2 days per week; days may be arbitrarily chosen by the physician or the patient).

4. The physician considers that the patient should follow a certain diet and exercise schedule and sends the patient illustrative videos. The system notifies the patient of the indication to watch the videos and to follow the prescribed schedule. The system allows the physician to know whether or not the patient has watched the videos.

Patients Assisted by Persons Designated by the Social Services

Scenario: Patient in social frailty (living alone, without reference relatives) with mobility difficulties due to severe osteoarticular disease, regularly visited by a worker of the Social Services, who helps in doing the shopping and the household chores.

1. During the visits, the Social Services worker identifies situations that should potentially be communicated to the patient's family physician (e.g., development of skin lesions, onset of cognitive deterioration, behavioral alterations, physical worsening, etc.). Thus, the social worker joins the system or notifies the caretaker of such situations. The caretaker evaluates them and communicates the relevant ones to the physician.

Conclusions

Aging, Comorbidity, and Target Diseases

- Comorbidity and the effects thereof are more significant than aging *per se* in terms of adverse impact on health associated with the progressive aging of the population.
- Cardiovascular, chronic respiratory, and osteoarticular diseases have the greatest impact on the older people in terms of mortality, morbidity, dependency, and hospitalization.

Patient Scenario

- Currently, most telemedicine projects are exclusively aimed at monitoring a single disease such as heart failure or chronic obstructive respiratory disease. However, one of the characteristics of the older population is that they often suffer from more than one chronic, major illness (pluripathology). This means that telemedicine systems must be able to monitor several major diseases simultaneously.
- Telemedicine systems must be principally aimed at the secondary and tertiary prevention of the disease.
- The design of the involved devices should take into account relevant characteristics of the older population such as hypoacusism, vision impairment, and others. However, devices should not stigmatize patients, as this could significantly influence their acceptability. The *design for all* strategy should be kept in mind.
- The older population's demand for assistance or health care services may increase through reasons that are not strictly clinical but rather of a social nature. In this regard, telemedicine systems can be a useful tool for integration and cooperation between health care and social services.

Health Professional Scenario

- The important clinical information required to monitor the older population includes not only vital physiological signs (blood pressure, heart rate, etc.) but also information about their functional situation, affective state, and pain levels, among other data. This information can be gathered through questionnaires or scales normally used in clinical practice but applied in a telematic manner.
- Telemedicine systems must have great flexibility due to the wide variability in patients' clinical profiles and diseases. A patient's physician should be able to configure the system according to the patient's needs for devices and alert levels (*individualized medicine*).
- Assessment and submission of *raw* measurements obtained through the devices can result in information overload or raise false alarms among health providers. These systems should carry out a preliminary processing of the information gathered by sensors (e.g., through the use of medical algorithms), so that they only warn of relevant clinical situations. The caretakers should be able to add individual algorithms for the patient.

- The telemedicine system should be available continuously for patients on a 24/7 basis.
- These systems should be viewed not as replacing clinicians but as a tool to aid them in their work (*additional care*).

Health System Scenario

- There is a considerable potential market for telemedicine systems involving telecare and telehealth services.
- The perception of usefulness by clinicians and institutions is an important topic to be developed. Clinical trials have to be performed for evidence-based medicine.
- Implementing telemedicine systems could require significant organizational changes with regard to health systems: social and health care services integration, changes in clinicians' working methods, etc.

Other Requirements (Technical)

- For compatibility, the system should have extended interfaces.
- Especially for rural areas but also for mobility reasons, telemedicine systems should focus on mobile data transmission.
- To perform the balancing act of technical developments (design for all vs. including specific requirements of older people), usability tests with focus groups are recommended.

Acknowledgments

The authors would like to especially thank Kerstin Koehler, MD, and Oliver Deckwart from Zentrum fuer kardiovaskulaere Telemedicine GmbH, Berlin, Germany. They would also like to thank Antonio Yuste Marco, MD, from Fundacio Hospital Comarcal Sant Antoni Abat, Vilanova i la Geltru, Barcelona, Spain.

This work has been conducted within the eCAALYX project, which was supported in part by the Ambient Assisted Living (AAL) Joint Programme, a joint research and development funding activity by 20 European Member States and 3 Associated States, with the financial support of the European Community (EC) based on article 169 of the EC treaty. The eCAALYX Project Consortium included 11 member organizations in five European countries (http://www.ecaalyx.org).

References

AALIANCE. 2009. Ambient Assisted Living Roadmap. Available at https://connect.innovateuk .org/c/document_library/get_file?p_l_id=145400&folderId=609151&name=DLFE-4587.pdf (accessed October 17, 2012).

Anker, SD; Koehler, F; and William, TA. 2011. Telemedicine and remote management of patients with heart failure. *Lancet* 378 (9792): 731–739. doi:10.1016/S0140-6736(11)61229-4.

AOK Nordost. 2011. Offizieller Startschuss für brandenburgisches Telemedizin-Netz gefallen, press release. Available at http://www.aok.de/nordost/presse/Offizieller-Startschuss-f%C3%BCr -brandenburgisches-Telemedizin-Netz-gefallen-Dec%2010,%202011/detail/128/lastAction /list/page/6.

Bernard, M; Liao, CH; and Mills, M. 2001. The Effects of Font Type and Size on the Legibility and Reading Time of Online Text by Older Adults. Available at http://psychology.wichita.edu /hci/projects/elderly.pdf (accessed October 17, 2012).

Bernocchi, P; Scalvini, S; Tridico, C; Borghi, G; Zanaboni, P; Masella, C; Glisenti, F; and Marzegalli, M. 2012. Healthcare continuity from hospital to territory in Lombardy: TELEMACO project. *The American Journal of Managed Care* 18 (3): e101–e108.

Boult, C; Altmann, M; Gilbertson, D; Yu, C; and Kane, RL. 1996. Decreasing disability in the 21st century: The future effects of controlling six fatal and nonfatal conditions. *American Journal of Public Health* 86 (10): 1388–1393.

Brownsell, S; Aldred, H; and Hawley, MS. 2007. The role of telecare in supporting the needs of elderly people. *Journal of Telemedicine and Telecare* 13 (6): 293–297. doi:10.1258/135763307781644870.

Bruegel, RB. 1998. Patient empowerment—A trend that matters. *Journal of AHIMA/American Health Information Management Association* 69 (8): 30–33; quiz 35–36.

Chaudhry, SI; Mattera JA; Curtis, JP et al. 2010. Telemonitoring in patients with heart failure. *The New England Journal of Medicine* 363 (24): 2301–2309. doi:10.1056/NEJMoa1010029.

Cooper, C; Atkinson, EJ; Jacobsen, SJ; O'Fallon, WM; and Melton, LJ, 3rd. 1993. Population-based study of survival after osteoporotic fractures. *American Journal of Epidemiology* 137 (9): 1001–1005.

Demiris, G; Finkelstein, SM; and Speedie, SM. 2001. Considerations for the design of a Web-based clinical monitoring and educational system for elderly patients. *Journal of the American Medical Informatics Association: JAMIA* 8 (5): 468–472.

Department of Health (UK). 2011. Whole System Demonstrator Programme. Headline Findings— December 2011. Publication. Available at http://www.dh.gov.uk/en/Publicationsandstatistics /Publications/PublicationsPolicyAndGuidance/DH_131684 (accessed October 17, 2012).

Deutscher Ärztetag. 2010. Beschlussprotokoll des 113. Deutschen Ärztetags in Dresden.

Deutscher Ärztetag. 2011. (Muster-)Berufsordnung für die in Deutschland tätigen Ärztinnen und Ärzte—MBO-Ä 1997—in der Fassung der Beschlüsse des 114. Deutschen Ärztetages 2011 in Kiel.

Dong, H; Keates, S; and Clarkson, PJ. 2002. Accommodating older users' functional capabilities. In *A New Research Agenda for Older Adults, Proceedings of BCS HCI*, eds. Brewster, S and Zajicek, M. London: HCI BCS, pp. 10–11.

Edwards, R; and Englehardt, KG. 1989. Microprocessor-based innovations and older individuals: AARP survey results and their implications for service robotics. *International Journal of Technology and Aging* 2: 56–76.

Ellis, G; Whitehead, MA; O'Neill, D; Langhorne, P; and Robinson, D. 2011a. Comprehensive geriatric assessment for older adults admitted to hospital. *Cochrane Database of Systematic Reviews (Online)* (7): CD006211. doi:10.1002/14651858.CD006211.pub2.

Ellis, G; Whitehead, MA; Robinson, D; O'Neill, D; and Langhorne, P. 2011b. Comprehensive geriatric assessment for older adults admitted to hospital: Meta-analysis of randomised controlled trials. *BMJ (Clinical Research Ed.)* 343: d6553.

Empirica and Work Research Center (WRC). 2005. Various Studies on Policy Implications of Demographic Changes in National and Community Policies. LOT7: The Demographic Change—Impacts of New Technologies and Information Society. Final Report. Available at http://ec.europa.eu/employment_social/social_situation/docs/lot7_ict_finalreport_en.pdf (accessed October 17, 2012).

Ettinger, WH; Davis, MA; Neuhaus, JM; and Mallon KP. 1994. Long-term physical functioning in persons with knee osteoarthritis from NHANES. I: Effects of comorbid medical conditions. *Journal of Clinical Epidemiology* 47 (7): 809–815.

Everett, W; Kvedar, JC; and Nesbitt, TS. 2011. Telemonitoring in patients with heart failure. *The New England Journal of Medicine* 364 (11): 1079; author reply 1079–1080. doi:10.1056 /NEJMc1100395#SA3.

Fried, LP; Ferrucci, L; Darer, J; Williamson, JD; and Anderson, G. 2004. Untangling the concepts of disability, frailty, and comorbidity: Implications for improved targeting and care. *The Journals of Gerontology. Series A, Biological Sciences and Medical Sciences* 59 (3): 255–263.

Fuchs, J; Busch, M; Lange, C; and Scheidt-Nave, C. 2012. Prevalence and patterns of morbidity among adults in Germany. Results of the German telephone health interview survey German Health Update (GEDA) 2009. *Bundesgesundheitsblatt, Gesundheitsforschung, Gesundheitsschutz* 55 (4): 576–586. doi:10.1007/s00103-012-1464-9.

Gaßner, K; and Conrad, M. 2010. ICT Enabled Independent Living for Elderly. A Status-Quo Analysis on Products and the Research Landscape in the Field of Ambient Assisted Living (AAL) in EU-27. Available at http://www.aal-deutschland.de/deutschland/dokumente/ict_for_elderly _webversion.pdf (accessed October 17, 2012).

Giannakouris, K. 2008. Population and social conditions. Ageing characterises the demographic perspectives of the European societies. EUROSTAT. Statistics in focus 72/2008.

Gijsen, R; Hoeymans, N; Schellevis, FG; Ruwaard, D; Satariano, WA; and van den Bos, GA. 2001. Causes and consequences of comorbidity: A review. *Journal of Clinical Epidemiology* 54 (7): 661–674.

Glende, S; Podtschaske, B; and Friesdorf, W. 2008. Zielgruppenspezifische Produktentwicklung durch User Integration—Am Beispiel eines Mobiltelefons mit PC-Funktionalität für die Generation 55+. In *Produkt- und Produktionsergonomie—Aufgabe für Entwickler und Planer*, ed. Schütte, M. Dortmund: GfA Press.

Guralnik, JM. 1996. Assessing the impact of comorbidity in the older population. *Annals of Epidemiology* 6 (5): 376–380.

Hartley, J. 1994. Designing instructional text for older readers: A literature review. *British Journal of Educational Technology* 25 (3): 172–188.

Hawthorn, D. 2010. Possible implications of ageing for interface designers. *Interacting Computers* 12 (5): 507–528.

IKK Südwest. 2012. "IKK Herzstark" schenkt Versicherten mehr Lebensqualität, press release 4 April 2012. Available at http://www.ikk-suedwest.de/2012/04/%E2%80%9Eikk-herzstark% E2%80%9C-schenkt-versicherten-mehr-lebensqualitaet/.

Inglis, SC; Clark, RA; McAlister, FA et al. 2010. Structured telephone support or telemonitoring programmes for patients with chronic heart failure. *Cochrane Database of Systematic Reviews (Online)* 8: CD007228. doi:10.1002/14651858.CD007228.pub2.

INITIATIVED21. 2011. Digitale Gesellschaft. Available at http://www.initiatived21.de/wp-content /uploads/2011/11/Digitale-Gesellschaft_2011.pdf (accessed October 17, 2012).

INITIATIVED21. 2012. (N) Onliner Atlas 2012. Basiszahlen für Deutschland. Eine Typographie des digitalen Grabens durch Deutschland. Available at http://www.initiatived21.de/wp-content /uploads/2012/06/NONLINER-Atlas-2012-Basiszahlen-f%C3%BCr-Deutschland.pdf (accessed October 17, 2012).

Kamel Boulos, MN. 2009. UK telehealth and telecare scene in Q4 2009 (with emphasis on England). Report prepared for the eCAALYX EU project Consortium.

Karlamangla, A; Tinetti, M; Guralnik, J; Studenski, S; Wetle, T; and Reuben, D. 2007. Comorbidity in older adults: Nosology of impairment, diseases, and conditions. *The Journals of Gerontology. Series A, Biological Sciences and Medical Sciences* 62 (3): 296–300.

Kellaher L. 2001. Shaping everyday life: Beyond design. In *Inclusive Housing in an Ageing Society*, eds. Peace, SM and Holland, C. Bristol, UK: The Policy Press.

Klersy, C; De Silvestri, A; Gabutti, G; Regoli, F; and Auricchio, A. 2009. A meta-analysis of remote monitoring of heart failure patients. *Journal of the American College of Cardiology* 54 (18): 1683–1694. doi:10.1016/j.jacc.2009.08.017.

Koehler, F; Winkler, S; Schieber, M et al. 2011. Impact of remote telemedical management on mortality and hospitalizations in ambulatory patients with chronic heart failure: The telemedical interventional monitoring in heart failure study. *Circulation* 123 (17): 1873–1880. doi:10.1161/CIRCULATIONAHA.111.018473.

Koike, Y; Imaizumi, H; Takahashi, E; Matsubara, Y; and Komatsu, H. 1999. Determining factors of mortality in the elderly with hip fractures. *The Tohoku Journal of Experimental Medicine* 188 (2): 139–142.

Koot, VC; Peeters, PH; de Jong, JR; Clevers, GJ; and van der Werken, C. 2000. Functional results after treatment of hip fracture: A multicentre, prospective study in 215 patients. *The European Journal of Surgery = Acta chirurgica* 166 (6): 480–485. doi:10.1080/110241500750008808.

Kubitschke, L; Gareis, K; Lull, F et al. 2008. ICT & Ageing. European Study on Users, Markets and Technologies. Preliminary Findings. Available at http://www.ict-ageing.eu/ict-ageing-website/wp-content/uploads/2008/11/ictageing_vienna_handout_final2.pdf (accessed October 17, 2012).

Kubitschke, L; Müller, S; Gareis, K; Frenzel-Erkert, U; and Lull, F. 2010. ICT & Ageing. European Study on Users, Markets and Technologies. Final Report. Available at http://ec.europa.eu/information_society/activities/einclusion/library/studies/docs/ict_ageing_final_report.pdf (accessed October 17, 2012).

Leonardi, C; Mennecozzi, C; Not, E et al. 2009. Knocking on elders' door: Investigating the functional and emotional geography of their domestic space. In *Proceedings of the 27th International Conference on Human Factors in Computing Systems*, 1703–1712. Boston: ACM. Available at http://dx.doi.org/10.1145/1518701.1518963 (accessed October 17, 2012).

Lind, L; Karlsson, D; and Fridlund, B. 2008. Patients' use of digital pens for pain assessment in advanced palliative home healthcare. *International Journal of Medical Informatics* 77 (2): 129–136. doi:10.1016/j.ijmedinf.2007.01.013.

Mackie, RR; and Wylie, CD. 1988. Factors influencing acceptance of computer-based innovations. In *Handbook of Human-Computer Interaction*, ed. Helander, M. New York: Elsevier.

Malanowski, N; Özcivelek, R; Cabrera, M; and European Commission, Joint Research Centre, Institute for Prospective Technological Studies. 2008. Active Ageing and Independent Living Services: The Role of Information and Communication Technology. Available at http://www.umic.pt/images/stories/publicacoes2/JRC41496.pdf (accessed October 17, 2012).

McCreadie, C; and Tinker, A. 2005. The acceptability of assistive technology to older people. *Ageing & Society* 25 (1): 91–110. doi:10.1017/S0144686X0400248X.

Ministerio de Sanidad y Consumo. 2006. Conjunto Mínimo Básico de Datos 2005. Available at http://www.msc.es (accessed October 17, 2012).

Mollenkopf, H. 2006. Techniknutzung als Lebensstil? In *IT-basierte Produkte und Dienste für ältere Menschen—Nutzeranforderungen und Techniktrends. Tagungsband zur FAZIT-Fachtagung Best Agers in der Informationsgesellschaft*, eds. Kimpeler, S and Baier, E. Stuttgart: Fraunhofer IRB Verlag.

Mollenkopf, H; Marcellini, F; Ruoppila, I; Széman, ZT; and Tacken, M. 2005. *Enhancing Mobility in Later Life: Personal Coping, Environmental Resources and Technical Support—The Out-of-Home Mobility of Older Adults in Urban and Rural Regions of five European Countries*. Amsterdam: IOS.

Nevitt, MC; Cummings, SR; Kidd, S; and Black, D. 1989. Risk factors for recurrent nonsyncopal falls. A prospective study. *JAMA: The Journal of the American Medical Association* 261 (18): 2663–2668.

Nevitt, MC; Cummings, SR; and Hudes, ES. 1991. Risk factors for injurious falls: A prospective study. *Journal of Gerontology* 46 (5): M164–M170.

Percival, J; and Hanson, J. 2006. Big brother or brave new world? Telecare and its implications for older people's independence and social inclusion. *Critical Social Policy* 26 (4): 888–909. doi:10.1177/0261018306068480.

Peterson, PN; Shetterly, SM; Clarke, CL et al. 2011. Health literacy and outcomes among patients with heart failure. *JAMA: The Journal of the American Medical Association* 305 (16): 1695–1701. doi:10.1001/jama.2011.512.

Robert Koch Institute. 2009. *Gesundheit und Krankheit im Alter*. Berlin: Gesundheitsberichterstattung des Bundes.

Rogers, M. 2003. *Diffussion of Innovations*. New York: Free Press.

Schäfer, I; Hansen, H; Schön, G et al. 2009. The German MultiCare-study: Patterns of multimorbidity in primary health care—Protocol of a prospective cohort study. *BMC Health Services Research* 9: 145. doi:10.1186/1472-6963-9-145.

Scottish Centre for Telehealth and Telecare. 2009. Available at http://www.sctt.scot.nhs.uk/strategy .html. (accessed April 6, 2012).

Starfield, B. 2006. Threads and yarns: Weaving the tapestry of comorbidity. *Annals of Family Medicine* 4 (2): 101–103. doi:10.1370/afm.524.

Steventon, A; Bardsley, M; Billings, J et al. 2012. Effect of telehealth on use of secondary care and mortality: Findings from the Whole System Demonstrator cluster randomised trial. *BMJ (Clinical Research Ed.)* 344: e3874.

Stroetmann, KA; Artmann, J; Stroetmann, VN et al. 2011. European Countries on Their Journey towards National eHealth Infrastructures. Final European Progress Report. European Commission. Available at http://ec.europa.eu/information_society/activities/health/docs/studies/eh _strategies/ehealth-strategies_report012011.pdf (accessed October 17, 2012).

Stuck, AE; Siu, AL; Wieland, GD; Adams, J; and Rubenstein, LZ. 1993. Comprehensive geriatric assessment: A meta-analysis of controlled trials. *Lancet* 342 (8878): 1032–1036.

Takahashi, PY; Pecina, JL; Upatising, B et al. 2012. A randomized controlled trial of telemonitoring in older adults with multiple health issues to prevent hospitalizations and emergency department visits. *Archives of Internal Medicine* 172 (10): 773–779. doi:10.1001/archinternmed.2012.256.

The Information Centre. 2007. Health Survey for England 2005: Health of Older People [NS]. Available at http://www.ic.nhs.uk/pubs/hse05olderpeople (accessed October 17, 2012).

Valderas, JM; Starfield, B; Sibbald, B; Salisbury, C; and Roland, M. 2009. Defining comorbidity: Implications for understanding health and health services. *Annals of Family Medicine* 7 (4): 357–363. doi:10.1370/afm.983.

van Craen, K; Braes, T; Wellens, N et al. 2010. The effectiveness of inpatient geriatric evaluation and management units: A systematic review and meta-analysis. *Journal of the American Geriatrics Society* 58 (1): 83–92. doi:10.1111/j.1532-5415.2009.02621.x.

Vellas, BJ; Wayne, SJ; Garry, PJ; and Baumgartner, RN. 1998. A two-year longitudinal study of falls in 482 community-dwelling elderly adults. *The Journals of Gerontology. Series A, Biological Sciences and Medical Sciences* 53 (4): M264–M274.

Walker, NR; Norton, S; Hoorn, V et al. 1999. Mortality after hip fracture: Regional variations in New Zealand. *The New Zealand Medical Journal* 112 (1092): 269–271.

WHO. 1998a. WHO. A Health Telematics Policy in Support of WHO's Health-for-All Strategy for Global Health Development: Report of the WHO Group Consultation on Health Telematics, Geneva, December 11–16, 1997. Available at http://whqlibdoc.who.int/hq/1998/WHO _DGO_98.1.pdf (accessed October 17, 2012).

WHO. 1998b. World Health Statistic Annual.

WHO. 2011. Global Status Report on Noncommunicable Diseases 2010. Description of the Global Burden of NCDs, Their Risk Factors and Determinants. WHO. Available at http://www.who .int/nmh/publications/ncd_report_full_en.pdf (accessed October 17, 2012).

Wolff, JL; Starfield, B; and Anderson, G. 2002. Prevalence, expenditures, and complications of multiple chronic conditions in the elderly. *Archives of Internal Medicine* 162 (20): 2269–2276.

13

A Framework for Monitoring and Assisting Seniors with Memory Disabilities

Paulo Novais, Davide Carneiro, Ângelo Costa, and Ricardo Costa

CONTENTS

ABSTRACT Population aging brings increased social problems. Solutions for this new reality must be devised. Providing care services at home may benefit patients, health service providers, and social security systems and needs to be seen as a possible solution for those social problems. By maintaining the patient at home, in his or her own environment, care services costs can be diminished and, at the same time, the comfort and well-being of the person in need are significantly increased. To pursue this goal, we explore the advantages that ambient assisted living can bring to people in a home environment, focusing on the problems of health care services at home. Specifically, in this chapter, we present a framework focused on the monitoring and assistance of the elderly that are living alone, focusing on those elderly with memory disabilities. We believe that this approach will enable the challenges that the current trend of population aging poses to be tackled.

KEY WORDS: *ambient assisted living, ambient intelligence, simulation, monitorization, personal memory assistant.*

Introduction

The current trend of population aging, sustained by the current change in demographics, is an irrefutable truth that today's society does not seem to know how to deal with (UNFPA 2009). This phenomenon is more visible in developed countries, although developing countries will soon face the same problem (Holliday 1999). The following causes combined to lead this trend:

- Improvements in sanitation, housing, nutrition, and medical innovations, including new vaccines and the discovery of antibiotics, which contributed to a significant and rapid increase in life expectancy (Figure 13.1).
- Decrease in fertility rates (Figure 13.1), mainly due to improvements in women's education and a full integration of women into the formal labor market (World Health Organization 2000; United Nations 2001).

All these factors can be regarded as major breakthroughs in the evolution of our humanity. However, they also caused unbalanced societies with rapid growth in the proportion

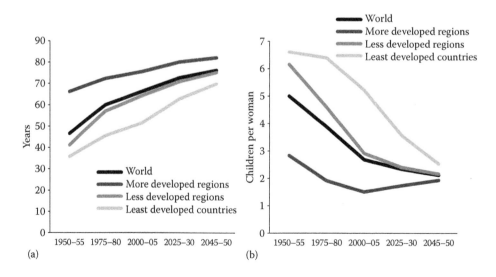

FIGURE 13.1
Life expectancy at birth (a); total fertility rate (b), 1950–2050. (From United Nations. 2001. World Population Ageing: 1950–2050. Available at http://www.un.org/esa/population/publications/worldageing19502050, accessed May 9, 2011.)

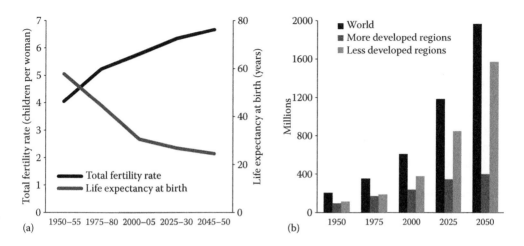

FIGURE 13.2
Total fertility rate and life expectancy at birth (a); population aged 60 or more (b), 1950–2050. (From United Nations. 2001. World Population Ageing: 1950–2050. Available at http://www.un.org/esa/population/publica tions/worldageing19502050, accessed May 9, 2011.)

of the population above 60 years old (Figure 13.2). This new reality raises concerns about whether or not a decreasing active population will be able at support the dependent part of the population (i.e., children and elderly). Looking at the old age dependency ratio, a measure that depicts the relation between active and elderly population, we notice that it will increase substantially by 2050 (United Nations 2001). This situation, more than economical costs, will bring along high social costs.

In fact, old age people frequently have special needs and require close and personalized daily monitoring by relatives or even professional caregivers, mainly due to health-related issues. Nowadays, two main trends can be identified here: either the elderly are left alone in their home or they moved into an elderly center. The first option can represent serious risks for the elderly and therefore is not desirable. The second option carries high economic costs that not every family is able to bear. Additionally, it is usually not the best option from the point of view of the elderly since they tend to show reluctance to be moved from their home. It should be possible for older people to age while maintaining their quality of life and their independence and still be able to deal with all the diseases and limitations that will arise from that fact.

A concept that addresses this subject is the one of active aging. According to the World Health Organization (2002), active aging is the process of optimizing opportunities for health, participation, and security in order to enhance the quality of life as people age. It is desirable that, while aging, people have an active role in the society: spiritual, educational, civic, cultural, or others.

This problem represents a real challenge for the social and security policies in the next few years, with the actual debate growing in intensity as decision makers around the world appear particularly worried about the apparent fatalism of government effectiveness to tackle this new reality. Generally, the only solution they present is to tax more the working population in order to support the rising costs associated with population aging (World Health Organization 2000). However, new cost-effective approaches must be devised to allow delivery of care and support to those in need, as this model will soon not be sustainable. Furthermore, it should also be taken into consideration that these people generally wish to continue living independently in their own home.

Following these ideas, in the last few years, we have witnessed the emergence of a promising approach: the provision of health care services in a remote way, directly to the home of the patient. This is evidently supported by a strong technological component. In this work, we describe an integrated health care provision system as a collaborative networked organization, where the different institutions that support care provision (e.g., hospitals, day/care centers, social security institutions, nursing homes, etc.) may operate as a long-term virtual organization. The various actors involved (e.g., the elderly and their caregivers, such as relatives, friends, neighbors, nurses, physicians, practitioners, etc.) could become part of a virtual care community platform that is able to monitor not only its users (people in need of care provision) but also their natural habitat (home environment). This approach is strongly related to the vision of ambient intelligence (AmI) (Aarts and Encarnacao 2006), or more specifically to ambient assisted living (AAL).

This work describes such an intelligent environment, developed with the aim of assisting and monitoring elderly people in their day-to-day lives. We believe that such an approach constitutes one possible solution to the above presented problem. It allows the patient to stay at home, saving public and private money, and, nevertheless, monitor their health status. Rather than describing the whole organization, in this chapter, we describe the developed AAL framework focused on the provision of care at home. It includes a monitoring solution for both in-home and on-the-move monitoring of the user, a simulation tool that allows the creation of specific scenarios developed for assessing and improving the whole framework, and a personal memory assistant (PMA) whose main objective is to assist users with memory disabilities to get through the day.

This chapter is organized as follows. In this section, we describe the problem addressed and the solution adopted, based on the contempt of AAL. In the section "The Growing Problem of Memory Loss," we analyze in more detail memory-related impairments caused by aging, followed by a high-level description of our framework VirtualECare and the related work. Then we move on to the central part of this chapter where we describe the components of the framework directly related to the user. More specifically, we will present its architecture and functionalities, the simulation tool, the monitoring solution, and the PMA. We will finish by pointing out some future lines of work and conclusions.

The Growing Problem of Memory Loss

Given the current changes in society, the elderly population is suffering from a state of loneliness and social exclusion that has never been seen before. In fact, while in the past families looked after their elder members, nowadays they barely have the time for it or they are simply not willing. In this evolution toward a more busy and stressful day-to-day life, society loses personal connections, and families, like neighbors and friends, become detached. Moreover, the promotion of individualism means that persons are more isolated and spend days or weeks without being in contact with their loved ones.

Additionally and considering elderly people, the problems related to degenerative diseases must be considered. In this chapter, we focus on memory-related problems due to old age and how to improve their quality of life (Tucker 1995). In terms of severity, memory loss has three stages identified by the medical community: cognitively impaired (the patient can perform normal daily experiences), mild cognitive impairment (the daily experiences of the patient are moderately affected; Figure 13.3), and severe cognitive impairment (a patient that

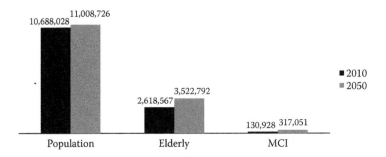

FIGURE 13.3
Graph of mild cognitive impairment in the Portuguese population. (From INE–Statistics Portugal. 2010. Anuário Estatístico de Portugal 2009. Available at http://www.ine.pt, accessed June 2011.)

needs constant supervision). Given the difficulties that a patient in the third state may have to even remember how to use a technological device, we state that the first and second stages are where the support of technology-based tools is more appropriate. The third stage represents a very serious condition in which the person is not autonomous anymore and needs constant supervision by appropriate and trained personnel.

Recent studies show that, on average, people start to lose cognitive abilities at the age of 50 (Charness 2008). This generally starts out as nonpatterned memory loss. This includes the typical "where did I leave my keys?" and tends to progress to more frequent episodes of memory loss. This evidently affects the way that persons live their daily life. With the aggravation of the problem, the daily routine becomes so affected that, in extreme cases, constant assistance of a caregiver is needed as patients cannot find their way home or even remember who they are, where they are, or what they are doing. Generally, a person in this situation will be moved to a nursing home, in which they will lose all their independence. Even worst, a significant amount of people suffering from memory disorders cannot afford the needed care and face a threatening scenario. Given that the population is aging at a significant rate, this problem can only be expected to get worse. There are studies pointing out that mental exercises are the best way to prevent further loss of memory (Geda et al. 2008). These exercises include question/answer memorization tests and everyday routine tests. These tests are created according to the daily collection of events of the user. Clues can be given that trigger submemories that relate to the events. The effects of memory loss cannot be undone and can only be slowed down. In that sense, these patients could always benefit from support in their daily life, either in the form of specialized personnel or technological solutions.

Moreover, memory impairments are more than not being able to access stored memories. In a study to test the creativity and the development of new ideas, the Harvard University (Geda et al. 2008) revealed that people who are debilitated in long-term memory are also severely debilitated in terms of creativity. This means that a person with severe memory disability has trouble generating new ideas, an ability also known as envisioning. As a consequence, the blockage of creativity decreases the ability to project new activities. The *cause and consequence* ability is also lost since when a person cannot remember the consequences of previous actions, he or she cannot predict the consequence of a similar action now taking place. All this results in an inability to make plans, making it hard to plan the day or to remember the plans throughout the day (Corchado et al. 2008).

All that being said, the main problem addressed in this work concerns memory disabilities: to assist the user in planning their day-to-day schedule and remember their plans.

In order to do it, we are exploring the concept of memory assistants, created to help users remember important memories they may have already forgotten. This can be done in very different ways, ranging from timed snapshots, to mind mapping software, and ending in event reminders. As we are tackling the specific problem of day-to-day planning, we implemented a dynamic agenda able to accept new events and to reschedule as necessary to accommodate them, considering several parameters (e.g., event priority, the person who generated the event). We are taking advantage of integration with an AAL framework in order to interconnect all stakeholders, including relatives, friends, and medical professionals. This way, the dynamic agenda may schedule events that include visits to doctors as well as some social time with an available friend or a dinner with a relative. In that sense, this tool may not only be seen as a memory assistant but also as a social enabler, fighting some of the worst effects of aging alone.

VirtualECare and Related Projects

The main objective of the VirtualECare Project (Novais et al. 2010) is to develop a framework that is able to monitor, interact, and provide its customers with constant health care services. This will interconnect not only health care institutions but also leisure centers, training facilities, shops, or patient relatives. The VirtualECare builds on a set of distributed modules, interconnected through a network, each one with a different role (Figure 13.4). The main modules as well as their functionalities are (Costa et al. 2009)

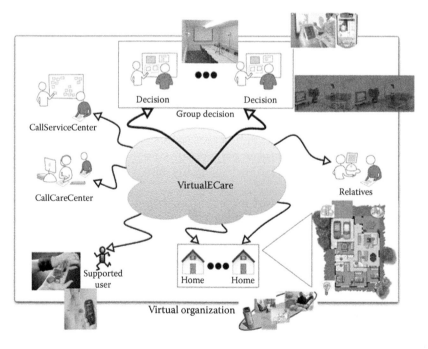

FIGURE 13.4
High level view of the VirtualECare framework.

- *Supported User*: Elderly people with special health care needs, whose clinical data are sent to the CallCareCenter and redirected to the Group Decision Support System. This user should be constantly monitored, inside and outside its environment, so the data must be provided in real time to the interested parties. It is the central component of the architecture, and all the other components must work together to ensure its safety and well-being.

- *Environment*: The natural environment of the elderly, enhanced with sensors, with the data being sent to the Group Decision Support System through the CallCareCenter, with the remaining being redirected to the CallServiceCenter. The data provided by this module must also be constantly available and analyzed. The environments can be, among others, the home of the user, a room of a hospital, an exterior environment, or a day center. The main actions of the other components toward the environment are to maintain the comfort and security parameters.

- *Group Decision*: This module is responsible for the long-term planning regarding the health care of the patients. It should be composed of specialized staff such as nurses and doctors as well as recommendation systems and tools for time- and space-distant meetings. Overall, this module should be able to plan all the issues related to visits to doctors and tests, automatically scheduling all according to the user's agenda.

- *CallServiceCenter*: Entity with all the necessary computational and qualified personal resources, capable of receiving and analyzing different data and taking the necessary actions according to them.

- *CallCareCenter*: Entity in charge of computational and qualified personal resources (i.e., health care professionals and auxiliary personnel), capable of receiving and analyzing the clinical data, and taking the necessary actions according to them. The user may interact with this service and request assistance or advice. In order to respond, the system may interact with other modules such as the Decision Support System.

- *Relatives*: This module includes individuals that may have an active role in the supervising task of their loved ones, being able to give precious complementary information about them and being able to intervene in a complementary way, in specific crises (e.g., loneliness). By being an important part of the equation, the relatives should also have access to the health status of the patient so that they are constantly aware of their situation.

In order for the Group Decision Support System to work, it has to collect the opinion of specialized staff (e.g., nurses, pediatrics, cardiologists). There is also the need to have a digital profile of the Supported User, allowing a better understanding of their special needs. In this profile, we can have several different kinds of relevant information, ranging from the patients' Electronic Clinic Process to their own personal preferences (e.g., musical, gastronomic) or even their own personal experiences, which can be used to better understand the needs or desires and thus take better decisions. In this scope, we are paying special attention to the acquisition of experiences of the user with the environment (e.g., actions, events) so that through its analysis, we can improve the actions of the framework.

This solution will help health care providers to integrate, analyze, and manage complex and disparate clinical, research, and administrative knowledge. It will provide tools and methodologies for creating an information-on-demand environment that can improve quality of living, safety, and quality of patient care (Costa et al. 2007).

Related Projects

In this section, we analyze other AAL projects in recent years that have followed a similar line of thought. This proves, on the one hand, the validity of this approach and, on the other hand, the growing interest of the scientific community in the field.

Amigo—Ambient Intelligence for the Networked Home Environment

This project was a consortium of 15 European companies who joined efforts to exploit the potential of the nowadays common home networks and improve people's lives. The idea was to benefit from the fact that almost all equipment comes with some kind of network connection. But still, there are lots of different standards that make more difficult their interoperability, this being their goal. This project ended in September 2004.

It is common that a house has several networks such as the electrical, Ethernet, or wireless networks. The Amigo project (Amigo Project 2004) interconnects these networks, thus enabling communication between all devices. Over this *Hardware* layer, Amigo implements services so that people's environments are empowered. From any point of the house or even from outside the house, people can change house parameters, watch the surveillance cameras, set their TV to record some program, etc. This is, in fact, the main purpose of the project: to empower the environment it is in, releasing people from boring activities as the person is the center of the system. This project used *home laboratories* across Europe including Philips Research's *HomeLab*, France Telecom's *Creative Studio Lab*, and the Fraunhofer Institute's *InHaus*.

Oxygen

The main objective of this project from MIT (MIT Artificial Intelligence Laboratory 2002) is to make technology as available everywhere as the air we breathe. Since the beginning, computers have been closed in rooms, and we had to get to them, interact with them using their means, and work with them the way they wanted, which means that until now, we have been living for the computers instead of the computers living for us. The MIT vision is that in the future, *computers* are available everywhere, so that everyone can use them and we do not need to carry our own devices. *Computers* will also be very generic, configurable to fit all our needs in every moment.

In order to do that, this project wants to make interactions between a person and a computer as natural as possible, using people's natural language or gestures. Computers will live for us, expanding our possibilities, simplifying our lives. They will learn our preferences, learn what we like, providing an even more natural interaction. They will be everywhere, watching our safety, automatically taking care of our needs, fetching information before we ask for it.

Several necessary modules have been developed for such a project to work. The Intelligent Room has a speech recognition system that receives and executes orders from people in the room. Imagine you are in a meeting; you can ask the room to read what is scheduled for today, show some video of the last meeting, show or read some document, etc. Another interesting technology is the Cricket/INS. This is a people location system inside a building that uses a badge carried by the people being traced. The main advance here is that the services someone is using follow the person as they travel from one room to another. Imagine you are listening to some music in your bedroom. When you walk into the living room, the system locates at each time where the nearest speakers are and automatically the sound starts playing there and stops playing in the bedroom. The same is possible for lights, air conditioning, TV, or any other service.

I.L.S.A.—The Independent Lifestyle Assistant

The main objective of this initiative from the University of Minnesota (Haigh et al. 2003) is to study the response of elderly to a monitoring computer system inside their houses and determine how such systems can help these people. They not only determine the main problems of elderly people living alone but also implement parts of a monitoring system in some test houses in real conditions. This application of AmI is good not only for the elderly living alone but also for their caregivers as everyone maintains its autonomy.

A group of sensors was placed in each house (11 houses during the half year) according to what was being monitored (behavioral patterns, medication taken, etc.). The information from the sensors was read and sent to a central site where it was studied. From here, alerts were emitted if the person in question did not take their medication or if the behavior during the day was very unusual. The main features implemented included passive monitoring (mobility, occupancy, sleeping patterns), cognitive support (like reminders), alerts and notifications, reports (summary reports of client behavior), and controlling remote access to information. Clients had a portable device from where they could check their agenda, change some system parameters, and even communicate with caregivers. This is a project that directly interacted with a specific public: elderly people living alone. This public of course has its own needs and creates specific problems or challenges that must be addressed, and that was the target of this project.

ReachMedia

This project from MIT (Feldman et al. 2005) consists of an RFID equipped wristband to provide us with on-the-move interaction with everyday objects. Usually, there is a lot of information related to the objects we deal with every day, mainly on the Internet, but it is normally only accessible through a computer. This project aims to present us that information wherever we are, in real time, without taking our attention from what we are doing.

The wristband contains an RFID reader that will read the information from RFID tags in objects close to our hands. After this, information is fetched from the Internet and presented to the user in some interface. At this moment, a phone is being used to fetch the information and the user listens to what is found. Imagine you are in a bookstore and you grabbed some book you want some information about. When your hand approaches the book's RFID tag, the system beeps notifying you that some services are available for that object. For a book, there could be reviews or ratings that some store or book specialist put online. You can then choose, while you are flipping through the book's pages, what you want to listen to about that book.

The navigation between several choices is also done using the wristband. As it is equipped with accelerometers, with small gestures of the wrist, the person can navigate through the several options for the object in question and select what to listen to. The uses for such a technology are many. When meeting people with the same wrist, we could know what their interests are, their hobbies, or what their personality is like. When shopping, we could know the characteristics of every product we grab (e.g., calories of food products) while we are walking and looking at other products instead of having to stop and read the product specification.

Telecare

The objective of the Telecare (Camarinha-Matos and Afsarmanesh 2001) project is to develop a configurable framework for assisting elderly people based on the integration of a multiagent and a federated information management approach. The results are services likely to be offered by emerging ubiquitous computing and intelligent home appliances, which are useful for elderly people. With this approach, the project expects to address issues such as elderly people being moved from their homes, providing them with autonomy and independence. To achieve these objectives, this project is based on telesupervision and teleassistance technologies. A virtual network is created, which connects the elderly home, the relative's office, the care or leisure centers, and a virtual shop, among others. It is through this virtual community that the elderly make use of the services. The project states that it is possible nowadays to create such a network that can provide cheap health care to elderly because of the current development of Internet-based infrastructures. The development of such projects is one important step toward countering the problems of aging population and possible elderly marginalization.

A Framework for Monitoring and Assisting Seniors with Memory Disabilities

The framework that is to be presented in this chapter is focused on providing support to the elderly with memory disabilities. In that sense, we will focus on the description of the components that directly deal with this problem. Four high-level components implementing four key functionalities will be described in this section. Firstly, we will describe a simulation tool that was developed to assess the behavior of the framework under specific or threatening scenarios. Based on the results obtained in the simulations, we were able to develop and improve the remaining components. We are then going to describe the monitoring module, responsible for constantly providing key information about the user and his/her surroundings. It operates in two main contexts: in-home monitoring (in which we focus on the quality of the environment and the user's activities) and on-the-move monitoring (in which we are interested on the positioning and location-based services). The third module is the PMA that has the main objective of assisting the user in planning and replanning the day-to-day schedule dynamically as well as remembering the plans. Finally, we will describe the learning module in which we are testing methodologies for evolving the framework to fit the needs and preferences of each specific user in an autonomous way.

Architecture

The development of architectures for AAL, as well as their specific framework, has particular requirements (Carneiro et al. 2010). The architecture for an assisted living environment must, first of all, be able to integrate a very heterogeneous group of devices and technologies. This means that the architecture must provide means for these components to coexist and to work together. It is therefore mandatory for the architecture to provide an information sharing mechanism independent of specific technologies or devices, which all different components can make use of. These architectures need also to be highly expandable because new technologies and new devices arrive on the market frequently. It is also expected to be easy to expand, i.e., it should be easy to add new components to the architecture without having to make changes to existing components or to the architecture itself. It is also important for such architecture to be scalable so that it can grow and accommodate new modules or even to be included in higher level architectures. Finally, considering all these features, we can also state that the architecture cannot be static since many changes can occur frequently. Therefore, the architecture should also be described as dynamic. We can summarize the main requirements for the implementation of an AAL architecture: dynamic, modular, expandable, flexible, scalable, and compatible.

Considering the framework, two main types of components can be identified. On the one hand, there are physical devices that exist in the environment (e.g., sensors, actuators, mobile devices, and computers). On the other hand, there are software components (e.g., knowledge base, decision support system, and planning). Evidently, all these different components must be interconnected. In order to successfully implement the architecture of the framework, we have combined the advantages of multiagent systems (MASs; Wooldrige 2002) with service-oriented architectures (SOAs; Alonso et al. 2004).

MASs are used to implement all the high-level decision and reasoning mechanisms. In fact, software agents are commonly used to implement social processes similar to those of humans, including negotiation, planning, or reasoning with incomplete information. On the other hand, SOAs are used in this context to create a middleware layer that allows transparent interconnection of all the devices. In effect, a system based on a SOA implements functionalities as a set of interoperable services that can be used without any prior knowledge about their implementation. This enables the interconnection of the physical devices and the sharing of their functionalities as interoperable services while hiding their eventual complexity and singularities. Combining software agents and interoperable services results in a highly modular approach as each functionality is packaged in one well-delimited bundle.

In order to implement the agent's community, we are using Jade (Java Agent Development Framework). Jade is a software framework that simplifies the implementation of MASs through a middleware that complies with the Foundation for Intelligent Physical Agents (FIPA) specifications. FIPA is a standards organization that promotes agent-based technology and the interoperability of its standards with other technologies. It develops specifications in different categories, including agent communication, agent transport, agent management, abstract architecture, and applications. Moreover, Jade also provides a set of graphical tools that support the debugging and deployment phases. It supports dynamic agent communities in the sense that the configuration can be changed at runtime by moving agents from one machine to another one, as and when required.

Concerning the development and lifecycle of the interoperable services, we are making use of the OSGi service platform (Chen and Gong 2001; OSGi 2003). This platform facilitates the componentization of software modules and applications and assures interoperability of applications and services over a variety of networked devices, providing specifications, reference implementations, test suites, and certification to foster a valuable cross-industry ecosystem. With OSGi we build applications as an infrastructure to support a generic, platform-independent framework. The resulting middleware layer provides services that expose the functionalities of the devices of the environment. Figure 13.5 depicts the high level organization of this architecture.

Simulation

Before implementing such a complex architecture, it is advantageous to create a simulation environment that allows for the system to be tested and assessed. We clearly need to

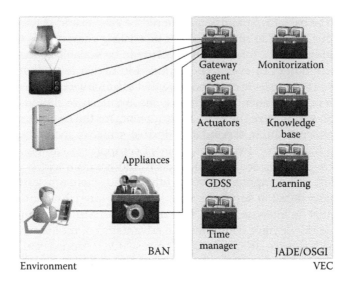

FIGURE 13.5
High level view of the architecture of the framework. On the left side, the appliances network is visible, as well as the user and his/her personal device. Both of these components connect to the gateway agent, which makes the bridge with the remaining members of the framework.

study the behavior of the system when specific cases occur, ranging from the reactive cases (e.g., react to a temperature change) to the more complex ones (e.g., there is no movement in the last room the person was spotted for a long period of time). We also want to know how the framework reacts in specific scenarios that are hard to occur or with harmful consequences, such as malfunctioning of some components or if all the alarms are firing at the same time. This is in fact one of the main advantages of simulation: it enables us to study specific scenarios that rarely occur but are possible, without having to face the consequences of them really happening.

The simulation comprehends a fully configurable home environment, the external surrounding environment, and the user as well as their actions, emotions, or movement patterns (Carneiro et al. 2008). Basically, the main factors that exist in a real home environment and influence the well-being and the safety of the users were considered during the development of the simulation tool. It is therefore possible to simulate temperature, luminosity, movement, humidity sensors; fire, flood, and gas alarm; vital signs of the user (which comprise heartbeat rate, body temperature, respiratory rate, and blood pressure); and an external weather station. Considering the devices and actuators in the environment, it is possible to simulate several kinds of home appliances, ranging from an oven or a coffee machine to the lights or the hi-fi. This is useful for determining which action the user is performing and in which room. It is also possible to simulate rooms with very different physical characteristics, defining not only their geometrical configuration but also the way that external environmental factors influence the home environment and consequently the well-being and the actions of the user.

The development strategy consisted of developing the simulation tool using OSGi. This means that the architecture and logic organization of the simulation tool are the same as those of the framework. By doing so, we optimize the last phase of the development of the framework since we only need to replace the components that simulate data by the ones that acquire them from the sensors in the environment. However, this has additional advantages. On the one hand, we have intermediary phases in which the framework has real and simulated components, allowing to test specific scenarios that already comprehend some real components. On the other hand, it allows us to test some aspects without actually acquiring the necessary devices. This results in a more reliable and stable development process since, one the one hand, the architecture of the framework is already defined and tested, and, on the other hand, we can gradually replace and thoroughly test each new component.

Simulating the Environment

The environment is the central component of the system. It is composed of different rooms, with different characteristics. The characteristics of each room (e.g., insulation, amount of glass, existence of window blinds, power of air conditioning) interfere with the environmental parameters inside the rooms. And of course, the environment inside the rooms directly interferes with our well-being and safety. In a sunny place, for example, the temperature inside a room will generally be higher if the amount of glass in the walls of that room is higher or the insulation is poor. Even the geometry of the house can influence the environmental parameters: the temperature or humidity in a room influences the temperature and humidity in rooms that share a door. The simulation of the environment is thus essential, and it is very important that it is fully configurable so that a wide range of different scenarios can be tested.

Thus, the first step on configuring a new simulation is to set up the configuration of the environment (Figure 13.6). In the light grey area, one can draw several rooms and dispose them in any possible way. When each room is drawn, it is assigned a name and its characteristics must be configured according to four key factors: the level of insulation, the

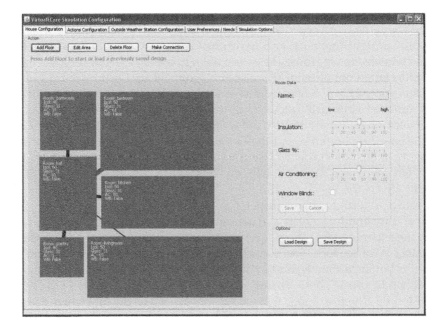

FIGURE 13.6
The simulation environment configuration. Some rooms are drawn and some connections between them are visible.

amount of glass that covers the walls, the power of the air conditioning, and the existence or not of window blinds. The insulation quantifies how significantly the external environmental variables influence the internal ones. The power of the air conditioning represents, in a general way, the capacity of interfering with the temperature of that room. This might happen by the action of some air conditioning device as well as any other heating or cooling device like central heating or a gas heater. The amount of glass in a room represents the amount of glass that covers its walls. This influences the temperature and the luminosity inside the room. If a room has a low percentage of glass, it will be less influenced by the outside temperature, since glass usually has a higher heat capacity than walls. The luminosity inside each room is also related to the amount of glass. Another important factor that influences the luminosity inside a room is the existence or not of window blinds on each window, and that is the last configurable parameter in a room. One may assume that in a room without window blinds, the luminosity depends only on the external luminosity and the state of the lights. On the other hand, if the room has window blinds, the luminosity would also depend on the position of the window blinds.

Additionally, in the simulation one can establish connections between rooms already drawn. These connections represent the doors between rooms and have the same function in the simulation. They are used in two different ways: to simulate the movement of the user inside the environment and to simulate the influence of the environmental parameters of each room on the neighboring rooms. Finally, it is also possible to save or load designs so that predefined designs can be used.

Simulating Sensors

For generating all the data concerning the environmental parameters, there is a group of different sensors that is being simulated. This includes a virtual outside weather station, equivalent to a real preassembled one. This weather station (as the real one) can provide information about the wind speed and direction, temperature, humidity, barometric pressure, rainfall, sunlight intensity, and lightning. This way, the simulation tool provides access to the knowledge regarding the external environment surrounding the user. This is useful as information not only for the user but also to be accessed by the Group Decision Support System or the PMA, when deciding on recommendations for the user. In fact, given the service-oriented approach followed, all the simulated data can be remotely accessed by external entities. In the simulation, the weather station has yet another very important role: it is the base for computing all the remaining environmental data. This means that the simulated parameters inside the environment depend firstly on the values of the same parameters outside, much like what happens in real life. The exact way that the external environment affects the inside environment depends then on factors like insulation and house exposure to sunlight, among others.

The temperature and luminosity virtual sensors are distributed along the environment to monitor these parameters. Their equivalents in the real environment are the DS18B20 and D2Photo 1-Wire sensors. The humidity sensors are used in the bathroom (to detect that the user is having a shower) and in the rest of the environment (to monitor air humidity for health purposes). These virtual sensors are equivalent to the TAI8540A 1-Wire Humidity Module. The fire, flood, and gas sensors as well as the movement sensor, on the other hand, are X10 based. The fire, flood, and gas sensors are used to detect threatening situations for the life of the user and are equivalent in functionalities to PR8307, PR8306, and PR8808, respectively. The movement sensor is used to determine in which room the user is equivalent to PR8070.

The simulation tool also generates data regarding the vital signs of the user, including the heartbeat, body temperature, blood pressure, and respiratory rate. These data are mainly intended to be used remotely by doctors or other services and to raise alarms in case of dangerous or abnormal readings.

The important question here is how to generate all these data in a realistic way, keeping in mind that we also want to create specific scenarios. In this simulation tool, it is thus possible to set the simulated values manually throughout the simulation (thus creating a specific scenario) or to let them evolve in a natural way. As said before, the base of the simulated sensors is the outside weather station, which means that the values inside depend on the values outside. It is thus only possible to manually configure the weather station sensors as the remaining ones depend also on the other parameters mentioned.

To implement scenarios, the simulation tool makes use of XML files. Each XML file contains the address and location of the simulated sensor and is followed by a list of pairs of the type <*tick, value*> that determine the instant *tick* of the simulation in which the sensor with a given address changes its value to *value*. Whenever a sensor bundle is started in the scenario mode, it searches for XML files that refer to any of the virtual sensors it controls and implements the desired behavior. The same methodology is used for any of the other sensors, differing only on the range and type of values that are according to the type of the sensor.

Let us now detail the second case, in which we do not want to set up static scenarios but instead let the values flow in a natural fashion. In this mode, values are generated using a Gaussian distribution, which is known to realistically shape natural phenomena. Thus, when configuring the simulation, in the *Outside Weather Station Configuration* tab, one may select for each simulated parameter the mean and the variation and that will define the weather that will occur during the simulation (Figure 13.7). It is thus possible to create relatively stable weather or, on the other hand, to create a weather configuration that can change rapidly and unexpectedly.

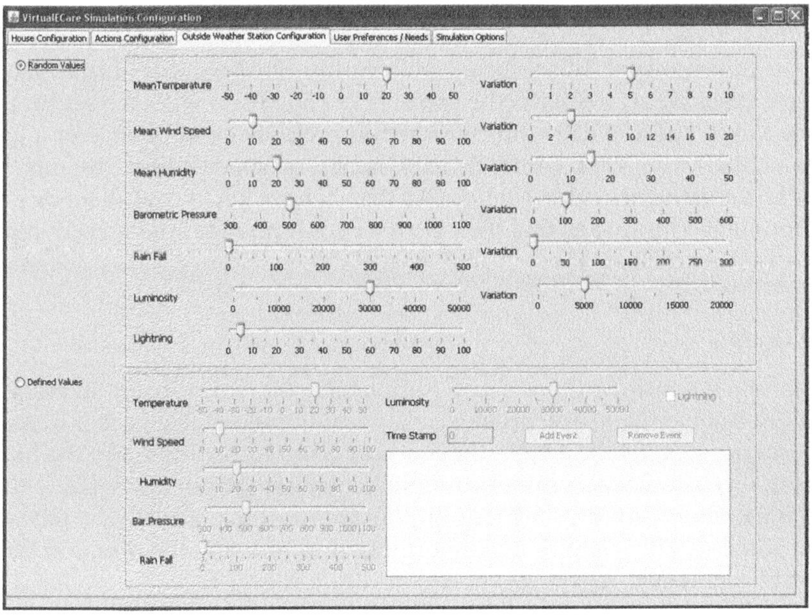

FIGURE 13.7
Configuration of the outside weather station.

Let us now detail how the data about the internal environment sensors are generated. The first step is to identify the main factors that stand between the outside environment and the inside environment in our homes, which have already been mentioned in the section "Simulating the Environment" (e.g., insulation, amount of glass), so the data generated depend on these factors. There are two additional factors that are taken into consideration by the simulation tool: the time factor and the number of adjacent rooms. In fact, taking as an example the temperature, it does not change immediately after a change in the state of the air conditioning. When we change the state of the air conditioning, the changes take a while to be noticeable so the time factor is used to add some delay to parameters like temperature or humidity. Luminosity, on the other hand, changes instantly so the time factor does not apply. As for the number of adjacent rooms, it is acceptable to state that the environment in a room is affected by the environment in the rooms that share a common door; on the other hand, it also affects the environment in all those rooms so this is another factor that must be considered.

Simulating Actuators

The actuators in the environment are responsible for controlling appliances and are also simulated by this tool, with the results of their use being visible in the environment. The tool provides the possibility to simulate lights, window blinds, coffee machines, hi-fi, televisions, and air conditioning systems. The simulated lights can be turned on or off or their brightness dimmed. The simulated window blinds can be pulled up or down. The coffee machines, hi-fi, and televisions can essentially be turned on or off. As for the simulated air conditioning, it can be turned on or off or its temperature adjusted. Moreover, the simulation tool allows for the states of all these virtual actuators to be checked, i.e., it is possible to have access to the position of the window blind or the actual temperature of the air conditioning system. Although this is possible in some recent real X10 modules, it is not possible in the older ones.

As with the sensors, the virtual appliances may be simulated in two different ways. It is possible to generate specific scenarios or to run in what we call normal mode. Using scenarios, the methodology used is the same as the one used with the sensors. An XML file is created for a specific X10 address, which represents an appliance of a given type, containing a list of valid X10 commands to be issued on specific time instants. Under the normal mode, the actuators behave much like they behave when controlled by a human in a real environment. This means that their state will only change after an action of the user, unless there is some malfunction.

Simulating Users

The users of the environment are a key component. Moreover, users interact with and change the environment and are, probably, the most unpredictable part of it. As an example, if the user decides to take a bath, they increase the temperature and the humidity on the bathroom. The simple fact of interacting with certain devices interferes with the environmental parameters: if the user turns on the oven to cook a meal, the temperature in the kitchen will rise. This justifies the importance of simulating the user and their actions inside the environment.

Concerning the actions, it is possible to simulate a wide range of standard actions that one generally performs inside a house (Figure 13.8). There are three different modes under which a user's actions can be configured: full random, bounded random, and planned.

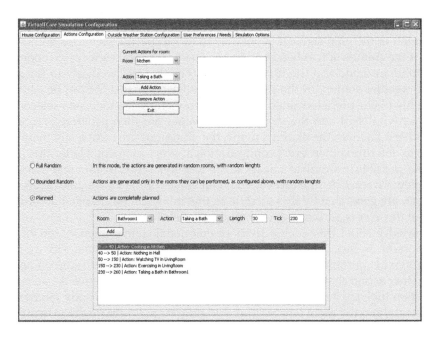

FIGURE 13.8
User actions configuration: planned mode is selected.

Under the full random mode, one has no control over the user's actions being performed inside the environment. The only restrictions are the user's level of activity (which dictates the rate at which new actions are generated when no action is being performed) and the maximum length of the action. The resulting behavior are random actions being performed in random rooms, with random lengths and starting at random moments throughout the simulation.

Under the bounded random mode, the actions are generated randomly, with random lengths, just like in the full random mode. However, under this mode, it is possible to configure which actions can be performed in which room. This mode allows for a more realistic simulation, without, however, having to worry about completely specifying what is going to happen in what tick and in which room. This mode is useful when we want more realistic scenarios with constraints such as the following: in the bathroom, the user can only take baths; and in the living room, the user can only watch television, listen to music, or perform exercise. Then, only these actions are generated in these rooms, although with random lengths.

The last mode is the one under which it is possible to completely specify the behavior of the user during the simulation. Under the planned mode, one can select which action will be performed in which room at each time and with what length. This way, it is possible to completely specify the routine of the user during the simulation. Figure 13.8 shows an example in which the planned mode is selected. When the simulation starts, the user will be cooking in the kitchen for 40 ticks. After finishing, the user will be in the hall doing nothing for 10 ticks. They will then be watching TV in the living room during 100 ticks and exercising in the same room for 80 ticks. At last, the user will be taking a bath during 30 ticks in the bathroom.

There are, however, more data being simulated concerning the user. As one of the objectives of the framework is to monitor the user's vital signs, these are also simulated mainly to test the inference mechanisms that try to evaluate the health status of the user. Using the simulation of the vital signs, it is possible to cause specific scenarios and observe the response of the framework. When configuring the user's vital signs, two modes are possible: the random mode and the planned mode (Figure 13.9). Similarly to the configuration of the weather station, in the first mode, the user's vital signs can be configured to run randomly inside predetermined values. When using this mode, one selects the mean value of each vital sign and the variance. The values are then generated according to a Gaussian distribution. In the planned mode, the vital signs are completely planned, and it is possible to determine their exact configuration at every moment. Under this mode, it is, for example, possible to simulate a heart attack in a given time instant and assess how the whole framework reacts to it. However, the final values of the vital signs are generally not the ones that are generated by this module as they may still be changed according to the activity that the user is performing or their emotional state.

The knowledge about how each activity or emotional state influences the vital signs is really important. In fact, by knowing that a given or emotional state activity influences some vital sign in a certain way, the framework can advise the user to stop doing it or even to take another action that causes a better configuration of vital signs. As an example, in the simulation tool, the action *exercise* increases the heartbeat, the body temperature, the respiratory rate, and the room temperature and humidity. Therefore, if the heartbeat is too high and the user is exercising, the framework may advise them to stop or even go to rest so that the heartbeat can slow down.

Additionally, some more information about the users can be simulated. The user's activity level determines the rate at which new actions are generated when no action is being performed. The user's level of richness is used by the framework as a parameter in the decision-making process. As an example, when the framework must decide on which action to take when the temperature rises past a given level, it may lower the window

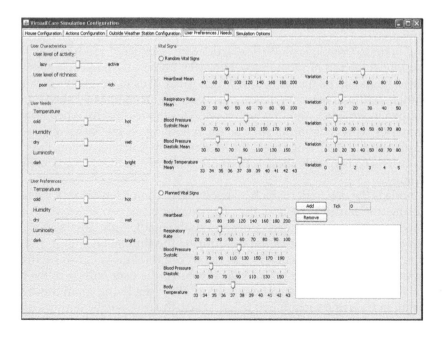

FIGURE 13.9
Configuration of the user's vital signs.

blind or turn on the air conditioning. The most effective action would be to turn on the air conditioning. However, if the user's level of richness is low, the framework could choose to act on the blinds. As for the user's needs and preferences, the use is similar. When the framework acts on the environment, all these factors are weighted to try to find the optimal solution that provides both comfort for the user and an adequate environment. In order to improve the decisions based on these factors, learning mechanisms were implemented, as will be seen next.

Running the Simulation

After fully configuring the simulation, some additional options can be set such as the simulation speed or length. A log file can be saved according to the desired verbosity that can later be analyzed. When the simulation starts, an OSGi controls its execution. This bundle controls the length of each tick and, in this way, the speed of the simulation. At each tick, the control bundle requests from all the other bundles of the simulation the simulated values for the current tick and displays them on a GUI (Figure 13.10). It also provides a simple interface for interacting with the simulation, which allows the simulation-related parameters to be changed. However, the most interesting aspect is not the interface itself but the fact that all these simulated data are available to be used by other modules as will be seen next, allowing testing of the framework under specific circumstances.

Monitoring

The monitoring of users is paramount when it comes to their security. In that sense, this framework aims at constant monitoring of users both when they are in their home environment and when they are outside. The monitoring module has been developed and improved with the experience collected from the simulation platform. It is composed of the following components: the database, the sensor manager, the sensor monitor, the

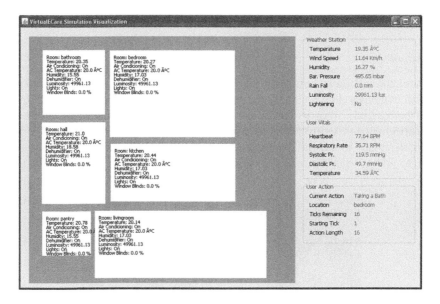

FIGURE 13.10
Visualization and control of the simulation.

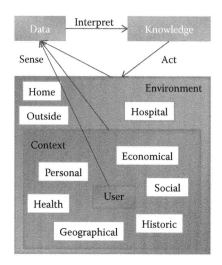

FIGURE 13.11
Data flow in the monitorization module.

sensors, and the decision making. Figure 13.11 depicts the general idea of the monitoring module: using a wide range of sensors, the framework interprets the user and their surroundings (i.e., its context) and then acts back on the environment, as necessary. This may encompass information about the environment, other persons present and the relations between them, economical context, historic context, and geographic context, among others. These data are of utmost importance for describing the user and their environment. When interpreting them, one can infer knowledge after which actions are performed on the environment according to the knowledge generated and the user's preferences and needs. The monitoring module has an architecture that is equivalent to that of the simulation tool. This allows the tool to complement the monitoring module with data that we have not accessed yet or to create specific scenarios that mix real data with simulated.

In-Home Monitoring

To implement the in-home monitoring module, different sensor networks are being used according to purpose (Figure 13.12). Specifically, for environmental monitoring, 1-Wire sensors are being used. In order to be able to manage the sensor network, the sensor manager application was added to the framework. Using the sensor manager, it is possible to assign a given sensor to a room, to move sensors between rooms, to remove sensors from the rooms, to add or remove sensors from the database, or to read detailed information

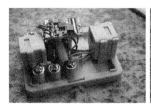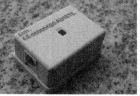

FIGURE 13.12
Luminosity sensor installed inside a small plastic box with its address visible.

about each sensor. It constantly checks for new sensors in the network and issues warnings every time a new one is detected, as well as if some sensor in use in a room is not reachable. Conditional searches are also supported, such as searching for all alarming sensors. It was developed as a bridge between the system administrator and the database that stores all the information about sensors (e.g., type, location), making the configuration of the sensor network easier.

The monitoring module is also an important addition to the 1-Wire technology as it transforms a regular 1-Wire network into a plug-and-play 1-Wire network, adding a whole new range of possibilities. On the one hand, it makes it much easier to configure the 1-Wire network: one has just to lay down the cable and connect the sensors, which is also very easy to do since they are built into plastic boxes with the respective connectors. As the administrator goes on connecting new sensors, the module detects them and queries the user about their physical location and intended use, being at this point possible to associate them to a room. It also detects when, for some reason, some registered sensor is not reachable, querying the administrator about maintaining it or not on the database.

Another component that builds the in-home monitoring module is the actual monitoring of the values read from the sensors. This component is responsible for providing the values of different sensors to the platform in the form of interoperable OSGi services. To do it, the component provides the functionalities of the sensors (e.g., get temperature, get luminosity, program set point) in the form of interoperable OSGi services, which can then be transparently used by the remaining framework. It knows how to communicate with each type of sensor and converts the information received from them into information that can be accessed by any other component of the system. This way, it is possible to hide the singularities of each type of sensor, making it easier and faster to develop further applications that use 1-Wire sensors. This component also implements some basic functionalities for monitoring the values of the sensors, constantly checking their values and alarming states. However, this information is made available to the framework and its monitoring is very important for another component, the Group Decision Support System.

Finally, a user interface was created that implements easy access to all the services implemented by the monitoring module. This interface is an OSGi bundle that interacts with the sensor manager and sensor monitor using all the services provided. It is therefore possible to manage and monitor the sensors as well as to view detailed information about their functionalities. However, the important part is not this interface but the possibility of the remaining framework remotely accessing the values of the sensors and thus the state of the environment.

On-the-Move Monitoring

To only monitor a user inside their own environment is a significant limitation as the external environment is by far the more risky one, especially when one is considering users with memory disabilities. For that reason, the EMon (Embodied Monitoring) module was added to the framework. EMon's objective is to make monitoring so portable that it may, eventually, be worn by the user the same way they wear a watch or a necklace. Using such a device, the user can be accompanied and monitored while they are on the move, increasing their self-assurance, autonomy, and security. Although there are already some devices in the market with the objective of monitoring their users while they move, none of them provides a complete and integrated solution. Some are simple GPS-based locators while others monitor one or some vital signs (Figure 13.13).

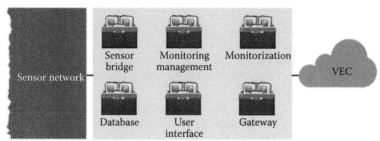

Environment   Monitoring

FIGURE 13.13
High-level organization of the monitoring module, making the bridge between the sensor network and the VirtualECare framework.

In this approach, we seek an integrated device that can provide a full range of important information to describe the context of the user and make it so small that it can comfortably be carried by its users. What we expect to achieve is that AAL environments are no longer static, mandatorily associated to a single physical location, but can instead move while their users move, following them wherever they go.

We are aware that, given the technological constraints, a device with such features is not yet possible to develop: although the needed devices become smaller every day, they are still too big to be integrated in a single device that can be worn comfortably. However, we developed a prototype that was integrated into the framework that allows us to start maturing and testing these ideas, proving that the concept is valid.

In order to implement it, some target key functionalities were established. One of the most important and the first one to be considered given the domain of the problem is the user's location. If the framework has information, in real time, about the location of the elderly, it can efficiently react in case of an emergency. Moreover, useful location-based services can be provided to the elderly, including suggesting nearby interesting places according to preferences or providing directions to nearby services (e.g., hospital, police). Another important feature is to inform the elderly about nearby friends, relatives, or users of the framework with the same interests with whom they eventually would like to interact. This functionality is integrated with the PMA and is described in the section "Personal Memory Assistant."

In order to implement this group of features, we are using a PDA's Global Positioning System (GPS) integrated module, together with software developed to implement some of the said features. The software is responsible for constantly reading the NMEA strings from the GPS receiver and providing them to the framework. Among the functionalities implemented by this software, we can mention the record of the path traveled by the elderly, the current position, or the smallest path to walk to a predetermined location. All these functionalities are implemented using Google Maps and Google Earth APIs.

Another important functionality, especially when considering the health of the elderly, is evaluation of the quality of the surrounding environment. This quality may be given in terms of factors like airborne pollutants, humidity, or temperature. The conviction that the monitoring of the environment around the elderly is paramount for ensuring their safety and well-being is also shared by D'Amato et al. (2002). The importance of the air quality is even higher when we consider elderly with diseases like asthma, bronchitis, or cancer (Oberdörster 2000). Having this in mind, we decided to incorporate into the prototype sensors that could provide the framework with information about the environment. The

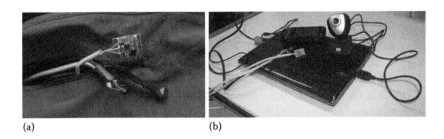

(a)   (b)

FIGURE 13.14
Sensors embedded in the sleeve of the user's jacket (a) and the prototype of EMon with its components connected: a netbook, a PDA, a webcam, and two sensors (b).

main objective is for the framework to be able to warn the user if they are in a place where the environment is not safe or recommended, according to their conditions. In that sense, EMon has been equipped with some sensors that may be embedded in the sleeve of the elderly's jacket (Figure 13.14).

Finally, the last implemented functionality worth mentioning is the ability to take pictures with associated positioning information. This may have several important advantages. On the one hand, the GPS is not always accurate in an urban environment, especially when used around obstacles that can prevent the signal from being received in the best conditions (e.g., high trees, buildings). The picture can therefore help to determine the exact location of the elderly in case of need (e.g., by identifying landmarks, stores, streets), acting as a complement to the GPS module. On the other hand, the user can also take photos that, together with the positioning information, will help them remember their routine and build their daily memories at the end of the day. In order to implement this functionality, a webcam was added to the prototype.

In order to allow the connection between EMon and the framework, OSGi services as well as web services are being used over a mobile data connection. The central device of EMon is a netbook. It provides support for all the other modules and is responsible for running the OSGi platform and the web services as well as for connecting all the devices. Two of the bundles running in this platform are the GPS and the 1-Wire bundles. The first one is responsible for constantly reading NMEA strings and parsing them. The second one regularly reads the values of the sensors. These two bundles provide as services the values read so that the framework can have easy access to that information. In the case of the sensor values, they are simply sent to the VirtualECare platform. As for the values of the GPS bundle, they can be used for three main purposes: to obtain the last known position of the user, to calculate a walking path to the destination, and to access the recorded path of the user.

The whole prototype is still too big to be carried comfortably (Figure 13.14). However, it is a proof of concept that has already allowed us to test and validate the approach, especially its integration with the whole framework. We believe that, as technology evolves, these devices will become smaller and similar approaches will allow the implementation of mobile AAL environments.

Personal Memory Assistant

Given the problem of memory disability in the elderly population addressed before, in this module, we are searching for a technology-based solution that can support the user in the tasks of planning their day-to-day schedule. In that sense, a PMA (Wu and Baecker

2005) was devised: the iGenda (Costa et al. 2011). The iGenda module was developed upon the concept that memory loss should not affect the comfort of the everyday routine, the security of the relatives, and the tranquility of a planned day. To develop this module, we have taken into consideration recent studies (Tucker 1995; Geda et al. 2008) on the consequences of memory loss and possible ways of attenuating them. Basically, the iGenda can be seen as an intelligent distributed event manager and dynamic agenda that builds on three main components (Figure 13.15) and a user interface depicted ahead. It implements and allows the reception of new events and schedules them into the agenda. In this process, there may be conflicts and it may be needed to reschedule preexisting events. This task can be quite difficult for a person with memory disabilities, especially in cases in which the planning ability is already affected. It is thus autonomously undertaken by the framework, taking into consideration parameters like the role of the person scheduling the event or its priority. Moreover, iGenda also implements a playful activities enabler whose main objective is to fill empty slots in the agenda of the users with cultural or social activities, in an attempt to counter the effects of loneliness. With the same objective in mind, it is also possible to share agendas between users, relatives, and friends, allowing the framework to plan joint activities. Among other minor functionalities, the iGenda can also send notifications to the user with different degrees of importance. This module, together with the already described monitoring modules, builds a powerful solution that allows not only monitoring the user's status but also assistance and support to be provided. Let us now depict each of its three building blocks.

The core of the iGenda PMA is the agenda manager (AM). It is responsible for managing all the incoming and outgoing messages. It also controls the lifecycle of the remaining components. The AM is responsible for assessing the degree of importance of each message received, based on concepts like the role of the sender or degree of importance of the content. According to the degree of importance inferred, the AM will take the appropriate course of action to implement the respective behaviors. The AM also has access to the database of users, which arranges users access to content, making use of this information to select the appropriate agenda to share given events of a user. Moreover, this information is also used to determine which users may make changes (e.g., add an event, modify an existing event) to the agenda of a given user. This typically includes persons directly involved in the daily life of the user such as medical personnel, family, or friends.

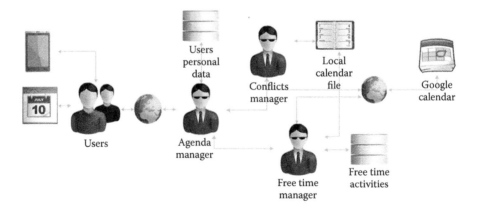

FIGURE 13.15
Overview of the architecture of the PMA.

In order to implement the remaining functionalities, the AM interacts with the conflicts manager (CM) and the free time manager (FTM). The first is in charge of scheduling all the incoming events and resolving eventual conflicts by means of a logic inference engine implemented in Prolog, while the second implements methods for occupying the free time of the user with cultural or social activities.

The CM in fact, plays, an important role as conflicts between events are very common. As a consequence, generally one or more appointments must be rescheduled. In order to schedule appointments, several parameters are taken into consideration. This includes the priority of the event (e.g., an appointment with the doctor has a high priority), the preferences of the user, or even the person or persons scheduling or participating in the event. The priority of the task is understandably the most important parameter.

Several scenarios are therefore possible. When a new event is scheduled and there is no conflict (e.g., no overlap of events), the event is simply scheduled in the agenda of the user. When there is a conflict, two main scenarios are possible: conflicts involving events with the same or with different priorities. If the new event has a degree of priority lower than the already scheduled event, the CM will search for a nearby free slot. If it exists, it will try to schedule it on that slot (by questioning all the involved parties about the minor change). Otherwise, it will notify the user that is scheduling the appointment about the impossibility of doing it on that time. On the other hand, if the priority of the new event is higher, the CM will try to reschedule the already scheduled appointment to a nearby free slot. If it is possible, the old event is moved and all the involved users are notified. Otherwise, the old event is deleted in order to schedule the new one with higher priority. In the scenario of both events having the same priority, the user is questioned about its preferences concerning the events in conflict. In such a scenario, the preference of the user is learned by the system, with the objective of later applying such a decision autonomously or, at least, suggesting it to the user. Finally, another different operation can be performed by the CM, concerning events whose durations can be changed (e.g., a walk in the park, playing cards with the friends). If a conflict exists involving at least one event of this type, the duration of the event can be changed so that it is possible to accommodate the new one minimizing the changes in the agenda. This is depicted in Figure 13.16. On the left side, the original agenda is shown, with a visit to the park scheduled on the 21st of April. This event is shortened in order to accommodate a visit to the doctor, which has a higher degree of priority (depicted by the color on the right of the event).

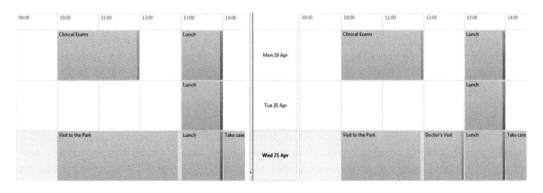

FIGURE 13.16
Modifying an existing event to accommodate the one with higher priority.

In order to increase portability and compatibility, the CM can deal with and provide information about the calendars under different formats, including iCal (ICS) and Google Calendar. This way, users can utilize already available tools for calendar editing and management currently existing in the paradigm of cloud computing. This results in an easy and seamless integration of these already usual tasks in our day-to-day routine with the framework. By following this approach, we also want to take advantage of the growth in the use of mobile devices that include native support for these cloud applications. Specifically, we are targeting the Android mobile system, which has most of Google's services embedded in the core of the operating system. A framework that supports compatibility with these formats allows its users to interact with it in an already familiar way using tools that already form part of their day-to-day lives.

In order to add support for events with multiple persons (e.g., a dinner with relatives, an appointment with the doctor), the concept of shared calendars has been created. Shared calendars must be distinguished from regular calendars because they have unique characteristics. Besides supporting multiple users, one must be aware that not all users that are invited will be attending the event. Moreover, one must also take into consideration that this kind of event generally has lower priority than personal events.

Basically, the functionalities implemented by the CM module develop around the issue of event scheduling, dealing with the issues of eventual events overlapping and the need to resolve those conflicts based on concepts such as event priority. In order to resolve these conflicts, the framework may need to reschedule existing events. In order to do it, the CM also encompasses a notification system that allows a message to be sent to all the implied parties.

The AM also interacts with the FTM in order to fill eventual spaces in the user's daily agenda. This is done with several objectives in mind. On the one hand, the idea is to fill the day of the user with activities outside of the home so that they always have something planned, keeping their minds active. This is important as most elderly people spend significant parts of their time alone at home. On the other hand, we also want to add a social component, with agendas trying to create events in which users can participate together, in an attempt to counter the effects of loneliness. All this, we expect, will significantly increase the quality of life of the elderly and definitely contribute to active aging. The development of the FTM has, in fact, as the main objective, to propose activities that make the users move, stimulating their mind and body.

To implement this, the FTM has access to a database that describes the preferences of each user regarding daily activities. This means that initially users have to state which are their regular activities and rank them according to their preferences, allowing the framework to create a profile about each user. Based on that profile, the framework will suggest group or individual activities to its users. Moreover, the framework will also collect information about user feedback. That is, for each activity suggested, the framework will interpret the feedback from the user in an attempt to perceive eventual changes in the preferences of the user, which are natural as time goes by. This information is then used to modify the mechanisms that select the free time activities, in a constant attempt to shape them to the user's preferences.

According to this information, the FTM defines distribution functions that will determine the frequency according to which events are selected. The process of selecting a new activity for filling in an empty space in an agenda goes as follows. First of all, activities are preselected from the user's database of preferences according to their length: only activities that have a length that allows them to fit in the empty space are preselected. Then, an activity is selected according to a probability distribution function.

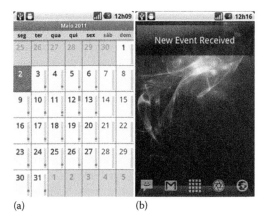

(a)   (b)

FIGURE 13.17
Two screenshots of the usability of iGenda. (a) Agenda of the user; (b) reception of a new event.

In the case of multiperson activities, the process is slightly more complex as it involves the need to check and validate several calendars. In order to implement this, the FTM must therefore cooperate with the CM and the AM. While the first will be responsible for checking and resolving eventual conflicts, the second will be responsible for contacting all the implied users and notifying them about the possible changes that will be performed on their personal agendas, so that they can have the necessary information to accept or reject the new activity.

Basically, this module has, as the main objective, to boost the activities of the users, with a significant social component that aims to get relatives or people with similar interests together. Moreover, it also collects feedback from the users so that the activities proposed can shape eventual changes in their preferences. The learning mechanisms are detailed shortly.

Finally, the iGenda PMA is also composed of a user interface (Figure 13.17), thought to be minimal and easy to use, mainly considering its target users (Picking et al. 2010). In that sense, the main point of interaction with the system is the preferred calendar management applications of the user. Thus, the user has only to indicate the file corresponding to their calendar and then they may edit it using whatever application they want to. The application remains in the background, monitoring any changes that the user performs on the calendar and notifying the framework accordingly. Also, the application receives events from the framework, adds them to the respective calendar file, and notifies the user of a new event, after which the user can visualize it in their favorite application.

Learning

AAL environments can be seen as a group of services being provided to their users with the aim of supporting their day-to-day living. Nowadays, when users need a given service, they must consciously request it. This may pose obstacles, depending on people's degrees of impairment or on the way that services are requested. Having this in mind, in this framework, we are following a different approach. We are building a service environment in which services have a description that is rich enough for the environment to select the best service to deal with a given event on each occasion. The objective is that the environment is able to detect when a given action is needed, activating the corresponding service without any interaction on the part of the user. In order to implement it, we are looking at learning mechanisms that are able to understand how the user usually acts and then implement similar behaviors in an autonomous way (Carneiro et al. 2009). This is no simple task, mainly because each user is a unique case, with their own preferences and needs: a good decision in the context of a given user may not be as good in the context of another user (Augusto et al. 2007).

The first important step to achieve the maximization of the user's satisfaction by means of autonomous services is to develop a rich service description. In fact, it is not hard for a human to decide between turning on the light and pulling up the window blind when the luminosity inside the room is low. However, we are able to do so because we have our own description of the features and possible consequences of each action, which we gained in past similar experiences. We are aware that lights are generally more effective in increasing the luminosity but are also more energy consuming, while window blinds consume no energy but may not be as effective in increasing the luminosity, depending on factors like the size of the window or the external luminosity. In fact, when we make this kind of choice, we are in a process of analyzing costs versus profits, although we do it so naturally that we do not even realize it. These decisions are based on the description of the services that we have built in our mind and keep updating with our ongoing experiences. As an example, as more efficient lights arrive on the market, we update our representation of the cost of using them and gradually use them more often or more easily than before.

In order to define a complete service description, it is first necessary to identify which are the main parameters that we consider when we select a service in our own houses. In that sense, we divided the description into two sets of properties: functional and nonfunctional properties. Functional properties describe properties that relate directly to what the service does or to the actions that will be performed when the service is used. This is important in order to evaluate the possible consequences of using a given service. Nonfunctional properties describe constraints or principles that must be met in order for the service to be available.

Moreover, a closed set of words that is enough to describe the services present in a common environment is also needed. This set of words must be easily expandable in order to be able to describe new services that are eventually added. These words are organized into three groups:

- *Alarms*: These words identify an event in a room. It can be a fire alarm, a high or low state alarm (e.g., temperature above a given threshold), an intrusion alarm, or the user pressing the panic button, among others.

- *Actions*: Words under this group identify actions that a service can take. Actions can include a call to the firefighters or to a relative, turning on or off the heat, or moving a window blind, to name just a few. These actions in fact represent other service invocations that are autonomously used when the service is requested. These methods may encapsulate calls to services or devices in the environment.

- *Descriptions*: Words under this group give a meaning to the remaining ones. As an example, the word *uses* denotes that a given service wants exclusivity over a resource; the word *needs* denotes that a given service needs to use a resource; and the word *against* denotes that a given service is intended to be used in the occurrence of a given alarm.

Services are also organized into three categories, according to their purpose. Thus, they can be classified as security, health, or comfort services. This organization was also devised with the objective of addressing a common challenge in these kinds of environments: cycles. To exemplify this, let us imagine the occurrence of a fire alarm. The usual reaction of an intelligent environment is to activate the sprinklers. A likely consequence of this action is the activation of the flood alarm. When this happens, the system identifies the sprinklers as being the source of the flood alarm and decides to turn the sprinkler off. This will aggravate the fire problem, which will once again activate the fire alarm, and so on.

In the presented framework, the solution to this problem relies on a mechanism to compare the importance of the services (based on their categories), a way of comparing services inside the same category and the previously mentioned service description. Following the same example, the sprinkler and flood alarms are in the same category: security. However, it makes sense to consider that a fire alarm is more important than a flood alarm, since it may potentially cause more damages more quickly. In that sense, a service against a fire event would have more priority than a service against a flood one. So, the service description is used to indicate which resources each service locks and which are required.

If we applied this approach to the above-mentioned example, the fire alarm would request the lock of the power and the sprinkler resources and would obtain them even if they were locked by another service since the fire alarm is the service with the highest priority. It would then activate the sprinkler. When the flood alarm went on, it would try to gain control of the sprinkler but, as it is locked by a service with higher priority, this would not happen and the service request would be blocked by the service environment. This is the kind of problem that we aim to address with this approach.

In the example mentioned above, the selection of the services is not too complex since it involves quite simple decisions. In fact, in our everyday life, when we are faced with life-and-death scenarios, the mechanisms involved are generally very simple and of fast response. The same happens here.

However, in home environments, there are decisions that may involve many more variables. Retrieving the example of what to do when the luminosity drops, there are several factors that may influence the decision: we may consider the power consumption of each service, the effectiveness, our willingness to save energy or the amount of money that we are prepared to pay on the electricity bill, the external luminosity, and the time until being dark outside, among others. In our everyday life, we make these decisions without even noticing that we are weighting all these parameters. And in fact, most of the times, we are not exactly weighting them at all. We usually decide fast because we rely on past cases, i.e., when faced with a familiar situation, we do not go through all the pros and cons: we usually do what we have already done with success in the past.

When using machinery to take such decisions, several aspects must be taken into consideration. First of all, a computer must evidently take a decision, either by weighting all the pros and cons, applying rules, using optimization functions, or considering past cases. However, each of these methods has its own advantages and disadvantages. Considering optimization functions or rules, the main problem is that they are static. That is, we may spend some effort to define the best optimization function or the correct rules, but then, if the preferences of the user change, they are useless as they do not reflect them anymore. On the other hand, weighting all the pros and cons every time a decision must be made can be significantly time consuming, which is especially undesirable when fast decisions must be taken.

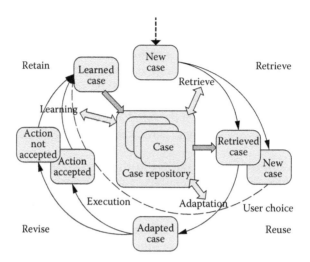

FIGURE 13.18
Case-based reasoning model used, based on the one presented by Aamodt and Plaza (1994). (From Aamodt A., Plaza E., *AI Communications*, 7(1):39–59, 1994. IOS Press.)

Considering all of this, we argue that such systems should not be static but instead adapt to their users. According to this, we developed the framework around the idea that it should learn the preferences and habits of the user and, when it is sure enough that in a given case the user would take a given action, the framework itself takes the action. In order to implement this, we rely on a case-based reasoning (Aamodt and Plaza 1994) model (Figure 13.18).

The learning process is triggered by an alarm. An alarm is the occurrence of a predetermined event such as the value of a sensor going past a given threshold. Whenever there is an event, a new case is created. A case contains a snapshot of the state of the environment at that moment as well as the actions that the user takes to deal with the alarm. A complete case, as when it is stored in the knowledge base, contains the following information:

- *Room*: the ID of the room in which the alarm occurred
- *Alarm*: the alarm that the case refers to
- *Service*: the service used by the user to solve the alarm
- *Value*: a value that denotes the success of this case when used by the system
- *Time*: the instant of time at which the alarm occurred
- *Sensors*: the information about all the sensors in the room and the weather station sensors

The process goes on as follows. When an alarm occurs, the framework searches the knowledge base for cases that contain the same alarm and are similar to the case just created. The measure of similarity is higher when the values of the sensors are closer and when the room is the same. After selecting the most similar case, two things can occur: the case is similar enough so that the action in the case can be taken by the system with a high degree of confidence on the success, or it is not that similar and the user interaction is requested.

The first scenario denotes that there is a high confidence on the case and it is reasonable to assume that the user would take a similar action if they had to choose. When this happens, the case may either be directly used or it may have to be adapted. Adapting cases is relatively common and may happen, as an example, in scenarios in which the alarm is the same and the values of the sensors are very similar but the room is different. In such cases, it is reasonable to assume that the user would take the same action that they took in a different room.

Every time the framework takes an action that influences the environment, a process starts in which the behavior of the user is analyzed for a few moments. This process's objective is to determine if the action just taken by the framework is the correct one in the correct time. If during a predetermined period of time the user takes no action that counters the effects of the action that was automatically taken by the framework, the value of the case increases. This is an indication that the case is valid and reflects the preferences of the user, being in a better position to be selected in future iterations. On the other hand, if during that period of time the user takes an action, it must be analyzed. Two things can be inferred from the user's behavior. If the user simply cancels the action that the system took, it means that the case is correct, i.e., the action performed was the correct one, although the instant at which it occurred is not. As a consequence, the framework changes the values of the thresholds of the respective alarm. As an example, let us imagine the occurrence of a high temperature alarm in a given room, after which the framework decides to turn on the air conditioning. If, after a few moments, the user turns it off, that may mean that the user wants the air conditioning to be turned on only when the temperature is a little higher. As a consequence, the limit of the temperature alarm for that room is increased slightly and the value of the case is slightly decreased, as it was not successful.

Let us now imagine that the user, besides canceling the action taken by the framework, takes another action that has the same objective of the canceled action. This may indicate that the time at which the alarm occurred is correct, although the action selected may not be correct. As an example, we can think of the framework turning on the lights because the low luminosity alarm was activated, after which the user turns the lights off and moves the window blinds up. The actual effects of such a behavior on the framework are that the value of the case applied is decreased slightly, and a new case is added to the knowledge base, which contains the state of the house and the action taken by the user.

There may also be the scenario in which there are no cases with a sufficient degree of similarity. Under such scenarios, the user interaction is requested. The framework selects the services available in the service environment that are suited to resolve the alarm and requests input from the user in order to perceive what they would like to do. Given the target users, services are presented to the user with minimal information, with an intuitive image describing them (Figure 13.19). This kind of interface is thought mainly to be used

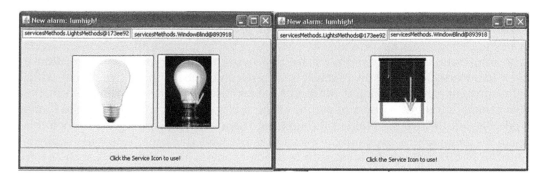

FIGURE 13.19
User can select among three services to deal with the high luminosity alarm.

in tactile portable devices, making the service selection a very easy process for the user. Moreover, it is also very convenient for users with some physical disability as they can interact with the environment through the interface, without having to move around the home. When the user clicks on the image of a service, the framework adds the information about the action taken by the user to the new case and the case is added to the knowledge base. At last, the action is executed by the framework.

This service selection model has many advantages for the user; the most important being that it is not static. It constantly adapts to the users, mimicking their preferences. This means that after some time, each implementation will be unique: a personalized environment. More than that, the environment will keep evolving with the user's constant interaction. This means that even if the user's preferences change, the system will gradually adapt, without external interaction or explicit configuration. That would not happen if, instead of using this approach, one used optimization algorithms or rule-based systems, since they would have to be changed according to the preferences of the user. Moreover, this is also an approach that allows collection of user preferences and habits in a noninvasive way, constantly evolving with each interaction without the awareness of the user.

Future Work

The framework presented here supports a wide range of services targeted at assisting the users in a home environment, specifically elderly users with some degree of disability, such as memory disabilities. Following the same approach, we are continuing to develop additional services to be added to the framework.

We are considering the development of a fall detection mechanism. It is based on a mobile device empowered with an accelerometer and a compass. The main objective is to empower the framework with the ability to detect the falls of the users in order to increase their security. Furthermore, we are also aiming at decreasing the response time to react to alarming situations. This functionality, together with those already presented, is being developed in line with the concept of the virtual home. Our main aim is to develop a virtual representation of the home of the users with as much information as possible so that the remote decision-taking mechanisms (encompassing relatives, decision support systems, and medical personnel) can take better decisions based on more information.

A second line of development is being carried out concerning Personal Memory Assistance. The main objective of this line of research is to make use of the already available GPS information provided by EMon in order to improve and empower iGenda. With information about location, we are improving the event allocation algorithm in order to include the approximate travel time between the locations of two events, which at the moment is not considered. Moreover, we are also using the real-time information about the location of the users to empower the social enabler component of the framework. Specifically, we are interested in getting friends or relatives together, when they are in the geographical proximity of each other and have free time. This will usually be centered in filling small duration gaps between events with social events such as having a coffee or a walk in the park. With these two new services, we expect to continue empowering the framework with functionalities that will make the life of their users better.

Conclusions

Ambient intelligence is the result of the intersection of a group of different fields. One of the most important is without a doubt artificial intelligence. In fact, some authors even consider ambient intelligence as a subfield of artificial intelligence. In that sense, there are many aspects in which techniques and methodologies from artificial intelligence have important contributions. Moreover, these techniques are nowadays applied not with the aim of automating tasks, as was envisioned in the past, but with the aim of supporting the user's daily routines, as envisioned by Aarts and Grotenhuis (2011).

One of the most important aspects concerns planning. In a few words, planning is about defining a sequence of activities that will lead to an expected consequence. In fact, planning is still one of the most complex activities, mainly because it involves the analysis of many (usually conflicting) variables, depending on the complexity of the problem. However, it is very important as it is one of the pillars of intelligence. Without planning, an intelligent environment is unable to foresee the consequences of a given course of action and is thus unable to take correct decisions. Therefore, when developing intelligent environments, one should not only consider the ability to draw plans as well as the ability to redraw them dynamically, in light of changes in the context of interaction. Artificial intelligence traditionally implements planning in the form of optimization algorithms, like using genetic algorithms, ant colonies, or particle swarm optimization.

As shown in this chapter, another very important subject in this context is the one of learning. In fact, an intelligent environment should be able to learn in order to be able to adapt not only to the needs of their users but also to the natural evolution of their preferences. This learning should be done in a seamless way, without questioning the user at all times. In that sense, learning in intelligent environments usually takes place simply by observing the users and their routines. With learning mechanisms, it is therefore possible to develop environments that are dynamic. In this field, artificial intelligence has important contributions, e.g., through the use of artificial neural networks, data mining, case-based reasoning, or decision trees.

The interaction between the user and the environment is another aspect in which artificial intelligence has an important means of contribution. This interaction should be natural, centered on the users and their natural means of communication. In intelligent environments, this implies the development of context-aware interfaces, able to adapt to changes in the state of the environment or even in the state of the users. The contribution of artificial intelligence in this field focuses mainly on the topics of affective and social computing.

Finally, another important topic that stems from the development of this framework is at the level of the actuation. In fact, an intelligent environment must be able to influence not only the environment of the users but also the users themselves. In this field, the main topics are the use of actuator networks or even robotics. Ultimately, artificial intelligence will contribute with highly specialized autonomous robots that will assist users in managing the environment and in performing their tasks. Robots empowered with a social or affective facet are also envisioned, which will provide support at the emotional level.

In the development of this framework, several aspects have been taken into consideration that can be seen as a contribution to the state of the art of ambient intelligence. First of all, we follow an approach that sees ambient intelligence as a MAS. The main advantage of this is a logical organization of the architecture that is easy to reconfigure by adding new modules with new functionalities. This is very important, especially when we are considering a domain such as that of intelligent environments, which are very dynamic, and in which new components can be added or removed at any time. Moreover, this approach also allows advantage to be taken of the features of software agents because of the ability to plan and take decisions in an autonomous way.

Concerning the architecture of the environment itself, during the development of the framework, it became evident that the best approach relied in conjugating the advantages of MASs with ones of SOAs. In that sense, the framework makes use of the OSGi service platform to create a service environment that acts as a middle layer, ensuring compatibility between all the different devices. Jade, on the other hand, is used as the agent platform in which higher-level decision-making mechanisms are implemented. Both technologies are highly modular, allowing the development of dynamic environments in which components can be easily added or removed. The main contribution at this level concerns the interoperability between agents and services, which at first sight would seem to be different approaches but, as was proved, can be seen as complementary.

Another important contribution of this work is at the level of learning. In fact, the development of environments that are able to learn and adapt to their users is one of our main concerns. Specifically, we make use of the preferences, needs, desires, actions, or even the emotional response of the user as arguments for learning mechanisms whose main objective is to allow the framework to learn how to manage the environment by observing the user. One of the main concerns is that this learning minimizes the interaction with the user, being as discreet as possible.

All these insights result in intelligent environments that are dynamic and highly focused on the user's preferences and needs. Following this approach, we believe that some of the social challenges of current population aging can be tackled. Specifically, we believe that such frameworks will not only provide specialized and personalized health care services but also have an important contribution to avoid the loneliness and other aging-related issues, resulting in a better quality of life and more active aging.

Acknowledgments

The work of Davide Carneiro is supported by a doctoral grant by the Fundação para a Ciência e a Tecnologia (FCT, Portuguese Foundation for Science and Technology; SFRH/BD/64890/2009). The work of Angelo Costa is supported by a research grant by the FCT within the project PTDC/JUR/71354/2006 and PEst-OE/EEI/UI0752/2011.

References

Aamodt A., Plaza E. (1994). Case-based Reasoning: Foundational Issues, Methodological Variations, and System Approaches. *AI Communications*, 7(1): 39–59.

Aarts E., Encarnacao J. (2006). *True Visions: The Emergence of Ambient Intelligence*. Springer, New York.

Aarts E., Grotenhuis F. (2011). Ambient Intelligence 2.0: Towards Synergetic Prosperity. *Journal of Ambient Intelligence and Smart Environments*, 3: 3–11.

Alonso G., Casati F., Kuno H., Machiraju V. (2004). *Web Services Concepts, Architectures and Applications, Data-Centric Systems and Applications Series.* Springer, New York.

The Amigo Project. (2004). Amigo—Ambient Intelligence for the Networked Home Environment. Short Project Description. Available at http://www.hitech-projects.com/euprojects /amigo/ (accessed May 9, 2011).

Augusto J.C., McCullagh P., McClelland V., Walkden J.-A. (2007). Enhanced Healthcare Provision through Assisted Decision-Making in a Smart Home Environment. In *Proceedings of the 2nd Workshop on Artificial Intelligence Techniques for Ambient Intelligence (AITAmI'07),* pp. 27–32.

Camarinha-Matos L., Afsarmanesh H. (2001). Virtual Communities and Elderly Support. In *Advances in Automation, Multimedia and Video Systems, and Modern Computer Science,* eds. Kluev V.V., D'Attellis C.E., Mastorakis N.E. pp. 279–284. WSES Press, New York.

Carneiro D., Costa R., Novais P., Machado J., Neves J. (2008). Simulating and Monitoring Ambient Assisted Living. In *Proceedings of the ESM 2008—The 22nd Annual European Simulation and Modelling Conference.*

Carneiro D., Novais P., Costa R., Neves J. (2009). Case-based Reasoning Decision Making in Ambient Assisted Living. In *Proceedings of the IWAAL—International Workshop of Ambient Assisted Living,* eds. Omatu S., Rocha M.P., Bravo J., Fernández F., Corchado E., Bustillo A., Corchado J.M. LNCS 5518, pp. 787–794. Springer-Verlag, Berlin.

Carneiro D., Novais P., Costa R., Neves J. (2010). Developing Intelligent Environments with OSGi and JADE. In *Artificial Intelligence in Theory and Practice III,* ed. M. Bramer. Series: IFIP International Federation for Information Processing, pp. 174–183. Springer-Verlag, Berlin.

Charness N. (2008). Aging and Human Performance. *Human Factors: The Journal of the Human Factors and Ergonomics Society,* 50: 548–555.

Chen K., Gong L. (2001). *Programming Open Service Gateways with Java Embedded Server Technology.* Prentice Hall, Upper Saddle, NJ.

Corchado J.M., Bajo J., de Paz Y., Tapia D.I. (2008). Intelligent Environment for Monitoring Alzheimer Patients, Agent Technology for Health Care. *Decision Support Systems,* 44(2): 382–396.

Costa A., Novais P., Corchado JM., Neves J. (2011). Increased Performance and Better Patient Attendance in an Hospital with the use of Smart Agendas. *Logic Journal of the IGPL,* 20(4): 689–698.

Costa R., Novais P., Machado J., Alberto C., Neves J. (2007). Inter-organization Cooperation for Care of the Elderly. In *Integration and Innovation Orient to E-Society,* eds. Wang W., Li Y., Duan Z., Yan L., Li H., Yang X. Series: IFIP International Federation for Information Processing. Springer-Verlag, Berlin.

Costa R., Novais P., Lima L., Carneiro D., Samico D., Oliveira J. et al. (2009). VirtualECare: Intelligent Assisted Living. In *Electronic Healthcare,* ed. D. Weerasinghe. Series Institute for Computer Sciences, Social Informatics and Telecommunications Engineering, pp. 138–144. Springer-Verlag, Berlin.

D'Amato G., Liccardi G., D'Amato M., Cazzola M. (2002). Outdoor Air Pollution, Climatic Changes and Allergic Bronchial Asthma. *European Respiratory Journal,* 20: 763–776.

Feldman A., Tapia E., Sadi S., Maes P., Schmandt C. (2005). ReachMedia: On-the-Move Interaction with Everyday Object. In *Wearable Computers. Proceedings of the Ninth IEEE International Symposium.* Ambient Intelligence Group, MIT Media Laboratory.

Geda Y., Roberts R., Knopman D., Petersen R., Christianson T., Pankratz V. et al. (2008). Prevalence of Neuropsychiatric Symptoms in Mild Cognitive Impairment and Normal Cognitive Aging: Population-based Study. *Archives of General Psychiatry,* 65: 1193–1198.

Haigh K., Kiff L., Myers J., Guralnik V., Krichbaum K., Phelps J., Plocher T., Toms D. (2003). *The Independent LifeStyle Assistant: Lessons Learned.* UK: Honeywell Laboratories.

Holliday, R. (1999). Ageing in the 21st century. *The Lancet,* 354(Suppl.):SIV4.

INE—Statistics Portugal. (2010). Anuário Estatístico de Portugal 2009. Available at http://www.ine.pt (accessed on June 2011).

MIT Artificial Intelligence Laboratory. (2002). Oxygen—Pervasive, Human-Centered Computing. MIT Laboratory for Computer Science. Available at http://www.oxygen.lcs.mit.edu /Publications/Oxygen.pdf (accessed May 9, 2011).

Novais P., Costa R., Carneiro D., Neves J. (2010). Inter-Organization Cooperation for Ambient Assisted Living. *Journal of Ambient Intelligence and Smart Environments*, 2(2): 179–195.

Oberdörster G. (2000). Pulmonary Effects of Inhaled Ultrafine Particles. *International Archives of Occupational and Environmental Health*, 74: 1–8.

OSGi. (2003). *OSGi Service Platform, Release 3*. IOS Press Amsterdam, The Netherlands.

Picking R., Robinet A., Grout V., McGinn J., Roy A., Ellis S. et al. (2010). A Case Study Using a Methodological Approach to Developing User Interfaces for Elderly and Disabled People. *The Computer Journal*, 53(6): 842–859.

Tucker G. (1995). Age-Associated Memory Loss: Prevalence and Implications. *Journal Watch Psychiatry*. New Jersey, USA.

UNFPA. (2009). State of World Population.

United Nations. (2001). World Population Ageing: 1950–2050. Available at http://www.un.org/esa /population/publications/worldageing19502050 (accessed May 9, 2011).

Wooldrige M. (2002). *An Introduction to Multiagent Systems*. John Wiley & Sons, New Jersey.

World Health Organization. (2000). Social Development and Ageing: Crisis or Opportunity? Presented at the Geneva 2000 Forum, Switzerland. Available at http://www.who.int/ageing /publications/development/alc_social_development.pdf (accessed May 9, 2011).

World Health Organization. (2002). Active Ageing: A Policy Framework. Presented at the *Second United Nations World Assembly on Ageing*, Madrid, Spain.

Wu M., Baecker R. (2005). Participatory Design of an Orientation Aid for Amnesics. In *Proceedings of the SIGCHI Conference on Human Factors in Computing Systems*, pp. 511–520. ACM, New York.

14

Ambient Assisted Living—From Technology to Intervention

Paulo Freitas, Paulo Menezes, and Jorge Dias

CONTENTS

ABSTRACT   This chapter aims to present and discuss a prospective study on technological systems for people with cognitive disabilities. It will provide an analysis of technological solutions for care of dementia illness, and of intelligent systems of assistance for improving quality of life in a preferred living environment. A deep analysis of the current state of the art will be presented. From the analysis of this prospective study, emerging and flexible solutions to assess the progression of signs and symptoms related to the physical and mental health of the patient are presented as novel approaches for earlier detection of dementia diseases. The intention is to contribute with an overview of information and communication technologies (ICT) solutions for better prediction, prevention, and support through long-term trend analysis of basic daily behavioral and physiological data, building on unobtrusive sensing and advanced reasoning with humans in the loop.

KEY WORDS: *ambient assisted living, dementia, information and communication technologies, sensors, long-term assessment, user information, regulatory policies, security rules, privacy rules, human rights.*

Introduction

New European population projections for 2008–2060, published by the European Office for Statistics (Eurostat 2008), have recently underlined that the number of elderly persons will quickly increase. The number of deaths projected from 2015 onward is estimated to outnumber births in the EU27, and in 2060, it is estimated that the number of people older than 80 years of age will be almost three times more than the current situation. These statistics demonstrate a demographic change and the aging of the European population. Consequently, it will lead to a growing number of older people living alone at their homes with the need for (intensive) care and to an aging workforce in general. These will lead to a strong investment in new care services and new research activities, services, and products securing and enhancing their health, safety, entertainment, and communication needs. Considering that this trend will also be accompanied by a rapid growth in the number of persons with physical and cognitive disabilities, it is clear that the problem of providing health care and assistance for these persons will become more and more important, crucial sometimes, from a social and an economic point of view.

It is possible to find in the existing literature content with statistical data that show projections on the future demographic state at the European level (Eurostat 2008; Gabner and Conrad 2010) and that support the social and demographic trends previously mentioned. Analyzing Figure 14.1, it reveals a significant increase in the number of people over 65 years of age along the coming decades; the figure then refers to the years 2035 and 2060 to compare this growth. In the European Union (EU), established by the current 27 countries comprising the union, an increase in the number of people in this age group by 8% and by about 13% in 2035 and 2060, respectively, is expected to happen. On the other hand, Figure 14.2 shows, for the same years 2035 and 2060, a forecast rise of 3.5% and 7.7%, respectively, of people aged over 80 years. The report (Eurostat 2008) ends with the presentation of statistical data that point to a continuous increase during the coming years of the number of elderly, who are dependent on health care and require special needs. These data are shown in Figure 14.3. By analyzing Figure 14.3, one may conclude that from 2008 to 2060,

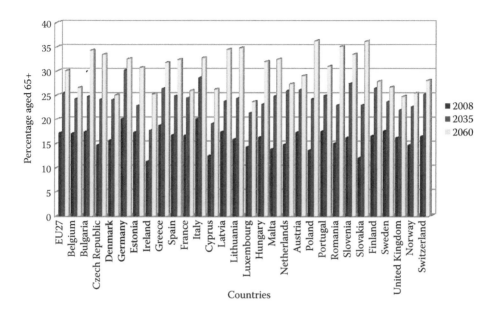

FIGURE 14.1
Percentage of people over 65 years.

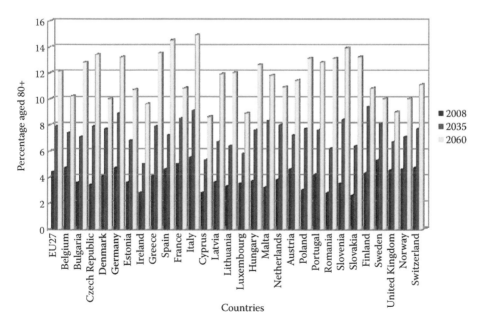

FIGURE 14.2
Percentage of people over 80 years.

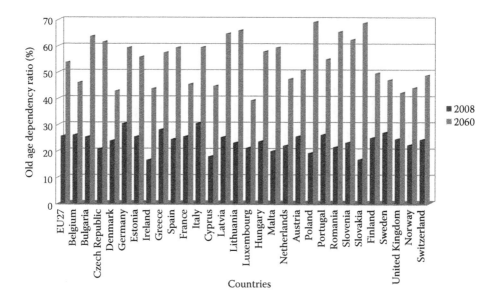

FIGURE 14.3
Old age dependency ratio (%).

the number of aged people dependent on health care provision, taking into account primary and secondary care, will double considering the average of the EU members.

These figures revealed by Eurostat show the urgency of finding solutions to ensure better living conditions and prolong the period of independence, autonomy, and social participation of European populations. These social trends will lead to dramatic challenges for health care systems, state pension schemes, and employers alike, but at the same time, they will offer research innovation in scientific areas, new approaches, and also business opportunities for technology providers in the development of information and communication technologies (ICT) and in the field of ambient assisted living (AAL). Actually, the range of possible applications of ICT in the health sector is enormous. Technology has progressed significantly and many estimate that ICT implementation can result in care that is higher in quality, safer, and more responsive to patients' needs and, at the same time, more efficient (appropriate, available, and less wasteful). The complementary area of AAL refers to intelligent systems of assistance for a better, healthier, and safer life in the preferred living environment and covers concepts, products, and services that interlink and improve safety, care support, and social environment. It aims at enhancing the quality of life (the physical, mental, and social well-being) for everyone (with a focus on elderly persons) in all stages of their life. AAL can help elderly individuals to improve their quality of life, to stay healthier, and to live longer, thus extending their active and creative participation in the community. Recognition of situations and awareness about the activities for users in their environment are a core function for AAL applications. The results obtained in this area might help in modeling, preventing, and classifying situations like falling, lying on the floor, physical immobility, monitoring activities of daily living, occupation of spaces at home, locomotion, system interoperability, fusion signals, pattern recognition, multicriteria approaches for decision support, and other possibilities. All the improvements in each of these scenarios are an important step toward the development of solutions that are more effective and safer to allow the subsequent design of new mechanisms, products, and even services in order to improve the quality of life of people that need care provision.

Currently, there are technological systems for many purposes to support the activities of health care, such as telemedicine systems, electronic health records, fall detection applications, game activities, robotic systems, home automation, security systems, and techniques for behavior analysis, among others (Broek et al. 2009). All of these systems, which are available as products and services, have great potential to be an important support tool in the execution of daily tasks, prevention and safety, and registration of clinical data of the final users.

However, the differences in cultures, lifestyles, and specific needs that can be found in communities in several countries demonstrate the necessity to develop technological solutions in a user-centric perspective (Gabner and Conrad 2010). This perspective promotes the development of new approaches to be able to become more suitable to the surrounding environment of users, taking into account their preferences, usability, specific requirements for the interaction process with the systems, and requirements and factors that lead to demand for health care. From this perspective, people with special needs, especially with cognitive disorders such as dementia, require systems tailored to their daily activities in order to serve as an important support to improve independence, quality of life, and well-being. Indeed, dementia care provision is a focus of attention for medical and pharmacological research areas, and also for technological fields. Current communities rely on the progress of such areas to give an effective answer to the increasing number of onset dementia cases. Moreover, the European projections indicate that the number of diagnosed dementia cases continues to increase (Mura et al. 2010). Figure 14.4 provides statistical data related to this projection from which it is possible to conclude that there maybe an estimated increase in cases of dementia of around 93% between 2010 and 2050.

The number of diagnosed dementia cases proves to be growing and will indeed have a strict impact on today's social community and lifestyle, and will require changes in economic and social structures, demanding and looking for new schemes to support good quality levels for living. The rise in the incidence of mental disabilities and the increase in the elderly population are a major cause for high social, economic, and personal costs, becoming a growing public health concern. Early and accurate identification of individuals who are at high risk of developing dementia and other chronic diseases is regarded as a research priority. This identification followed by effective interventions may significantly contribute to reducing the prevalence and incidence of dementia diseases, improving the quality of life of both the patients and their caregivers, and making a more efficient use of the resources needed to provide adequate institutional and home health care. The process

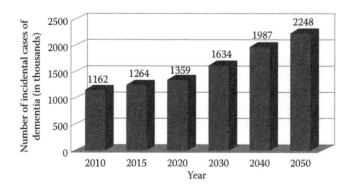

FIGURE 14.4
Projections of the annual incidental cases of dementia.

of early identification assumes even greater importance knowing that there are already treatments to help slow down disease progression, and prevention strategies including lifestyle change (Hendrie 1998; Roberson and Mucke 2006). Furthermore, there are studies (Petersen et al. 2005) suggesting that medical therapies might reduce the risk of dementia development, and the growing availability of symptomatic therapies has the potential to delay progression of mild cognitive deficits.

In fact, there are scientific works that point out the benefits of delaying the onset and retarding the progression of dementia diseases, for example, Alzheimer's disease (Brookmeyer et al. 2007). Considering the design modeling presented in Brookmeyer et al. (1998), these studies show the results of evaluating four different scenarios, each one consisting a reduction in the age-specific incidence rate from 2005 onward by a factor of 5%, 10%, 20%, and 50%. These scenarios correspond to delays of 0.4, 0.8, 1.6, and 4.8 years, respectively, in the onset of Alzheimer's disease. The conclusions reflect a drastic impact in the number of prevalence dementia cases; in the first scenario, if interventions could reduce the age-specific incidence rate of Alzheimer's by 5% in 2005, delaying the onset of the disease by around 5 months, then relative to current projections,

- By 2020, there would be 4583 (3.5%) fewer cases of Alzheimer's.
- By 2040, there would be 9462 (4.8%) fewer cases of Alzheimer's.
- By 2050, there would be 11,100 (4.8%) fewer cases of Alzheimer's.

Regarding the most optimistic scenario, if interventions could reduce the age-specific incidence rate of Alzheimer's by 50% in 2005, delaying the onset of the disease by around 5 years, then relative to current projections,

- By 2020, there would be 46,568 (35.2%) fewer cases of Alzheimer's.
- By 2040, there would be 96,690 (48.5%) fewer cases of Alzheimer's.
- By 2050, there would be 113,611 (48.7%) fewer cases of Alzheimer's.

The benefits of predicting and retarding the progression of dementia diseases are enormous. Several works have been presented that propose new approaches to support and provide possible solutions to achieve this goal. The DESCRIPA Study (Chatzigiannakis et al. 2007) presents an evaluation over 3 years of a set of clinical criteria for further analysis of which variables best predict dementia, in particular, Alzheimer's disease. The study by Gaddah and Kunz (2003) evaluates diagnosis criteria for mild cognitive impairment (MCI) incorporating changes in activity level and cognitive functioning. Functional impairment in people at risk of dementia has been studied to understand the indicators associated with the disease's progress (Al-Jaroodi et al. 2009). Other techniques for measuring the progression of Alzheimer's are being tested using scales such as the Mini-Mental® Status Examination (MMSE®; Kjaer 2007) and tests for memory impairment analysis (Buschke et al. 1999). A comparison of various methods for predicting and screening Alzheimer's disease is available in the work of Saeed and Waheed (2010), which points out the strengths and weaknesses of each one.

Detecting the presence of symptoms or signs of a disease does not require that formal diagnostic criteria be met. For dementia and its most common cause, Alzheimer's disease, screening methods are a means to identifying the critical cognitive impairments or daily living dysfunctions that signify the earliest manifestation that can be recognized feasibly. On this matter, technology is required to assume an increasingly important role in promoting better screening methods, prediction indicators, prevention activities, and daily support for people with dementia. Dementia care supported by ICT solutions is an emerging trend in the social and health care sectors. Currently there are a vast number of European and national research activities in the field of AAL involving various technology areas and innovative technology approaches. However, a common vision among all these entities should be achieved. It is needed to develop technology focused on user needs and take into account some issues in the design and development of new technological systems for this target group. In particular, it should be borne in mind that most end users have cognitive and physical abilities, making it hard for them to learn, use, and accept new devices and interfaces. Moreover, during the design phase of AAL solutions, one must also be aware that the location of assistance can vary considerably depending on the user and on the daily activities. Examples are as follows:

- Different living locations, like the family home, home for seniors, supported or sheltered housing or apartment, nursing home, etc.—depending on the needs of the primary user.
- Mobile locations, e.g., walking, cycling, driving your car, being a passenger in a car or taxi or public transport.
- Visiting locations such as family homes, workplaces, or public spaces, e.g., shops or museums.
- Location of people who are involved in caring for people who belong to the primary target group. Such factors lead to the consideration of the need to support clients in a person-centered way (geared toward the primary user at different locations and taking the situation into account, e.g., with respect to environmental sensors at various locations) and to support caregivers in a more task-oriented way.

It is on this basis, as described so far, that the subject of this chapter is founded and focused. Within this topic, the concepts of middleware platforms and decision support systems (using multicriteria models), and how they can be adapted for novel AAL solutions, are explored. Throughout this chapter, ICT systems and scientific approaches to assess users' state and health progression as an informal indicator for the decision-making support in the process of diagnosing dementia diseases are analyzed and their strengths and weaknesses discussed. Furthermore, the advantages and disadvantages of these technologies will be discussed, giving some directions and trends for future research and development. This chapter will address concepts, R&D projects, products, and services able to provide early detection and adaptive support to change individual needs related to chronic diseases (e.g., increased risk of falls, depression, sleep deprivation, or cognitive decline, lying on the floor; physical immobility; monitoring activities of daily living; occupation of spaces at home; locomotion; tracking; the recognition of situations; awareness about the activities of the user in their environment using sensor data), and to support timely involvement of the social environment (carers and family) of people with dementia. Also, the major challenges when designing new systems for health care that are especially focused on dementia will be discussed throughout this chapter. Major challenges to be addressed include self-learning solutions, which can share contextual information with other artifacts (like sensors) in the surroundings of the user; innovative multimodal user interaction, taking into account the capabilities of the users; user requirements for novel interfaces; and user case scenarios.

This chapter is organized as follows. Initially, it presents an overview of methods, systems, and research projects focused on proposing new solutions for monitoring and tracking disease progression of dementia. Subsequently, it discusses some current challenges that should be addressed in the definition and design of ICT systems. The "Introduction" covers some psychological factors that become barriers to acceptance of new technologies by seniors, presentation standards, and guidelines for the development of interfaces. The remaining of this chapter is divided in three parts: (1) research and technological advances that feature solutions in terms of behavior analysis, reasoning, and recognition of user activities ("State of the Art on Techniques, Methods, and Systems for Dementia Screening, Prediction, and Retard"); (2) regulations and codes of ethics in the area of AAL ("Regulations and Ethics"); and (3) conclusion with general findings of our study along with future research expected scopes ("Existing and Future Solutions for Privacy in Personal Data").

State of the Art on Techniques, Methods, and Systems for Dementia Screening, Prediction, and Retard

Identification of individuals that are at a high risk of dementia has focused on the concept of MCI, which is considered to be an intermediate state between normal cognitive aging and dementia. Models of dementia risk prediction have been developed for use across the older population. The aim of screening models is to classify individuals into various risk categories (such as low, moderate, and high) so that decision rules can be followed (Stephan et al. 2010). For example, a low-risk diagnosis would enable support in the decision not to intervene and would provide some guidelines to encourage activities and adopt adequate lifestyles. A diagnosis of moderate risk would prompt preventive actions such as reexamination or a supervision period, while a diagnosis of high risk would trigger intervention (Barnes et al. 2010). There are different approaches to assessing the risk of progression to deeper stages of dementia associated with the mental and physical states of the person. These models have mainly retrieved data from neuropsychological testing and sociodemographic variables, including age, sex, and education. Moreover, there are categories where each model fits by the way it combines various data types (Stephan et al. 2010), in particular multistage screening approaches, a combination of demographic and neuropsychological measures with health or genetic variables, health and vascular risk indices, cognitive profiles, and multidementia subtype preclinical groupings.

Neuropsychological methods are employed traditionally as an important aid to diagnose dementia. These methods are based on assessments that include standard tests of alertness, attention, memory, language, visual–spatial skills, and reasoning, e.g., the Mini Mental State Examination (MMSE), the Clinical Dementia Ratio (CDR), the Global Deterioration Scale, the Blessed Dementia Scale, the Consortium to Establish a Registry for Alzheimer's Disease (CERAD), the Alzheimer's Disease Rating Scale, the Alzheimer's Disease Cooperative Study—Activities of Daily Living Inventory, and Disability Assessment for Dementia. Many others can be found in Psychiatric Rating Scales for Alzheimer's Disease and Dementia (2010).

Other techniques to predict future mental states are biological measures, also known as biological markers. They include cerebrospinal fluid constituents such as amyloid beta or tau (Stefania et al. 2006), positron emission tomography (PET) that visualizes brain metabolism, structural and functional methods using magnetic resonance imaging (MRI), etc. So far, these methods perform the prediction on a statistical but not individual level and thus were not validated as diagnostic procedures (Korczyn and Aharonson 2007). However, the use of biological markers presents some problems:

- They are not totally reliable or accurate for diagnosis of Alzheimer's disease as the same pattern findings are found in other conditions.
- Some procedures are invasive, can be uncomfortable, and are not without risk, i.e., lumbar puncture test.
- The high costs involved and the limited availability of the instruments used, such as MRI and PET scanners, will prohibit large-scale use of these methods.

The screening methods discussed previously require trained personnel for their administration and interpretation. This might result in inconsistencies when applied by different administrators and limits the administration to the professional clinical setting. Moreover, these assessments are applied using questionnaires, which raise the subjectivity issue when the patient or the caregiver is answering them. Also, those tests cannot be repeated on the same patient within short intervals because of learning effects, and this limits their ability to be repeated when doubt exists about the validity of a test result.

Technology can be a key element in the treatment and support of patients at home or in the hospital. Future treatments for care will become more flexible and interconnected, including home care, stationary care, and acute medical treatment. This not only involves individual care services and public and private institutions but also requires the use of new technology to enable the complex management of different players. New technologies are therefore potential enablers of modern future care and rehabilitation systems.

Research Activities and European Union Investments

The aging population requires new approaches in research that bring together diverse stakeholders, e.g., from care and medical institutions for senior citizens and from technology experts. Regarding the novelty of AAL as a research focus and the research funding for this subject, the picture has significantly changed in the meantime. The EU already understands the importance of technological projects in areas related to health care, well-being, personal safety, and social interaction. The work of Gabner and Conrad (2010) presents a long study on this topic. It presents several charts depicting the increase in investments in projects undertaking research and development activities related to ICTs for people's lives. To carry out those investments, the EU provides several funding schemes to encourage business entities, investigation and development organizations, universities, and other types of partners to build up consortia and elaborate projects with a well-defined value chain. For more focused information, the study by Marjo et al. (2007) offers a good overview of the ICT research landscape in Europe and presents existing funding schemes. This study also reflects the European policy trends and priorities where AAL is included on the list. Moreover, the EU prepared a document with a digital agenda (European Commission 2010) concluding that ICT has a crucial role to play in creating sustainable jobs and boosting Europe's economic growth, as outlined in the Europe 2020

Strategy, and so contributing to the economic recovery and long-term prosperity. The Digital Agenda for Europe (European Commission 2010) outlines seven priority areas for actions, and in one of those areas, the following is expressed: "applying information and communications technologies to address challenges facing society like climate change and the aging population (COM/2010/0245 f/2)." This document reveals the great importance of AAL and other related topics and how they are classified. The EU has started an AAL dedicated Joint Programme (AAL Joint Programme Funding 2011) with the Member States, and related advanced research as well as applications such as telecare and online support for social services will be reinforced.

These efforts to foster investment and leverage technological developments are making a direct impact on the number of European projects initiatives to deploy novel AAL products and systems, intended to be integrated as part of users' daily life.

Overview of AAL Projects

What follows is an overview of AAL projects funded by the EU. These projects are constituted by a consortium composed by institutions and companies from different Member States. The objectives and scopes of the projects will be described briefly below to give some examples of typical projects within the AAL research landscape.

- *COGKNOW*: The project COGKNOW (COGKNOW 2011) aims to provide a system to support people with debilitating symptoms of dementia and short-term memory loss. COGKNOW's system uses two devices: a flat-screen monitor for the home and a mobile smartphone. The in-home system can be set up to start issuing reminders during the entire day and to place control mechanisms to detect if the entrance door is opened. The smartphone has a built-in GPS sensor that allows the system to guide users if they become disoriented when they are outside the house. COGKNOW's system also has an elastic belt integrated that can monitor and record a person's physical movement and body posture in order to assist the users with rehabilitation exercises, and the system can be configured to automatically alert emergency services in the event of a fall.

- *AGNES*: The AGNES project (AGNES 2011) focuses on improving the mental and physical well-being of elderly people living alone at home, who often suffer the effects of social and physical isolation—including cognitive decline, low activity levels, and poor mood states. The project aims to use scientifically based knowledge on aging and innovative technology to intervene in the lives of target users, and the effects of these interventions on cognitive functioning and quality of life will be evaluated. The project will explore available technological solutions to exploit the power of social networks and the beneficial effect of social inclusion and activities on cognitive and mental processes.

- *eCaalyx*: The main objective of eCaalyx (enhanced complete ambient assisted living experiment; eCaalyx 2011) is to develop a health-monitoring solution that addresses chronic conditions in elderly people and provides reliable long-term, maintenance-free operation in a nontechnical environment to improve the elderly's quality of life by assessing their health risk, monitoring and controlling their health status, and teaching them how to manage their chronic conditions to continue to live independently at home. It includes a home system, a mobile system (wearable body sensors), and a caretaker site for medical professionals to monitor the patient and provide assistance if needed.

- *HOPE*: HOPE (2011) focuses its efforts to provide an integrated, smart platform that uses Zigbee technology in order to enable elderly people with Alzheimer's disease to use innovative technology for a more independent life, for access to information, and for monitoring their health. The major purposes of the project are to extend the time people can live at home by increasing their autonomy, self-confidence, mobility, and security; to prevent social isolation and to support maintaining the multifunctional network around the individual; and to support carers, families, and care organizations.

- *H@H*: The H@H (health at home) project (H@H 2011) aims to design, realize, and demonstrate a complete and integrated model of home care for a chronic patient. It aims at solving societal problems related to the provision of health care services for elderly citizens affected by chronic heart failure, providing them with wearable sensor devices for monitoring of pathophysiological cardiovascular and respiratory parameters and, at the same time, enabling the medical staff to monitor their situations at a distance and take action in case of necessity by the involvement of public and private health organizations.

- *HELP*: HELP (home-based empowered living for Parkinson's disease patients; HELP 2011) has the main objective of developing a system that is able to administer drug therapy in a controlled and either continuous or on-demand manner, to manage disease progression, and to mitigate symptoms in patients with Parkinson's disease. This system is a removable implant loaded with a configurable cartridge to administer a concise amount of drug, which will be absorbed by the body at a constant rate along the day.

- *ROSETTA*: The ROSETTA project (ROSETTA 2011) has its main objective focused on providing technological solutions for helping people with progressive chronic disabilities to retain their autonomy and quality of life as much as possible and support formal or informal carers. The technological system is composed of three main components: an advanced awareness and prevention service, which includes smart cameras for activity surveillance and also positioning by wireless beacons; an early detection system for monitoring patterns of behavior for detecting changes in chronic long-term conditions; and an elderly day navigator that includes reminders of activities of daily living and appointments, and simplified digital communication facilities.

- *HMFM*: The project HMFM (HearMeFeelMe; HMFM 2011) is designed for older people with visual impairments and provides an easy, simple, and intuitive way to access information and digital services in their home environment. The services allow users to locate and identify medicine packaging, listen to medication information and dosage instructions through audio, and receive instructions and reminders through an electronic medication plan.

- *COMPANIONABLE*: Without cognitive stimulation, the health condition level of elderly people with dementia decreases very quickly. This also is a challenge for care staff. To tackle this issue, the project COMPANIONABLE (Integrated Cognitive Assistive and Domotic Companion Robotic Systems for Ability and

Security; COMPANIONABLE 2011) targets at developing a smart home environment within the home of elderly people, which supports both the elderly patient and the care staff. Cognitive stimulation as well as medical organization will thereby be supported. The support systems will be evaluated by the elderly, their relatives, and further relevant stakeholders such as care staff. This system will also include a domestic assistance robot.

- *DOMEO*: The project DOMEO (Domestic Robot for Elderly Assistance; DOMEO 2011) aims to develop a robotic system that will allow cognitive and physical stimulation, helping elderly and disabled people to remain autonomous as long as possible and to stay longer and safer at home. Two robotics platforms are evaluated: RobuMate for cognitive stimulation and daily life assistance, and RobuWalker for walking assistance. They are connected with a remote medical center through a web interface helping caring personnel and relatives to better assist patients.

- *ALIAS*: ALIAS (2011) is a project with the main objective of designing and developing a mobile robot platform that has the capacity to monitor, interact with, and access information from online services. The robot is designed for people living alone at home or in care facilities such as nursing or elderly care homes. The goal is to provide assistance in daily life, to keep the user linked to wider society, and, in this way, to improve their quality of life by combating loneliness and increasing activities. The robot was design not to have manipulation capabilities.

- *MyHeart*: The main objective of MyHeart (2011) is to support citizens in preventing cardiovascular diseases through an appropriate lifestyle and early diagnosis. The approach is to integrate system solutions into functional clothes with integrated textile sensors (*biomedical clothes*). The process consists of performing diagnoses, detecting trends, and reacting to them. Together with professional services, the biomedical clothes create the MyHeart system, which will help to fight major cardiovascular disease risk factors and to avoid heart attacks.

- *AmIE*: The main objective of AmIE (ambient intelligence for the elderly; AmIE 2011) is the development and testing of a home platform, including nonintrusive sensing and vital signs monitoring combined with context awareness. The platform is intended to offer assistance services with the focus on individual adaptation. Its target is to improve the quality of life according to the individual's specific situation and in a nonintrusive and respectful way. The system is able to individualize its medical and home care assistance by adapting to the users' needs, preferences, and characters. In order to implement such an intelligent system, concepts for characterization models, rule engines and ontologies, and adaptive interfaces are used.

- *HEARCOM*: The HEARCOM project (hearing in the communication society; HEARCOM 2011) aims at reducing limitations in auditory communication of people who suffer from hearing impairment in order to allow them to keep on being members of a communication society. Although this project is not explicitly related to elderly people, it has been integrated into the AAL project list because hearing impairment is a typical disease of the elderly. The project addresses the development of different telescreening approaches of an individual's hearing ability. It also makes available different information about equipment already on the market and gives general information, for example, to family members. The objective involving the professionals is to support them with models, software tools, and demonstrations to estimate hearing devices in terms of their communication quality.

- *Go-myLife*: The Go-myLife (2011) project is focused on facilitating social interactions and readjust information and communications systems. The project undertook its developments to deploy a mobile social networking platform connected to disparate social networking sites allowing interactions with peers and families, as well as access to relevant geographically based information. The platform allows the users to adapt personalization schemes and security levels.

- *SilverGame*: The SilverGame project (SilverGame 2011) is dedicated to developing attractive and stimulating game-based multimedia applications that foster the social connection and interaction of elderly people with society and help them improve their physical and mental abilities with the system providing sensor-based feedback. The technological solution is based upon a central platform and virtual environment that allows the elderly to share their hobbies such as singing and dancing and helps them to stay in touch with other community members—with the goal being to transform these virtual interactions into real relationships and social inclusion.

- *WEL_HOPS*: WEL_HOPS (Welfare Housing Policies for Senior Citizens; WEL_HOPS 2011) undertook a large survey on the possibilities of independent housing for elderly people in six European countries. Its main objectives were to establish common guidelines for the design of senior citizens' homes and for the renovation of homes in which they live, to create a European Network of Experts to assess new schemes, and to promote the sharing of information and good practices. The study analyzes the needs of individuals by using interviews as well as best practices. It thus wants to give a realistic and consistent picture of the present situation of housing interventions for seniors and of their life quality relating to a on demand versus supply adjustment.

- *SHARE*: SHARE (Survey of Health, Ageing and Retirement in Europe) is primarily a data collection task force. The project developed a "multidisciplinary and cross-national panel database of micro data on health, socio-economic status and social and family networks of more than 85,000 individuals aged 50 or over" (SHARE 2011). The collected and analyzed data comprise various health indices (e.g., on self-reported health, health conditions, physical and cognitive functioning, health behavior, use of health care facilities), biological markers (e.g., grip strength, body mass index, peak flow), psychological variables (e.g., psychological health, well-being, life satisfaction), economic variables (current work activity, job characteristics, opportunities to work past retirement age, sources and composition of current income, wealth and consumption, housing, education), and social support variables (e.g., assistance within families, transfers of income and assets, social networks, volunteer activities). The survey has been conducted in several waves of data collection composed by a balanced representation of various regions in Europe.

Social interaction and communication are two elements that strongly influence the quality of life perceived by subjects. This is one reason why the number of projects and proposals for solutions is large across Europe. In addition to projects presented in more detail earlier, there are still many other initiatives with this objective, such as WeCare (2011), ELDER-SPACES (2011), HOPES (2011), PeerAssist (2011), and V2me (2011).

Several other projects are also supporting the wider deployment and commercialization of personal health solutions. The Medical Care Continuity (MCC 2011) and DREAMING

(2011) projects aim to assess the benefits of remote monitoring systems. Sensors around the home (including cameras) or worn by a patient are linked to a call center or health care professionals. If unusual circumstances are detected, the control center is alerted; with the aid of a decision-support system, professionals can initiate the most appropriate response.

The Range of AAL Products

Throughout this chapter, the term *product* is used as an equivalent word for different kinds of technological types, such as hardware systems, software, or services (traditional services performed by people and Internet services), and, in most cases, the products are integrated solutions. So far, there is no joint definition of an ICT-based AAL product for elderly people. In order to describe AAL services and products already available to sell on the market and to deploy in users' living spaces, it is essential to define the range of products that fit into the scope of *AAL products*. Moreover, AAL products very often integrate a wide range of technologies, comprising, for example, sensor technology, the Internet, innovative computer interfaces, mobile devices, bus communication systems, and control systems. Although several different technical components are often part of AAL products or systems, these components have not been developed especially for AAL solutions.

Product Groups

There is a wide range of possible AAL devices and elaborated solutions under study, which were classified according to their application areas. Based on IPTS (2006), it is possible to categorize technological products that enable elderly people to live independently. The following is a description of these categories.

Communication Devices

The devices classified under this group aim to provide a comfortable way to communicate, facilitate social activities, and provide various kinds of information to users. With all the problems associated with aging, such as visual and hearing disabilities, it is necessary that the suppliers of communication devices draw attention to those problems in order to develop suitable products such as visual telephone, specific Internet and e-mail applications, and computers containing devices for imaging or communication by symbols.

Compensation of Impairments

People with several diseases, especially elderly people, may develop, for example, diseases related to visual and hearing problems. Thus, there is an urgent need to find devices that compensate for the sensory deficiencies. Nowadays, these are overcome with devices like intelligent electric magnifiers and reading lenses, electronic communication aids, and associated information technological systems. Other technological solutions are designed to support and compensate for impairments related to cognitive disorders and physiological disabilities.

Consumer Electronics/Multimedia

In order to occupy elderly people's leisure time with activities and hobbies, and also to avoid the feeling of loneliness, nowadays, products and services using ICT are being developed and supplied to provide rich multimedia applications and entertainment activities. These types of products are being created with content that is suitable for the interests of elderly people, looking into the content provided and usability. Examples of these products may be multimedia applications and content specific to a respective age, ICT-based games, books and electronic newspapers, and Internet communities.

Safety and Security

Safety and security are key terms in AAL products; it is very important for the elderly to feel safe at home. In order to compensate for the loss of motor and mental skills, it is essential to supply technology to domestic areas to prevent accidents and to increase the sense of security. The increasing need for security is typically accompanied by the demand for security systems. Currently, there are already some security systems such as surveillance and locking systems as well as customized alarm systems (if a person has forgotten to turn down the cooker, for instance). However, these protection and safety products have not yet been developed for a large group of consumers.

Medical Assistive Technology

In order to support family members or teams of professional nurses in health care procedures provided daily for the seniors who need health care provision schemes, there is a specific type of product to support these kinds of scenarios, which are the medical assistive technologies. Some of these products are focused on medical applications and others require self-control by the patient, for example, concerning blood pressure and blood glucose. There are also other systems to help daily routines such as lifting or mobility aids, house cleaning, special bathroom technologies, and fall alarms.

Telemonitoring/Telemedicine

Telemedicine makes life easier for elderly people with certain disabilities or chronic illnesses allowing them to be monitored, advised, and treated in their home, in caregivers' facilities, or in other domestic environments. The main advantage of these products is that the patient to be monitored and treated does not need to travel to a medical institution, allowing an increase in patient autonomy, and in some cases, it was proven that there is a feeling of greater confidence and security. Information such as vital parameters can be recorded and transmitted to medical institutions through portable devices so specialized people can do the controlling and can intervene if needed.

Mobility

Usually, the decline in mental and physical abilities leads to the elderly losing their mobility. Simple and routine tasks like walking or driving a car can become very complicated, or worse, impossible, depending on the severity of the disease. In order to ensure that the welfare of the elderly is taken care of, it is very important to get devices that are able to restore or increase their mobility. These devices can be assistive devices that allow the elderly to drive a car or do sports or to simply manage wheelchairs or perform step lifts in order to enable them to move.

Smart Home/Daily Chores

For elderly people with several problems, it may be complicated to perform some trivial daily tasks like making the bed, cleaning the house, etc. In order to simplify that, products that are automated and intelligent devices and services that can perform those daily tasks or at least reduce the difficulty of doing them are needed, such as social and adapted robots, remote-controlled doors and gates, microwave or normal stoves with various sensors, or online services offering teleshopping or telebanking.

Challenges for ICT for User-Centered and Primary Care Community

Nowadays, life expectancy is increasing and with it the number of years that people live with disabilities. Therefore, it is expected that as the population grows older, the number of people living with some kind of limitations will also increase in the near future. These limitations that will cover more and more individuals will increase the risk of an older person becoming dependent on care from others. According to surveys done by entities such as SHARE (2011), 40% of people older than 50 have some kind of health problem that result in some degree of activity limitation, and almost 50% of the people have some kind of long-term health problem. As life expectancy increases and due to a decline in the age-specific mortality of the oldest old, constituted by people more than 80 years old, this age group has been shown to be the most growing age segment in most European populations. As age advances, people are more likely to suffer from several conditions that can harm the ability of independent living, for instance, cognitive impairment, visual and hearing impairments, and frailty due to disease (IPTS 2006).

The survey about disabilities, deficiencies, and the state of health (IMPACT 1999) summarized that some kind of disability is shown by 32.2% of older people. Within these 32.2%, there are 70% of people with some difficulty in performing daily activities, in which 47% of these show severe difficulties in doing so. These impairments detected in older people will have implications on the ability to accept and manage technological products or new services.

Analyzing this, it is very important to optimize and adapt all the devices and all the interactive processes to the state of health of each individual. To meet this objective, the most important limitations of sensory and cognitive capacities have to be reviewed and studied.

According to IPTS (2006), the primary mental health issues of elderly people are dementia, cognitive impairments, and loneliness, while the physical issues include low mobility level, impairment of vision, impairment of hearing, pain, sensory loss, fall-related injuries, adverse drug reactions, and chronic illnesses.

User Interaction Standards

This sections aims to provide a set of guidelines and phases based on the European standards ISO 9241 and ISO 13407. These ISOs enable new service providers and product developers to create new applications according to AAL users' requirements. Any application may fail or will not succeed if the user is not able to use it properly, so the design of service, application, or a piece of software that requires the interaction of a human user and may follow a systematic set of methods to reach such an interface is desirable. The definition of usability from ISO 9241 is "the extent to which a product can be used by specified users to achieve specified goals with effectiveness, efficiency and satisfaction in a specified context of use" (ISO/IEC 1998) in which the terms *effectiveness, efficiency,* and *satisfaction* are defined as follows:

- *Effectiveness*: The accuracy and completeness with which users achieve specified goals
- *Efficiency*: The resources expended in relation to the accuracy and completeness with which users achieve goals
- *Satisfaction*: Freedom from discomfort and positive attitude to the use of the product
- *Context of use*: Characteristics of the users, tasks, and organizational and physical environments

The European standard ISO 13407 (ISO/IEC 1999) defines four activities to design a product from the point of view of the human-centered design. These activities can be used to define, create, and evaluate AAL services, independent of the applications designed, user lifestyle, etc. The activities are given as follows:

1. Understand and specify the context of use. The designer may know the user (e.g., elderly with sign disability or elderly with movement impairments, health failure patients, etc.) and the environment of use (user's home, outside). Only in this case, can they propose an effective solution for the final user.
2. Specify the user and organizational requirements (e.g., how quickly a user is able to access whenever they want to use the application).
3. Product design solution. That means introducing the user interaction design in the application.
4. Evaluate designs against requirements.

Therefore, ISO 9241-10 (ISO/IEC 1998) defines seven principles for intuitive design of system dialogs:

1. Controllability. The user is able to maintain the focus of a goal over the whole course of the interaction process.
2. Self-descriptiveness. The interaction should be immediately comprehensible. Feedback to the user to achieve this goal (e.g., progress bar during loading of application).
3. Conformity with user expectations. The dialog should be designed according to the user's education, experience, knowledge, etc.

4. Error tolerance.

5. Suitable for the task.

6. Suitability for individualization. The interaction should be modifiable according to the user's needs and skills.

7. Suitability for learning. The interaction provides guidance and support to the user during the learning phase.

Incorporating these principles into the four previously described activities, designers should be able to define intuitive interaction models. In any case, this must only be a first approach that should be completed with defined user interface elements.

User Interaction Guidelines

This section focuses on elderly users' interaction schemes. The elderly are a very heterogeneous group, with different levels of technology knowledge (but generally cautious outlook to ICT), cognitive abilities, accessibility requirements, psychological and health status, as well as lifestyles. From the interaction point of view, this focus group poses an enormous challenge in user interface design (Zwick et al. 2005). Many people over the age of 60 have difficulties using ICTs and consider the standard user interfaces of the devices confusing and difficult to understand. These fears and their common belief that they are too old to learn make it very difficult for them to explain what their real requirements are. The guidelines of Human Computer Interaction and User-Centered Design are valid also for designing user interfaces for the elderly. As for any other user groups, in what concerns elderly people, the usability of an application depends on its appearance and the user's satisfaction in using the application. The designers should avoid using wrong interface designs that cause formation of inappropriate mental models for elderly people.

What follows is a set of *good* practices in user interaction design for elderly people (ISO/IEC 1999; Hawthorn 2000; ISTAG 2004; Zwick et al. 2005).

1. Memory loss associated with age refers to the normal decline of memory due to aging. As a consequence of this process, elderly people are less able to cope with a complex list of instructions. The interaction should be designed to reduce the load on memory, e.g., with short messages or avoiding long lists of instructions.

2. Contrary to young people, some older users are not motivated to use ICT, so the effort required to accept the technology should be reduced. It is likely that they will have to spend a lot of time learning how the hardware works before they can use the application; therefore, to make the interaction easier for elderly users, the complexity should be reduced.

3. Concentration and cognitive ability are decreased in elderly people, so a simple interface is important in order not to waste their concentration on understanding the interaction process.

4. Elderly people require more time to process the information they read, so the designer should always place the most important tasks first.

5. Elderly people may have problems in transferring their experience to a new context. The computer system should repeat the traditional model that elderly people are used to managing (e.g., a calendar).

6. The dialog user system should be natural, so that the designers should select the appropriate model of interaction according to the location, the device, the individual, etc. In the case of elderly users, speech and vision are the most natural forms of communication, especially by multimodal forms of interaction. Feedback is important to the users, so it should be delivered by different interaction modes (visual, auditory, and haptic). Large target size facilitates reading and mouse (or finger) clicking. In the case of sound message (useful in alarms or warnings), lower sound frequencies are more appropriate for elderly users.

7. Auditory signal or instructions are only temporarily available, so it may be most appropriate for alarms or to draw attention; text is most appropriate to those users with lower cognitive abilities.

Every interaction model should be designed following the issues of user privacy and user control.

Middleware Frameworks for Health Care Provision

Generally, middleware is expected to hide the internal workings and the heterogeneity of a system, providing standard interfaces, abstractions, and a set of services that depend largely on the application. The scientific work presented by Chatzigiannakis et al. (2007) provides a discussion about the meaning of *middleware*, although it focuses on the frameworks for wireless sensor networks (WSNs). Nowadays, extensive research and development is being carried out on sophisticated middleware platforms that provide conditions to accelerate new systems integration, supporting interoperability for data and applications functioning and for new service deployment. Thus, new middleware architectures keep on emerging. Since AAL solutions consist of several quite often independently developed systems that come from multiple suppliers or providers, interoperability is an important issue and relies on the use of standards. Indeed, interoperability is a key factor in the success of middleware designed for the AAL area.

Recent articles have reported about middleware research and analysis focused on specific areas of technological development. The work by Gaddah and Kunz (2003) has provided a general overview of the most relevant mobile middleware systems. It presents several research projects that have been initiated to address the requirements and technological aspects of mobile distributed systems. The paper concludes that conventional and traditional middleware platforms fail to provide the appropriate support for modern mobile applications. The paper by Al-Jaroodi et al. (2009) presents a survey focused on security middleware that is particular to pervasive and ubiquitous environments. It provides a discussion about the approaches used in security middleware and their properties when applied in pervasive and ubiquitous environments. In the work of Kjaer (2007), a survey of a chosen set of context-aware middleware architectures is presented and their characteristics and use are classified according to their proposed taxonomy. Baldauf et al. (2007) have focused their work on providing an overview of various context-aware systems. They presented different existing middleware and server-based approaches to ease the development of context-aware applications. Moreover, in the work of Saeed and Waheed (2010), context-aware features still are the main attention. In their work, Saeed and Waheed (2010) initially defined a set of criteria to be assessed on the platforms under review, including fault tolerance, adaptability, interoperability, architectural style, discoverability, location transparency, and aspect-oriented composition. After a description of each platform, summary tables are presented to compare their features with the criteria previously defined. Surveys based on middleware for WSNs are available, and they provide an overview of features, advantages, and drawbacks. Hadim and Mohamed (2006) present a set of challenges to design successful middleware layers for WSNs. Based on these challenges, several types of middleware for WSNs are evaluated and compared, and a summary table is provided comparing each defined challenge with each platform. With the same objective, the work of Molla and Ahamed (2006) specifies a set of challenges and presents a comparative study of several state-of-the-art middlewares for sensor networks. The paper by Henricksen and Robinson (2006) presents a survey and analysis of different middleware approaches such as event-based, tuple space, service discovery, and database solutions, highlighting the open research challenges. Furthermore, this paper points to some future directions of what requirements will be expected in the middleware for WSNs. In the work of Chatzigiannakis et al. (2007), another survey centered on WSNs is presented. It provides a perspective to the categorization of middleware, the design issues and requirements, and a discussion about the future trends for these types of platforms. Other surveys providing overviews of middleware applied in other specific areas and discussing new technological approaches are available. The paper by Wang et al. (2010) addresses the concepts and architecture of event-based middleware. Furthermore, it presents research and development results of projects of this type of middleware, discussing the adopted architecture, implementation strategy, and application. The subject of the study by Bernard (2006) is middleware that integrates different types of sensors and distributed systems. This paper presents new requirements for middleware design and a discussion about the main challenges that have to be addressed in developing new middleware approaches, and as a conclusion, the paper points out new perspectives for middleware research and development. The authors of RUNES Consortium (2005) made a detailed survey of middleware platforms for mobile, embedded, and sensor systems. They conclude that during the design and development phases, the major efforts are on adaptability, but when the platform is released, this adaptability feature remains static. Moreover, this work concludes that no single middleware platform addresses all the nonfunctional requirements. However, none of the existing work investigated the current state of research on design and development of middleware for health care and, more specifically, middleware that provides tools for helping on signaling dementia indicators. Furthermore, we explore different relevant middleware projects in the health care area.

Technologies that are designed to be implemented in a user's home or in an institutional care provider environment are typically based on behavior analysis and vital signs logging. Middleware can provide a layer for different and heterogeneous applications, communicate, use the platform services, and take advantage of existing synergies with other products. There are European projects that have, as a result, functional prototypes of middleware that enable interoperability between new applications and provide support services in the area of health care. Many of these services, which are an integral part of the platforms, provide functionalities to developed applications and leverage the speed of development. In the context of the proposed work to be discussed in Chapter 15, it is important to choose the platform that gives more guarantees to successfully achieve the objectives. The remainder of this section surveys solutions and approaches to evaluate advantages and drawbacks, and presents technological features.

- *MonAMI*: MonAMI is a five-year project that started in 2006 (MonAMI 2011). Its objective is to provide a set of services to elderly and disabled persons living at home, demonstrating that those people will benefit by using appropriate technology. Moreover, MonAMI tries to demonstrate viable ways (socially and economically) of how to join together heterogeneous technologies to provide and to facilitate inclusive access for elderly and disabled citizens. However, to the best of our knowledge, there is no service available that is specific to help people with dementia issues, in particular performing a long-term analysis of the evolution of people's disabilities. Therefore, MonAMI can be a good platform to integrate health care services, but currently, it does not present a feasible solution or supporting processes for dementia-related diseases.

- *myURC*: The myURC framework (Zimmermann et al. 2004; myURC 2011) intends to provide a standardized and versatile user interface description for devices and services, to which any universal remote console (URC) can connect to discover, access, and control a remote device or service. The proposed standard is an approach to allow users to interact with networked devices and services in their own environments, integrating different types of interfaces. These features allow developers to provide better services for health care using the most adequate sensors or other equipment and to create dynamic systems that better fit the users' requirements. myURC is cross-platform, compatible with any operating system or device, and there is good supporting documentation with examples of how to use myURC. Therefore, the myURC framework leverages the development of applications that can be designed for eHealth. However, this platform only provides mechanisms to support services and guarantee the interoperability between them, and does not offer particular solutions for chronic illnesses.

- *OpenAAL*: OpenAAL (Wolf et al. 2010) is a popular middleware that was a result from the SOPRANO Project (SOPRANO 2011). A paper published during the SOPRANO project (Wolf et al. 2008) points out the objective of the platform. The openAAL middleware has the objective of becoming a flexible system that enables the provision of IT services for elderly people, especially those that suffer functional impairments. This framework is built on top of OSGi (Lee et al. 2003), which is responsible for integration and communication between services. OSGi provides to openAAL a service-oriented infrastructure where new system components can be added, updated, and exchanged. Additionally, openAAL provides generic services that support new service development with common features such as data collecting and abstracting about the environment, workflow-based specifications of system behavior, and new service discovery based on semantics. Therefore, the platform provides supporting mechanisms for service developers and many features for external device management. It is released under the Lesser General Public License (LGPL) and is cross-platform, and the community behind openAAL provides support and updated documentation. Despite all the features that openAAL incorporates and the interoperability between different applications, it does not present a concrete approach to support services for chronic illness care.

- *PERSONA*: PERSONA (PERSONA 2011) is middleware based on a message brokering approach with the objective of guaranteeing that two services or components can exchange data using a predefined ontology. The middleware provides a set of communication buses dedicated to different types of data: an input bus for dispatching captured user inputs, an output bus for the generated system outputs, a context bus for event-based messages, and a service bus for intercomponent communication. Moreover, PERSONA provides a set of services for different focuses of activities (daily activities, social participation, safety and security, and mobility), which can be used by the end users. More related with the scope of this paper, PERSONA has a specific service named the Long-Term Analyzer, which creates models of behavior of an assisted person in a certain period of time. Then the objective of this service is to compare two or more periods and detect potential changes in the quality of life of the assisted person, and that may indicate the existence, or a tendency, of diseases in the initial phase. Any kind of source of information (wearable sensors, mobile devices, behavior analysis, etc.) can be used in PERSONA to create a model of the behavior of the assisted person for a certain period of time. This specific service is very close to the objective of this paper. However, as will be discussed in Chapter 15, a more accurate analysis cannot be sustained without a comparison with a basis that confirms which kinds of changes in human behaviors are significant for specialized diagnoses, and that are a direct consequence of the progress of dementia diseases. Finally, PERSONA provides freely the project's documentation and an open-source version of the middleware, which are good properties for new service developers.
- *AMIGO*: The AMIGO project (AMIGO 2011) is structured as a service-oriented architecture with service composition strategies. This platform aims at enabling ambient intelligence for the networked home environment. The AMIGO system architecture was designed to be an open networked home system that could integrate heterogeneous devices dynamically. Additionally, the AMIGO system integrates a set of user services to improve its usability and attractiveness. The scope of this platform is to support new service development for users' home environment automation, focused on providing technology for people's well-being. Therefore, the main target of AMIGO is not related to the development of service support for health care, despite some technologies integrated in the platform that could be adapted for other purposes.
- *MPOWER*: The MPOWER project (MPOWER 2011) developed middleware based on a service-oriented architecture allowing the deployment of distributed and integrated services. The focus of MPOWER is to provide services that can support elderly and cognitively disabled people's everyday activities. This focus matches with the scope of this paper, but despite MPOWER offering relevant services to create new applications, it does not integrate adequate mechanisms to develop new services for people suffering from dementia-related diseases. The initial services that are integrated with MPOWER are sensor management, communication, security, information, and management.
- *UniversAAL*: The UniversAAL project (UniversAAL 2011) is an ongoing project that aims to produce an open platform that provides a standardized approach. This has the support from other middleware and projects so that it can mix a set of results coming from those projects and produce a step forward in the development of an open and standard platform for the AAL market. All the documentation and other technical results will be available during the project lifecycle.

This section aims to present an overview of middleware and platforms that provide a set of services for health care support. This work has its main direction set on presenting solutions and new approaches for bridging the technology with disabled people affected by dementia diseases. The overview of platforms presented and discussed previously concerns the analysis of technological frameworks about what they have implemented and the discussion about the provision of supporting services, tools for new applications, and the availability of mechanisms designed for the specific requirements that elderly people need.

ICT Systems and Decision Support Models for Assessment Alarm of Dementia Progression

Developing an effective technique for screening and predicting dementia diseases has been a long-term goal for distinct areas of scientific research, clinical medicine, pharmacology, genetics, neuropsychological assessment, and even the technology field. The purpose of this section is to provide an overview of technological systems that have been adapted for people with special needs with regard to their mental health, and that can act as supporting tools for care activities. Particularly, the focus of the overview is about middleware platforms that are already available for developers and end users, comparing their advantages and drawbacks to discover the approaches they take to address various challenges associated with the special needs of the users, and also to know how they have succeeded or failed in doing so. Furthermore, during the analysis, particular attention is given to available characteristics, features, services, and tools to help or support the process of predicting dementia diseases or provide reports for further medical analysis.

Reasoning Tasks in AAL

A core function of AAL systems is awareness and perception of the activities of the user and the current situation in their environment. The reasoning tasks not only include the analysis of daily activities and surrounding conditions but also the detection of emergency situations, which need an immediate alarm signal and a response reaction. The requirements for reasoning tasks are to reliably, and in some cases quickly, detect and classify the current situations where the user is involved based on input data typically provided by sensory sources, which must always be considered as imprecise and need to run through a process to be structured in a human readable form. To achieve highly reliable systems, they must be designed to fuse multiple heterogeneous source streams. Moreover, the output information from reasoning tasks is an important source for the analysis procedure of the user's mid-term and long-term behavior to assess the development of their physical and psychosocial status. The reasoning systems must be adaptable to varying environments and users.

In systems and approaches for reasoning tasks, there are entity elements (Floeck and Litz 2008; Lõõbas et al. 2010) that may include a person, a device, a location, or a software application. Entities are characterized by attributes, e.g., location, noise level, light intensity, temperature, and humidity. Recent approaches (Kurschl et al. 2009; Hristova et al. 2008; Monekosso and Remagnino 2010) have described this information using models because they improve the separation of concerns of application logic from structural characteristics. Designing frameworks based on the model approach improves interoperability, extensibility, and reuse in software applications. Issues brought out by reasoning models due to their complexity still have to be resolved, and to improve reasoning techniques, the models used must be extended and additional background knowledge must be considered (Sun et al. 2006; Nick and Becker 2007). Model evolution is a further challenge.

Behavior Analysis and Activity Recognition

Human-activity recognition is a broad field of research. Multisensor platforms, constituted by accelerometers, radio-frequency identification (RFID) tags, vision sensors, laser-based products, reed switches on doors and cupboards, etc., and some worn on different parts of the body and others integrated in the house infrastructure, have been presented as solutions for the recognition of such activities as falling, walking, running, and climbing up stairs. A comparison of different types of sensing modalities for activity recognition was presented in the works of Rodrigues et al. (2010) and Sim et al. (2010).

In recognizing situations and behavior, a differentiation is made between critical situations whose detection must be performed in an online analysis of the information streams provided by the sensor infrastructure, in which a quick system response is a key requirement, and mid- and long-term behavior, which is monitored and does not require online analysis.

The computation of reasoning tasks for the recognition of situation, environment conditions, and users' behavior can be differentiated in different levels of semantic abstraction. Under the scope of AAL, in the literature, the following levels are currently identified: physical activity understanding, behavior classification, specific actions, and complex processes.

The characteristics of physical activities are evaluated to describe the general activity toward the modes of locomotion (e.g., sitting, standing, walking, or lying), and the user's location within the environment, on the room level, on the level of functional areas in the environment, or in spatial relation to the objects in the environment. Regarding the analysis of medical conditions, changes in the user's behavior and in vital data must be deduced and evaluated. From analyzing trends in the user's activities and vital data, deterioration in the physical health status can be derived. In addition, recent research shows that there are common changes in some behaviors that are strongly correlated with the deterioration of the mental state of people (Small et al. 1997; Ravaglia et al. 2008). These two factors reveal the great importance of behavior analysis techniques for AAL systems in order to provide quality information about the user needs in terms of health care. Normally, the approach used to detect changes in a user's behavior is to compare and evaluate the daily life activities that the user shows during the day against a predefined *normal* behavior in order to infer the changes. Specific actions performed by the user are inferred from punctual observations, describing interactions of the user with the environment (e.g., opening the front door and leaving the house) or specific events in motion (e.g., falling, stand-up-and-go, walking).

However, human daily living activities follow a planned sequence of action steps, which are executed in order to fulfill a certain objective. This sequence of steps is a complex process of analysis of the existing technologies that have been used in the design of AAL systems. To monitor these processes, multiple actions and events must be correlated with respect to their temporal ordering. Also, it is necessary to take into account that the complexity for modeling, recognition, and classification of these processes increases due to the fact that the same person often performs the same activity differently, and also different people perform the same activity differently.

Challenges for Activity Recognition

The complexity of the reasoning task increases by the complexity of modeling the activities and the environment conditions, and, on the other hand, by the amount of heterogeneous information that must be fused. Nowadays, challenges for activity recognition (Aggarwal 2005) still exist that must be addressed in future work. One of the common challenges is that human activities suffer variations in their execution, even while keeping the same conditions and the same environment, and being performed by the same people. Consider the activity of cleaning the living room; a user can perform the task quickly or in an extended way at different times of the month. Moreover, different users perform the same task in different ways. These personal differences in carrying out activities affect the type and order in the steps that are performed, as well as the length of time in which the user spends on this activity. Besides this, the reasoning system must also be able to adapt to interpersonal differences in carrying out activities, as each person shows individual characteristics in their behavior.

Another challenge for the research in activity recognition field is the human ability to perform several tasks during a certain period and changes in the user's plans leading to some activities remaining incomplete.

Design Requirements and Technical Approaches

Designing Requirements

When designing reasoning systems, one should address a set of requirements for the appropriate development of an activity recognition algorithm. A common and very well-known requirement is that one must be able to handle the system even with imperfect information. Any system designed for a reliable diagnosis and for situation recognition has to take this aspect into account when combining multiple data sources. This issue comes from the fact that the information in the real world is subject to various causes of imperfection like missing data, credibility of information sources, and error in measurement.

Another requirement to be considered is the need to control information according to their temporal order. A complete analysis of human behavior has always taken into account the temporal sequence of events in order to assess more complex situations. Moreover, besides taking into account the requirements described previously, reasoning systems must be scalable to manage the integration of different highly expressive models and must be capable of describing complex situations, for example, human abilities.

Other requirements can be identified such as the nonfunctional necessity to perform an online analysis and execution of the tasks. Some issues may arise inherent to this requirement; for example, the computational demand tends to grow as the complexity of the algorithm and also the quantity of data to be processed increases. As usual, a compromise must be made between the response time and the computational complexity of the system.

Finally, we have identified one more requirement. To achieve higher adaptability levels, reasoning systems should be able to handle self-adaptive models, adjusting the parameters and configurations by learning the user's activities and interactions with the system. These models may require a training phase to be adapted to a specific environment or to specific user needs. However, just this feature may not be enough to completely cover all the necessities for reliable analysis, so that a model based on *a priori* knowledge, for example, the medical instructions, may be incorporated to introduce initial knowledge for the system.

Technical Approaches for Reasoning Systems

In this section, we present technical approaches used so far in the literature for designing reasoning systems. The reasoning approaches discussed in this section can be compared by their knowledge representation scheme and by the type of semantics used. We start by analyzing the rule-based reasoning approach. Huang and Miles (1996) describe in detail this paradigm, and Storf et al. (2009) present a multiagent-based activity recognition framework to recognize characteristic activities of daily living. Indeed, this approach does not affect the computational complexity of reasoning, but as rule bases, it cannot be checked for consistency in an automated way, so that the definition and extension of complex models become difficult and error-prone. Furthermore, rule-based reasoning is well-suited to online analysis and is also scalable to handle large amounts of data. However, rule-based reasoning has some negative points. It gives no inherent support for reasoning of incomplete data or the handling of uncertain information (probabilistic information), and it does not support temporal orders due to the model itself. There is the possibility of adding new models and extensions to specify these needs, but this leads to an increase in the complexity of the overall system.

Case-based reasoning is an approach based on an analogy scheme; this means that, for solving new problems, it takes the solutions of similar past problems. The work presented by Ni et al. (2003) discusses this approach and presents an integrated version based on rule-based reasoning. Zhou et al. (2011) propose a case-driven model for AAL to sense, predict, reason, and act in response to the elderly activities of daily living in a home environment. The system architecture is composed by synthesizing various sensors, activity recognition, and case-based reasoning, along with assistance customized knowledge. Unlike what happens with the rule-based approach, this one is able to handle incomplete data as well as uncertain data as an input for classification. Temporal ordering of input information cannot be considered in this approach. Regarding the scalability property, this model does not efficiently handle complex and integrated models as the overall system becomes quite complex. The expressiveness of models is considered high, as no generalization in the description of the classified cases is made, and each new case is evaluated with respect to previously acquired cases. In general, case-based reasoning is suitable for carrying out online analysis.

Description logic-based reasoning is suitable for reasoning of incomplete information and also for dealing with uncertainties and temporal constraints (Sun and Hao 2010). This approach provides detailed information models, and its consistency can be checked automatically. However, a trade-off between the complexity of the system and the computational effort must be made, because for an online analysis, when handling large amounts of data, this approach is revealed to be unsuitable.

The Bayesian networks are a probabilistic reasoning approach to handling incomplete information and to treating uncertain information sequences. This approach is scalable, and no explicit support for temporal reasoning is given in the classical mode. Despite being an efficient reasoning approach for online analysis, the Bayesian networks are probably unsuitable for representing complex situations or even human behavior compared with other technical designs. Several works have been presented demonstrating the applicability of Bayesian networks for human behavior monitoring. A different hierarchical approach was proposed by Park and Aggarwal (2004) using event hierarchy, where Bayesian networks were employed to understand two-person interactions. In the work of Shi et al. (2004), the propagation networks (a form of dynamic Bayesian networks) and the discrete condensation algorithm are introduced to classify and recognize sequential activities. In the work of Zhu et al. (2010), a Bayesian framework is proposed to integrate motion sensor data and the location information from a vision system for human daily activity recognition. The problem of considering two different data sources for the model is addressed.

Markov models have been frequently used for modeling human motions as they efficiently abstract time series data and can be used for both subsequent motion recognition and generation. Yin and Bruckner (2010) applies a hidden Markov model, the forward algorithm, and the Viterbi algorithm to build a person's daily activity model. The author has addressed the problem of receiving data in a nonuniform way due to the changes of the activities of the user. As Markov models are more restricted in their expressiveness than Bayesian networks, they will not be the fittest approach for recognizing complex scenarios. For online analysis, this approach is suitable, as very efficient and easy-to-implement algorithms already exist (Yin and Bruckner 2010).

We have tried to cover the most common approaches used in the literature for reasoning systems. Furthermore, Ahad et al. (2008) present other approaches, for example, principal component analysis methods, image-based rendering, motion-flow history, and analysis of spatiotemporal features.

Ongoing developments show that no single approach exhibits all the properties required for reasoning in AAL applications. The current state of the reasoning systems leads us to conclude that the best approach would be a modular reasoning layer enabling the combination of different reasoning approaches.

Technologies to Monitor Cognitive Decline

It is estimated that half the senior population have cognitive problems, requiring the presence of care, in which half of them with an age over 85 exhibit symptoms that characterize Alzheimer's disease (Morris et al. 2003). From mild decline to severe dementia, cognitive decline is one of the biggest threats to independence and quality of life, while making it an expensive disease to monitor and treat. This section intends to provide an overview of existing technological solutions that can address these problems through monitoring and assisting patients with cognitive decline and providing support to their caregivers. These systems provide features to assess patients' behavior in specific tasks and hence evaluate cognitive decline. Based on activity recognition, and by analyzing changes in behavioral patterns over time, it is possible to provide early warnings of dementia. Indeed, many research groups point out the importance of assessing variations (in both short and long term) in patterns of behavior and movement that can be indicative of symptoms of early dementia (Kaye 2008). Matic and Osmani (2009) proposed a framework, in order to recognize activities of patients with cognitive impairments, that fuses the data from vision sensors with RFID information. They have tested this system in two different scenarios, and the conclusions demonstrate that the system was able to measure the subject's behavior change over time and the variability of cognitive functions. Dante Tapia and Juan Corchado presented a distributed multiagent system with the aim of strengthening the assistance and health care for patients with Alzheimer's. The main features of the system include reasoning and planning mechanisms, and the use of context-aware technologies to acquire information from users and their environment. This system is focused on providing tools for securing, monitoring, and automating medical staff's work and patients' activities. The presented results obtained in real scenarios demonstrate that the system improved the efficiency of health care tasks.

Wu et al. (2007) described a method for an activity recognition system based upon automatically acquired models of activities and the objects involved. Using RFID tags to generate events when a tagged object is manipulated during an activity, and video streams to be correlated with these events, the system uses this signal to be modeled by Bayesian networks and it is used as a training signal to automatically acquire object models. With the results obtained in a realistic kitchen setup, and considering a scenario involving 16 activities and 33 objects, the activities were recognized successfully in 80.97% of the video frames using an automatically learned object model, and objects were recognized in 73.30% of the frames. Bayesian networks are also applied by Castro et al. (2007) and Elisle et al. (2002) as a modeling tool to support the assessment of Alzheimer's disease. These works take as a basis for comparison a set of databases with standardized assessments such as CERAD and with the scores of the MMSE.

Joshi et al. (2009) presented a study that demonstrates the applications of machine learning as well as neural networks methods for classifying dementia states. The authors have demonstrated that these methods can improve the classification accuracy of current screening tools, such as the MMSE and the Functional Activities Questionnaire.

Ramanujam et al. (2011) and Tandona et al. (2006) proposed a methodology for the assessment of the cognitive level for Alzheimer's disease using the neural networks method. The method takes as input the same data as the MMSE and classifies a patient by analyzing every input. The system learns from the observed data, and the results in the paper demonstrate that the system improves as the amount of training data increases.

Jimison et al. (2004a,b) have adapted a standard computer game to monitor and analyze the accuracy of the users' movement when interacting with the game. The focus group was elders at risk for dementia in order to monitor their capacity on performing a task that involved significant strategic planning. Based on this analysis, the game difficulty could be adjusted and it allowed detecting meaningful individual cognitive trends.

Lin et al. (2008) presented an information platform for care organizations to manage a dementia patient's symptoms for family members and to facilitate the reassessment process, particularly applying MMSE and CDR questionnaires. This system allows care personnel to easily, through an information system, update the cognitive state of the patients. Moreover, the work by Lin et al. (2008) presents a technological approach based on RFID and mobile phone technology to prevent dementia patients from entering hazardous areas or getting lost.

Physical activities are also subject to study to understand changes in behavior patterns of people with Alzheimer's disease, more specifically by performing the correlation between heart rate and levels of physical activity (Tamura et al. 1997). The results of this work showed that there was no correlation between the severity of intellectual deterioration and the degree of behavior disintegration in dementia patients. Moreover, as a result, the elderly shifted smoothly between activities, while the dementia patients showed sudden fluctuations of activity.

The cognitive decline of diseases such as dementia can be prevented through stimulation activities. Several works proposed solutions and approaches to facilitate the contact with family members and the monitoring of elders' activities, promoting outdoor activities with friends by providing guidelines and feedback to the user. Telemedicine is a wide area of research activities with products and services already available to be installed at home by the users (Jasemian 2008; Moreno et al. 2009). Other research activities (Meza-Kubo et al. 2009) take advantage of information technology and communication systems to provide the users new ways of interacting with friends and family, such as the deployment of social networks suited to the requirements of this specific group of people.

Regulations and Ethics

Considering the widespread availability of scientific knowledge and the technological achievements in the AAL area, there are remaining issues that developers, designers, and end-users should be concerned with when thinking of a new product, service, or any kind of solution for AAL purposes, which are ethic rules, policy regulations, security, and privacy. According to Schülke et al. (2010), the main concern is that privacy information may be misused or usurped. Therefore, a balance between privacy and protection must be assumed by the technological provider. Moreover, Schülke et al. (2010) presented the hierarchy of values, which include the following:

1. *Principle of nonharm*: No harm shall be done to anyone using technology.
2. *Principle of autonomy*: Use of technology is in accordance with the wishes, desires, and values of users.
3. *Principle of welfare*: Demands the maximization of possible advantages, minimizes disadvantages, and improves the situation of others.
4. *Principle of equality*: Dictates at least a formal prohibition of irrelevant differentiation and fair provision of resource(s).

The ICT environment has largely facilitated the global transmission and exchanging of personal data, and it has become much easier to acquire and share private information. ICT has triggered calls for the definition of specific requirements to ensure that users have a right to privacy in a controlled mode. As a result, many countries have enacted legislation for data protection to provide privacy rights to individuals by restricting the manner in which personal information is used by any kind of organization. Information systems need to be controlled and secured if they are to be reliable. When designing security controls, the following factors should be addressed:

- *Prevention*: A security control to prevent security accidents, errors, and breaches must be considered.
- *Detection*: Detect when an unauthorized event by the system has been verified. This kind of event could be a security violation or a restricted area has been accessed.
- *Data recovery*: In cases of data corruption or the hardware breaks down, it is important to be able to recover lost data and information.

Existing and Future Solutions for Privacy in Personal Data

The issues of data access, storage, and analysis have been looked at in a number of areas, and technical solutions exist that can be applied to health care to increase privacy and security in a multiuser setting. Meingast et al. (2006) presented a set of existing solutions: role-based access control, encryption systems, and authentication mechanisms. The role-based access control is the model for advanced access control that allows the definition of access levels for different types of users. Encryption systems can be used to ensure the security of the data, and authentication mechanisms can be used to ensure that the data are being generated from the expected person/entity.

However, Marci Meingast et al. (2006) point out some directions for future work in some areas that can be improved, such as the definition of data mining rules and technological measures, privacy rules for patients at home, and the definition of clear attributes for role-based access.

Medical Data Protection Regulations

To keep up with the above challenges, European countries have adopted legislation in tune with technological progress and the requirements of the market. These initiatives have started the adoption of a new regulatory framework on electronic communications and information systems. Regarding medical data protection, Directive 2001/20/EC of April 4, 2001 establishes specific provisions regarding the implementation of clinical trials on human subjects, in particular, Article 3 (protection of clinical trial subjects) and Article 5 (clinical trials on incapacitated adults who were not able to give informed legal consent forms and specific instructions for how trials should be planned and conducted). Concerning the protection of personal data, including medical information, Directives 95/46/EC and 2002/58/EC, as well as the national data protection laws implemented accordingly, establish regulatory guidelines for the protection of individuals with regard to the processing of personal data and the free movement of such data, and the processing of personal data and the protection of privacy in the telecommunication sector, respectively. The application of the national regulations concerning processing of personal data varies in the member states, within the general limits established by the directives mentioned. Directive 95/46/EC is the reference text, at the European level, on the protection of personal data. It sets up a regulatory framework within the EU, which seeks to achieve a balance between a high level of protection for the privacy of individuals and the free movement of personal data. To do so, the directive sets limits on the collection and use of personal data and demands that each Member State set up an independent national body responsible for the protection of these data. This directive applies to digital data and traditional paper files with the user profile and records.

The regulatory means for databases can be found in Directive 96/9/EC, which aims to provide copyright protection to databases. The objective of the directive is to provide

- Copyright protection for the intellectual creation involved in the selection and arrangement of materials
- Protection for any kind of investment (time, energy, human resources) in the obtainment, verification, or presentation of the contents of a database

Concerning the processing of personal data and the protection of privacy in the electronic communications sector, the directive contains provisions such as for the Member States to keep connection data for the purposes of police surveillance, rules for sending of unsolicited e-mail, regulations for the usage of cookies, and the inclusion of personal data in public directories. This directive also specifies requirements to ensure that users can trust the services and that they use them for communicating electronically. In the following, we present a brief description of these requirements.

- Providers of electronic communications services and equipment must ensure that the personal data are accessed by authorized persons only, protecting personal data from being destroyed, lost, or accidentally modified, and ensuring the implementation of a security policy on the processing of personal data.

- Assurance of the confidentiality of communications made over a public electronic communications network. The user who stores his or her information must first be informed of the purposes of processing his or her data.

- Except for cases in which the users have given their consent, traffic data and location data must be erased or made anonymous when they are no longer required for the conveyance of a communication or for billing. Some special cases, such as investigations or safeguarding national security, are specified in which protection of data may be removed.

- Users must give their prior consent before unsolicited communications are addressed to them. However, exceptions are provided.

- The directive states that users must give their consent for information to be stored on their terminal equipment, or that access to such information may be obtained. In order to do this, users must receive clear and comprehensive information about the purpose of the storage or access.

- Each of the users must give prior consent in order for their telephone numbers, e-mail addresses, and postal addresses to appear in public directories.

Conclusion and Future Trends

AAL aims to create a background of safety and care by means of technological solutions that enable better living conditions, new methods of communication, and new supporting schemes for personal care, which are able to adapt to the physical, cognitive, and sensory needs and demands of individuals.

Our work presents a comparative study and analysis of the current state of scientific and technological developments in the area of AAL. This chapter presents a set of specific and concrete approaches that tackle a problem that is affecting advanced countries increasingly: the continuous growth in the number of people with dementia. Screening, prediction, and retard are key concepts to address and deal with this inevitable advance in the number of diagnosed cases and with the increased costs in social systems. The technology has an important role in the area of health care provision and is increasingly assuming a critical position as a tool for the support of those involved in the processes of care provision, as primary and secondary care, and as informal care. We conclude that technological solutions can provide better living conditions and new forms of communication and interaction, and are important in stimulating the adoption of healthy lifestyles. In fact, in what concerns the problem of dementia, we present a set of scientific activities and tests in real scenarios with different solutions as promising approaches to achieve significant advances in this area. The results of the studies presented throughout this chapter show that there are clear advantages in adopting new technologies as a complement to traditional procedures in the provision of health care and the monitoring of people with dementia.

We expect that the next trends will pass through the development of new approaches that integrate existing solutions and combine various signals and data to obtain more reliable conclusions.

References

AAL Joint Programme Funding Official web link. 2011. http://www.aal-europe.eu/ (accessed July 3, 2011).

Aggarwal, J. K. 2005. Human activity recognition—A grand challenge. Paper presented in Proceedings of IEEE Conference on Digital Image Computing on Techniques and Applications. Cairns, Australia.

AGNES. 2011. http://www.agnes-aal.eu/site/ (accessed May 9, 2011).

Ahad, M. A. R., J. K. Tan, H. S. Kim and S. Ishikawa. 2008. Human activity recognition: Various paradigms. Paper in International Conference on Control, Automation and Systems. Seoul, Korea, October 14–17.

ALIAS. 2011. http://www.aliasproject.eu/ (accessed May 20, 2011).

Al-Jaroodi, J., A. Al-Dhaheri, F. Al-Abdouli and N. Mohamed. 2009. A survey of security middleware for pervasive and ubiquitous systems. Paper presented for the International Conference on Network-Based Information Systems. Indianapolis, December 8.

AmIE. 2011. http://www.indracompany.com/en/sostenibilidad-e-innovacion/proyectos-innovacion /amie-ambient-intelligence-for-the-elderly-8109 (accessed May 20, 2011).

AMIGO Project. 2011. http://www.hitech-projects.com/euprojects/amigo/ (accessed June 6, 2011).

Baldauf, M., S. Dustdar and F. Rosenberg. 2007. A survey on context-aware systems. *International Journal of Ad Hoc and Ubiquitous Computing* 2(4):263–277.

Barnes, D., K. Covinsky, R. Whitmer, L. Kuller, O. Lopez and K. Yaffe. 2010. Dementia risk indices: A framework for identifying individuals with a high dementia risk. *Alzheimer's Dementia* 6:138–141.

Bernard, G. 2006. Middleware for next generation distributed systems: Main challenges and perspectives. Paper presented on the International Workshop on Database and Expert Systems Applications. Krakow, October 16.

Broek, G., F. Cavallo, L. Odetti and C. Wehrmann. 2009. *Ambient Assisted Living Roadmap*. Berlin: AALIANCE Office.

Brookmeyer, R., S. Gray and C. Kawas. 1998. Projections of Alzheimer's disease in the United States and the public health impact of delaying disease onset. *American Journal Public Health* 88:1337–1342.

Brookmeyer, R., E. Johnson, K. Ziegler-Graham and H. M. Arrighi. 2007. Forecast-ing the global burden of Alzheimer's disease. *Alzheimers Dement* 3:186–191.

Buschke, H., G. Kuslansky, M. Katz, W. F. Stewart, M. J. Sliwinski, H. M. Eckholdt and R. B. Lipton. 1999. Screening for dementia with the memory impairment screen. *Neurology* 52(2):231–238.

Castro, A., P. R. Pinheiro and M. Pinheiro. 2007. Applying a decision making model in the early diagnosis of Alzheimer's disease. *Lecture Notes in Computer Science* 4481:149–156.

Chatzigiannakis, I., G. Mylonas and S. Nikoletseas. 2007. 50 ways to build your application: A survey of middleware and systems for wireless sensor networks. Paper presented for the IEEE Conference on Emerging Technologies and Factory Automation. Patras, January 24.

COGKNOW. 2011. http://www.cogknow.eu/ (accessed May 19, 2011).

COMPANIONABLE. 2011. http://www.companionable.net/ (accessed May 20, 2011).

COM/2010/0245 f/2. Communication from the Commission to the European Parliament, the Council, the European Economic and Social Committee and the Committee of the Regions. A Digital Agenda for Europe.

DOMEO. 2011. http://www.aal-domeo.org/ (accessed May 20, 2011).

DREAMING. 2011. http://www.dreaming-project.org/ (accessed May 20, 2011).

eCaalyx. 2011. http://ecaalyx.org/ (accessed May 19, 2011).

ELDER-SPACES. 2011. http://www.ftb-net.com/elder-spaces.html (accessed May 20, 2011).

Elisle, P. B., L. Joseph, D. B. Wolfson and X. Zhou. 2002. Bayesian estimation of cognitive decline in patients with Alzheimer's disease. *The Canadian Journal of Statistics* 30(1):37–54.

European Commission. 2010. Report a digital agenda for Europe. Prepared by European Commission Information Society and Media. Brussels. Available at http://www.ec.europa.eu/information _society/digital-agenda/documents/digital-agenda-communication-en.pdf (accessed May 25, 2011).

Eurostat. 2008. Population projections 2008–2060—From 2015, deaths projected to outnumber births in the EU27 Almost three times as many people aged 80 or more in 2060, by Tim Allen, Eurostat Press Office. Available at http://www.europa.eu/rapid/pressReleasesAction.do?reference=STAT/08 /119&format=PDF&aged=0&language=EN&guiLanguage=en (accessed June 14, 2011).

Floeck, M. and L. Litz. 2008. Activity- and inactivity-based approaches to analyze an assisted living environment. Paper presented on the Second International Conference on Emerging Security Information, Systems and Technologies, SECURWARE '08.

Gabner, K. and M. Conrad. 2010. Report ICT enabled independent living for elderly. A status-quo analysis on products and the research landscape in the field of Ambient Assisted Living (AAL) in EU-27. Prepared by Institute for Innovation and Technology of Germany. Available at http://www.ec.europa.eu/information_society/newsroom/cf/redirection.cfm?item_id=5797 (accessed June 15, 2011).

Gaddah, A. and T. Kunz. 2003. A survey of middleware paradigms for mobile computing. Carleton University Systems and Computing Engineering Technical Report SCE-03-16. Available at http://www.sce.carleton.ca/wmc/middleware/middleware.pdf (accessed June 16, 2011).

Go-myLife. 2011. http://www.gomylife-project.eu/ (accessed May 20, 2011).

H@H. 2011. http://www.health-at-home.eu/ (accessed May 20, 2011).

Hadim, S. and N. Mohamed. 2006. Middleware for wireless sensor networks: A survey. Paper presented for the First International Conference on Communication System Software and Middleware. New Delhi, India, January.

Hawthorn, D. 2000. Possible implications of ageing for interface designers. *Interaction with Computers* 12:507–528.

HEARCOM. 2011. http://www.hearcom.eu/main.html;jsessionid=9F95824787FEC2BA7E5BF607 FE9564AC (accessed May 20, 2011).

HELP. 2011. http://www.help-aal.com/HELP/index.php?seccion=9 (accessed May 20, 2011).

Hendrie, H. C. 1998. Epidemiology of dementia and Alzheimer's disease. *The American Journal of Geriatric Psychiatry* 6(2 Suppl 1):S3–S18.

Henricksen, K. and R. Robinson. 2006. A survey of middleware for sensor networks: State-of-the-art and future directions. Paper presented in Proceedings of the International Workshop on Middleware for Sensor Networks. New York.

HMFM. 2011. http://ttuki.vtt.fi/hmfm/index.html (accessed May 20, 2011).

HOPE. 2011. http://www.hope.be/ (accessed May 19, 2011).

HOPES. 2011. http://www.hopeproject.eu/ (accessed May 20, 2011).

Hristova, A., A. M. Bernardos and J. R. Casar. 2008. Context-aware services for ambient assisted living: A case-study. Paper presented on the First International Symposium on Applied Sciences on Biomedical and Communication Technologies, 2008. ISABEL '08. Aalborg, December 16.

Huang, Y. and R. Miles. 1996. Relevance rule based reasoning. Paper in Proceedings of Conference on Collaboration in Intelligent Systems Technologies. November 15.

IMPACT. 1999. Increasing the IMPACT of assistive technology. Available at http://www.fontys.nl /impact/1_Introduction.pdf (accessed June 3, 2011).

IPTS. 2006. User needs in ICT research for independent living, with a focus on health aspects. Available at fiste.jrc.ec.europa.eu/pages/documents/WSREPORT-finaldraft.pdf (accessed June 3, 2011).

ISO/IEC 13407. 1999. Human-centred design processes for interactive systems, ISO/IEC 13407; 1999 (e).

ISO/IEC 9241-14. 1998. Ergonomic requirements for office work with visual display terminals (VDT) S-Part 14 menu dialogues ISO/IEC 9241-14:1998(E).

ISTAG. 2004. *Report on Experience & Application Research. Involving Users in the Development of Ambient Intelligent.* Edited by European Communities. Luxembourg: Office for Official Publications of the European Communities.

Jasemian, Y. 2008. Elderly comfort and compliance to modern telemedicine system at home. In *Pervasive Computing Technologies for Healthcare.* Tampere, January 30–February 1.

Jimison, H., M. Pavel, J. McKanna and J. Pavel. 2004a. Unobtrusive monitoring of computer interactions to detect cognitive status in elders. *Information Technology in Biomedicine* 8(3):248–252.

Jimison, H. B., M. Pavel, J. Pavel and J. McKanna. 2004b. Home monitoring of computer interactions for the early detection of dementia. In *Annual International Conference of the IEEE Engineering in Medicine and Biology Society* 6:4533–4536. San Francisco, September 1–5.

Joshi, S., P. Deepa Shenoy, K. R. Venugopal and L. M. Patnaik. 2009. Evaluation of different stages of dementia employing neuropsychological and machine learning techniques. In *International Conference Advanced Computing*, December 13–15, 154–160.

Kaye, J. 2008. Home based technologies: A new paradigm for conducting dementia prevention trials. *Alzheimer's Association* 4(1 Suppl 1):S60–S66.

Kjaer, K. E. 2007. A survey of context-aware middleware. Paper presented for the Proceedings of the 25th Conference on IASTED International Multi-Conference: Software Engineering, Innsbruck, Austria.

Korczyn, A. and V. Aharonson. 2007. Computerized methods in the assessment and prediction of dementia. *Current Alzheimer Research* 4:364–369.

Kurschl, W., S. Mitsch and J. Schoenboeck. 2009. Modeling situation-aware ambient assisted living systems for eldercare. Paper presented on the Sixth International Conference on Information Technology: New Generations, 2009. ITNG '09.

Lee, C., D. Nordstedt and S. Helal. 2003. Enabling smart spaces with oSGi. Paper presented on the IEEE Conference on Pervasive Computing.

Lin, C. C., P. Y. Lin, P. Lu, G. Y. Hsieh, W. L. Lee and R. Lee. 2008. A healthcare integration system for disease assessment and safety monitoring of dementia patients. *IEEE Transactions on Information Technology in Biomedicine* 12(5):579–586.

Lõõbas, I., E. Reilent, A. Anier, A. Luberg and A. Kuusik. 2010. Towards semantic contextual content-centric assisted living solution. Paper presented for the IEEE International Conference e-Health Networking Applications and Services (Healthcom). Lyon, July 1–3.

Meingast, M., T. Roosta and S. Sastry. 2006. Security and Privacy Issues with Health Care Information Technology. Conference: Annual International Conference of the IEEE Engineering in Medicine and Biology Society - EMBC, pp. 5453–5458.

Marjo, U., P. Janne and N. Hannu. 2007. Report European ICT R&D landscape: Report on national priorities and programmes. Prepared by Finnish Funding Agency for Technology and Innovation. Available at http://www.umic.pt/images/stories/publicacoes/cistrana_eu_ict_report.pdf (accessed May 20, 2011).

Matic, A. and V. Osmani. 2009. Technologies to monitor cognitive decline. In *1st Workshop Technologies to Monitor Cognitive Decline.* Trento, Italy.

Medical Care Continuity (MCC). 2011. http://www.ec.europa.eu/information_society/activities /health/in_practice/eten/index_en.htm (accessed May 20, 2011).

Meingast, M., T. Roosta and S. Sastry. 2006. Security and privacy issues with health care information technology. *Conf Proc IEEE Engineering in Medicine and Biology Society* 1:5453–5458.

Meza-Kubo, V., A. L. Morán and M. D. Rodríguez. 2009. Intergenerational communication systems in support for elder adults with cognitive decline. Paper presented at the International ICST Workshop on Technologies to Counter Cognitive Decline. London, England, March 31.

Mini-Mental® State Examination (MMSE®). Psychological Assessment Resources (PAR). http://www4.parinc.com/products/product.aspx?Productid=MMSE (accessed January 2015).

Molla, M. M. and S. I. Ahamed. 2006. A survey of middleware for sensor network and challenges. Parallel Processing Workshops. *ICPP 2006 Workshops. 2006 International Conference* 6:228.

MonAMI Project. 2011. http://www.monami.info (accessed June 8, 2011).

Monekosso, D. N. and P. Remagnino. 2010. Behavior analysis for assisted living. Paper presented on the IEEE Transactions Automation Science and Engineering.

Moreno, P., M. Hernando, A. de Poorter, R. Pallares and E. J. Gómez. 2009. IP multimedia subsystem technology for ambient assisted living. *Computer Science* 5597:257–260.

Morris, M., J. Lundell, E. Dishman and B. Needham. 2003. New perspectives on ubiquitous computing from ethnographic study of elders with cognitive decline. *Ubiquitous Computing* 2864:227–242.

MPOWER Project. 2011. http://www.sintef.no/mpower (accessed June 6, 2011).

MyHeart. 2011. http://www.hitech-projects.com/euprojects/myheart/ (accessed May 20, 2011).

myURC. 2011. http://www.myurc.org (accessed June 6, 2011).

Mura, T., J. A. J. F. Dartigues and C. Berr. 2010. How many dementia cases in France and Europe? Alternative projections and scenarios 2010–2015. *European Journal of Neurology* 17:252–259.

Ni, Z. W., S. L. Yang, L. S. Li and R. Y. Jia. 2003. Integrated case-based reasoning. *Machine Learning and Cybernetics* 3:1845.

Nick, M. and M. Becker. 2007. A hybrid approach to intelligent living assistance. Paper in 7th International Conference on Hybrid Intelligent Systems. Kaiserslautern, Germany, September 17–19.

Park, S. and J. K. Aggarwal. 2004. Semantic-level understanding of human actions and interactions using event hierarchy. Paper in Computer Vision and Pattern Recognition Workshops, *CVPRW '04. Conference* 12:12.

PeerAssist. 2011. http://cnl.di.uoa.gr/peerassist/ (accessed May 20, 2011).

PERSONA Project. 2011. http://www.aal-persona.org/ (accessed June 6, 2011).

Petersen, R. C., R. G. Thomas, M. Grundman, D. Bennett, R. Doody, S. Ferris, D. Galasko, S. Jin, J. Kaye, A. Levey, E. Pfeiffer, M. Sano, C. H. van Dyck, L. J. Thal and Alzheimer's Disease Cooperative Study Group. 2005. Vitamin E and donepezil for the treatment of mild cognitive impairment. *The New England Journal of Medicine* 352(23):2379–2388.

Psychiatric Rating Scales for Alzheimer's Disease and Dementia. 2010. Available at http://www.chicagomanualofstyle.org/tools_citationguide.html (accessed May 16, 2011).

Ramanujam, S., N. Purohit and N. Bhoir. 2011. Assessment of cognitive level for Alzheimer's using neural networks. In *Conference on Intelligent Systems, Modelling and Simulation*. January 25–27, 13–18.

Ravaglia, G., P. Forti, A. Lucicesare, N. Pisacane, E. Rietti, M. Bianchin and E. Dalmonte. 2008. Physical activity and dementia risk in the elderly—Findings from a prospective Italian study. *Neurology* 70(19 Pt 2):1786–1794.

Roberson, E. D. and L. Mucke. 2006. 100 years and counting: Prospects for defeating Alzheimer's disease. *Science* 314(5800):781–784.

Rodrigues, G. N., V. Alves, R. Franklin and L. Laranjeira. 2010. Dependability analysis in the ambient assisted living domain: An exploratory case study. Paper in Fourth Brazilian Symposium on Software Components, Architectures and Reuse. Salvador, Bahia Brazil. September 27–29.

ROSETTA. 2011. http://www.fp7rosetta.org/ (accessed May 20, 2011).

RUNES Consortium. 2005. Survey of middleware for networked embedded systems. Deliverable D5.1. Available at http://www.ist-runes.org/docs/deliverables/D5_01.pdf (accessed June 6, 2011).

Saeed, A. and T. Waheed. 2010. An extensive survey of context-aware middleware architectures. Paper presented for the IEEE International Conference on Electro/Information Technology. Normal, October 28.

Schülke, A. M., H. Plischke and N. B. Kohls. 2010. Commentary Ambient Assistive Technologies (AAT): Socio-technology as a powerful tool for facing the inevitable sociodemographic challenges? *Philosophy, Ethics, and Humanities in Medicine* 5:8.

SHARE. 2011. http://www.share-project.org/data-access-documentation.html (accessed May 20, 2011).

Shi, Y., Y. Huang, D. Minnen, A. Bobick and I. Essa. 2004 Propagation networks for recognition of partially ordered sequential action. Paper in Proceedings of Computer Vision and Pattern Recognition 2:862–869.

SilverGame. 2011. http://www.silvergame.eu/project (accessed May 20, 2011).

Sim, K., G. Yap, C. Phua, J. Biswas, A. P. Wai, A. Tolstikov, W. Huang and P. Yap. 2010. Improving the accuracy of erroneous-plan recognition system for activities of daily living. Paper in International Conference on e-Health Networking Applications and Services. Lyon, July 1–3.

Small, G. W., P. V. Rabins, P. P. Barry et al. 1997. Diagnosis and treatment of Alzheimer's disease and related disorders: Consensus statement of the American Association for Geriatric Psychiatry, the Alzheimer's Association and the American Geriatrics Society. *The Journal of the American Medical Association* 278(16):1363–1371.

SOPRANO Project. 2011. http://www.soprano-ip.org/ (accessed June 6, 2011).

Stefania, A., A. Martoranaa, S. Bernardinid, M. Panellab, F. Mercatic, A. Orlacchioa and M. Pierantozzib. 2006. CSF markers in Alzheimer disease patients are not related to the different degree of cognitive impairment. *Journal of the Neurological Science* 251:124–128.

Stephan, B., T. Kurth, F. Matthews, C. Brayne and C. Dufouil. 2010. Dementia risk prediction in the population: Are screening models accurate? *Nature Reviews Neurology* 6(6):318–326.

Storf, H., M. Becker and M. Riedl. 2009. Rule-based activity recognition framework: Challenges, technique and learning. Paper in Pervasive Computing Technologies for Healthcare, 1–7.

Sun, F. and S. Hao. 2010. Knowledge reasoning system architecture based on description logic. Paper in International Conference on Electrical and Control Engineering. Wuhan, June 25–27.

Sun, H., V. De Florio and C. Blondia. 2006. A design tool to reason about ambient assisted living systems. Paper presented on the Sixth International Conference on Intelligent Systems Design and Applications, 2006. ISDA '06. Jinan, December 11.

Tamura, T., T. Fujimoto and T. Togawa. 1997. Quantitative assessment of behavior in dementia patients by continuous physical activity monitoring. In *Proceedings 19th International Conference IEEE/EMBS*. Chicago, October 30–November 2.

Tandona, R., S. Adaka and J. A. Kayeb. 2006. Neural networks for longitudinal studies in Alzheimer's disease. *Artificial Intelligence in Medicine* 36(3):245–255.

UniversAAL Project. 2011. http://www.universaal.org/ (accessed June 6, 2011).

V2me. 2011. http://www.v2me.org/web/page.aspx?sid=5987 (accessed May 20, 2011).

Wang, T., W. Xu, J. He, R. Chen and W. Gu. 2010. A brief survey of event-based middleware. Paper presented on the International Conference on Computer Engineering and Technology. Chengdu, June 17.

WeCare. 2011. http://www.wecare-project.eu/ (accessed May 20, 2011).

WEL_HOPS. 2011. http://www.interreg3c.net/sixcms/detail.php?id=8107&_map24sid=&_searched =&_currfloaterlang=en (accessed May 20, 2011).

Wolf, P., A. Schmidt and M. Klein. 2008. SOPRANO—An extensible, open AAL platform for elderly people based on semantical contracts. Paper presented on the 3rd Workshop on Artificial Intelligence Techniques for Ambient Intelligence (AITAmI'08), 18th European Conference on Artificial Intelligence (ECAI 08). Patras, Greece.

Wolf, P., A. Schmidt, J. P. Otte, M. Klein, S. Rollwage, B. König-Ries, T. Dettborn and A. Gabdulkhakova. 2010. OpenAAL—The open source middleware for ambient-assisted living (AAL). Paper presented on the AALIANCE Conference. Malaga, Spain, March 11–12.

Wu, J., A. Osuntogun, T. Choudhury, M. Philipose and J. M. Rehg. 2007. A scalable approach to activity recognition based on object use. In *IEEE 11th International Conference on Computer Vision*. Rio de Janeiro, October 14–21, 1–8.

Yin, G. Q. and D. Bruckner. 2010. Data analyzing and daily activity learning with hidden Markov model. Computer Application and System Modeling (ICCASM), *International Conference* 3:380–384.

Zhou, F., J. Jiao, S. Chen and D. Zhang. 2011. A case-driven ambient intelligence system for elderly in-home assistance applications. *IEEE Transactions on Systems, Man, and Cybernetics—Part C: Applications and Reviews* 41(2):179–189.

Zhu, C., Q. Cheng and W. Sheng. 2010. Human activity recognition via motion and vision data fusion. Paper in IEEE Signals, Systems and Computers. November 7–10.

Zimmermann, G., G. Vanderheiden, M. Gandy, S. Laskowski, M. Ma, S. Trewin and M. Walker. 2004. Universal remote console standard—Toward natural user interaction in ambient intelligence. Extended Abstracts for the 2004 Conference on Human Factors in Computing Systems. New York, ACM Press.

Zwick, C., B. Schmitz and K. Kuehl. 2005. *Designing for Small Screens*. Lausanne, Switzerland, AVA Publishing SA.

15

Innovative Solutions for Inclusion of Totally Blind People

Michał Choraś, Rafał Kozik, Salvatore D'Antonio, Giulio Iannello,
Andreas Jedlitschka, Klaus Miesenberger, Luca Vollero, and Adam Wołoszczuk

CONTENTS

ABSTRACT   In this chapter, we present innovative solutions to support social inclusion of totally blind people. We propose to use a dedicated harness and mobile devices (e.g., smartphones) to support instrumental activities of daily living (IADL). Moreover, we present innovations in computer vision algorithms, multisensor data fusion, situational awareness, ontology, and risk assessment as well as innovations in resilient personal telecommunications.

KEY WORDS: *computer vision, object recognition, obstacles detection, decision support, visually impaired people.*

Introduction

Nowadays, it is extremely difficult for totally blind and visually impaired people to live a normal life in terms of interacting with society. Most often, such people are excluded, and they interact only in the special well-known environments created for them (e.g., special schools).

Although various technological approaches have been proposed, none of them comprehensively addresses assistance for daily activities and social inclusion of totally blind and visually impaired people. Currently available solutions focus mainly on one specific kind of support, e.g., navigation. Moreover, various technical solutions lack usefulness and ease of use because they are not oriented according to the specific requirements of blind users and are therefore not accepted by them.

Our goal is to provide a multisensor-based, distributed service framework for inclusion of visually impaired and totally blind people through daily assistance (e.g., traveling aid) and executing everyday routines.

Therefore, in this chapter, we propose a number of innovative solutions to facilitate social inclusion of blind people. In particular, the following aspects are presented:

- System architecture
- Innovative portable devices and human–machine interfaces
- Computer vision algorithms
- Innovations in multisensor data fusion (DF)
- Innovative situational awareness, ontology, and risk assessment
- Innovations in wireless personal telecommunications solutions

Moreover, real-life scenarios and services are presented. Sample cases and results are demonstrated. The overall impact of the proposed solutions on inclusion of blind people is discussed. Conclusions are given thereafter.

Context and Background

Partial or full vision impairment has been reported as being a huge factor for exclusion. For example, the ratio of visually impaired and totally blind people currently employed (and actively working) is significantly low. According to Refs. [1] and [2], ca. 314 million people are visually impaired worldwide, 45 million of them are blind, and an average of 3% of Europe's inhabitants experience loss of sight.

In Europe, the average unemployment rate of blind and visually impaired persons of the working population is more than 75% [3]. However, those blind or visually impaired people who are working are concentrated in unskilled and lower-paid jobs. For example, in Kuyavia and the Pomerania region in Poland, it is estimated that less than 15% of blind people have a regular job. Those who are employed usually have jobs that are not related to their skills and knowledge.

There are several factors contributing to this problem, including:

- Inadequate rehabilitation plans
- Lack of self-motivation caused by high unemployment rate and limited (or poor) government support
- Lack of (limited access to) schools adapted for blind persons
- Limited access to (and high costs of) rehabilitation facilities
- Limited number of facilities adapted for blind persons

The problem is even greater, since in many European countries, public facilities (bus or train stations, museums/cinemas, government buildings) are not adapted for blind people.

The Eurostat report [4] showed that access for people with visual disabilities to services such as public transport, sport events, workplaces, universities and schools, restaurants, and cultural events is significantly more difficult than for people with other impairments (e.g., deaf or physically or intellectually disabled people). According to this report, visually disabled people perceive access to buildings, services, and events in Europe as being fairly difficult to very difficult. Furthermore, traditional means for supporting people suffering from vision impairment like guide dogs or echolocation-based canes are still hardly accessible. For example, in the case of guide dogs, there is a huge amount of time required for both the animal and the human to cooperate and understand each other.

Nowadays, only a small percentage of blind people have such well-trained dogs (e.g., in Poland, according to data from the Polish society of blind people, only 3% of totally blind people over 16 years of age have guide dogs). The Polish society of the blind can provide only 8–10 dogs a year, while special nongovernmental foundations can provide only one dog every 2 years.

Existing Solutions for the Visually Impaired

Current vision-based solutions dedicated for blind people can be categorized into two distinct groups. The first group engages single-camera sensors, while the second commonly engages two (or more) cameras. Multicamera-based approaches generally aim at reconstructing the 3-D shape of the observed scene and provide the user with additional information about the terrain shape (e.g., curb detection). Moreover, these approaches allow for real-time foreground and background separation, since triangulation of two (or more) views allows measurement of a distance to a particular object. However, these solutions require at least two camera sensors (attached and calibrated). After the depth segmentation process, postprocessing is common for single-view and multiview approaches. These usually engage both computer vision and machine learning algorithms. Commonly, texture features are extracted from video streams (or from still images) and correlated with some knowledge in order to identify, classify, or detect particular objects. The majority of the known approaches stop video processing at this step simply by informing the user of the name and/or location of detected objects, while more sophisticated ones engage a data model or prior knowledge to understand the scene and the context. Single-view approaches usually engage pattern recognition and machine learning algorithms to recognize objects. The majority of algorithms serve single-object detection (e.g., dedicated to find a particular class of objects), while some are aimed at identifying a wide range of objects. Typical single-object detectors allow for recognition of such objects as doors [5,6], pedestrians [7], or staircases [8]. Usually, such solutions are considered by blind persons as an additional source of information during travel. The majority of such solutions are implemented by using efficient real-time computer vision algorithms (e.g., Haar-like features and rapid AdaBoosted cascades of filters [9,10]); therefore, smartphone deployable versions of these applications are often available. A similar class of solutions dedicated for blind people are so-called screen readers. These solutions are focused on finding text in a cluttered background and presenting it to a blind person in audio form. Commonly, these systems allow identifying of the names of the streets and buses or presenting the content of LED/LCD screens. Ref. [11] presents an assistive application for detecting the text in images of natural scenes. The algorithm is based on the gray-level co-occurrence matrix (GLCM) for texture coding. Due to relatively low computation requirements, such solutions are usually dedicated for mobile phones.

To recognize or detect a wide range of diverse objects, typical smartphone capabilities are insufficient. Therefore, in such systems a client–server architecture is often adapted. Usually, the phone is used for video streaming while the remote server performs more computationally expensive tasks. Particularly, the LookTel system [12] engages video streaming over 3G to perform object recognition and presents the results using a text-to-speech engine. The server side engages robust scale-invariant feature transform (SIFT) video content descriptors to query the databases and identify objects. The system is also capable of detecting video frames containing text and transforming it to voice. An example of LookTel functionality is called Money Reader. A similar system for the visually impaired is proposed in Ref. [13]. The system, named GroZi, is a grocery shopping assistant. It allows the user to scan the shelf for items on a shopping list. For rapid object recognition, speeded up robust features (SURF) descriptors and multiclass naive Bayes classifiers are adapted.

Another class of solutions that are useful for visually impaired people are so-called simultaneous localization and mapping (SLAM) algorithms. Such localization and mapping applications focus on a sparse set of landmarks that are tracked, and their position is estimated. The map is maintained as a set of landmarks located in 3-D space. Given the landmarks, the camera trajectory is estimated. Only a subset of all the landmarks is observed from each camera position. Using these observations, the most probable landmark's 3-D coordinates and camera poses are estimated. Common methods that address this kind of problem adapt extended Kalman filters (EKFs) or different variants of bundle adjustment. In Ref. [14], the authors presented a system that uses sparse landmarks for blind user localization. The proposed system was tested in several outdoor and indoor scenarios. The localization is based on information obtained during the learning phase, where at first, the environment is recorded with a camera, and then its 3-D structure is estimated with an offline structure form motion algorithm. The blind person's position is estimated on the basis of the current frame, which is matched with a 3-D model built during the learning phase. The advantage of the proposed system is that it does not stigmatize the blind person, since the camera is mounted on the chest and the processing unit (in this case, a laptop) is hidden in a backpack. However, as stated in Ref. [15], a set of landmarks (rendering the map) could be too sparse for tasks in autonomous navigation, path planning, obstacle avoidance, etc. Therefore, the authors of Ref. [15] propose a dense stereo localization and mapping algorithm that estimates a dense 3-D map representation. They demonstrate the algorithm's effectiveness in an urban environment. A different approach to this problem was presented in Ref. [16], where the authors proposed hidden Markov models (HMM) position estimation based on GIST and SURF texture features for user localization. The context in this approach is recognized thanks to a map combined with prior knowledge of the visual appearance of particular localizations.

The reason behind adopting multicamera (typically stereo) solutions for computer vision systems is additional knowledge about the depth of the observed scenes. It is possible to measure the distance to a particular object through stereo matching and simple triangulation. It is extremely useful for rapid foreground and background segmentation, which has further impact on overall system effectiveness. Without prior knowledge of object localization, the region of interest (ROI) where texture is analyzed usually covers the whole image (which is a common drawback for single-view approaches). For stereo vision approaches, texture processing is typically applied starting from the nearest object and is usually stopped at a particular depth (commonly no further than several meters from the camera sensor). Obstacle detection is an essential capability for the safe guidance of a blind person, especially in an urban environment. Most of the existing stereovision techniques for obstacle detection rely on the planar ground assumption. Such an example of stereovision application is presented in Ref. [17], where authors proposed solutions that help blind people avoid obstacles. In this approach, a 3-D scene model is mapped to an acoustic image, where obstacles are assigned unique acoustic signals. However, as stated in Ref. [18], in urban environments, the real-time requirement and the range of distances that must be considered imply that the planar assumption is too restrictive. In order to enhance the reliability of the obstacle detection task, the authors of Ref. [18] do not model urban roads as rigid planes but as quasi-planes, whose normal vectors have a predictable constraint. In Ref. [19], the authors proposed a method for analyzing the terrain with a depth map obtained from a stereovision camera. The application is developed to cooperate with a camera mounted on a wheelchair. This allows mounting of a camera close enough to ground level. Therefore, the depth can be measured more precisely. In Refs. [20] and [21], the authors proposed a stereovision system that aims at detecting the obstacles that are localized at head level. The system also allows for environment mapping and blind person localization. In order to provide the system with such capabilities, the authors proposed a sparse set of features combined with a depth map obtained from a stereovision camera. Using this information, the sparse 3-D structure of the scene is built. The structure is tracked in subsequent frames, and the position of the blind person is estimated. The advantage of the proposed system is that it does not stigmatize the blind person. A head-mounted stereovision camera is used in Ref. [22]. The authors of this paper claim that such placement of the sensor allows the blind person to scan the environment more comfortably. Moreover, such placement allows the system to detect a wider range of obstacles (e.g., not only at the head level). The proposed algorithm engages a depth map in order to build the traversability map of the environment.

A different class of solutions are applications that engage a single camera with structured light (so-called red green blue depth [RGB-D] cameras). In Ref. [23], the authors proposed a wearable RGB-D camera–based navigation system for the visually impaired. The navigation system is expected to enable the visually impaired to extend the range of their activities compared to that provided by conventional aid devices, such as white canes. In order to extract information about the position of the blind users, the authors incorporated visual odometry and feature-based SLAM into the system. The application builds a vicinity map based on dense 3-D data obtained from the RGB-D camera. In order to provide the visually impaired with 3-D traversability information, path planning is performed. The 3-D traversability analysis helps the blind person to avoid obstacles in the path.

Proposed Architecture

In order to facilitate inclusion of blind people, we propose the general architecture presented in Figure 15.1.

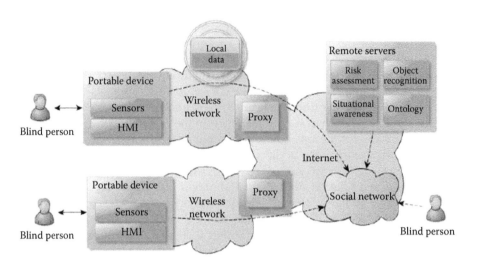

FIGURE 15.1
General architecture of the proposed solution.

The proposed architecture follows the cloud concept, allowing blind users to share experiences and information through a social network. The network will allow blind persons to post information about particular dangerous or friendly places or past experiences to the community of connected people. Remote servers will be capable of handling such data. Moreover, portable device will also read the *local data*, which will be broadcast by remote devices (vending machines, dispensers, etc.) via radio/wireless channels.

We plan to go much further beyond state-of-the art and current support solutions, by using vision-based sensors (e.g., cameras) and other sensors integrated into a dedicated harness.

We advance the state of the art, for example, using the *guide me to* service, which guides a blind person from one point to another, detecting and helping to avoid obstacles. The blind person will be able to select a destination point (e.g., rehabilitation and training center), and the system will plan the shortest route from the current location by using GPS localization capabilities.

The proposed system will be capable of avoiding the nearest and colliding objects (detected by computer vision algorithms). Having information of the context (GPS, location, objects recognized by computer vision algorithms), further detectors will be used (like walking path edge tracking, fast movement detectors, etc.), contributing to enhanced situational awareness of the blind person.

During travel, the proposed system will find the nearest bus or train station, parse the timetable, recognize the bus number, and find the entrance. In an environment unknown to the blind person, the proposed system will complement guide dog duties, like finding free seats or exits. Moreover, we propose a self-adaptive, learning system. The blind user might ask the system for guidance to the closest bakery, and the system will propose the optimal route and help avoid obstacles (e.g., a construction site). Our proposed innovation is to use social networking to learn that construction works started recently and to advise the blind user to choose another bakery due to safety reasons (e.g., because of the construction site, it would be necessary to cross a road with lots of traffic at this time). We propose innovative ICT solutions to facilitate social inclusion of the blind on several layers:

- Sensing layer, based on intelligent cameras (computer vision algorithms) and other sensors integrated in the dedicated harness
- Communication layer, based on resilient wireless personal telecommunication
- Risk assessment and situational awareness layer, based on semantic notations, correlation, and reasoning algorithms
- Interaction layer for the end user, based on innovative nonvisual interfaces

The proposed solutions progress beyond the state of the art in support for blind people in the following aspects:

- We propose to use smartphones and to use a dedicated harness as devices supporting blind people.
- We suggest devices that will not stigmatize a blind person (thus enabling social inclusion).
- We focus on building vision-based situational awareness (not on simple object avoidance and recognition).
- We propose to use social networks for blind persons in order to empower information exchange.
- Our solution will be implemented for user-friendly portable devices.
- The proposed devices will use resilient wireless personal networks.
- The proposed devices will have interfaces dedicated for interaction with blind persons.

Proposed Portable Device Solutions

Currently, most vision-based devices developed in previous projects (e.g., FP6 CASBliP) use cameras mounted on special helmets and a processing unit in the backpack [24].

Such an approach is not accepted by end users and will stigmatize the blind person. We aim at using/designing user-friendly devices such as nonvisible cameras and smartphones. Our goal is to provide solutions that will not stigmatize a blind person (as presented in Figure 15.2).

Moreover, it is our goal to support amodal information representation in the system and, based on this, multimedia presentation and multimodal interaction, which allows an adaptation following profiles of a diverse set of end user needs and preferences.

Mobility and independence resulting from the ability to freely and confident move within an outdoor environment are the most common challenges for blind people. Therefore, we propose to integrate the proposed solutions (sensors, algorithms, services) to run on the following portable devices:

1. Smartphone or similar handheld device
2. Dedicated harness (with wearable sensors and actuators)

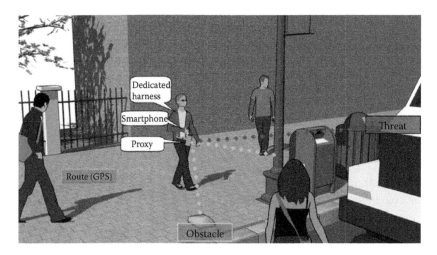

FIGURE 15.2
Blind person with the proposed man machine interface (MMI) devices (smartphone and dedicated harness).

It will also be possible to use them together in order to help a blind person since the smartphone and the dedicated harness will communicate using wireless technologies (e.g., wireless sensor network [WSN], Bluetooth, Wi-Fi).

- Smartphones have the following characteristics:
  - Widely available
  - Communication (wireless local area network [WLAN], Universal Mobile Telecommunications System [UMTS], 4G, Bluetooth, etc.)
  - Sensors (cameras [e.g., 5MPix], G sensor),
  - GPS
  - Services
  - Sonification/voice
- Dedicated harnesses have the following capabilities (Figure 15.3):
  - Wearable sensors
  - Mini cameras

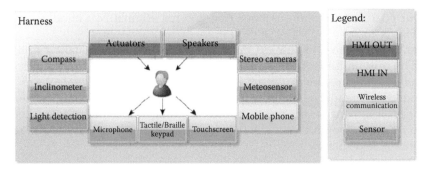

FIGURE 15.3
Dedicated harness components.

- Compass
- Inclinometer
- Meteosensors
- Light sensor
  - Communication (WLAN, UMTS, 4G, Bluetooth, etc.)
  - Microphone and speakers
  - Innovative interaction with blind users (actuators)
- Tactile
- Vibration
- Thermal (Peltier cells)

The main component of the harness will be a set of cameras that enable gathering of information on context (where, who, how many, etc.), obstacles, and threats (dynamic obstacles such as an approaching vehicle). The stereovision and audio data will not be processed locally. They will be sent (e.g., via the smartphone) to remote servers to be processed for object recognition, risk assessment, situational awareness, etc.

The harness itself will be equipped with the control unit for basic local data processing. In order to provide as much relevant environment (local) information as possible, the harness could also be equipped with a multisensor system consisting of a compass and inclinometer for information about where a person is facing and body position (so the system may detect when a user falls, sits, or lays down and react properly); a meteorological sensor for gathering weather information; and a light sensor to measure the intensity of illumination (which would give quickly information on entering dark and confined spaces such as tunnels or halls). All the components of the harness will utilize components off the shelf to provide high modularity and reconfiguration capability as well as cost-effectiveness of the solution.

Innovations in Human–Machine Interfaces for Interaction with Blind People

To enable effective interaction between the user and the harness, the ergonomic human–machine interface (HMI) will be implemented in the harness. The HMI will communicate with the user via the senses of touch and audition. The proper filtration and separation of incoming information is essential for the user to avoid an excess of messages. That is why the different innovative sensing channels will be used to inform or alert the user. A vibroactuator may inform a user of threat proximity, speakers would provide verbal messages or ping signals when a static obstacle is close by, and Peltier cells on the inside of the harness would provide thermal information. It is also important for the user to configure the harness with respect their personal preferences. The harness would allow the user to assign the stimuli to selected functionalities (for example, using thermal information as an indicator of distance to destination).

A smartphone and a wearable harness will not stigmatize a blind person; they will be transparent for other people. It is an important factor since such a solution will not create additional barriers and will enable social interaction.

The proposed solutions aim at covering an ergonomic principle for hardware and software design (e.g., TC 159/SC 4 [25], ISO/TS 16071:2003 [26]) and, in particular, accessibility requirements (ISO/TS 16071:2003, W3C/WAI), which are very important.

Innovations in Computer Vision–Based Support of Blind People

Much research has been done on the deployment of computer systems supporting visually impaired people in their interaction with the environment. Most of these solutions are based on computer vision techniques, and they can be categorized into two distinct groups:

- Solutions relying on a single video sensor (SVS)
- Solutions based on multiple video sensors (MVS)

SVS and MVS share similar approaches in data preprocessing: filtering and low-level segmentation are usually performed on every image composing the video under analysis.

Filtering aims at enhancing images and removing distortion and noise, while low-level segmentation is designed to roughly extract objects from images, classifying an image's pixel into two groups: foreground (pixels of interest) and background.

Typical low-level segmentation algorithms are designed to be fast in order to promptly provide data to users or to other systems for further processing. Based on the specific task, data preprocessing is performed on a frame basis or on a sequence basis. Sequence-basis elaboration is more demanding on processing and memory, but it is usually more reliable.

After segmentation, postprocessing is common for both SVS and MVS approaches. Postprocessing usually involves computer vision and machine learning algorithms. Features (e.g., textures or shapes) are extracted from segmented images and correlated with some a priori knowledge in order to identify, classify, or detect particular objects.

Typical single-object detectors allow for recognition of objects such as doors [1–6,24,27–33], pedestrians [7], or staircases [8]. Their implementation is based on efficient real-time computer vision algorithms (e.g., Haar-like features and rapid AdaBoosted cascades of filters [9,10]) viable for smartphone implementation. Some examples of object detection are shown in Figure 15.4.

The adoption of MVS is motivated by the ability of obtaining additional information about the depth of the observed scene (examples are shown in Figures 15.5 and 15.6). Stereo

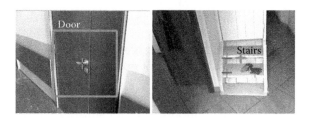

FIGURE 15.4
Examples of applications dedicated for real-time object recognition.

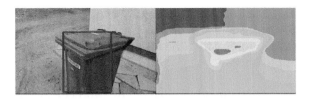

FIGURE 15.5
Example of obstacle detection (left image, red rectangle) using depth map segmentation (right image).

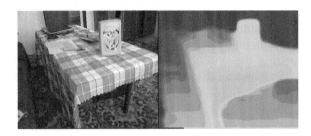

FIGURE 15.6
Example of depth map obtained in real time with a stereovision camera.

matching and simple triangulation allow for measuring the distance to a given object. This may allow for applications that help people in reaching objects and in avoiding obstacles while moving in unknown environments [17]. Moreover, in multisensor imaging, the same object is detected from multiple sources, and this increases system reliability. However, processing multiple video streams has a computational burden that may make this solution unviable for portable devices.

To identify or detect a wide range of objects and to support MVS, a typical smartphone's capabilities are insufficient. Therefore, in such systems, a client–server architecture is required. Usually, the mobile is used for video streaming and for simple computer vision tasks with real-time constraints, while the remote server performs computationally expensive and delay-tolerant tasks. The major limitation of such systems is the data processing model. The mobile and the server follow light cooperation patterns: the processing steps are split among them and completed independently. The mobile is in charge dispatching the processing task and collecting and presenting the results. The server provides reliable on-demand services for processing images or image sequences. This solution is effective in most prototypical cases. However, this processing model is too stiff in most practical situations, especially when serving people with visual impairments [12].

In real scenarios, computer vision applications need to be fast and reliable, and in their implementation, the developers need to solve a trade-off between these two requirements. The tuning between speed and reliability is difficult, and it requires a close match with the expectations of users. In the context we consider, in order to best fit the requirements of blind people, computer vision applications need to be modular, distributed, progressive, and proactive. Distributed solutions allow for supporting both delay-sensitive and reliability-sensitive applications. However, good distributed solutions need a clear modular organization in processing and communications units. In order to be fast and reliable in data processing, the same task can be completed concurrently by two modules, the former providing an approximate solution for fast feedback and the latter yielding more reliable information that can be merged, later, with that previously presented (progressive processing). Eventually, application responsiveness can benefit from proactive processing, forecasting the next user requests and precomputing results that the user may want to know.

Innovations in Multisensor DF for Support of Blind People

DF is the process of combining information gathered from different sensors (sensor fusion networks [SFNs]) with the aim of producing a more comprehensive and unified model of the object or the event of interest that has been observed [34,35].

DF is a process requiring the synergy of several elaboration steps: sensing, signal processing, estimation, and decision. DF techniques can be categorized into three groups:

1. Low-level fusion (LLF)
2. Intermediate-level fusion (ILF)
3. High-level fusion (HLF)

In LLF, the DF process combines the same type of raw data to produce a new, more informative, raw data set [36,37]. In ILF, processed features from several data sources are combined together in a feature map [38,39]. Eventually, in HLF, the decisions from several systems operating on a subset of sensors are combined (statistical methods, fuzzy logic, etc.) in order to provide a global description/decision [40,41].

Data sources managed by the applications of interest are heterogeneous in nature regarding data quality and information content. They will require novel ad hoc solutions to extract the most appropriate context information from incoming data for the benefit of accurate semantic reasoning. DF processing capabilities can be embedded into an architecture supporting blind people according to the model sketched in Figure 15.7.

Figure 15.7 shows the application model for devices and its connections with remote resources (processing or data). In the model, local data sources are embedded sensors or wireless connected sensors providing a local view of the environment surrounding the user. Data from those sources are synchronized and adapted in a standard representation form for local processing. Local processing relies on local information, or it can benefit from the availability of remote resources. A processing/resource STUB provides an interface that hides remote connections and resource search and retrieval processes.

The local sensor fusion within the wearable equipment could be applied to enable reliable monitoring of the environment and the user with emphasis on detecting potentially dangerous situations. Detection of the events when the user falls is possible by combining the image from the camera with acceleration data from the inclinometer. The same combination enables predicting possible collisions with objects in the environment and enhances constructing the 3-D model of the environment (by providing some information about the camera motion between consecutive frames by the inclinometer). The fusion of the data from the camera and microphone enables speaker detection and tracking the head of the speaking person and, in consequence, being able to determine the context of the conversation (if the speaker is looking at the user or someone else, or if the speaker is pointing at something).

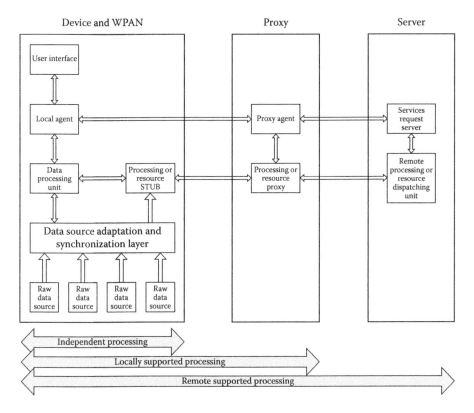

FIGURE 15.7
Distributed architecture for data fusion and processing.

The remote processing of data is supported to increase the level or reliability of the applications and in order to provide, whenever useful, monitoring capabilities for checking user safety. Moreover, the remote collection of data acquired by several users can be used for developing new inclusion applications. For instance, the system can merge data from multiple users and make them aware of the environment and of other users moving in the same context.

Innovations in Situational Awareness, Ontology, and Risk Assessment for Support of Blind People

The presence of an obstacle in front of the user does not provide complete awareness of all threats connected to that object. In the real world, there are complicated relationships between objects. These relations can cause threats only if two or more objects appear together.

Also, *social interactions* of the blind person have to be enriched with context information and situational awareness.

Different objects in the environment, through their visual appearance, influence human behavior (e.g., traffic lights or signs). Therefore, object recognition through computer vision is a crucial task. However, to have full situational awareness, prior knowledge is required to recognize the context and to collect all data parts (Figure 15.8). Such context knowledge can be maintained in an ontology. An example showing how situational awareness could be applied is shown in Figure 15.2. Recognition and object sensing are partial observations coming from the real world (computer vision algorithms). These are used to infer further information (to understand the context). Commonly detected objects like cars, pedestrians, or crossings introduce threats. This information has to be combined with information about user activity (like the goal of travel). For example, the system may have prior information about localization of the specific pedestrian crossing (in case it is not detected by camera sensors). Moreover, such data could be correlated with information about further objects (particularly those not *seen* by sensors) in a given range. All these information sources correlated together allow the building of situational awareness and preparation of a threat mitigation plan (see Figure 15.9) that would help the blind person reach the travel destination safely.

The ontology is focused on risk assessment in order to build situational awareness. The more threats are introduced in the environment, the higher the risk is. Risk may be decreased or eliminated by a particular reaction (like avoiding collision). According to the

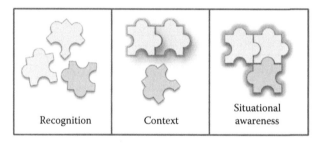

FIGURE 15.8
Situational awareness through context recognition.

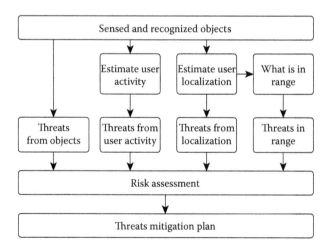

FIGURE 15.9
Situational awareness flow chart.

ontology, threats are introduced by physical properties (features) of objects. Particularly, a moving car is more dangerous than a parked one. Moreover, there are different relations. (e.g., traffic lights and pedestrian crossing) between objects that also introduce threats.

Innovations in Resilient Wireless Personal Telecommunication Support of Blind People

Personal-based communication includes both the data exchange among the sensors of personal equipment and the data transmission between the WSN proxy and the remote servers. Technologies to support these communication requirements have been widely investigated in recent years.

Global systems for mobile communications (GSM)/general packet radio service (GPRS), UMTS, and WLAN are solid solutions that allow long-range wireless communication. Recently, new technologies such as Long Term Evolution (LTE) and IEEE 802.16 (WiMAX) have been designed to ensure ultrawide-band (UWB) wireless communication.

Concerning personal communication equipment, we are observing a growing interest in technologies related to the wireless body area networks (WBANs) [42–45], especially in the area of wearable biosensors for health monitoring. Such infrastructure consists of lightweight, small-size, and ultralow-power sensors for monitoring human physiological activities.

Although several protocols and algorithms have already been proposed for the WSNs, from which the WBANs derive, the peculiarities of this new technology make it not completely compliant with the WBAN requirements.

Several research activities focus on the data security issue in WBAN [46–49]. Due to the security-sensitive information that is stored and exchanged and the security vulnerabilities affecting sensors, solutions for ensuring data confidentiality, dependability and integrity, and authentication are needed. A common approach concerns the use of data encryption and authentication mechanisms for guaranteeing that information is securely stored and transmitted.

Another important challenge for the WBAN technology concerns energy efficiency. The use of small-size sensors with limited battery lifetime requires proper development of policies and mechanisms that can reduce the energy consumption of the sensors. Many works have been proposed aiming at increasing the energy efficiency of the WBANs [50–52]. These solutions involve both the MAC layer and network layer protocols.

One of the main objectives is to propose innovative solutions in the area of wireless communication technology by challenging, in particular, issues related to quality of service (QoS), security, reliability, and resiliency.

QoS Management in 802.11 Wireless Networks

The scenario foreseen by the proposed solution where the user's device communicates with a remote server for further processing of the information (images and videos) captured by the camera clearly imposes additional requirements on the proposed solution architecture. Indeed, in order for the information returned by the server to be really useful, it is necessary that such information is delivered as quickly as possible. One of the major roots of the latency experienced by a client is the delay introduced by the communication network. The proposed solution will thus design techniques to prioritize the traffic generated by and destined to the devices of visually impaired people such that they experience the required QoS. In particular, the proposed solution will focus on wireless LANs operating according to the IEEE 802.11 standard, given the worldwide spread of WLAN hot spots and the availability of Wi-Fi interfaces on most of the newest mobile phones.

In 2005, the 802.11e amendment to the 802.11 standard introduced support for QoS in wireless LANs. Two variants have been introduced: Enhanced Distributed Controlled Access (EDCA) and Hybrid Coordination Function (HCF) Controlled Channel Access (HCCA). EDCA, like the basic distributed coordination function (DCF), provides a contention-based channel access, while HCCA introduces contention-free periods. In both cases, the access point (AP) is in charge of controlling the admission of flows into the network. In the case of EDCA, four different access categories (background, best effort, video, and voice) are defined, and each station negotiates with the AP the maximum amount of time it can use the channel in a certain time interval to transmit packets of a given access category. In the case of HCCA, each station negotiates with the AP the amount of time it will be granted for exclusive use of the channel (no contention).

The goal is to investigate the performance of the two QoS mechanisms under different conditions (different traffic loads, different requirements, etc.) and determine which mechanism is better suited to the needs of the application. Also, a technique will be developed to identify the parameters used by the mobile phone in the negotiation with the AP (each station has to provide the AP with a specification of the amount of traffic it needs to transmit).

Real-Life Application, Scenarios, and Services

A visually impaired person will be provided with a device capable of getting medium–high-quality images/videos of surrounding objects and scenes, and of effectively transmitting them to a service provider. Similar devices with only local capabilities already exist and are going to be made available on the market—they provide limited capabilities to extract useful information for the user from the images like text reading, object classification, etc.

The user, besides exploiting available local device capabilities, may send images and videos to a remote server that returns a description of recognized objects and scenes. The server may take advantage of both greater processing power and access to virtually unlimited information repositories to extract as much useful data from the raw information received. An example of such a situation is the need for scene understanding (e.g., determining if, in the scene, there is a river, a building, a gate, a car, etc.). Scene understanding will be performed by measuring the similarity of the current scene with images in a large annotated database. Information from further sensors integrated in the portable device (e.g., GPS, radio-frequency identification [RFID] reader) will enrich the information returned to the user by making use of information fusion approaches aiming at an increased understanding of the environment. After receiving feedback, e.g., in the form of an audio stream or through other communication channels accessible to visually impaired people, the user may cooperatively interact with the server (only if the user wishes to—such a process will be transparent) to further explore the environment and get even more exploitable information, e.g., they may guide the information extraction algorithms, providing themselves high-level annotations about the context, or the server might ask the user to get new raw information that better matches the processing capabilities of the information extraction system.

A list of concrete situations where these functionalities could be exploited is given in the following:

- While in *unknown, outdoor, and uncontrolled* environment, the system detects the presence of people in the scene and their number, sex, and activity (movements, proximity, conversation, etc.) and provides feedback to the user so as to improve their interaction capabilities with other people. For instance, while approaching a public transportation vehicle, a wearable device reports through an earphone if the bus is crowded or almost empty or other information useful to characterize the vehicle. Likewise, after the person gets on the bus, the device reports the main characteristics of the people traveling (sex, age, what they are doing, etc.). The device can also answer specific questions: Why have people on the left raised their voice? What is happening in front of me? (When, for example, some unusual sound just raised the curiosity of the end user.) Has the bus stopped because there is too much traffic or because the traffic lights turned red?

- Considering the case where the user is sitting in a *park or outside a cafe*, possibly in a small town, where it is likely that they may meet people they know, the device will inform the user that some person is approaching them, whether the person is known or not, and of their general appearance (a visual database concerning known people needs to be associated with each user).

- While GPS provides localization *outdoors*, it is still necessary to know a user's orientation in many situations to guide them towards a certain target or give more meaning to proximity information retrieved through databases containing information on shops, restaurants, museums, etc. Orientation information will be autonomously reconstructed by matching images acquired by the portable device with visual information contained in a database (e.g., Google Street View).

- *Going out* to a restaurant: as mentioned by end users, simple daily activities (such as going out to a restaurant) may cause many problems. The proposed system will provide solutions that can find empty tables/seats and provide information about items left on the table (e.g., by previous customers), possible obstacles, the way to the washroom, and hints (menu) using social networking, etc.

- University scenario with *blind students*: localization services, route planning service, guidance to the lecture hall, obstacle detection, finding of items and places (e.g., library, bus stop), recognition of the known students (e.g., from one's group) and lecturers, social networking, etc.

- *Going out* to the special cinema: recently, there have been efforts to organize special cinemas for blind people with the human lector not only reading the dialogue but also describing the scenes. We will provide needed support for the blind to go out to such cinemas. With the proposed solution, a blind person will be able to ask for the cinema schedule, cinema location, and optimal route at any time.

Most of these examples refer to situations where the visually impaired person can autonomously acquire context information through the proposed services without the help of other (normal-sighted) persons.

This may promote social interaction of the visually impaired person who is no longer constrained to ask everything of other people but may ask more specific questions to satisfy their curiosity to know more about their interlocutor.

The services that are enabled by the proposed innovations are listed as follows:

- Localization (standard rough GPS position estimated by mobile or smartphone and reinforced by computer vision and prior knowledge)
- Contextual localization (Google Maps or other map-based information, computer vision–based recognition and understanding)
- Obstacle/threat detection (computer vision–based recognition and understanding connected to ontology)
- People counting/people behavior characterization (computer vision)
- Street text recognition (computer vision connected with ontology)
- Risk analysis (situational awareness, ontology)
- Route planning (GPS, maps, route planning applications, social networking, self-adaptation)
- Finding places and items (computer vision connected with ontology, situational awareness)
- Empty seat/table finder (computer vision)
- Adaptation of system to user (historical user experiences and decisions connected with knowledge in ontology)
- Guiding/warning (nonvisual stimulation of user via dedicated actuators)

In the next section, some demonstration cases regarding some of the described scenarios and services are presented.

Demonstration Cases and Sample Results

In this section, the following scenarios and services are demonstrated and described: free seat detection, door detection, navigation in an unknown place, and threat detection.

Computer Vision–Based Free Seat Detector

Finding a free seating place in an environment unknown to a blind person is a challenging task. In this scenario, a blind person enters the room having the proposed system. From the touchable screen of the smartphone, the blind person can choose *free seating place*.

The environment is scanned with the stereovision camera. The simplified map of the room is shown in Figure 15.10, Tables 15.1 and 15.2.

FIGURE 15.10

Simplified map of the room with free seating places (gray filled boxes). The gray filled circle indicates the blind person.

TABLE 15.1

System in Operation: Seat Detection

Frame Sequence	Description
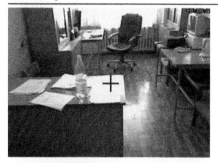	First frame
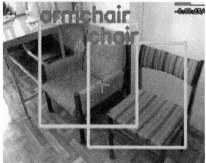	Succeeding frames (right side of the room). Two places are suggested by the system. Beeping sounds is assigned (and/or special vibrations are used) to these two seat candidates, and the blind person can easily locate the objects.
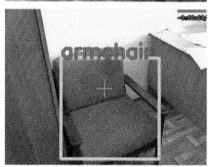	Left side of the room. The armchair is suggested by the system. Again, beeping sounds and/or vibrations are assigned to help the blind person locating the object.

TABLE 15.2

System in Operation: Free Seat Detection

Frame Sequence	Description
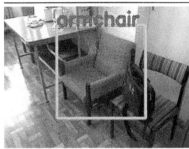	Right side of the room. Only one seat is suggested by the system. The occupied one is not signalized.
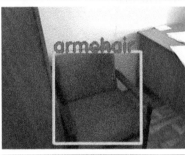	The armchair standing on the left side is signalized as free.

Computer Vision–Based Free Seat Detector (One Is Occupied)

This scenario is a modification of the previous one. The modification is that one of the seats is occupied. The situation is shown in Figure 15.11, where the cross indicates the occupied place.

Door Detection (Adverse Conditions)

Locating the appropriate door in a room is also a challenging task for a blind person (Table 15.3). The task is even more complicated when the blind person is moving across the hall. The map where the scenario takes place is shown in Figure 15.12.

Without the system, a blind person is forced to count the doors. However, as can be noticed (Figure 15.13), there are also notice boards in the hall, which look like doors.

FIGURE 15.11
Location of the seats (gray filled boxes)—one (crossed) is occupied.

TABLE 15.3

System in Operation: Doors Detection

Frame Sequence	Description
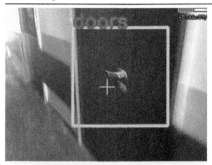	Firstly, the door is detected. It can be noticed that the door is detected even if the image is slightly blurred due to the camera motion.
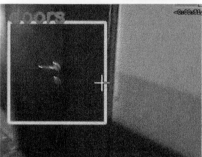	The second door is detected.
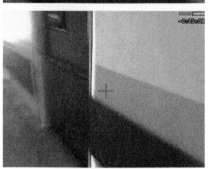	The notice board is not classified as a door (neither from a far nor from a short distance).
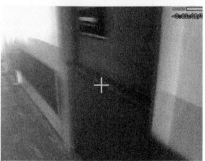	

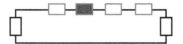

FIGURE 15.12
The plan of the office hall. Gray boxes indicate office doors, while the gray filled box indicates a notice board.

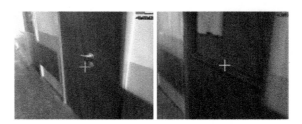

FIGURE 15.13
The difference between the notice board and an office door is small and hard to distinguish with touch.

Recognizing the notice board without prior knowledge could be difficult, since the door and the board are of the same height and width and both have a characteristic wooden edge.

This demonstrations aims at showing that the system can easily recognize the doors with computer vision techniques. Moreover, the system can count the doors and perform camera tracking for accurate camera position localization.

Navigation in an Unknown Place

Unknown places can be very stressful for the blind person. However, many of these, such as training centers, shopping malls, streets, hotel rooms, etc., can be easily annotated and semantically described. Moreover, taking advantage of social networks, both blind persons and their relatives can post their opinion about a particular place, threats, facts, etc.

The following demonstrates how the proposed system can help the blind person to move around an unknown environment, which is an example hotel room where a blind person spends some time during training. Commonly, for that person, an assistant would be assigned, and their responsibility is to take the blind person around the apartment and explain *what is where is what*. With the proposed solution, a blind person can explore the apartment on their own in a shorter time.

Threat Detection

Threat detection differs slightly from the object recognition cases described in the previous demos. First of all it, is more critical and requires a special approach (Tables 15.4 and 15.5).

If a dangerous object is not recognized in time, it may expose a blind person to serious injuries. What is more, a threat detector requires more sophisticated communication between the server and the local machine.

In particular, the system must information on a small set of dangerous objects that are likely to appear in the location where the blind person moves. Such a detection schema allows the preservation of the main system functionalities in the case where the communication channel (due to some technical reason) is unavailable or slows down.

TABLE 15.4

System in Operation: Object Recognition

Frame Sequence	Description
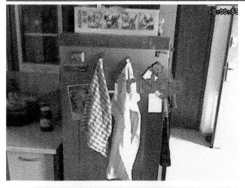	The fridge is detected. A spoken message is played by the system, and/or vibrations are used. Thanks to the stereovision camera, the distance can be measured. If the distance to an obstacle is too short, an appropriate warning message is generated.
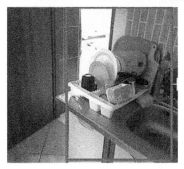	The sink is detected.
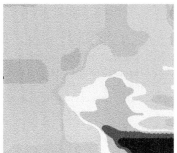	Gray boxes indicate colliding objects (top). An alert is generated. At the bottom, there is a depth map. Black color indicates short distance, while hatched pattern, long distance.

(Continued)

TABLE 15.4 (CONTINUED)

System in Operation: Object Recognition

Frame Sequence	Description
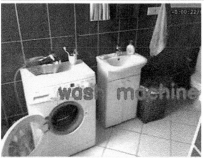	The washing machine is detected.
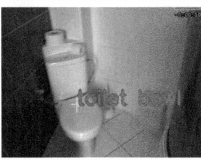	The toilet bowl is detected.

TABLE 15.5

System in Operation: Threat Detection

Frame Sequence	Description
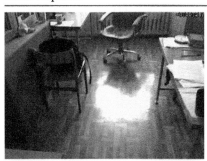	Initial frame. No dangerous objects are found.
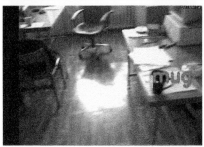	The mug is detected. The information is passed to the reasoning engine. It uses the ontology to infer. It maintains information that the mug may contain hot content that could expose the blind person to injury. The warning notification is played, and/or vibrations are used.

(Continued)

TABLE 15.5 (CONTINUED)

System in Operation: Threat Detection

Frame Sequence	Description
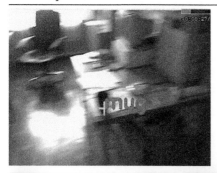	The mug is tracked.
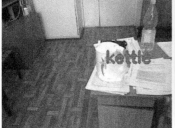 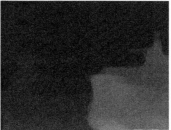	The kettle is detected. It is also classified as a dangerous object in the threat ontology. A warning message is played. Using the depth map, it can be inferred that the object is standing on corner of the table. This situation may be assigned high severity value since it is more likely that the blind person might spill the content when moving towards the obstacle.
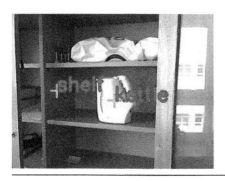	This situation is assigned lower severity value since the kettle is recognized together with the shelf where the kettle is supposed to be kept. Therefore, adjusting the system threshold for warning generation, the blind person might be informed only about severe threats if needed.

This demo shows some examples of dangerous object detection capabilities. The scenario concerns an indoor office environment. There are two dangerous objects: kettle and mug.

Indoor/Outdoor Obstacle Detection and Avoidance

Examples of obstacle detection are shown in Figures 15.14 and 15.15, respectively. In both cases, for visualization purposes, the presence of an obstacle (that is likely to cause a collision with the blind person) is marked with a black rectangle. For blind persons, information about the collisions is signaled with short beeping tones. That kind of source of information allows the blind person to have better awareness regarding traversability. As shown in Figure 15.15, the proposed algorithm can also successfully operate in an outdoor environment.

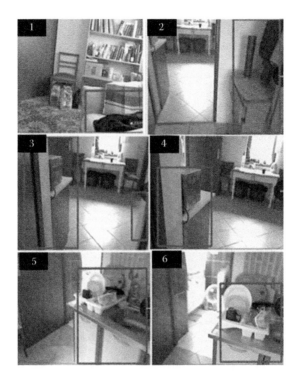

FIGURE 15.14
Indoor obstacle detection.

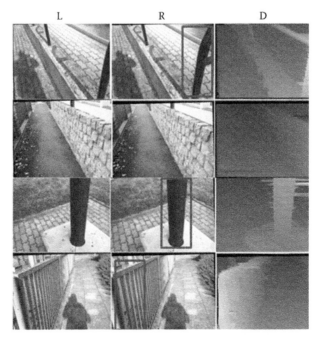

FIGURE 15.15
Outdoor obstacle detection.

Impact of the Presented Solutions on Inclusion of Blind People

Our propositions are fully compliant with the new EC Disability Strategy 2010–2020, published on November 15, 2010. In this document, the European Commission adopted a new strategy to break down the barriers that prevent persons with disabilities from participating in society on an equal basis. This strategy will try to improve the conditions of people with disabilities (also visually impaired and blind persons) and guarantee their rights for the next 10 years. One of the key pillars of this strategy assumes that disabled people will be able to make decisions about their lives and to execute daily activities in a fully independent manner.

Four main areas of action according to the EU strategy are as follows:

1. Providing unlimited access to goods and services
2. Increasing employment rates
3. Providing educational opportunities
4. Preventing social exclusion of disabled people

The strategy for the years 2010–2020 can be considered a continuation of the 2003–2010 EU Disability Action Plan, with similar assumptions and areas of actions.

The proposed solution is also compliant with the United Nations Convention on the Rights of Persons with Disabilities from May 2008.

The proposed solution enables all four of the mentioned areas, leading to social inclusion of blind people.

The proposed solutions aim at encouraging blind people to leave their homes and get along in unknown outdoor environments. They will also have significant influence on blind people's situations by enabling them to take up jobs, go out, and actively live in society.

The proposed solution is to provide guide dog capabilities. Guide dogs are the best help for blind people; however, only a small percentage of blind persons have such well-trained dogs. The cost of guide dog training is very high, while the proposed solutions will be cheap and accessible. The proposed solution will enable social interaction and inclusion, while unfortunately, a guide dog is often a problem and a barrier. As reported by a Polish TV news station, blind people with guide dogs are often not let in to markets, etc. [53].

The proposed innovations will increase social inclusion, safety, and independence of blind people. Nowadays, blind people, when moving in an unknown environment, depend solely on their senses, a guide dog, or company. The last two are often not available because of either high cost or lack of time, resulting in limited social inclusion, i.e., a blind person does not feel comfortable in an unknown area and thus tends to avoid related challenges, but also opportunities.

Moreover, proposed solutions aim at stopping/decreasing the *someone else* social factor. Now, very often, society labels blind persons as *someone else* (often unconsciously), which leads to avoiding social contact with blind people and social exclusion of such persons. It is worth mentioning that none of the solutions stigmatize a blind person and, in the long term, they are thought to be almost seamless. In general, the proposed solutions will impact inclusion of blind people by providing better mobility, more safety, new services, and better interfaces.

Conclusions

In this chapter, we presented innovative solutions for inclusion of totally blind people.

In particular, the major contributions of this chapter are as follows: an original system architecture, innovative portable devices and human–machine interfaces, computer vision and stereovision algorithms, innovations in multisensor DF, innovative situational awareness, ontology and risk assessment, as well as innovations in wireless personal telecommunications solutions.

Moreover, we discussed real-life scenarios and services. Sample cases and results were also demonstrated.

The proposed solutions aim at increasing inclusion of totally blind people and providing new services. However, the proposed innovations dedicated for blind people could also help people with other disabilities:

- People with other disabilities: the proposed innovations will provide innovation in mobility aid, risk assessment, communication, and interfaces.
- Deaf people: the proposed innovations will provide much-needed innovation in interaction with deaf people since we will not focus on audio/voice interfaces. We will provide innovative information distribution channels and interfaces (e.g., tactile). The proposed device (dedicated harness) can also be used by deaf people.
- Elderly: most solutions and services can be used by the elderly to help in daily living activities and independent mobility.

Acknowledgments

We would like to thank end users for their help and suggestions for our ideas, especially the Polish Society of the Blind in Bydgoszcz, Poland, and the Association for the Welfare of the Deafblind in Warsaw, Poland.

References

1. World Health Organization. WHO Fact Sheet N°282, May 2009. Available at http://www.who.int/mediacentre/factsheets/fs282/en/ (accessed May 26, 2011).
2. European Blind Union (EBU). Key facts and figures concerning blindness and sight loss. Available at http://www.euroblind.org/resources/information/nr/215 (accessed May 26, 2011).
3. Action For Blind People. Facts and figures about issues around sight loss. Available at http://www.actionforblindpeople.org.uk/news/media-centre/facts-and-figures,893,SA.html (accessed May 26, 2011).
4. Eurobarometer 54.2. European Commission, 2001.
5. Yang, X., and Tian, Y. Robust door detection in unfamiliar environments by combining edge and corner features. In *Proceedings of 12th International Conference on Computers Helping People with Special Needs (ICCHP)*, 2010.

6. Chen, Z., and Birchfield, S. Visual detection of lintel-occluded doors from a single image. In *IEEE Computer Society Workshop on Visual Localization for Mobile Platforms (in association with CVPR)*, Anchorage, Alaska, June 2008.

7. Gray, D., and Tao, H. Viewpoint invariant pedestrian recognition with an ensemble of localized features. In *ECCV '08: Proceedings of the 10th European Conference on Computer Vision*, 2008.

8. Wang, S., and Wang, H. 2D staircase detection using real AdaBoost. In *Proceedings of the 7th International Conference on Information, Communications and Signal Processing*, IEEE Press, Macau, China, pp. 376–380, 2009. 978-1-4244-4656-8.

9. Viola, P., and Jones, M. Rapid object detection using a boosted cascade of simple features. In *Proceedings IEEE Conf. on Computer Vision and Pattern Recognition*, 2001.

10. Chen, X., and Yuille, A.L. A time-efficient cascade for real time object detection. In *1st International Workshop on Computer Vision Applications for the Visually Impaired* (in association with CVPR 2005), June 2005.

11. Hanif, S.M., and Prevost, L. Texture based text detection in natural scene images—A help to blind and visually impaired persons. In *Proceedings of the Conference and Workshop on Assistive Technologies for People with Vision and Hearing Impairments: Assistive Technology for All Ages (CVHI-2007)*, Granada, Spain, August 28–31, 2007.

12. Sudol, J., Dialameh, O., Blanchard, C., and Dorcey, T. LookTel—A comprehensive platform for computer-aided visual assistance. In *Computer Vision and Pattern Recognition Workshops (CVPRW), 2010 IEEE Computer Society Conference on*, pp. 73–80, 2010.

13. Winlock, T., Christiansen, E., and Belongie, S. Toward real-time grocery detection for the visually impaired. In *Computer Vision and Pattern Recognition Workshops (CVPRW), 2010 IEEE Computer Society Conference on*, pp. 49–56, 2010.

14. Treuillet, S., Royer, E., Chateau, T., Dhome, M., and Lavest, J.-M. Body mounted vision system for visually impaired outdoor and indoor wayfinding assistance. In *Conference and Workshop on Assistive Technologies for People with Vision and Hearing Impairments Assistive Technology for All Ages CVHI*, 2007.

15. Lategahn, H., Geiger, A., and Kitt, B. Visual SLAM for autonomous ground vehicles. In *International Conference on Robotics and Automation (ICRA)*, 2011.

16. Liu, J.J., Phillips, C., and Daniilidis, K. Video-based localization without 3D mapping for the visually impaired. In *Computer Vision and Pattern Recognition Workshops (CVPRW), 2010 IEEE Computer Society Conference on*, pp. 23–30, 2010.

17. Strumiłło, P., Pełczyński, P., Bujacz, M., and Pec, M. Space perception by means of acoustic images: An electronic travel aid for the blind. In *ACOUSTICS High Tatras 06—33rd International Acoustical Conference—EAA Symposium*, Štrbsk Pleso, Slovakia, October 4–6, pp. 296–299, 2006.

18. Yu, Q., Araujo, H., and Wang, H. Stereo-vision based real time obstacle detection for urban environments. In *Proceedings of ICAR 2003 The 11th International Conference on Advanced Robotics*, Coimbra, Portugal, June 30–July 3, 2003.

19. Coughlan, J., and Shen, H. Terrain analysis for blind wheelchair users: Computer vision algorithms for finding curbs and other negative obstacles. In *Proceedings of the Conference and Workshop on Assistive Technologies for People with Vision and Hearing Impairments: Assistive Technology for All Ages (CVHI-2007)*, Granada, Spain, August 28–31, 2007.

20. Saez, J.M. First steps towards stereo-based 6DOF SLAM for the visually impaired. In *IEEE Conf. on Computer Vision and Pattern Recognition (CVPR)*, San Diego, CA, 2005.

21. Saez, J.M., and Escolano, F. Stereo-based aerial obstacle detection for the visually impaired. In *European Conference on Computer Vision (ECCV)/Workshop on Computer Vision Applications for the Visually Impaired (CVAVI)*, Marselle, France, 2008.

22. Medioni, G., Pradeep, V., and Weiland, J. Robot vision for the visually impaired. In *CVAVI10, IEEE International Conference on Computer Vision and Pattern Recognition (CVPR)*, 2010.

23. Lee, Y.H., and Medioni, G. RGB-D camera based navigation for the visually impaired. In papers from the USC Computer Vision Group, 2011.

24. Available at http://casblipdif.webs.upv.es/ (accessed May 26, 2011).

25. Ergonomic principles. Available at http://www.iso.org/iso/iso_catalogue/catalogue_tc/catalogue_tc_browse.htm?commid=53372 (accessed May 26, 2011).

26. ISO/TS 16071:2003. Available at http://www.stc-access.org/2008/04/18/iso-standards-for-usability-accessibility-software-documentation/#iso16071 (accessed May 26, 2011).

27. Available at http://www.mobileaccessibility.info/_ndphones-results.cfm (accessed May 26, 2011).

28. Available at http://www.codefactory.es/en/products.asp?id=326 (accessed May 26, 2011).

29. Available at http://www.rnib.org.uk/shop/Pages/ProductDetails.aspx category=phones product ID=HM3501 (accessed May 26, 2011).

30. Available at http://www.loadstone-gps.com (accessed May 26, 2011).

31. Available at http://www.ubergizmo.com/15/archives/2009/08/braille phone concept.html (accessed May 26, 2011).

32. Available at http://www.defense-update.com/products/f/_w-atd.htm (accessed May 26, 2011).

33. Available at http://telecom.esa.int/telecom/www/object/index.cfm?fobjectid=12843 (accessed May 26, 2011).

34. Hu, H., and Gan, J.Q. Sensors and data fusion algorithms in mobile robotics. Technical report: CSM-422. Department of Computer Science, University of Essex, United Kingdom, 2005.

35. Wilfried, E. An introduction to sensor fusion. Research report 47/2001. Institute fur Technische Informatik, Vienna University of Technology, Austria, 2002.

36. Zhou, Y., Leung, H., and Blanchette, M. Sensor alignment with earth-centered earth-fixed coordinate system. *IEEE Transactions on Aerospace and Electronic Systems* 35(2):410–418, 1999.

37. Raol, J.R., and Girija, G. Sensor data fusion algorithms using square-root information filtering. *IEE Proceedings—Radar, Sonar and Navigation* 149(2):89–96, 2002.

38. Goshtasby, A.A., and Nikolov, S. Image fusion: Advances in the state of the art. *Information Fusion* 8:114–118, 2007.

39. Zitova, B., and Flusser, J. Image registration methods: A survey. *Image and Vision Computing* 21:977–1000, 2003.

40. Stover, J.A., Hall, D.L., and Gibson, R.E. A fuzzy-logic architecture for autonomous multisensor data fusion. *Industrial Electronics, IEEE Transactions on* 43(3):403–410, 1996.

41. Koch, W. On Bayesian tracking and data Fusion: A tutorial introduction with examples. *Aerospace and Electronic Systems Magazine, IEEE* 25(7):29–52, 2010.

42. Cao, H., Leung, V., Chow, C., and Chan, H. Enabling technologies for wireless body area networks: A survey and outlook. *IEEE Communications Magazine* 42(12):84–93, 2009.

43. Pantelopoulos, A., and Bourbakis, N.G. A survey on wearable sensor-based systems for health monitoring and prognosis. *IEEE Transaction on Systems, Man, and Cybernetics, Part C: Applications and Reviews* 40(1):1–12, 2010.

44. Chen, M., Gonzalez, S., Vasilakos, A., Cao, H., and Leung, V. Body area networks: A survey. *Mobile Networks and Applications (MONET)*, 2010.

45. Ullah, S., Higgins, H., Braem, B., Latre, B., Blondia, C., Moerman, I., Saleem, S., Rahman, Z., and Kwak, K. A comprehensive survey of wireless body area networks. *Journal of Medical Systems*, 36:1065–1094, 2010.

46. Li, M., Lou, W., and Ren, K. Data security and privacy in wireless body area networks. *IEEE Wireless Communications*, 17:51–58, 2010.

47. Jang, C., Lee, D., and Han, J. A proposal of security framework for wireless body area network. In *Proceedings of International Conference on Security Technology—SECTECH '08*, 2008.

48. Raazi, S.M.K.-u.-R., Lee, S., and Lee, Y.-K. A novel architecture for efficient key management in humanware applications. In *Proceedings of International Joint Conference on INC, IMS and IDC—NCM'09*, 2009.

49. Raazi, S.M.K.-u.-R., Lee, H., Lee, S., and Lee, Y.-K. BARI: A distributed key management approach for wireless body area networks. In *Proceedings of International Conference on Computational Intelligence and Security—CIS'09*, 2009.

50. Jovanov, E. A survey of power efficient technologies for wireless body area networks. In *Proceedings of International Conference of the IEEE Engineering in Medicine and Biology Society*, 2008.

51. Kutty, S., and Laxminarayan, J.A. Towards energy efficient protocols for wireless body area networks. In *Proceedings of International Conference on Industrial and Information Systems—ICIIS*, 2010.
52. Shankar, V., Natarajan, A., Gupta, S.K.S., and Schwiebert, L. Energy-efficient protocols for wireless communication in biosensornetworks. In *Proceedings of IEEE International Symposium on Personal, Indoor and Mobile Radio Communications—PIMRC'01*, 2001.
53. Available at http://www.tvn24.pl/2116129,12690,0,314,1,wyrzucili-niewidoma-ze-sklepu,wideo .html (accessed May 26, 2011).

Section IV

Business Models and Study Cases

16

A Business Model for Ambient Assisted Living Solutions

Henrique O'Neill and José Duarte Realinho

CONTENTS

ABSTRACT   Ambient assisted living (AAL) stresses the importance of advanced information systems and communication technologies to satisfy the requirements of an ever-growing elderly population in areas like personal support, health care, and home care. This chapter presents a collaborative network business model that aims to bring together the distinct contributions of the different providers that are needed to offer these products and services. The model is being developed as a management decision-making support framework in the scope of the Ambient Assisted Living for All (AAL4ALL) project, aiming to highlight the stakeholders' benefits in joining this ecosystem. However, the recommendations presented may also be useful for those entities aiming to provide AAL products and services to the senior citizens' sector.

KEY WORDS: *ambient assisted living, Canvas framework, collaborative networks, business strategy model.*

Introduction

The health care and social care sectors in developed countries are facing major challenges arising from a set of factors such as the ageing population, the sharp increase in the number of people who suffer from chronic illnesses, the shortage of skilled human resources, the reduction of financial resources, increased regulation, and intense global competition.

Like many developed countries, Portugal also faces the challenges of population ageing. As depicted in Figure 16.1, there is a tendency for the base of the age pyramid to decrease over time, while the top tends to become larger, reflecting an increasing number of elderly people.

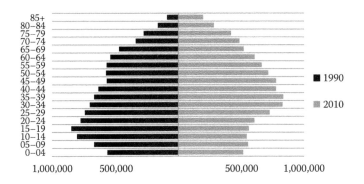

FIGURE 16.1
1990 and 2010 age pyramids. (Adapted from PORDATA, Estatísticas, gráfico e indicadores de Municípios, Portugal e Europa [Online], http://www.pordata.pt/, 2012.)

According to provisional data of the 2011 census, 19% of the population living in Portugal are over 65 years of age, and a mere 15% are less than 15 years old (Censos 2011). The ageing ratio of the population is 129, meaning that there are 129 elderly for every 100 young people. In 2001, this ratio was 102. The old age dependency ratio is 29, meaning that there are 29 elderly dependents for every 100 workers. In 2001, this ratio was 24.

Together with the ageing of the population, the issues of loneliness and elderly abandonment arise. Referring again to the predefinitive 2011 Census data, published in February 3, 2012, by the National Statistics Institute (INE), about 60% of the elderly living in Portugal live alone (400,964 people) or in the exclusive company of another elderly person (804,577).

It should also be noted that, according to the World Health Organization, chronic diseases are the major cause of death worldwide, representing 63% of all deaths (WHO 2013).

Nevertheless, these challenges create new opportunities for primary health care and social care service providers.

One way of addressing these challenges is undoubtedly bringing to light the potential of information and communication technologies (ICTs). However, the individual and atomized approaches that characterize the offer in this domain have not yet fulfilled expectations, despite the high level of technology and innovation incorporated in each of them.

The recurrent use of ICT as an answer to this challenge has justified the promotion of several actions, including the creation of the Ambient Assisted Living Joint Programme (AAL JP 2012). However, the AAL Association also itself identifies a set of barriers that hinder the successful implementation and deployment of ICT solutions in this domain: (1) the technology appears to be overly complex for the majority of its users; (2) in the European Economic Area, privacy and personal data protection laws are varied, and their disparity does not support the generalization of new or existing solutions; (3) the absence of a social standard (primary care standards regarding ambient assisted living [AAL]) that would permit the prescription and reimbursement of these solutions; and (4) the lack of a clear and well-defined business model.

To address these issues, this chapter emerges with the objective of presenting a business model for primary care regarding basic AAL services. An effective offer of AAL solutions requires the bringing together of a diversified set of providers able to blend products and services in the areas of health care, home care, and personal development (social and personal relations, psychological support, education and training, coaching, etc.) with information technology (IT).

To assemble such a set of competences and skills requires the setup and management of a collaborative network (Camarinha-Matos and Afsarmanesh 2005) involving all stakeholders—users, caretakers, and products and service providers—able to identify the business opportunities, to translate user requirements in suitable products, to foster synergies among potential partners, and to minimize the negative effects of rivalries.

The model has been developed in the scope of the Ambient Assisted Living for All (AAL4ALL) project and aims to set up the benefits the distinct stakeholder will have by joining the ecosystem (Figure 16.2).

AAL Stakeholders

To become successful, any business has to provide satisfactory answers to its stakeholders' needs. A stakeholder is a person, a group of individuals, or an organization with an

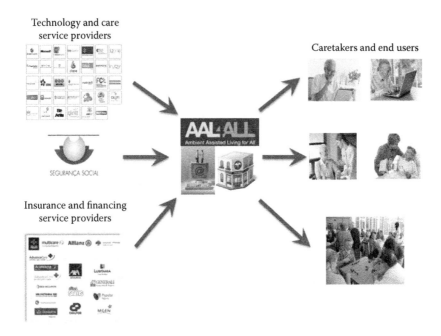

FIGURE 16.2
The AAL4ALL collaborative network.

interest in a particular business outcome, that is directly involved in its accomplishment or that is affected by the changes that are required for its implementation (Ward and Daniel 2006).

So, to start building a business model it is essential to identify and analyze the different stakeholders and how they will be affected by the business outcomes. Particular attention must be paid to the firm's customers (Marzo et al. 2007).

The AAL4ALL project has selected four different categories of stakeholders in the area of ICT for ageing, in line with the findings of other authors (BRAID Project 2010; Wright 2010). These are as follows:

- Private users of ICT for ageing solutions including senior and impaired citizens as well as informal caregivers, such as family members or friends (Primuscare 2012)
- Professional users of ICT for ageing solutions, including health care professionals, social care providers, nursing homes, or other service providers, such as housing associations. This group may also include *mobility* providers, such as senior tourist operators or public transportation services
- Suppliers of ICT for ageing solutions, comprising public and private research organizations as well as firms doing business in telemedicine or telecare, providers of the IT infrastructure, or small and medium-size technology service providers
- Other agents such as sponsors of ICT for ageing solutions, policy makers, social institutions and insurance companies, public administrations, standardization organizations, civil society organizations, or media

There are different relationships between these groups of stakeholders. For instance, the professional users of ICT for ageing solutions have a business-to-consumer (B2C) relationship with the group of private users, by selling their service solutions to this group. In another way, the professional users buy the ICT for ageing solutions from their technical suppliers.

Business Model Conceptual Background

Although the term *business model* is often used, it is possible to find several distinct definitions and perspectives about this concept, suggesting the lack of consensus that exists in the literature (Zott et al. 2010).

According to Lambert and Davidson (2013), the business model serves as a tool to analyze and communicate strategic choices. It is seen as a manifestation of strategy and articulates how a firm creates value, the internal sources of the firm's advantage, and how the firm will capture value.

To correctly describe the firm, a generic business model needs to address elements such as value proposition, i.e., the benefits the product or service brings to the customers; the firm's supply chain, describing the suppliers' relationship with the firm; the customer interface i.e., the firm's relationship with its customers; and the financial requirements concerning the incomes and the costs of the business (Boons and Lüdeke-Freund 2013).

Business Model Patterns

Specific aspects of some distinct business model patterns may be applicable in the context of the AAL health care and the social care sectors (Ferreira and Cunha 2006).

Unbundling Business Model

In an attempt to handle the complexity of vertically integrated businesses, the *unbundling* business model looks at the business activities across three basic types of components: customer relationship, innovation in products, and infrastructure. As each type has different economic, competitive, and cultural imperatives; the three types can coexist within a single society, but they are usually *unbundled* into separate entities to avoid unnecessary conflicts or *trade-offs*.

Long-Tail Business Model

Long-tail business models concentrate on selling less of more: The focus is on providing a great deal of niche products, each of which might not be sold with relative frequency. The combined sales of niche items can be as profitable as a traditional model where a limited number of bestsellers collect the most revenue. Long-tail business models entail few inventory costs but need strong platforms that allow niche content to be readily available to consumers interested in purchasing those products.

Multisided Business Model

Multifaceted business models congregate two or more distinct but interdependent groups of consumers. The platforms supported by this model only provide business value to a particular consumer group if the other consumer groups are also present. This model creates value by facilitating interactions between the different groups. The value of a multi-faceted platform increases in so far as it attracts more users and creates a synergetic effect.

Freemium

In a freemium business model, at least a substantial segment of consumers can benefit from a continuous free supply of offers. Different patterns enable the supply of offers with no additional costs. Another part of the business model or another segment of consumers funds the nonpaying consumers.

Open Business Model

Open business models can be used by companies to create and capture value through systematic collaboration with external parties. This can happen either from the outside inwards, by exploring external ideas within the company, or from the inside outwards, by providing to external partners ideas or assets that are dormant within society.

ICT-Based Business Models

According to Osterwalder and Pigneur (2010), in the areas of ICT, there have been countless types of business models adapted to the varying needs of individual companies or customer types. The authors identify the following models.

Dealer Model

This model occurs when there is a commercial trade between a given wholesaler and retailer, which is conducted electronically. This happens only when electronic data are exchanged: the company only sells via their website or an online catalogue, or via stores that function as online and offline distribution channels.

Brokerage Model

Companies that adopt this type of model are considered facilitators and market magnifiers because they enable transactions to occur, facilitating the contact between potential buyers and sellers. In general, the trader is entitled to a commission on the transactions that are carried out on their website, which has costs well below those charged by offline channels.

Subscription Model

Digital products can be sold through a subscription model. Consumers pay a periodic subscription fee in order to use a service or to access information. Owing to the high level of competition, sometimes, there is content and information with added value that is offered free of charge to consumers. This might cause consumers to generally expect to get information on the Internet for free. However, some of the most prestigious brands began charging their customers for certain services in electronic format that were already available in other formats with the general acceptance of the customers. This approach led to websites sharing information free of charge, and for a membership subscription, customers are able to access premium information. The adoption of this model is still viable seeing as there is a growing amount of information on the Internet, frequently leading consumers to prefer paying for information that is more objective. Various websites also make it possible for customers to pay exclusively for the content that suits their interests.

Manufacturer or Direct *Model*

This model allows manufacturers to directly serve the end user, eliminating middlemen and reducing the distribution channel and increasing efficiency. This enables a greater number of end consumers to be served in a more direct manner. This factor encompasses a better understanding of the preferences, tastes, and needs of different consumers, by offering a top-quality service. Manufacturers should take into account whether there is a *cannibalization effect* between the two services, which may lead to the occurrence of problems and conflicts between the two distribution channels (online and offline).

Community Model

Virtual communities may be defined as places that bring together people with a common set of interests or needs. While functioning as information transmitters, there are other functions that should be highlighted. The feasibility of this model is based on loyalty because members often adopt an emotional stance and devote much time to participating in the community. Revenues are derived from the sale of products and services, advertising, or voluntary contributions, related to the community shared topics. The Internet helps the development of broader communities because it allows people who live in different parts of the world to exchange ideas, knowledge, and information, as opposed to more restricted face-to-face gatherings.

Health and Social Care Business Models

In the field of telemedicine, there has been no compelling commercial success, although several pilot projects have been developed. This phenomenon can be explained by different factors (Österle and Osl 2010): consumers clearly benefit from face-to-face services, and there is some resistance to pay for access to the same type of services when offered online. Although providers may benefit from telemedicine solutions, the volume of business is marginal, and the technological interfaces and business procedures are often unfamiliar to them. The acquisition and integration of supplies requires technical expertise and the assurance of quality by the service integrator.

The same author identifies that key success factors for service integrators are as follows: the critical mass of consumers; the need for consumers not to be charged access fees; the need for service providers not to be charged flat rates; building trust with consumers through ratings and user reviews; focus on the consumers' points of interest; and creating benefits for all the members of the value chain.

Phillip Osl et al. (2008) define a checklist to guide the development of collaborative business models in the field of AAL. This checklist highlights the key success factors for a business to operate in AAL, focusing on the supply of its products and services, its processes and organization, and its marketing and revenue model. Regarding the supply of products and services, emphasis is given to the importance of fully grasping the demands of consumers. Nevertheless, there should also be ample supply of products and services and a modular construction of these products and services that will meet consumer demands and maintain the flexibility of supply. An adequate level of user configurable automation, allowing the extraction of information in the least intrusive way possible, must also be considered. In terms of processes and organization, the author defines the need for a comprehensive vision of the skills of all partners involved. Apart from avoiding any conflicting responsibilities, the role of the partners should be clearly defined, and that information should be set out in a legal contract. The organizational and technical interfaces should be defined in a concrete way as well as the mechanisms for scalability. A coordinator for the infrastructure network should be named. Long-term cooperation with all partners should be maintained, or at least, there should be clearly defined reaction mechanisms in the event of an abrupt end to collaboration, and collaboration risks for the network should be discussed. Lastly, network coverage should be verified and should meet consumer needs. Regarding marketing, the author regards it as necessary to have a clear and shared view of the value of the solutions offered to consumers; that the message conveyed is politically correct and relates to consumers' needs in the way they prefer; and that all the sales channels for the target consumer group are used. In the revenue model, the author identifies as important the definition of a flexible revenue model to address the different needs of consumers, together with ensuring that each partner has a realistic view of the revenue for themselves and others. Maintaining a list of prices for internal and external offers previously accepted and approved by all partners, and an agreement in relation to the distribution of risk across the network, eventually secures harmony on the revenue model level.

There is a need to seek, to develop, and to innovate in activities that can bring new products or solutions to the market, in less than 3 years after the completion of the project. It is essential that a business model for the sustainable development of these solutions exist. Business models must conceptualize the proper framework and involve different actors/ stakeholders that may generate value for the network. In this context, several projects arise as, for instance, those within the AAL JP (Ambient Assisted Living Joint Programme 2011).

For the scope of the AAL JP, the business model developed should not only involve companies and business partners but also take into account the creation of solutions that provide economic value, social value, and other types of value. This is because one must take public sector organizations and nonprofit organizations into account in the development of AAL business models. It is essential that they bring socioeconomic benefits to end users and take the partners' return on investment into account. In this case, more general lines of business should be developed, seeing that the most extensive development should be done during the preparation of business plans.

A business model needs to help find answers to several key questions about the firm (Wheelen and Hunger 2008). Who are the different stakeholders of the value chain? From the customers' viewpoint, the questions to be answered include the following: Which product/service is being provided? Who will purchase the product/service being provided (market segments)? What problems do these solutions solve, or what are the benefits for users? What is the added value of the developed products/services in comparison with what is currently on the market? Who can pay for it? How does the firm make money?

A business model also aims to help in answering the following logistics type of questions: How does the firm deliver its product or service? How will the product be sold? Who will provide it? What is the estimated cost of production? What is the estimated size of the market?

Considering the need to integrate distinct competencies, the model should also enable description of the following: Who are the consortium members that are involved in the value proposition for consumers? What is the role of the different partners in the implementation of the product/service? Do the partners have experience in the market/a position in the market? How do the partners derive benefits of the project's results, especially financially? What external stakeholders are required so that the proposed solutions can be implemented successfully? What are the risks and market barriers?

Finally, it is necessary to mention that the technologies and market evolutions require the business model to be dynamic, able to continuously control and monitor the firm's environment and behavior (Ferreira and Cunha 2006), and its implementation must be an ongoing and iterative process (Shafer et al. 2005).

The main concerns of the literature on business models is the shaping of people and of the activities in order to generate value for the organization, while in the case of health care and social care, the main context relates to the contribution to society (Valeri et al. 2010). Thus, when a business system is created in this context, the main concern is to identify the value that is generated for the distinct stakeholders: the patients, caretakers, medical doctors, psychologists, nurses, etc.

Developing a business model linked to health care and social care should take into account intangible elements, both internal and external, and only then should it consider the monetary requirements. The internal elements aim to improve health and social services, namely, the reduction of medical errors, decreasing the length of hospitalization, improving the image of health services, or a better quality of life. Externally, the social benefits are considered, such as reducing transport costs and time for healing provided by services such as telemedicine, or decreasing patient anxiety and stress.

Therefore, particular attention should be given to cost-effectiveness during the development of business models, never forgetting that the nonfinancial aspects must be considered and quantified. For this to happen, special attention should be paid to the following: personal limitations; the operating system and the maintenance tools, on the part of the user; time available for training; the limitation of formal and informal costs, including the development cost for increased usability; and acceptance performance levels.

Health Information Exchange Business Models

Particular attention must be paid to the health information exchange requirements. A health information exchange is a multistakeholder organization that enables or oversees the business and legal issues involved in the exchange and use of health information, in a secure manner, for the purpose of promoting the improvement of health quality, safety, and efficiency (Deloitte Center for Health Solutions 2006). Services essentially consist of clinical data exchange, e-prescriptions, push services, and radiology imagery.

Physician and Payer Collaborative

These companies are created by health care and paying customers in a given geographical area. They can take on the role of nonprofit organizations or for-profit organizations, but their main purpose is the exchange of mutual benefits between doctors and clients.

Health Care Unwired

The operational/clinic capabilities model extends traditional services with the aim of increasing access to information and reducing costs (Price WaterHouse Coopers 2010). These services can be carried out at long distance through monitoring health and well-being, which avoids the need for professionals to travel and reduces costs to users/hospitals. It is a way of monitoring and centralizing control and facilitates interaction.

The customer product/services model is based on consumer needs and is related to services that may be provided or are already provided through mobile devices. Examples are the monitoring of well-being and health, ongoing follow-ups, access to information in a timely manner with alerts, etc.

Business Legal Background

Business models have emerged in various forms, mostly based on several constraints, such as tax laws, monetary incentives, and control factors (e.g., representation of the community's interests or the interests of more restricted groups). They are usually related to the coordination of groups or are involved in developing solutions and/or implementing infrastructures. The legal background of business models may consider the following.

For Profit

For profit organizations are created with private funding and have very defined financial objectives, seeing their purpose and operations as based primarily on financial benefits.

Not for Profit

In this case, the business model is designed to help patients and communities in terms of service provision. These firms may be exempt from some state taxes as they try helping to reduce the drawbacks related to funding and fees and to provide credit and special incentives to end users.

Public Utility

These are companies that are created and maintained with the assistance of state/federal funds and provide their services to the state/federal governments. In this case, the major difference lies with the funding of these organizations.

AAL Business Model

In the scope of the AAL4ALL project, a business model aiming to identify and assess the benefits of the ecosystem from the perspective of the distinct stakeholders is being developed.

To enable a common understanding among all the stakeholders and project partners, the ecosystem business architecture was defined based on a widely used tool, the Canvas business model framework (Osterwalder and Pigneur 2010). This tool addresses four key business areas—clients, offer, infrastructure, and economical viability—and enables the detailing of nine business categories (Table 16.1):

Customer Segments

Based on stakeholder analysis, five different customer segments were identified in the AAL4ALL ecosystem. Each customer segment was classified according to its distinct value

TABLE 16.1

The Canvas Business Model Categories

Business Category	Description
Customer segments	The groups of people the firm aims to serve according to its business domain.
Value proposition	The products and services the firm offers aim to satisfy the requirements of its target customers.
Channels	The way the company influences its customers for communication, distribution, and sales purposes.
Customer relationships	Define the types of business relations the firm aims to establish with its customers, which may be personal or supported by automatic means.
Revenue streams	Represent the cash received from the customers, i.e., what distinct customer segments are willing to pay for the firm's products or services.
Key resources	Include the most important assets required for business development (physical, financial, intellectual, or human).
Key activities	These are the business processes required for the firm to operate.
Key partners	Alliances or partnerships with other firms, aiming to optimize their business outcomes.
Cost structure	Includes the distinct cost types the firm incurs to sustain its activity.

propositions, its needs, and its role in the ecosystem. The most important customers that have been identified are as follows: seniors and people with disabilities; informal caregivers, including family members and friends; formal health caregivers represented by nurses and doctors; health care service providers, referring to firms from the public, private, or social sectors, such as health centers, hospitals/health units or clinics; and social care service providers, also from the public, private, or social sectors, represented by professionals belonging to nursing homes, day centers, or home care institutions.

Value Proposition

A broad value proposition addresses the generic requirements of the different customer segments. The most important value proposition of AAL is to increase the quality of life of senior citizens, providing more autonomy, self-confidence, and independence for people inside their homes; to reduce the response time in case of emergency, to offer home care in a permanent way, and to facilitate access to health care services and social support; to create a set of solutions for increasing quality of life, available to a large group of users, at a competitive price; and to simplify access to and exchange of health information about the products and services, for a more efficient answer to the elderly citizens' needs.

From a clinical point of view, it is also important to facilitate the follow-up by the health care professionals, providing the best-quality health care information, and facilitating access to the patient's health records. To increase accessibility, comprehension and access to personal health diagnosis, in a fast and easy way, through electronic devices is also worth mentioning.

The requirements of specific customer segments must also be considered. For the formal caregivers, the business aims to do the following: to provide medical professionals and institutions with the required tools to improve the quality and efficiency of health care and, at the same time, to reduce its costs; to improve the coordination and information flow between all involved organizations; and to provide the tools and resources that ensure a better follow-up and monitoring of the senior patients or to enable a broader range of services to be provided through connection to a support center.

For the informal caregivers, the business proposition aims to provide the required tools to support permanent and efficient elderly care, reducing the associated effort, increasing the levels of security, and reducing the levels of anxiety of the elderly and of their relatives.

For the public and private institutions of the health system, the business proposition focuses either on reducing the expenses in human resources costs or on enabling improvement of the service level with the same costs. It also aims to provide access to certified AAL services and products benefitting from all the advantages that they carry, such as medical devices with specifications for interoperability, etc.

Channels

The AAL business will adopt TV, web, or mobile generic channels to reach its customers. This requires the development of applications and/or content that offer the possibility for acquisition, follow-up, and status assessment of products and services. Public and private health care and social care institutions, through the family and/or specialty doctors and nurses, may be considered to endorse the most adequate products and services according to their patients' needs. A commercial call center (outsourced) will be also available to present the AAL products and services or to clarify any doubts. This platform will be made available to any key partner institution or brand, enabling confidence to be transmitted to the target customers. Physical stores or specific areas integrated on the distinct partners' premises will also be considered, enabling personal contact (face to face), which promotes confidence and proximity between the client and the ecosystem.

To reach seniors and informal caregivers, the following channels will be considered: nursing homes, day centers, home care institutions, and private health care service providers. If the client already has any kind of service (e.g., home support), these institutions can provide any of the products and services made available by the ecosystem partners and get a monthly payment from the client. A fleet of mobile units (e.g., cars or vans) may be used to contact isolated clients (persons or institutions) to demonstrate all the advantages of the ecosystem product and services in a friendly and warm way.

The interactive channels (e.g., telephone, Internet, TV), which enable the customer to know the AAL solutions, watch videos, answer questions, and subscribe to the service, may be set up with the support of communication service providers. Other channels may be established through partnerships with companies that supply medical equipment or by promoting the solutions in professional medical conferences, exhibitions, and marketplaces. The formal caregivers and health system institutions may be reached through the health care professionals as they know the benefits of the AAL products and services and may suggest their use to their patients.

Customer Relationship

Distinct means will be adopted to enhance personal relationships with the members of the distinct customer segments. A personal assistant, highly trained in social care and dedicated to a small group of clients, enables continuous monitoring of customers, clarifying any doubts, and providing permanent contact, through the AAL call center or in the store (like a family doctor). Technical support on the products and services may be provided by trained professionals, able to help in the acquisition process, clarifying doubts or giving advice about the best solutions according to specific customer requirements.

Customized online services (applications or content) that can be used to communicate with the clients, in an automatic and fast way, like health reminders and marketing electronic leaflets, will also be adopted.

To answer to the specific requirements of formal caregivers and health care and social care institutions, a technical contact center (outsourced) will be available to support the AAL products and services and to clarify any customer doubts.

Revenue Streams

The business revenue will result from the sales of products and services. The acquisition of equipment (communication platform or devices) or services will finance the business operations. Depending on the value of the product, the support of financial partners (banks, insurance companies) may be necessary to enable renting or leasing the equipment. As in a modular system, services can be enhanced in several ways, so packages can be offered with basic, intermediate, or premium configurations, enabling the customer to subscribe to what best suits their needs. Paid publicity and advertisement services may be made available to providers in distinct channels, enabling the enhancement of awareness of their solutions and brands to potential customers. The certification process of the AAL products and services will be another source of revenue to maintain and improve this institution and its services.

Key Resources

Resources are required to set up the business infrastructure, the certification institution, and the business processes able to strengthen the products and brand position on the market. A commercial contact center will be needed to promote, follow up, and assess the acquisitions of products and services by the clients. A technical contact center will support the caregivers in clarifying doubts and giving advice. A website and an e-business platform, with B2C, business-to-business (B2B), and consumer-to-consumer (C2C) functionalities, will be used to enhance the dissemination, presentation and/or sales of products or services. Key resources also include specialized service platforms (health care, social care, e-learning), providing the management services required to coordinate the communications infrastructure that supports the AAL solutions (e.g., managing emergency signals associated with monitoring sensors) as well as services for online appointments (video calls).

Key Activities

To provide high-quality customer service is a key business driver. This requires development and enhancement of the AAL products and services by closing the links with customers and the synergies among suppliers. Key business activities include developing personalized service for each client through the distinct channels; providing close support; and creating empathy between the AAL brand, the professionals, and the users. To develop contracts and partnerships and to constantly increase the portfolio of products and service providers, as well as the customer base, become paramount to the success of the business. This requires defining accurate selection processes concerning product certification and partners' participation in the ecosystem, aiming to keep the best partners and providers to improve the credibility and visibility of the AAL brand. To set up and to continuously improve business processes will be necessary to understand customers' needs and to improve their level of satisfaction.

Key Partners

The AAL key partners include providers of products and technologies, health care and home care providers, telecommunications service providers, or leisure and education service providers. Home support service providers may be able to facilitate technology adoption and to provide a closer follow-up service and solutions assessment. Public health institutions may assume an important role in promoting this concept and the products and services, as well as in enhancing trust in the ecosystem image. Financial partners are necessary to provide clients with more affordable payment forms, like monthly renting, thus avoiding the need to purchase a product that may be expensive. Banking service operators (e.g., PayPal or SIBS) will be useful in supporting online acquisitions and subscriptions. Insurance companies may enable the acquisition of products and services, through health care plans. Technological partners, such as data centers, will be very important in hosting the application platforms and exchanging information and data between the different kinds of health care solutions the client can use. The distributors of products/services in the medical field may enable AAL to reach more specialized customers.

Cost Structure

The most important costs inherent to the business model are related to the implementation and maintenance of the website and e-business platforms; the commercial and technical contact centers; the telecommunication services; the distribution of the different solutions to the stores or clients; the data center usage or acquisition; and the quality assessment, tests, and usage trials. The operational costs for service delivery also include the marketing costs, like publicity, dissemination of the products to the potential clients, the customer relationship follow-up, and the product/service certification.

Table 16.2 summarizes the AAL business model key characteristics as identified by the AAL4ALL project.

Strengths, Weaknesses, Opportunities, and Threats Analysis

The implementation of an AAL collaborative network business model faces important challenges. This suggests trying to foresee the main opportunities and threats the business will have to face. On the internal side, the strengths as well as the weaknesses that differentiate this network from its competitors may also be identified (Lynch 2006).

Tables 16.3 and 16.4 present a strengths, weaknesses, opportunities, and threats (SWOT) analysis of the AAL4ALL ecosystem. The external analysis presents the opportunities and threats to the AAL market (Table 16.3), whereas the main strengths and weaknesses of the ecosystem are identified through an internal analysis (Table 16.4).

TABLE 16.2

AAL Business Canvas Representation

Key Partners	Key Activities	Value Proposition	Customer Relationships	Customer Segments
• AAL4ALL Partners • Providers of products and technologies • Health and home care providers • Telecommunications service providers • Leisure and education providers • Financial partners • Insurance companies • Home support service providers • Public health institutions • Data centers • Distributors of products/services in the medical field	• Develop a personalized approach to each client through the distinct channels • Increase the number of contracts and partnerships • Define and rigorously select the processes concerning product certification and partner participation in the ecosystem • Guarantee the quality of the logistic processes and of customer support • Understand the level of satisfaction and needs of the customers • Develop AAL4ALL products and services	• To increase the quality of life • To decrease the response time in cases of emergency • To create a set of solutions available to a large group of users • To simplify the access and exchange of health information • To facilitate clinical follow-up by the health care professionals • To increase the accessibility and access to as well as comprehension of personal health information • To provide professionals and institutions with the tools to improve the quality and efficiency of health care and to reduce the associated costs	• Personal assistant • Customized help • Customized electronic services • Technical contact center	• Seniors and people with disabilities • Informal caregivers (family, friends) • Formal caregivers (nurses, doctors) • Public health system (health centers, public hospitals/health units) • Private health system (private hospitals/health units, clinics)

(Continued)

TABLE 16.2 (CONTINUED)

AAL Business Canvas Representation

Key Resources	Value Proposition	Channels
• AAL4ALL brand and certification institution • Commercial contact center • Technical contact center • Communication structure to support AAL4ALL services • Website and e-business platform • Health services support lines	• Improve the coordination and information flow between all involved organizations • Provide the tools and resources that ensure a better follow-up and monitoring of senior patients • Provide a range of services connected to a support center • Provide informal caregivers with the required tools to support the elderly permanently and efficiently • Reduce physical and human resources in health institutions	• Physical stores and mobile units • TV, web, mobile • Public and private health care institutions • Commercial call center • Nursing homes, day centers, home care institutions • Communication platforms • Directly to health professionals • Companies supplying medical equipment • Medical conferences and exhibitions

Cost Structure	Revenue Streams
• Website and platform maintenance for the clients and partners • Commercial contact center • Telecommunication services • Transport of the different solutions to stores or clients • Information storage or data center usage or acquisition • Development of the prototypes, quality tests and clinical trials, production costs, and services provided • Marketing costs	• Product sales • Service subscription • Publicity and advertisement initiatives • Maintenance contracts of some equipment or services • AAL4ALL certification institution

TABLE 16.3

SWOT Analysis for the AAL4ALL Environment

	Opportunities	Threats
External	Demographic trends, namely, ageing population	End users' lack of financial capacity
	Technology trends	Uncertainty about the social security system
	Increased support for development programs on health	having become unsustainable
	Increasing acceptance of new technologies, especially by the elderly	Reduced likelihood of social support
	Lack of uniformly accepted solutions	Computer science and technology *illiteracy* in a good part of this population segment
	Lack of objective study on the real needs, which leads to solutions that are seldom adapted to suit the end user	Physical and motor difficulties leading to frustration when using technological products and resulting in disengagement from such products
	Tendency to reduce the length of hospitalization	Fragmentation of reimbursement and certification systems
	Tendency towards increased prevention and closer, ongoing monitoring of users and formal and informal caregivers	Lack of interoperability between ICT systems
	Increased number of people facing extreme solitude	Greater fragmentation in the markets pertaining to new technologies
	Computerization of health services	Legal aspects: compliance with standards, certification, and regulations
	Increased social responses	Inflexibility of the National Commission for Data Protection (CNPD)

TABLE 16.4

SWOT Analysis for the AAL4ALL Environment (Strengths and Weaknesses)

	Strengths	Weaknesses
Internal	Provide improved autonomy, self-confidence and mobility	Production costs are still high
	Promote a healthier lifestyle	Some solutions are too technologically driven and difficult to use
	Understand the lifetime preferred environment for anyone, at home	Heavy reliance on particular communications and energy infrastructures
	Increased safety, especially of those who possess limitations	Difficulty in ensuring comfort, volume, and autonomy
	Increased efficiency and productivity of resources	Hard cooperation between the different partners
	Extended working life	Customers with low life expectancy rates
	Integration with telecommunications companies, which already have an extensive network infrastructure connected to households	Difficulty in reaching out to customers through a direct channel
	Highly recognized ecosystem partners	Difficulty in establishing customer loyalty
	Various ways of capturing and acquiring clients	Size of the project, which may hinder supervision and control
	High range of products and services	Need to establish partnerships with large private health groups
	Different means of purchasing goods and services (economic benefits)	Lack of technical convergence
	Pioneers in the implementation of an ecosystem that will bring together various solutions that function in interoperability	
	Ensuring confidentiality of the information produced	
	Certification and interoperability of products	
	Products tailored to customer needs	

Conclusions

The dissemination and adoption of AAL solutions among senior citizens requires the complementary contribution of product and service providers in the areas of health care, home care, leisure, and education or flexible work. This chapter presents a business model and the management guidelines for a collaborative network that aims to bring together these contributions. The identification of stakeholders and the assessment of their requirements was an initial step that enabled detailing the business architecture. The Canvas framework was used to describe the customer segments, the value proposition, and all the other business categories.

A more detailed analysis was done from the suppliers' perspective to stress the benefits the AAL4ALL partners may have by joining the ecosystem.

A collaborative network seems a promising approach to set up the AAL4ALL ecosystem in the near future, when the research project results will be mature enough to reach the marketplace. The framework presented in this chapter is an initial contribution to start building the vision of such a collaborative network in the AAL4ALL project environment. Although it is an interesting option from a conceptual point of view, the practical details impose significant challenges to the implementation of a collaborative network. These challenges rise in domains like technology, management, and organization as well as personal and business behavior.

The technological challenges arise from the need to address such a broad set of distinct application environments—health care, social care, home care—and satisfy very specific functional requirements according to the end users' needs, in particular, in terms of usability and interoperability. The AAL4ALL project aims to address this issue by providing a certification process for the AAL products and services that wish to join the ecosystem, contributing to meeting the high standards the ecosystem aims to provide for their customers.

From a managerial and organizational point of view, the model presented in this chapter proposes a coordination unit for the AAL4ALL ecosystem whose mission will be to encourage collaboration between customers and suppliers, thus fostering a marketplace for AAL products and services. To facilitate access to AAL solutions, several web platforms will be made available to the providers, to promote their services and products among their customers and users, in domains like e-commerce, e-learning, e-health care, and e-social care.

However, the implementation of the collaborative network requires the partners to be able to cooperate in a deep way. And this becomes one of the most critical factors for the successful implementation of the business model.

Cooperation is not the most usual attitude among private firms and business people, who usually see the market place as a competitive arena. Even nongovernmental or nonprofit private organizations in the social sector tend to compete for the limited resources that are made available.

However, the demographic trends impose a new paradigm where cooperation assumes a special role, as a way to answer to the needs of an ever-growing elderly population, which simultaneously faces a reduction in the financial resources that are available for social care.

To encourage cooperation between AAL products and services suppliers becomes a key challenge for the success of the AAL4ALL ecosystem and a key objective of the coordination unit previously mentioned. The business model proposed in this chapter aims to provide an answer to these challenges, which are also shared by most entities aiming to thrive in the AAL solutions sector.

Future Work

The next step will be to develop a detailed business strategic plan, where development scenarios and an implementation program will be described, aiming to materialize the preliminary proposals of the business model.

Acknowledgments

The authors would like to thank the Portuguese Quadro de Referência Estratégica Nacional and Compete programs that have sponsored the AAL4ALL research project. They also want to show their gratitude to the AAL4ALL partners, in particular, those involved in the business model specification: Citeve (Graça Bonifácio); Faculdade de Ciências e Tecnologia–Universidade Nova de Lisboa (Luis M. Camarinha-Matos, Ana Inês Oliveira, Filipa Ferrada, João Rosas); Exatronic (Mariana Neto Costa); FhG (Filipe Sousa); Inovamais (Gil Gonçalves); Intellicare (Soraia Rocha, Ana Leitão); and Microsoft (Lucas Garcia, Guilherme Esmael).

References

Ambient Assisted Living Joint Programme. (2011). Call for Proposals 2011—AAL-2011-4.
Ambient Assisted Living Joint Programme. (2012). ICT for Ageing Well. Retrieved from http:// www.aal-europe.eu/about/objectives/ (accessed June 12, 2012).
Boons, F., Lüdeke-Freund, F. (2013). Business models for sustainable innovation: State-of-the-art and steps towards a research agenda. *Journal of Cleaner Production* 45, 9–19.
BRAID Project. (2010). Report on mechanisms for stakeholder co-ordination. Retrieved from http:// auseaccess.cis.utas.edu.au/sites/default/files/BRAID%20D3%20-%20Mechanisms%20Final .pdf.
Camarinha-Matos, L. M., Afsarmanesh, H. (2005). Collaborative networks: A new scientific discipline. *Journal of Intelligent Manufacturing* 16, 439–452.
Censos. (2011). Retrieved from http://censos.ine.pt.
Deloitte Center for Health Solutions. (2006). Health Information Exchange (HIE) Business Models: The path to sustainable financial success. Chicago, IL: Deloitte Center for Health Solutions. Retrieved from http://www.providersedge.com/ehdocs/ehr_articles/Health_Info_Exchange _Business_Models.pdf.
Ferreira, R. F., Cunha, C. A. (2006). *Estratégia e Negócio Electrónico*. Porto, Portugal: SPI—Sociedade Portuguesa de Inovação.
Lambert, S. C., Davidson, R. A. (2013). Applications of the business model in studies of enterprise success, innovation and classification: An analysis of empirical research from 1996 to 2010. *European Management Journal* 31, 668–681.

Lynch, R. (2006). *Corporate Strategy*, 4th Edition. Upper Saddle, NJ: Financial Times/Prentice Hall.

Marzo, M., Pedraja, M., Rivera, P. (2007). The customer concept in university services: A classification. *International Review on Public and Non Profit Marketing* 4 (1/2), 65–80.

Osl, P., Sassen, E., Österle, H. (2008). A Guideline for the Design of Collaborative Business Models in the Field of Ambient Assisted Living, Ambient Assisted Living, Proc. 1. Deutscher AAL-Kongress, VDE, Verlag, Feb. 2008, Paper 2.3.4.

Österle, H., Osl, P. (2010). The Crux with the AAL Business Models, AAL Forum, Odense.

Osterwalder, A., Pigneur, Y. (2010). *Criar Modelos de Negócio*. Lisboa: Publicações Dom Quixote.

PORDATA. (2012). Estatísticas, gráfico e indicadores de Municípios, Portugal e Europa. Retrieved from http://www.pordata.pt/ (accessed June 12, 2012).

Price WaterHouse Coopers. (2010). *Healthcare Unwired*. Health Research Institute. Retrieved from http://www.pwc.com/us/en/health-industries/publications/healthcare-unwired.jhtml (accessed March 27, 2010).

Primuscare (2012). Retrieved from http://primuscare.com/cuidados-informais-ou-formais (accessed March 27, 2012).

Shafer, S. M., Smith, H. J., Linder, J. C. (2005). The power of business models. *Business Horizons* 48, 199–207.

Valeri, L., Giesen, D., Jansen, P., Klokgieters, K. (2010). Business Models for eHealth. European Commission DGINFSO ICT for Health, pp. 11–15. Retrieved from https://www.myesr.org/html/img/pool/business_models_eHealth_report.pdf.

Ward, J., Daniel, E. (2006). *Benefits Management: Delivering Value from IS and IT Investments*. Chichester, UK: John Wiley & Sons, Ltd.

Wheelen, T., Hunger, D. (2008). *Strategic Management and Business Policy: Concepts and Cases* (Vol. 11). Upper Saddle, NJ: Pearson Prentice Hall.

WHO. (2013). World Health Organization. Retrieved from http://www.who.int/topics/chronic_diseases/en/ (accessed December 20, 2012).

Wright, D. (2010). Structuring stakeholder e-inclusion needs. *Journal of Information, Comunication and Ethics in Society* 8 (2), 178–205.

Zott, C., Amit, R., Massa, L. (2010). *The Business Model: Theoretical Roots, Recent Developments, and Future Research*. Barcelona: IESE Business School.

17

Social Innovations and Emerging Business Models in the Field of Ambient Assisted Living: Reflection on a Pilot Project

Katrin Schneiders and Ralf Lindert

CONTENTS

ABSTRACT   The article considers ambient assisted living (AAL) from an integrated social sciences and economic perspective. Technologies and services based on AAL offer a wide range of new possibilities for use in residents' own home environment, which reached public attention as the so-called third health site. Cross-linked living is on no account limited only to the integration of modern information and communication technology (ICT) into people's homes but also extends to the social linkage of different industries, technologies, and their relevant actors in order to overcome the interfaces between the involved areas. So far, in Germany, only a few innovative AAL projects have been transferred successfully into continuous operation after the expiry of the project phase. Their implementation is accompanied by many challenges, e.g., insufficient service orientation, low acceptance within the target group, and the lack of business models. Innovative services under the concept of *smart and independent living* can be referred to as an innovation at the interface between technology and social issues. The reasons for these problems are, of course, manifold. Our thesis therefore is that the problems during the process of implementation are attributed to the lack of coordination of social, technical, and economic issues and interests. The case study *service4home* that we sketch can be seen as an attempt at a multidisciplinary social, technical, and economic innovation.

KEY WORDS: *business models,* the home *as the third health care site, housing industry, social innovation, social services, diffusion, potential analysis, welfare mix, care, home care, interface management, demographic change.*

Introduction

The article considers ambient assisted living (AAL) from an integrated social sciences and economic perspective. The current discussion on this subject is mostly technology oriented. Under the influence of demographic shift, the German health system will meet its financial limits in the foreseeable future. Thus, people's home environment in addition to inpatient and outpatient care has reached public attention as the so-called third health site. But so far, in Germany, only a few innovative AAL projects have been transferred successfully into continuous operation after the expiry of the project phase. Their implementation is accompanied by many challenges, e.g., insufficient service orientation, low acceptance within the target group, and the lack of business models. Therefore, spotlights of the analysis are on economic and sociologic considerations for innovative service offerings under the concept of *smart and independent living*, which can be referred to as an innovation at the interface between technology and social issues. Especially, technologies and services based on AAL offer a wide range of new possibilities for use in residents' own home environments for the target group, mostly elderly people. Cross-linked living is on no account limited only to the integration of modern information and communication technology (ICT) into people's home (environments) but also extends to the social linkage of different industries, technologies, and their relevant actors in order to overcome the interfaces between the involved areas. After addressing (1) social innovations and (2) identified emerging business models in the field of AAL, the authors combine both perspectives together to identify obvious interdependencies and to demonstrate the need for an integrated approach. By using a case study of a service agency, which can be seen as an attempt at a multidisciplinary social, technical, and economic innovation, the authors describe several steps in the implementation of an AAL pilot project. The information gained by means of continuous monitoring and identified variations between the plan and actual parameters during the evaluation of the pilot phase, also taking into consideration the results of the preliminary study, allows a critical review of the actual status, of both social innovations and appropriate business models, for successful implementation of social services at the health care site *at home*.

Demographic Change, Age-Appropriate Living, and *Service4home*

Demographic change and its impact on society and the economy are, perhaps, currently one of the most greatly discussed socioeconomic trends in Germany and many other Western European states. Although the changes to the population's age structure have been known for decades and have been comprehensively documented in the form of statistics, an extensive political and societal discussion in Germany regarding the issue only started several years ago. Following years of suppression—in part due to Nazi Germany's population policies—the topic has now made it into the public and political domain. However, there has been a certain change in perspective in recent times. Up until only a few years ago, the aging of society was almost exclusively considered as a threat and a burden for the positive future development of the economy and society. The increasing number of elderly people, especially the drastically rising number of very old people and those in need of care, was seen not only as an almost insurmountable challenge for the social security systems but, at the same time, as a sign of the important reasons behind the decline of innovation.

Demographic Change as an Opportunity

This perception of prospects for the aging society began changing only a few years ago. The deficit theory, which, for a long time, had dominated the discussion, was pushed aside in favor of highlighting expertise and potential. It is increasingly emphasized that a longer life expectancy should be seen as a success for society, politics, and the economy. On the other hand, politics and the economy are more frequently realizing that the specific interests of elderly people are a good basis for generating demand and increasing both turnover and employment through products and services that are geared toward the needs of the elderly generation (Heinze et al. 2011).

If demographic change is regarded as a challenge, and not as a threat, then the focus falls on new alliances between various actors and their readiness to network the diverse areas of knowledge. In light of the fact that the *baby boom generation*, which boosted the population, will become senior citizens over the next few years, the innovation opportunities that accompany demographic change need to be explored. Germany is still on the *right side* in a demographic sense (Kaufmann 2005), but as the *pioneering country* of declining birth rates, it is, to a certain extent, called upon to go down new paths in order to activate the potential of the aging society (Bischoff and Brauers 2006). For the housing sector, this basically means turning away from the classic view of housing provision and taking the insights offered by innovation research seriously. The interaction between various technologies and services offers up interesting new perspectives. This view has been a topic for discussion in comparable countries for quite some time, and there is a series of interesting projects with regard to the potential and networking structures in the areas of both health care and living (de Jong 2007). It is not only studies on the future that talk of living as a central raison d'être and a growing utilization of housing space. As a general rule, the older a person gets, the greater the amount of time they spend at home (Schneiders 2010). As a person's physical and mental capabilities generally change with age, environmental factors for their own well-being are becoming increasingly important (Wahl and Oswald 2010). Physical vitality correlates with an easier adjustment to favorable and unfavorable environmental factors. This means that a physically healthy person notices no deficit when faced with factors such as a living environment containing barriers. However, these unfavorable conditions have a negative impact on the lifeworld and well-being of elderly people with decreased mobility, if their daily routine can only be carried out with a great deal of effort. The result of age-related factors is simply that people's *spatial radius of action becomes smaller* (Backes 1998; Saup and Reichert 1999). The living area therefore occupies a central position in the daily life of elderly people; it is a place where they communicate, enjoy their social life, and spend their free time. The home, being considered in the context of a public space, increasingly becomes the focal point of their lives. This has also been proved by the findings of time–budget studies looking into elderly people's daily routines (Little 1984; Engstler et al. 2004).

Housing for the Elderly—A Business Area with Substantial Potential

In Germany, no more than 5% of people aged over 65 currently live in old people's homes (BMVBS 2011). All of the studies into elderly peoples' housing wishes and needs show that the overwhelming majority of them want to remain in their familiar living environment as long as possible, even when they need assistance and care (BKK Bundesverband 2009; Philips 2010; KKH-Allianz 2011; TNS Emnid 2011). The composition of elderly people's living and housing environments is therefore of significant importance in terms of social, economic, and employment-related perspectives, and can be considered an area of business with enormous future potential.

A significant amount of newly constructed flats in Germany have been designed to be suitable for disabled and elderly people. The area of constructional housing adaptation measures has been expanded. Housing construction companies in particular, as well as advisory professions such as architects and social workers, are highly involved in this area. Constructional features are, however, only one facet of high-quality housing that is suitable for elderly people (BMVBS 2011). In addition, there are also the demands for the infrastructural setup of the housing environment with regard to public facilities and services, as well as the social environment.

Close-to-Home Social Service Offers Not Yet Implemented across the Whole of Germany

While various architectural solutions and technical equipment have been developed in line with the constructional requirements for housing suitable for the elderly, which are increasingly subject to legal norms and quality standards, models for the integration of close-to-home and social service provision are still in their infancy. However, high-quality living for elderly people, particularly with regard to the onset of mobility restrictions, is only guaranteed when there is a service provision that meets their requirements. In addition, although measures in the living area, whose strategic development is predominantly driven forward by AAL (for information on AAL, see the work of Tang and Venables 2000; VDE

2007; Mukasa et al. 2008), are at a high level of development in technical terms, they have not been implemented to a great degree (Gersch et al. 2010; Heinze et al. 2011; Lindert 2011a).

Furthermore, the development of a workable business model is identified as one of the main challenges in the implementation of such innovations. It seems to be essential to also consider, as early as the premarket phase, both the ability of the conception and development of AAL operation scenarios to be economically marketed after the project phase has expired and the required value creation and business model architectures. This is particularly the case for areas that are characterized by high levels of state regulation as well as a public or parafiscal cost-bearing structure, and in which the people's individual willingness to pay (currently) plays only a subordinate role. Other aspects are also closely linked to this: insufficient service orientation, lack of acceptance in the target group, (disproportionately) high specific investments in ICT, and finally, underestimated diffusion barriers for those involved in the diffusion process. As part of the development of a business model, friction also arose, which can be traced back to the varying action orientation or forms of organization of the actors involved. Calculating prices for individual services became difficult when several service providers with different legal forms (private commercial as well as free charitable/nonprofit) were involved in the provision of services. There were also legal issues related to labor and liability, whose importance and response were very differently weighted or interpreted depending on action orientation or organization type. The welfare mix, which is repeatedly propagated in German and international research into social policy, fails partly due to these organizational and institutional hurdles.

Services for an Ageing Society

Social services, which have been enjoying a positive development since the 1970s, have particularly contributed to a labor policy–related increase in importance for service activities on the whole in Germany. The market for social services is today considered a *mega market* (Schramm 2007). Social services in a more specific sense include the sectors of health care, social care, care for children and young people, education, and assistance for people with special circumstances. According to the latest estimates, between 8 and 10 million people are employed in this field. Expenditure in this segment accounts for just under 20% of the gross domestic product (GDP) (Meyer 2008). According to conservative estimates, over half of the total volume of social services provided in Germany now concern services for elderly people (Heinze et al. 2011).

The social services sector for elderly people is characterized by a high level of heterogeneity. Social services, in a more specific sense, can thus always be part of the discussion surrounding important sociopolitical services for people that aim to alleviate or overcome specific immaterial situations of assistance and needs in the context of social risks and problems (Bäcker et al. 2010). Contrary to corporate and production-oriented services, social services are always directly aimed at natural people (people-related services) or indirectly aimed at people in their particular household environments (household-related services).

Social Services—A Multifaceted Sector

Health care services (primarily in the field of treatment, therapy, rehabilitation, and care), child care, education, and counseling can be considered people-related social services. In addition, there are also more household-related social services, i.e., services that serve to help people live their daily lives at home in an independent way and which are provided for (mainly elderly and/or disabled) people who are no longer able to do so or for those who appreciate them as supportive convenience services. This entails cleaning services, shopping services, accompanying and visiting services, food services, and security services (Schneiders 2010).

Even though being old cannot simply be equated with a requirement for assistance and support, there is empirical evidence for structural age-related immaterial social risks and problems with the resulting increased need for social services (Kuhlmey and Schaeffer 2008; Heinze et al. 2011). This is predominantly the case for people who are old or very old. When multimorbidity—i.e., suffering from numerous illnesses at the same time and the resulting decreased functions—increases, the chronification of severe illnesses increases, as does the risk of the person needing care at an exponential rate. The cases of depression and dementia also increase. At the same time, the number and the proportion of one-person households increase (*singularization of old age*) (DESTATIS 2011). In addition, social contacts and networks with social-support functions decrease, whereas (health-related) mobility restrictions increase. On the whole, the need for assistance and support for *daily activities* increases, and as result, increases the risk of elderly people not being able to maintain an independent lifestyle. Nonetheless, the overwhelming majority of elderly people are not affected by the typical age-related social risks. If one takes 65 as a threshold, for instance, then this currently applies to only between 15% and 20% of people aged 65 and above. However, if one considers people aged 80 and above, then the strongest growth rates in this regard are to be expected (Rothgang 2008). In this respect, the demographic trend of people reaching old age can be considered as the real driving force behind the need for social services in the area of assistance and care-oriented services (Schneiders and Ley 2010).

From a sociopolitical perspective, social services for elderly people can be split into the following categories:

- Measures to ensure integration
- Measures to support an independent life style
- Measures when assistance and care are required (Naegele and Gerling 2007)

Social Services Greatly in Need, but Demand Remains Low

It may now be assumed that there is a comprehensive, quality-assured service provision only with regard to care services, primarily due to the reimbursement possibilities through care insurance. A large number of housing companies have been trying since the 1990s to establish additional service provision for their elderly tenants in particular. These activities were often stopped due to a lack of demand. Whereas the need for people- and household-related services has been proven time and time again through various studies, the willingness to pay remains too low to be able to establish an appropriate service offer that is at least economically viable (Schneiders and Eisele 2006, 2007; Schneiders 2010; Schneiders and Ley 2010).

Over the course of the demographic and simultaneously occurring sociocultural change, the need for household-related services is developing further across generations. The number of couples without children and single people is constantly on the rise (DESTATIS 2011). At the same time, a pluralization of lifestyles is perceptible: same-sex partnerships, multilocal family structures (where family members often live far apart due to work), and patchwork families are becoming increasingly common (Peuckert 2008). Against this backdrop, family support structures for elderly people are becoming less reliable and need to be complemented with or replaced by other informal and/or formal assistance or service systems. It is therefore not only elderly people but younger generations as well that are dependent on extrafamilial support services. As a result of more women pursuing careers, successfully combining career and family is only possible with reliable formal and informal assistance systems. For couples without children and single people, household-related and close-to-home services mean a substantial increase in quality of life and time, when it has been agreed that household-related services, such as letting workpeople into the home and supervising them, help with shopping, cleaning services, etc., can be provided during their work-related absence. With regard to the motivation behind using household-related services, people needing the service can be split into two groups. The first comprises people who make use of the service due to time constraints. The second includes people who do not have the ability to carry out these activities themselves. With people getting older and the age-related restrictions they face, it is this second group of people that is becoming more important (BMFSFJ 2005; Geissler 2010).

Increasing Need for Household-Related Services

A result of the current demographic development is the risk of elderly and morbidly ill people becoming isolated, particularly those who do not have children. Even today, roughly 10% of people aged 70–85 say that they have nobody who can help them around the home. This societal development of decreasing familial networks will benefit the demand for social, health care-, and household-related services. The rising number of elderly people with specific needs and consumption structures will lead to increasing expenditure for personal and household-related services. At present, public funding in the area of household-related services in particular remains underdeveloped or even in decline (particularly since the introduction of care insurance). This gives rise to market opportunities for commercially run initiatives (BMFSFJ 2005). Voluntary and professional services in the field of caring for and looking after old people will become more important in the long-term (Kohli 2000; Link 2003). Even now, social and household-related services are considered a growth market from a labor-policy perspective (Heinze 2009; Schneiders 2010; Heinze et al. 2011).

High Level of Interest, Low Willingness to Pay

The extent to which elderly people need or want housing-related services is the subject of much debate. As early as 1997, Heinze et al. observed that a large part of the 55- to 75-year olds polled expected to need a multitude of housing-related and other social services in the future. The spectrum of the services mentioned ranged from cleaning services for the home and building to support for shopping, food services, and physical care to free-time services. Only a fraction of the people polled at the time were, however, actually making use of the said services. Only demand for household-related services, such as cleaning and winter services, reached notable levels. In addition, the amount of money set aside for such services was very low; the overwhelming majority of tenants named a personal maximum budget of EUR 100 per month (Heinze et al. 1997).

This growing economic importance of the service sector has led to intensive research in this field in recent years. Nonetheless, research into services (even that conducted by the German research association DFG) is, on the whole, very weak. It has become clear from the existing research activities that services, much like material goods, need to be developed in a more systematic and target- and result-oriented manner than has hitherto been the case (Herrmann et al. 2005).

A further development arises through demographic change. The birth rate has been stagnant at a level below the mortality rate for years. Although the population deficit has, so far, been offset by immigration, the declining trend will not be able to be stopped in the future. Demographic effects are already impacting the housing market (Schneiders 2010). It is therefore also in the interest of companies that build homes to keep the quality of housing and general housing satisfaction at a constantly high level, in order to act now to counteract the level of vacancies there are likely to be in the future. Elderly people in particular have been increasingly considered as an interesting group of tenants in recent years (Schneiders 2001, 2004, 2010; Schneider et al. 2002; Narten and Scherzer 2007). Many of them are still the *first occupants* in houses constructed in the 1950s and 1960s, which have not undergone constructional or technical work to fulfill the specific needs of elderly people (Schneiders 2010).

High Level of Housing Satisfaction among Elderly Tenants

It is primarily tenants who have built up a longstanding connection with their living environment who express less desire to improve it. In this context, ecogerontological research observes the so-called residential satisfaction paradox, which is closely tied to intensive personal feelings of belonging to one's own living environment (see *Erinnerungslandschaften* [landscapes of memory] in the work of Wahl and Oswald 2007) and states that elderly people are positive and happy about their living situation even if it is not in line with their current situation regarding needs and life.*

It is only when they find themselves in acute deficiency or disability situations, or in direct comparison to possible attractive housing alternatives, that their level of residential satisfaction falls.

Elderly people not only appear to be positive, largely undemanding tenants to housing associations, but they also form an important group of tenants in a qualitative sense: "Senior citizens are mostly reliable tenants, and are not expected to make too much noise or cause damage by vandalising property. They are also ascribed better morals with regarding to paying rent. It is also to be hoped that elderly tenants will stabilise the neighborhoods" (Schneiders 2010).

Elderly Tenants as Stabilizing Factors for Neighborhoods

It is not only housing associations that benefit from satisfied elderly tenants in the long term, as elderly people's satisfaction with their own housing situation can have positive effects on their general satisfaction with life. According to European studies, living independently in their own homes in an inner-housing living environment that they are accustomed to supports both the objective aspects of housing as well as subjective housing experiences, which are, in turn, linked to feelings of autonomy and comprehensive well-being (Wahl and Oswald 2007). Elderly people who are able to continue living in their familiar housing environment exhibit significantly lower levels of depression, feel more

---

* Over 84% of the 45- to 85-year olds consider their living situation to be *very good* or *good*, despite objectively measurable differences regarding living conditions (see Wahl and Oswald 2007).

independent when carrying out daily activities, and have a stronger feeling of belonging to their housing environment, regardless of cultural–societal framework conditions.

A generally satisfying living situation not only can have an extremely positive effect on life expectancy but also potentially prevents age-related depression, which, as a problem with a high number of estimated unreported cases, should not be underestimated. If an elderly person has a positive outlook on life, they will, on average, live for 7.5 years longer than elderly people who have lost their purpose in life. Early prevention and the activation of neural reserves are of fundamental importance in this regard (Priebe 2006; Kruse 2008).

Residential Quarters as a Place for Intergenerational Exchange

It is to be expected that extrafamilial assistance relationships will be of growing importance in the future due to changing and differentiating family structures. Even today, elderly people receive a relatively large amount of extrafamilial informal assistance from friends and acquaintances. Studies into the amount of such support services show that between 11% and 20% of all elderly people requiring assistance (need to) rely on support from people who are not part of their family. Nonetheless, informal extrafamilial assistance often remains restricted to intragenerational exchange, i.e., the young help the young, and the old help the old. Accordingly, both the Enquete Commission Demographic Change and the German government's reports on the situation of the elderly call for voluntary social commitment to be developed in a way that is more oriented toward an *exchange market* between generations and are thus formulating a sociopolitical need for action (BMFSFJ 2006).

Exchange groups or exchange markets represent an example of the organization of extrafamilial voluntary assistance relationships.* Nonetheless, practical experiences of the last few years have shown the following:

- They often do not make it past project status, as there is a lack or insufficient amount of professional and reliable management concepts.
- There are usually no solutions for cases when there is no suitable informal services offer to meet the demand for services.

Exchange groups also often fail due to the complicated running and management of the system components. In addition, this is mostly carried out by very few highly committed people who, after a certain period of time, show signs of fatigue. Additionally, a part of the services that elderly people would like to make use of cannot be offered by voluntary commitment. This concerns services that require people to have particular skills, that are very time consuming, and the provision of which are of existential importance to elderly people looking to make use of the said services. For example, a large part of the care in a specific sense and the health care services thus cannot be provided by voluntary efforts.

Welfare Mix in Service Production

Against this backdrop, the welfare mix concept is drawing an increasing amount of attention in both academia and the public (Evers 2005; Schneiders 2010). Regarding the welfare mix, it is assumed that social service production should be split between the spheres of

---

* In an exchange group or exchange market, it is predominantly services, and occasionally goods, that are exchanged between members without the use of legal forms of payment (see exchange groups from a conceptual perspective in Offe and Heinze 1990).

community, state, and (private) economy, whereby various service providers have specific strengths and weaknesses that need to be optimally utilized to optimize welfare production. The combination of these various service providers does, however, require a high level of management and coordination. This is where the service4home project comes in.

Service Coordination through Digital Pen and Paper Technology

Through the use of microsystems technology (MST), new products and processes in many sectors can be developed, or existing ones can be improved. Nevertheless, MST should not be overrated, since technical innovations are always only effective if they function in conjunction with the economy, society, and politics (Pfirrmann and Astor 2006).

The technology employed in the DiabCare/Homecare/CareOnline systems, which is based on special MST, has been very successfully implemented in logistics and health care management. In the research field of sociotechnical service provision for the elderly, it is primarily MST from the AAL field that is used. At present, there is only a small number of test projects. These projects were developed with the aim of examining existing and future needs and then being transformed into marketable concepts. They also offer the opportunity to investigate various technology and service concepts in a real-life scenario and research how MST can be used in an affordable and sustainably feasible way.

Services to Support Independent Lifestyles for Elderly People

There is much to be said for comprehensive sociotechnological efforts to enable elderly people to remain living in their accustomed environment for as long as possible. Newer alternatives to *standard living arrangements* have only been adopted by a very limited amount of elderly cohorts. Only 2% of people aged over 65 (roughly 150,000–230,000 people) currently live in assisted housing. The number of elderly people aged over 65 who live in social housing units and accessible assisted living facilities is currently estimated at around 9000–10,000 people. Nonetheless, this is becoming a growing trend, meaning that this type of housing can be cautiously considered to have growth potential for the future (Wahl and Oswald 2007). An international study (Cutchin et al. 2003) found that important factors for the acceptance of new housing alternatives included a combination of the extrafamilial social activities on offer, personal safety and accessibility in the living environment, and the feeling of being a part of the place of residence (place identity).

Technical Innovations to Support Living Independently

It needs to be mentioned in this context that the potential regarding the adaptation of the living areas of private people (particularly those of an advanced age) is currently only being exploited at a rudimentary level. Only 22% of the German people taking part in the Enabling Autonomy, Participation, and Wellbeing in Old Age: The Home Environment as a Determinant for Healthy Aging (ENABLE-AGE) study said that they had heard of such measures and corresponding financing options. Less than 9% said that they had already adapted their living areas. It became clear in an international comparison that only an extremely small portion of German people aged over 65 have made use of the technical assistance resources and general adaptation measures that are currently available. There is currently a good indication that access to appropriate living area adaptations and technological innovations is highly dependent on personal initiative and initiative acted out in the direct environment (Wahl and Oswald 2007).

A multilayered field of action is strongly developed on a regional and local level through the creation and expansion of complimentary service offers, in which resources that have been hitherto largely underused or civil assistance potential needs to be developed. This entails various service offers such as neighborhood assistance, household services, repair services, help with shopping, assistance to maintain communication and contact (especially for single people), and service provision to care for people suffering from dementia and to provide respite for family members who perform care services for the person concerned.

One of the prerequisites for the implementation of this kind of low-level service provision is that no direct competition with professional service providers, such as tradespeople or cleaners, is created, thus not putting any regular labor contracts in danger. These low-level services are offered by volunteers, who are usually paid a small allowance for their work by the people they do it for. Examples of these types of offers and services include the following:

- Within the home and in the household: small repair/maintenance tasks around the home, help with easy and difficult tasks around the house (e.g., cleaning windows; spring-cleaning; cleaning the curtains and hanging them back up; making the bed; doing the washing, hanging it up to dry, ironing, etc.; doing the dusting; cleaning the floor/carpets; shopping for everyday items; preparing food or delivering it; doing the washing up; cleaning the hallway; emptying rubbish bins; etc.)

- Work on the house: sweeping or clearing the walkway between the door and the street, sorting out the rubbish and disposing of it, cleaning the balcony and terrace, doing work in the garden such as mowing the lawn, pruning trees, etc.

- Mobility: pickup and delivery service (food, drinks, etc.); providing transport for people (going with them to doctors appointments etc.); visiting services (maintaining contact with people, organizing free time); accompanying them on trips; taking care of their animals; visiting church or the cemetery

Successful Implementation of the Welfare Mix Requires Coordination

There are already the first signs of services for day-to-day tasks in many areas, but there is often a lack of coordination and allocation of the various offers and comprehensive service provision. In order to be able to offer the appropriate service provision and structures at a local level, certain prerequisites need to be created, such as the following:

- An appropriate implementation concept that incorporates the potential of all service providers of the welfare mix

- Voluntary helpers who receive adequate specialist guidance, training, constant monitoring, and support

- Set standards regarding the minimum amount of time (e.g., a minimum of 20 h) that the voluntary helpers are required to receive general training and regular additional training

- Suitable facilities for care groups

As a rule, the costs for these services are covered privately. However, in certain exceptional cases, it is possible for the costs to be covered by higher-level funding providers.

According to the findings of a study conducted by the GfK market research company, elderly citizens have great interest in various household-related services (GfK 2002).

Elderly people mostly expressed their desire for an emergency call center, a care service, and cleaning and household assistance. The latter was most often preferred by respondents aged between 70 and 79. A further 30% of the same age group mentioned their needs for shopping services, food services, or being accompanied to the doctor or public authorities. Around 20% of respondents were in favor of service offers such as transportation services, washing services, help in the garden, and assistance for small repair/maintenance tasks. Compared to a first poll in 1999, it is primarily the demand for shopping services and household assistance that has increased.

It could be ascertained in this context that the level of monthly costs for household-related services that people over 50 would be willing to pay varies greatly. Around 40% say that they would, in principle, be prepared to pay a monthly fee of EUR 50–125. Almost a quarter of the respondents, however, would only be prepared to pay a maximum of EUR 50 for said services. A further 4% said that they would, in general, be willing to go up to EUR 350 a month.

Tenants' Obligatory Duties the Most in Demand

It is particularly significant that elderly people expressed an above-average interest in service provision but that their willingness to pay for the services is below average. For cleaning services around the home, they are prepared to pay around EUR 30 per month, and for food services, roughly EUR 45. The polls also showed that the majority of elderly people can still count on the support of their familial and/or neighborhood networks, and thus have not been able to gather personal experience with commercial service provision and the costs of these (Schneiders and Eisele 2007).

According to the findings, one can assume a certain discrepancy between expressed wishes and real use. Further possible causes for such a discrepancy could be that there is not actually any great need for such services, that there is a high level of inaccessibility to the services on offer, and that people are generally unaware of the local services that are on offer and their possible uses. Tenant surveys conducted by InWIS found that around 40% of the respondents were, in principle, prepared to pay for both so-called obligatory duties for the tenant (cleaning services for the hallway, winter services) and other services such as repair/maintenance support services. Their willingness to pay an appropriate amount of money for these services depends on age and income. It is therefore unsurprising in this context that elderly people express a high level of interest in various service offers, as this population group is, at times, already dependent on these services due to the increasing onset of physical impairments. However, the 30–45 age group also expresses a high interest in a diverse service offer, and the willingness to pay in this age group is at its highest (Schneiders and Eisele 2007; Schneiders and Ley 2010).

The Welfare Mix Concept

Welfare production in Germany is primarily carried out by the state (local councils, public-sector companies, etc.); the community (family, social networks); association-related actors (primarily welfare associations); and the private market (companies, freelancers). A pluralism of welfare production has developed in recent decades between these sectors. A significant part of welfare production informally takes place as part of primary social networks. However, professional services in the private area, against the backdrop of the societal change of familial and network structures as a result of demographic change, are increasingly becoming in demand. These services can be provided by both individual people and welfare associations. The boundaries between the individual areas of welfare production are fluid, meaning that it must be stated that the current composition of the welfare mix is more the result of contingencies and the distribution of power than a result of careful consideration of the advantages and disadvantages of the specific composition of services. This gives the concept of the welfare mix the advantage that within it, the potential of elderly people can be incorporated as well (Schneiders 2010).

Civil Involvement Key to Welfare Production

Social networks represent the integration of people into social relationships and ties. This is visualized through networks in which individual people represent the interconnection points and their relationships among one another form the connecting lines between these points. Individuals are integrated into society through their involvement in social networks, and at the same time, they receive information regarding social expectations, validation, and abstract and material support through daily interaction. Family, relatives, and friends are understood to be the primary social network and also the primary social system. The mutual support and assistance is, in a certain sense, carried out incidentally and is embedded in day-to-day life (Heinze et al. 1988).

As the primary social networks are often stretched to their limits with regard to assistance for elderly people, the activation of civil involvement, from both an economic and societal perspective, represents a concrete factor for fine-tuning within welfare production. The term *civil involvement* incorporates various concepts such as volunteer work, self-help, political participation, political protest, civil disobedience, and voluntary social activities and is oriented toward a new conceptual context. Civil involvement is equivalent to social involvement through the underlying principles of organized volunteer work and general volunteering. The citizen invests time for a charitable cause that benefits the community. Civil involvement acts as a sort of collective or umbrella term for a wide spectrum of various forms of volunteer work and voluntary social involvement, which is mostly offered free of charge by associations, trade unions, clubs, churches, and welfare care establishments (Heinze and Olk 2001).

Volunteer work is, by definition, a more narrowly defined term and is understood as a subarea of civil involvement. Voluntary commitment is often discussed in the context of involvement in associations and traditionally comprises the areas of social welfare associations (e.g., Arbeiter-Samariter-Bund), welfare associations (e.g., Diakonie, Caritas), churches, and sports clubs. Traditional volunteer work is characterized by three aspects: It is organized by associations (often welfare associations), it primarily recruits middle-class citizens, and it is characterized by societal core values, such as the Christian *love thy neighbor* and class solidarity. The *new* volunteer work, however, is characterized more by a connection of social attitudes, personal involvement, the desire for personal fulfillment, and the political willingness to change (Heinze and Strünck 2000).

Innovative Solution Strategies Are Essential

Due to the institutional processes of change in recent years, the services sector has developed into a growth market, which, in the future will also increase in importance with regard to the increasingly aging society. However, there are still currently tangible reservations in the field of service offers for the elderly and very old against professionally provided services in the household-related area. Organization-oriented service provision is currently failing, which is also due to cost disease. As a result, model projects, which bring together accessible living with service offers, which are partly provided in the form of volunteer-based involvement and run through the use of modern information technology (IT) and communication media, are examples of an innovative solution strategy in the face of demographic change and the cost disease toward professionally provided service offers. It is particularly those combinations of service offers that combine accessible housing with a specific service offer that fulfill the increasing demand for independent living in old age (Schneiders 2010; BMVBS 2011). The aforementioned cost disease can be explained, on the one hand, with the current restrained willingness to pay for appropriate service offers in the field of social economy among predominantly elderly target groups. There are also other aspects that have so far restricted the development and establishment of sustainable business models. The implementation of applications supported through AAL technologies, such as the aforementioned service agency as an element of cross-linked living, can barely be carried out by a single provider as part of a fully integrated business system. This is down to the two challenges mentioned previously, among other things. As at times, completely new (combinations of) resources and expertise are required for the social and health care system, these are often not found collectively in a preexisting institution. The economic principles of economies of scale and scope promote a task-sharing structure of specialists working cooperatively in existing or newly developing value creation structures. In this regard, changes to existing sector architectures are to be expected, and specific examples of these may already be observed. The area of living is playing an ever-more-important role in the development of innovative services in combination with MST and new communication technology (GdW 2007). The target groups for AAL applications are essentially very broad, and therefore a restriction to certain age groups is unnecessary. Nonetheless, many projects in Germany at the moment focus on an elderly target group. AAL applications can help to enable elderly people, especially with the onset of age or illness-related restrictions, to fulfill their wish to remain in their own homes (Heinze and Ley 2009; BMVBS 2011).

Incorporating Voluntary Involvement

The signing of a franchise agreement between housing companies and social service providers or the founding of not-for-profit societies is possible as a special form of cooperation. This type of cooperation is still relatively rare in Germany and leads to a shift in the role of the housing company. While it acts only as a mediator in the Bielefeld model, and as a rule, acts separately from social service providers in a business sense, economic integration as part of the society or franchise model is significantly closer. This type of cooperation is, for instance, currently being implemented by SOPHIA, a holding company that has arisen from a research project between the Joseph-Stiftung foundation in Bamberg and the University of Bamberg, and which awards licenses to housing companies to build regional SOPHIA service centers. The founding of regional associations in the form of society models is also possible, as franchise models are not advantageous or practical for every company due to tax reasons. Another feature of the SOPHIA concept is the incorporation of civil involvement. The participating tenants are embedded in a social network, which is made up of both professional and voluntary workers and into which the circle of relatives and friends can be integrated. Every participant at SOPHIA is allocated their own mentor, whose job involves being personally available to residents and making direct contact with them. The house emergency call is used as the primary technical component, even though other more advanced technical components (such as video communication through the television) are also possible (Heinze and Ley 2009).

In summary, it may be said that the incorporation of MST into the field of housing has, so far, hardly been implemented into regular operation. Even though the technical possibilities have meanwhile been fully developed, there is a lack of market-ready solutions that can be implemented in business models. In order to counteract this problem, a work package concerning business model development was planned from the start in the service4home project.

Identifiable Business Models for Innovative Approaches in the Area of Cross-Linked Living and AAL

In an economic sense, business models are a necessary prerequisite for evaluating the diffusion process of the technology in general and assessing the characteristic utilization scenarios for concrete business systems as the individual realization of generalized business model types (Gersch et al. 2010). The objective of a qualitative explorative study was the identification of the first basic types of economic activity in the AAL area (Lindert 2009; Gersch et al. 2010). A multistep iterative approach, from exploration and deduction to data collection and analysis, was selected. Based on this approach, typical characteristics of new business models in the area of ambient assisted living were identified. They were then able to be condensed into a typology of identified basic forms of economic activities, which are to be found on the primary and secondary health care market (Gersch et al. 2011a). Using the partial model approach, which serves to systematically characterize business models, is well suited for a detailed description of individual business models. The six partial models offer, through their individual perspectives, structured access to the differentiation of further analyses (Gersch 2004; Wirtz 2010; Gersch et al. 2011b).

The market model describes the relevant market, which is made up of the demand groups considered relevant, the (direct, but also indirect) competitors, and the relevant framework conditions. Based on this model, the characteristics of the designated package of services to satisfy the needs of the individual demanders are substantiated in the service offer model. The service creation model determines business system architecture to realize the service offer. It sets out which subactivities are necessary to realize the service offers and which resources and input factors are required. As part of the *make or buy consideration* regarding the vertical range of manufacture of a business system that is deemed appropriate, it is decided which of the subactivities that are considered necessary should or need to be carried out by third parties (specialists) and which will be realized in the internal business system. The procurement and distribution model is responsible for the coordination of the upstream and downstream value creation levels. The organizational and process structure of the business system, as well as conceivable cooperation with (perhaps several) activities, is set out in the organization and cooperation model. The capital model primarily considers the monetary aspects of the business system. It analyses the financial resources expected through the streams of revenue and the current as well as future capital requirements (Gersch et al. 2011b).

Service4home: Coordination and Networking

Against this backdrop, the project service4home—Dienstleistungskoordination durch mikrosystemtechnisch gestützte Informationseingabe (service4home—coordination of services through information input supported by technical microsystems)—looked into the issue of how living areas need to be structured in order to be in line with the demands and wishes of the future generation of elderly people, and at the same time keep service provision and care structures affordable (Schneiders et al. 2011; Lindert 2011a). The project assumes that both technical and social innovations in this regard are needed in order to develop sociotechnical systems that fulfill the aforementioned complex demands (Howaldt and Jacobsen 2010). In technical terms, the project relies on the use of MST to find out information and generate data from private households, which are then passed on to service providers via a service agency. The project is supported as a research association in the *innovation and services* support program of the German Federal Ministry of Education and Research (BMBF).

The Service4home Agency—Pilot Operation from Fall 2010 to Summer 2011

A substantial component of the service4home project lies in carrying out an analysis of the potential, which, unlike the usual tenant/customer questionnaires, aims to look into the wishes and needs related to services as well as the actual demand and the willingness to pay (regarding the results of this analysis into potential in accommodation, see Schneiders and Ley 2010). A service portfolio and a business model for a services agency were developed for the project based on this potential analysis. The concept was implemented between autumn 2010 and summer 2011 in a residential area in Grumme, Bochum, in a pilot project as part of the project funding. The basic considerations of elderly people regarding housing wishes and service needs were then presented. This was then linked to an overview of exemplary projects, within which the integration of modern information and communication possibilities in the housing area and their use for service processes had already been investigated. It was clear that in these projects, in addition to the technical implementation, the orientation of the service portfolio (providers and some service providers) toward the needs of the target group was of key importance to the success or failure of service agencies.

As part of the service4home project, a social, technical, and economic model was developed for the management of services within a residential area. The aim is to improve quality of life for everyone, but above, all elderly residents, through the provision of services and the activation of intergenerational exchanges in a residential area. As part of the project, a service agency was established to act as an interface between the involved service partners and the customers, i.e., those requiring the services. It takes on the coordination and management of personal and household-related services. The concept, which was developed in cooperation with the project partners, was able to be tested as part of a 10-month model project phase and modified as required. The conceptualization process was also used as a basis for theory and was taken as a reference model for other fields of application.

A special system of digital *microsystem writing technology* (digital pen and paper technology for short) is used to generate, coordinate, and transfer the data that are required for the service processes. The device used is in the form of a multifunctional pen, and the user fills in values on a special paper document. A camera is integrated into the pen, and it digitally saves what the user writes and then automatically sends the data via a transmitter unit to a service center. The advantage of using such technology is that the pen is a medium that can be used ad hoc (Schneiders et al. 2011). Elderly people without experience in how to use complex technical devices can enjoy the benefits of the digital technology.

During the 6 months of testing, the demonstrating project has shown acceptance within the target group. The technique was not only accepted by elderly people but was also easy to handle. The evaluation has demonstrated that even the service portfolio was valued to be appropriate by the target group. Nevertheless, during the project period, it was not possible to acquire the number of customers that was needed to ensure economical operation. The evaluation results indicate that the main reason is the lack of economic potential in the model area. Besides this, it is also a consequence of the German version of a welfare state, where the social services are usually provided by charities, but publicly, not privately funded, mostly by social insurance.

It is thus evident that the introduction of the AAL also has to take into account the institutional embeddedness (Ruddat et al. 2012).

Conclusion/Outlook

Due to the aging process of the general society, sociotechnical service offers are developing as test cases for Germany as a hub of innovation. Even though the potential is there, the market is facing the fascinating option, at least from the perspective of Germany as a hub for a certain activity, of establishing itself as a *lead market* for socioeconomic innovations for elderly people in one of the *oldest* populations of the world (Heinze 2009; Heinze et al. 2011).

Residential Area–Based Approaches Leading the Way

In this context, the inclusion of not only the individual local housing situations but also the entire residential or city area, the inhabitants and social networks are of particular importance in a future-oriented perspective. Safety and independence for elderly people are becoming central topic areas and offer various approaches for innovative service concepts. The pilot projects that have been carried out in this area for years with a substantial amount of effort have so far lacked broad acceptance on the part of the benefactors and the end customers. A possible reason behind the practical failure of the projects to date might be their overly strong orientation on what is technically achievable and at the same time inadequate consideration of the actual preferences, needs, and interests of the potential users (Heinze 2009). Service offer structures, which are less oriented toward technology but instead are more focused on the practical interests of the elderly, whereby they combine private, part-private, and public service providers and welfare producers that are in line with the requirements of the welfare mix, now need to be tested and expanded.

Caring for elderly people in their private homes opens up new opportunities not only for service companies, but also for housing and property companies (Lindert 2011b). It is predominantly service packages that are for day-to-day management and are oriented toward household-related services that can contribute to elderly people remaining in their own homes and leading an independent life (BMFSFJ 2005). The implementation of sociotechnological service offers from voluntary and professional providers does, however, require the management of complex and heterogeneous networks and interests. The use of MST can play a supporting role in this respect (Gersch et al. 2011b).

Demographic Change as an Innovation Opportunity

A trend that has been driven forward in the last few years, by the BMBF, among others, is the development of so-called ambient assisted living concepts. With the help of technical support, various measures have been integrated in this area, which are aimed at improving quality of life both in and outside of the home. The developed technologies can also be transferred over into other fields of application, and on the other hand, new products and possible uses can arise, as well as social/organizational forms for further target groups. Due to its demographic characteristics, the Ruhrgebiet (Ruhr area) can act as a *German laboratory* in the search for solution possibilities for the pan-German composition of the challenges posed by demographic change.

In the sense of possible cost savings and, at the same time, possible improvements of quality levels of care (the findings of further health care and socioeconomic added value analyses are not yet complete), AAL can represent a very useful innovation for the provision of services for elderly people. The implementation of this is, however, connected to numerous obstacles, as previously demonstrated, and rigidity, which needs to be overcome, due to the systemic character of the German social system. In the same respect, although these obstacles can decelerate the diffusion of AAL and the innovative approaches that the technology serves, they can also, at the same time, be protective in a way, if rigid structures of labor division and business model types have evolved in this sector. The window of opportunity to expand these structures (and an advantageous position) and to play a part in reshaping them is currently open. The first attempts for improved cooperation between individual actors from the housing industry and service providers, as well as benefactors such as health funds, are evident. This process can be driven forward through the use of new technologies. The business system that was conceptualized in the service4home project represents, in this context, only an example of the broad company-related interest in AAL. In this respect, it can serve as evidence that actors from the most diverse sectors are currently discovering this opportunity and are prepared to face the business-related risks.

References

Bäcker, G., Naegele, G., Bispinck, R., Hofemann, K., and Neubauer, J. 2010. *Sozialpolitik und soziale Lage in Deutschland 2. Gesundheit, Familie, Alter und Soziale Dienste*. Wiesbaden: VS Verlag für Sozialwissenschaften.

Backes, G. M. 1998. Alternde Gesellschaft und Entwicklung des Sozialstaates. In *Altern und Gesellschaft. Gesellschaftliche Modernisierung durch Altersstrukturwandel*, eds. W. Clemens, and G. M. Backes, 257–286. Opladen: Leske + Budrich.

Bischoff, S., and Brauers, S. 2006. SeniorTrainer. Das Erfahrungswissen älterer Menschen nutzen. In *Länger leben, arbeiten und sich engagieren. Chancen wertschaffender Beschäftigung bis ins Alter*, eds. J. U. Prager, and A. Schleiter, 151–164. Gütersloh: Verlag Bertelsmann Stiftung.

BKK Bundesverband. 2009. Schwerpunktthema Pflege. *BKK Faktenspiegel*, June. Available at http://www.bkk.de/fileadmin/user_upload/PDF/Faktenspiegel/Aktuelle_Ausgaben/Schwerpunktthema Pflege.pdf (accessed May 17, 2011).

Bundesministerium für Familie, Senioren, Frauen und Jugend (BMFSFJ). 2005. *Fünfter Bericht zur Lage der älteren Generation in der Bundesrepublik Deutschland. Potenziale des Alters in Wirtschaft und Gesellschaft. Der Beitrag älterer Menschen zum Zusammenhalt der Generationen*. Berlin: Bericht der Sachverständigenkommission.

Bundesministerium für Familie, Senioren, Frauen und Jugend (BMFSFJ). 2006. *Trendberichte zur Seniorenwirtschaft in Deutschland*. Dortmund.

Bundesministerium für Verkehr, Bau und Stadtentwicklung (BMVBS). 2011. *Wohnen im Alter. Marktprozesse und wohnungspolitischer Handlungsbedarf*. Berlin: Forschungen, 147.

Cutchin, M. P., Owen, S. V., and Chang, P.-F. J. 2003. Becoming "at Home" in Assisted Living Residences: Exploring Place Integration Processes. *The Journals of Gerontology Series B: Psychological Sciences and Social Sciences* 58:234–243.

de Jong, R. 2007. Re-Inventing Civil Society: The Role of Dutch Social Housing Organisations. Paper presented at the Social Services of General Interest in the European Union Conference, Brussels.

DESTATIS. 2011. *Demografischer Wandel in Deutschland. Heft 1: Bevölkerungs- und Haushaltsentwicklung im Bund und in den Ländern.* Wiesbaden: Statistisches Bundesamt.

Engstler, H., Menning, S., Hoffmann, E., and Tesch-Römer, C. 2004. Die Zeitverwendung älterer Menschen. In *Alltag in Deutschland, Beiträge zur Ergebniskonferenz der Zeitbudgeterhebung 2001/2002 am 16./17. Februar in Wiesbaden, Analysen zur Zeitverwendung, Bd. 43,* ed. Statistisches Bundesamt, 216–246. Wiesbaden: Statistisches Bundesamt.

Evers, A. 2005. Mixed Welfare Systems and Hybrid Organizations: Changes in the Governance and Provision of Social Services. *International Journal of Public Administration* 28:737–748.

GdW Bundesverband deutscher Wohnungs- und Immobilienunternehmen e.V. 2007. *Vernetztes Wohnen. Dienstleistungen, Technische Infrastruktur und Geschäftsmodelle.* Hamburg: Hammonia Verlag.

Geissler, B. 2010. Der private Haushalt als Arbeitsplatzreservoir? Zur Akzeptanz und Abwehr von Haushaltsdienstleistungen. *WSI Mitteilungen* 63:135–142.

Gersch, M. 2004. Versandapotheken in Deutschland—Die Geburt einer neuen Dienstleistung. Wer ist eigentlich der Vater? *Marketing-ZFP, Special Issue Dienstleistungsmarketing* 26:59–70.

Gersch, M., Lindert, R., and Hewing, M. 2010. AAL-Business Models: Different Prospects for the Successful Implementation of Innovative Services in the First and Second Healthcare Market. In *Proceedings of the AALIANCE European Conference on AAL*, Malaga, Spain. Available at http://www.aaliance.eu/public/aaliance-conference-1/papers-and-posters/8_2_fu-berlin (accessed June 28, 2011).

Gersch, M., Goeke, C., and Lindert, R. 2011a. AAL-Geschäftsmodelle—Gelegenheitsfenster für die Akteure im Gesundheitswesen. In *Versorgungsforschung für demenziell erkrankte Menschen*, eds. O. Dibelius, and W. Maier, 167–173. Stuttgart: Kohlhammer.

Gersch, M., Hewing, M., and Lindert, R. 2011b. Geschäftsmodelle zur Unterstützung eines selbstbestimmten Lebens in einer alternden Gesellschaft—Communities, industrielle Dienstleister und Orchestratoren als Beispiele neuer Geschäftsmodelle im Bereich E-Health@Home. In *Dynamisch Leben gestalten. Lebensräume—Lebensträume*, Vol. 2, eds. M. Horneber, and H. Schoenauer, 159–177. Stuttgart: Kohlhammer.

Gesellschaft für Konsumforschung (GfK). 2002. *Wirtschaftstrendforschung. 50plus.*

Heinze, R. G. 2009. *Rückkehr des Staates? Politische Handlungsmöglichkeiten in unsicheren Zeiten.* Wiesbaden: VS Verlag für Sozialwissenschaften.

Heinze, R. G., and Strünck, C. 2000. Die Verzinsung des sozialen Kapitals. Freiwilliges Engagement im Strukturwandel. In *Die Zukunft von Arbeit und Demokratie*, ed. U. Beck, 171–216. Frankfurt a. M.: Suhrkamp Verlag.

Heinze, R. G., and Olk, T. 2001. Bürgerengagement in Deutschland—Zum Stand der wissenschaftlichen und politischen Diskussion. In *Bürgerengagement in Deutschland. Bestandsaufnahmen und Perspektiven*, eds. R. G. Heinze, and T. Olk, 11–26. Opladen: Leske + Budrich.

Heinze, R. G., and Ley, C. 2009. *Vernetztes Wohnen: Ausbreitung, Akzeptanz und nachhaltige Geschäftsmodelle.* Bochum/Berlin: Forschungsbericht.

Heinze, R. G., Olk, T., and Hilbert, J. eds. 1988. *Der neue Sozialstaat. Analyse und Reformperspektiven.* Freiburg i. Br.: Lambertus-Verlag.

Heinze, R. G., Eichener, V., Naegele, G., Bucksteg, M., and Schauerte, M. 1997. *Neue Wohnung auch im Alter.* Darmstadt: Schader Stiftung.

Heinze, R. G., Naegele, G., and Schneiders, K. 2011. *Wirtschaftliche Potenziale des Alters.* Stuttgart: Kohlhammer.

Herrmann, T., Kleinbeck, U., and Krcmar, H. eds. 2005. *Konzepte für das Service Engineering. Modularisierung, Prozessgestaltung und Produktivitätsmanagement.* Heidelberg: Physica-Verlag.

Howaldt, J., and Jacobsen, H. eds. 2010. *Soziale Innovation. Auf dem Weg zu einem postindustriellen Innovationsparadigma.* Wiesbaden: VS Verlag für Sozialwissenschaften.

Kaufmann, F.-X. 2005. *Die schrumpfende Gesellschaft. Vom Bevölkerungsrückgang und seinen Folgen.* Frankfurt: Suhrkamp Verlag.

KKH-Allianz. ed. 2011. *Pflege.* Forsa survey commissioned by KKH Allianz.

Kohli, M. ed. 2000. *Grunddaten zur Lebenssituation der 40-85-Jährigen deutschen Bevölkerung.* Ergebnisse des Alters-Survey. Berlin: Weißensee-Verlag.

Kruse, A. 2008. Psychologische Veränderungen im Alter. In *Alter, Gesundheit und Krankheit*, eds. A. Kuhlmey, and D. Schaeffer, 15–32. Bern: Verlag Hans Huber.

Kuhlmey, A., and Schaeffer, D. 2008. *Alter, Gesundheit und Krankheit: Handbuch Gesundheitswissenschaften.* Bern: Verlag Hans Huber.

Lindert, R. 2009. *Innovative (?) Geschäftsmodelle im Gesundheitswesen.* Invited speech at the Forschungstagung Marketing 2009, Berlin.

Lindert, R. 2011a. Business Models in the Field of Ambient Assisted Living (AAL)—Successful Interface Management as a Basis for Innovative Rehabilitation-Concepts at the Health Site "At Home". In *Proceedings of 3rd European Conference on Technically Assisted Rehabilitation (TAR) 2011*, Berlin: IGE.

Lindert, R. 2011b. Innovative AAL-Geschäftsmodelle—Chancen und Herausforderungen des demographischen Wandels aus ökonomischer Perspektive. Invited speech at the Annual Conference 2011 of the German Association for Demography (Deutsche Gesellschaft für Demographie e.V.—DGD), Bonn.

Link, W. 2003. Demographischer Wandel—Herausforderungen unserer älter werdenden Gesellschaft an den Einzelnen und die Politik. Eine Dokumentation in Auszügen aus dem Schlussbericht der Enquete-Kommission des Deutschen Bundestages. *Aus Politik und Zeitgeschichte* 53:B20/2003.

Little, V. C. 1984. An Overview of Research Using Time-Budget Methodology to Study Age-Related Behaviour. *Ageing and Society* 4:3–20.

Meyer, D. 2008. Systemwechsel in der Sozialwirtschaft: Ausschreibungen und personengebundene Budgets. *Theorie und Praxis sozialer Arbeit* 59:443–452.

Mukasa, K. S., Holzinger, A., and Karshmer, A. I. eds. 2008. Intelligent User Interfaces for Ambient Assisted Living. In *Proceedings of the First International Workshop IUI4AAL 2008*, Kaiserslautern: IRB Verlag.

Naegele, G., and Gerling, V. 2007. Sozialpolitik für ältere Menschen in Deutschland—Grundlagen, Strukturen, Entwicklungstrends und neue fachliche Herausforderungen. In *Das Recht der älteren Menschen*, eds. G. Igl, and T. Klie, 49–74. Baden-Baden: Nomos.

Narten, R., and Scherzer, U. 2007. *Älter werden—wohnen bleiben. Strategien und Potenziale der Wohnungswirtschaft in einer alternden Gesellschaft.* Hamburg: Hammonia Verlag.

Offe, C., and Heinze, R. G. 1990. *Organisierte Eigenarbeit. Das Modell Kooperationsring.* Frankfurt a. M./New York: Campus-Verlag.

Peuckert, R. 2008. *Familienformen im sozialen Wandel.* Wiesbaden: VS Verlag für Sozialwissenschaften.

Pfirrmann, O., and Astor, M. 2006. Trendreport MST 2020. Innovative Ideen rund um die Mikrosystemtechnik. Available at http://www.mstbw.de/imperia/md/content/mstbw/trendreport_mst_2020.pdf (accessed June 28, 2011).

Philips. ed. 2010. Philips Index for Health and Wellbeing: A Global Perspective. Available at http://www2.philips.de/index/2-Philips-Health-and-Well-Being-Index.pdf (accessed January 25, 2011).

Priebe, M. 2006. *Arbeitsmarkt und demographischer Wandel. Möglichkeiten betrieblicher Einflussnahme auf die Auswirkungen alternder Belegschaften.* Saarbrücken: VDM Verlag.

Rothgang, G.-W. 2008. *Psychologie in der Sozialen Arbeit 4: Entwicklungspsychologie.* Stuttgart: Kohlhammer.

Ruddat, C., Grohs, S., Heinze, R. G., Schönauer, A.-L., and Schneiders, K. 2012. New Players on Grazed Playing Fields. The Institutional Embeddedness of Social Entrepreneurship in Germany. Paper for the 2012 Espanet Conference, Edinburgh, September 6–8.

Saup, W., and Reichert, M. 1999. Die Kreise werden enger. Wohnen und Alltag im Alter. In *Funkkolleg Altern 2. Lebenslagen und Lebenswelten, soziale Sicherung und Altenpolitik*, eds. A. Niederfranke, G. Naegele, and E. Frahm, 245–286. Opladen: Westdeutscher Verlag.

Schneider, B., Eichener, V., Schauerte, M., Klein, K., and Kortenjann, B. 2002. *Zukunft des Wohnens. Perspektiven für die Wohnungs- und Immobilienwirtschaft in Rheinland und Westfalen*. Düsseldorf: Verband der Wohnungswirtschaft Rheinland-Westfalen.

Schneiders, K. 2001. Seniorenimmobilien—immer noch ein Zukunftsmarkt. *Die Freie Wohnungswirtschaft* 55:130–132.

Schneiders, K. 2004. Vermarktung von Seniorenimmobilien. Auswirkungen von Einkommensentwicklung und Eigentumsquoten. *Die Freie Wohnungswirtschaft* 58:191–192.

Schneiders, K. 2010. *Vom Altenheim zum Seniorenservice. Institutioneller Wandel und Akteurkonstellationen im sozialen Dienstleistungssektor*. Baden-Baden: Nomos.

Schneiders, K., and Eisele, B. 2006. Den Senioren auf der Spur: Aktuelle Befragungsergebnisse zu Wohn- und Dienstleistungswünschen älterer Menschen in Deutschland. *Die Freie Wohnungswirtschaft* 60:142–143.

Schneiders, K., and Eisele, B. 2007. Altersgerechte Wohnformen und Dienstleistungen—beliebt bei geringer Zahlungsbereitschaft. *Die Wohnungswirtschaft* 60:28–29.

Schneiders, K., and Ley, C. 2010. *Service4home: Dienstleistungen für eine älter werdende Gesellschaft*. Bochum: InWIS.

Schneiders, K., Ley, C., and Prilla, M. 2011. Die Verbindung von Technikakzeptanz, Dienstleistungsbedarf und strukturelle Voraussetzungen als Erfolgsfaktor einer durch Mikrosystemtechnik gestützten Dienstleistungsagentur. In *Mit AAL-Dienstleistungen altern. Nutzerbedarfsanalysen im Kontext des Ambient Assisted Living*, eds. D. Bieber, and K. Schwarz, 115–136. Saarbrücken: ISO-Verlag.

Schramm, M. 2007. Der Sozialmarkt im normativen Konflikt—Sozialethische Erörterung des Marktwettbewerbs in der Sozialwirtschaft. In *Markt und Wettbewerb in der Sozialwirtschaft*, eds. D. Aufderheide, and M. Dabrowski, 11–30. Berlin: Duncker & Humblot.

Tang, P., and Venables, T. 2000. 'Smart' homes and telecare for independent living. *Journal of Telemedicine and Telecare* 6:8–14.

TNS Emnid. 2011. Wohnwünsche im Alter. Available at http://www.dgfm.de/pdf-dateien/presse meldungen/2011/bau2011/Emnid _Wohnwuensche.pdf (accessed May 16, 2011).

VDE. 2007. *Intelligente Assistenzsysteme im Dienst für eine reife Gesellschaft*. Frankfurt a. M.: VDE Verlag.

Wahl, H.-W., and Oswald, F. 2007. Altern in räumlich-sozialen Kontexten: Neues zu einem alten Forschungsthema. In *Was bedeutet der demografische Wandel für die Gesellschaft? Perspektiven für eine alternde Gesellschaft*, eds. M. Reichert, E. Gösken, and A. Ehlers, 55–75. Berlin: LIT-Verlag.

Wahl, H.-W., and Oswald, F. 2010. Environmental perspectives on aging. In *International Handbook of Social Gerontology*, eds. D. Dannefer, and C. Phillipson, 111–124. London: Sage.

Wirtz, B. W. 2010. *Electronic Business*. Wiesbaden: Gabler.

18

The Living Usability Lab Architecture: Support for the Development and Evaluation of New Ambient Assisted Living Services for the Elderly

António Teixeira, Nelson Pacheco Rocha, Carlos Pereira, Joaquim Sousa Pinto, Miguel Sales Dias, Cláudio Teixeira, Miguel Oliveira e Silva, Alexandra Queirós, Flávio Ferreira, and André Oliveira

CONTENTS

ABSTRACT   The introduction of technology in the domestic environment is a reality. For the elderly, a significant percentage of the population, technology can have a positive impact on their quality of life. However, this can only be true if technologies for domestic environments are made accessible and usable by those staying at home. The Living Usability Lab (LUL) project aims to create conditions for the development and evaluation of innovative services for the elderly. Two of the main characteristics of the project are its attention to usability and design for all, and the exploration of next-generation networks. This chapter presents the conceptual architecture adopted for the living lab and the support architecture for development of new, complex ambient assisted living (AAL) services. The genesis of the living lab ecosystem is the aim to create an environment where developers and care professionals are able to create innovative AAL applications and services with ease and with access to a whole set of test groundings. To support our proposal, a new service for telerehabilitation—developed by the project—is used as a scenario within the proposed architectures.

KEY WORDS: *ambient assisted living, service-oriented architecture, e-health, ubiquitous computing.*

Introduction

Greater life expectancy is one of humanity's greatest triumphs. It is also one of our greatest challenges—global ageing will mean increased economic and social demands for all countries. At the same time, older people are precious, often ignored resources who make an important contribution to the fabric of our societies (WHO 2002).

Technology can have an important role in active and productive ageing, whether it is used to extend the lifespan, promote activity and participation of older adults, reorganize health and social support services, or simply disseminate information. Technological solutions can facilitate the daily life of the elderly; combat isolation and exclusion; and increase their proactivity, work capacity, and autonomy. Therefore, ambient assisted living (AAL) is a natural extension of the ambient intelligence paradigm (Mikulecky et al. 2008; Kung and Jean-Bart 2010), whose main objective is the integration of a broad rage of technologies—smart materials, microelectromechanical components, sensor technologies, embedded devices, ubiquitous communications, or intelligent interfaces—to proactively support people in their daily lives.

In our ageing society, AAL is defined as an "aim to extend the time people can live in a decent way in their own home by increasing their autonomy and self-confidence, the discharge of monotonous everyday activities, to monitor and care for the elderly or ill person, to enhance security and to save resources" (Steg et al. 2006). This aim demands a long-term research and development (R&D) effort, not only in terms of technological developments but also in integrating the existing technology, how to combine it, how to create new services joining technologies and services provided by humans, and how to make all this usable and acceptable to the elderly.

At home or in an institution, the elderly person has multiple needs requiring support from multiple health and social services. AAL solutions can impact the many different aspects of the life of old people at home: self-care; domestic activities; environmental monitoring and home automation (e.g., lights control) (Kim and Kim 2006); learning activities throughout life, recreation, and other community activities; notification and dispensing of medication (Dohr et al. 2010), rehabilitation (Eriksson et al. 2011; Peel et al. 2011); health education; monitoring state of health (Jara et al. 2009); personal security (Hsu and Chen 2010); and home security (including intrusion).

The Living Usability Lab Project

The Living Usability Lab (LUL) project is a joint academia–industry R&D initiative, started in January 2010, aimed at creating the conditions to develop and evaluate innovative services for the elderly (LUL Consortium 2010; Teixeira et al. 2011b). Nuclear to the project is its attention to usability, design for all, and the exploration of new opportunities afforded by next-generation networks.

Considering the high demands on overall AAL system quality and, consequently, on software and system engineering, user acceptance is an absolute necessity. Therefore, the early involvement of end users in the design process assumes great importance in meeting the actual needs of future users in their daily life.

Although the importance of user involvement and user participation in the design process has been recognized as essential, there is a need for further developments in daily practice, through the use of innovative strategies. A living lab can be defined as a research methodology that includes users by taking into account the microcontext of their daily activities. The creation of a living lab ecosystem can provide a significant boost to the development and testing of new technologies in near-real-life scenarios.

To enable the existence of a geographically distributed lab for new AAL service creation, evolution, and evaluation—our living lab—suitable architectures for the living lab and its development middleware (supporting creation and deployment of new services) are needed. This chapter describes both the conceptual architecture for the living lab and the architecture for the development of new, complex AAL services. The goal is to provide developers with the conditions to create AAL applications and services, using the proposed architecture as the basis, while having at their disposal a number of services that may help them achieve their business logics.

Chapter Structure

This chapter is structured as follows. The "Related Work" section introduces the evolution of AAL architectures and related state-of-the-art work, with representative examples. The "Living Lab Ecosystem Conceptual Model" section provides the living lab conceptual model, including explanations for each layer, from physical spaces to stakeholders. In the "LUL Architecture for New Service Development" section, we present the support architecture for the development of new services. The "LUL Services" section provides a more detailed view of the LUL services layer, including some examples and their objectives. In the "Examples of Architecture Application" section, an applicational example is described from its integration perspective within the living lab ecosystem and the support architecture—the telerehabilitation application. Finally, the "Conclusion" presents conclusions and some ideas for future research.

Related Work

A review of all existing architectures proposed for AAL over the years is outside the scope of this chapter. Nevertheless, to better introduce the adopted architectural options for LUL, information on current trends and mainstream approaches is presented, after a brief presentation of the evolution of AAL architectures in recent years.

AAL Architectural Reference Models

Today's AAL architectures are the result of an evolutionary process derived from their usage in smart environment contexts (Figure 18.1). The first architectural models were based on very specific rules in a somewhat *closed* perspective. In truth, although these solutions had high levels of reliability and functionality, the same cannot be said about their heterogeneity, which hampered their extensibility and compatibility with external devices (Aiello and Dustdar 2008).

A logical step was taken when new architectural models moved away from the closed, centralized model, bringing major advantages regarding the development of new solutions. These new models included the existence of central entities with which the devices could communicate, increasing the heterogeneity and scalability of solutions but causing performance problems in the original entities as the device network became more complex.

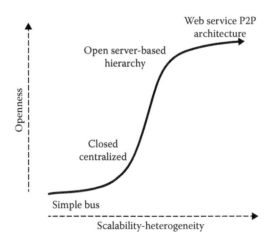

FIGURE 18.1
Evolution of AAL architectures. (From Aiello, M., 2006, The Role of Web Services at Home. Paper presented at the International Conference on Advanced International Conference on Telecommunications/Internet and Web Applications and Services. Retrieved from http://doi.ieeecomputersociety.org/10.1109/AICT-ICIW.2006.190.)

In response to this problem, new models evolved to a peer-to-peer approach where communications are performed via web services, opening prospects for future growth of the solutions. Fueled by the growing trend toward services as software components, the use of web services has become a very popular solution.

Web Services

Web services are defined by the World Wide Web Consortium (W3C 2004) as software systems constructed in order to support interoperability in the interaction between multiple machines across a network, independently of the platform or operating system being used.

From an architectural point of view, applications based on web services are composed of three components (Figure 18.2): the provider, the requestor (client), and the service registry (Huhns and Singh 2005).

Providers are entities that publish or advertise their services via the broker. Through the broker, clients can browse the services and invoke them if they wish. The connections between the various entities use web services standards, such as Web Services Description Language (WSDL), Simple Object Access protocol (SOAP), and Universal Description, Discovery and Integration (UDDI) (Papazoglou and van den Heuvel 2007).

Service-Oriented Architectures

Due to the existing heterogeneity in hardware and communication interfaces—especially between different vendors—a major challenge for today's architectures concerns interoperability.

This concern is particularly addressed by service-oriented architectures (SOAs) (Erl 2008). The SOA architectural model focuses on improving aspects such as efficiency, agility, and productivity by exposing business logics through services. SOA can be seen as a paradigm for exchange of value through services between active and independent participants, who have the legitimate right to use them, assuming that they adhere to the rules defined by policies and service agreements (OASIS 2011). Similarly, SOA is defined as a paradigm for organizing and using distributed capabilities through services that may be under the control of different entities. In other words, it represents the way the needs of one

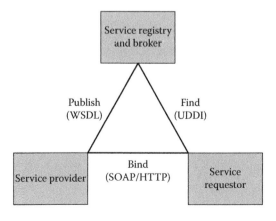

FIGURE 18.2
Architectural model of web services. (Adapted from Huhns, M. N. & Singh, M. P., *Internet Computing*, 9, 2005.)

stakeholder can be met using the solutions offered by others, based on the establishment of a trusting relationship between them.

From a more technical point of view, an SOA implementation in one organization differs from others by combining the use of technologies, products, application programming interfaces (APIs), and other support infrastructures.

Conceptually, an SOA is composed essentially of four layers (Thies and Vossen 2008):

- *Application layer*: includes legacy, customer relationship management (CRM), enterprise resource planning (ERP), and database systems.
- *Services layer*: includes architecture services, described in WSDL format.
- *Processing layer*: the services are composed using orchestration methodologies, such as Business Process Execution Language (BPEL).
- *Presentation layers*: responsible for providing architecture functionalities to different users or applications.

In addition, an SOA implementation aims to achieve good practice principles, such as the following (Balzer 2004):

- *Reuse, granularity, modularity*: developed services should be reusable before the existence of other scenarios; they should represent individual and autonomous modules in relation to the processing of a given instruction; more elaborated services should be constructed by composition or orchestration of the most basic services following a certain sequence.
- *Compliance to standards*: maximizing interoperability between services.
- *Identification, categorization, provision, delivery, and monitoring of services*: facilitating research by potential users and detection of abnormalities.

According to the same author, special focus should be given to other principles, such as the following:

- Separation of business logic from the underlying technology.
- Leveraging existing assets wherever an opportunity exists.
- Life cycle management.
- Efficient use of system resources—services developed should be concerned with performance and scalability.

This architectural style is of the utmost importance for AAL solutions, particularly in defining a structure for integrating devices and/or services that can be invoked, started, and stopped automatically and dynamically (Sun et al. 2009). The devices use the support platform to indicate their availability and are accessible to applications when needed to achieve business logics.

Cloud Computing

One of the fastest-growing concepts in recent years, cloud computing refers to the provision of services and applications over a distributed network, through virtualized resources that are externally accessible to users (Sosinsky 2011).

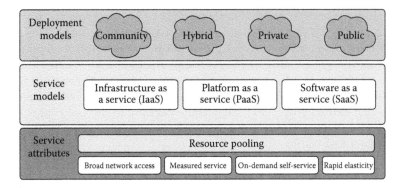

FIGURE 18.3
Models of *cloud computing* by NIST. (Sosinsky, B., *Cloud Computing Bible*, 1st ed. 2011. Copyright Wiley-VCH Verlag GmbH & Co. KGaA. Reproduced with permission.)

In cloud computing, two sets of distinct models can normally be found: implementation models and service models (Figure 18.3).

The implementation models are related to the location and administration of the cloud infrastructure:

- *Public cloud*: the infrastructure belongs to a particular organization, which sells its services for public use.
- *Private cloud*: the infrastructure is exclusive to a single organization, which will be responsible for its management or possible delegation to third parties.
- *Community cloud*: the infrastructure is organized to serve a common purpose or functionality to various organizations, which together, are in charge of its administration or delegation to third parties.
- *Hybrid cloud*: the infrastructure is a combination of the above, maintaining the characteristics of each but behaving like one.

On the other hand, service models consist of particular types of services that can be accessed in a cloud computing platform:

- *Infrastructure as a service (IaaS)*: provides virtual machines, virtual storage, virtual infrastructure, and other hardware resources. The infrastructure management is the responsibility of the service provider, leaving the client with the responsibility for other implementation aspects (operating system, applications, etc.).
- *Platform as a service (PaaS)*: provides virtual machines, operating systems, applications, services, development frameworks, and monitoring. The service provider manages the infrastructure, operating systems, and available software, while the client undertakes setup and management of its applications.
- *Software as a service (SaaS)*: provides a complete operating environment with applications, management tools, and user interface. The application is available to customers through an interface (typically a browser), and its purpose is solely focused on the insertion and management of data as well as interacting with the user. The infrastructure behind the client application is the responsibility of the service provider.

Simply, when we plan to migrate a system to the cloud and select a service provider, we are, in fact, renting or allocating a small part of a huge structure of servers, desktops, storage, or network capacity, avoiding administration concerns and reducing implementation costs (pay as you go). In addition, the cloud provides elasticity, ease of use, quality of service (QoS), reliability, and the simplicity of maintenance and growth (upgrade)—from a client's point of view. However, some organizations, with high investment capabilities in technology and skilled employees, raise some barriers to the use of the cloud, mainly due to concerns about the security and privacy of data and also about performance due to continuously generated traffic.

Service-Oriented Device Architectures

Lately, the emergence of numerous devices, with proprietary and specific communication interfaces, has increased the difficulty and cost of management in distributed platforms. Resulting from an adaptation of SOA, SODA intends to provide some level of abstraction to physical devices, simplifying external access to them (de Deugd et al. 2006).

Implementing a SODA implies the existence of three main components (Figure 18.4): a device adapter, bus adapter, and device service registry. The first abstracts the communication interfaces of the various devices, simplifying communication in the presence of devices with different interfaces. The second moves the data provided by the devices through the network protocols, mapping the abstract model of services for the specific mechanism links of the organization's SOA. Finally, the device service registry provides a way to search and access SODA services.

The applicability of this model is obvious in the context of AAL environments, being an alternative to consider for the integration of residential devices and actuators.

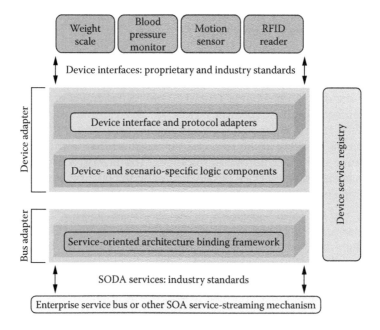

FIGURE 18.4
SODA architectural model. Radio-frequency identification (RFID). (From de Deugd, S. et al., *IEEE Pervasive Computing*, 5(3), 94–96, 2006.)

Peer to Peer

Known for their robustness, performance, and extensibility, peer-to-peer (P2P) systems consist of a complex network of autonomous nodes (peers), which can behave as both clients and servers.

The model presented in Figure 18.5 defines the terminology and the various layers of P2P networks (Subramanian and Goodman 2005): infrastructures, applications, and communications, supported by existing telecommunications networks. The first layer represents the infrastructures, which provide communication, integration, and translation functionalities between the technological components. The second layer contains the applications that use the available infrastructures, allowing communication and collaboration between entities in the absence of a central control. The third layer focuses on the phenomenon of social interaction, particularly in the formation of communities and the dynamics between them.

This model is advantageous in homogeneous environments, whose nodes have identical capabilities such as processing power, bandwidth, storage, and control. However, AAL environments are very heterogeneous, where nodes range from small sensors to powerful servers. Applying this model to these environments is possible in a subset of devices from identical classes. Its biggest advantage comes from its direct communication between nodes, eliminating the need for centralization and associated issues (Loeser et al. 2003; Becker 2008).

Event-Driven Architectures

In an event-driven architecture (EDA), the occurrence of an event is immediately disseminated to all stakeholders (people or automated systems), which evaluate it and act if necessary. Resulting actions may involve invoking a service, a business process, or the displaying of information (Michelson 2006).

According to the same author, there are three types of event processing, simple, continuous, and complex, used together in a mature EDA. The first is commonly used in a continuous work flow, in which an event triggers a certain action. The continuous style is commonly used in situations where the streaming of information is used for decision making. The complex style evaluates a set or series of events and then proceeds to a decision-making process, commonly implemented for detection and response to business anomalies, threats, and opportunities.

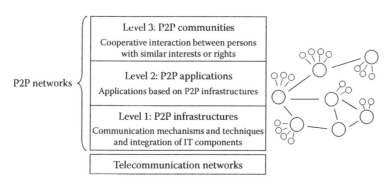

FIGURE 18.5
Levels of P2P networks. (From Subramanian, R. and Goodman, B. D., *Peer to Peer Computing: The Evolution of a Disruptive Technology*, Idea Group Publishing, 2005.)

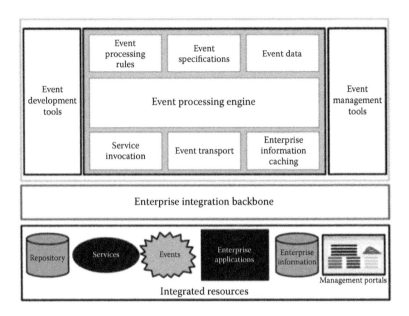

FIGURE 18.6
EDA components. (From Michelson, B. M., *Event-Driven Architecture Overview*, p. 8, Patricia Seybold Group, 2006.)

Figure 18.6 shows, schematically, the components of an EDA architecture, organized according to five categories: metadata (specification rules); event processing; tools (development or management of infrastructure); integration services (invocation and publishing of services, event transport channels, etc.); and finally, resources and targets (applications, services, business processes, databases, etc.).

With this model, systems can be constructed to facilitate a timely response to events—suited to situations in which environments are asynchronous and unpredictable (Becker 2008), such as the case of AAL. In these environments, with several sensors, this architecture can support different applications on decisions, for instance, emergency situations, in which an application response can only be calculated after analysis of an array of sensors, preventing a single sensor from triggering a nonexpected response.

Architectures in AAL Reference Projects

In recent years, many architectural paradigms have been suggested for AAL solutions. The previous section listed the most used and popular in the scientific community. Although these solutions are generic, in accordance with the purpose of each AAL project, architectures are commonly adapted and changed according to their evolution. In order to provide an insight into these implementations, relevant AAL projects are now presented, analyzed from an architectural approach.

Ambient Middleware for Context-Awareness

Ambient Middleware for Context-Awareness (AMiCA), is a project focused on the cloud, with a well-defined multilayer architecture with intelligent reasoning abilities and support for decision making. The development focuses on providing the high connectivity needed for dynamic environments, such as AAL environments (Lee et al. 2010). Use of the cloud aims to provide adaptable and efficient environments, facilitating, and speeding up the integration of new applications.

The typical requirements for developing middleware include aspects such as heterogeneity, mobility, scalability, and reliability of network communication. The AMiCA middleware platform (Figure 18.7) aims to satisfy all, providing support for the following: smart environments, sensitivity between contexts, dynamic discovery of available resources, transparency, asynchronous communication, component reusability, ambient adaptability and devices, minimal design, and distribution in the cloud.

The first layer of the architecture, with the various sensors, is separated from the other layers to enable the dynamic integration of various resources. The aggregator is used to join the data collected by the sensors, while the interpreter aims to transform the data into an understandable format for applications.

The next layer stores the information received by each context resource, so that responsible modules can infer user behavior information.

The application logic layer is responsible for managing (recording, researching, and invoking) the services available in the cloud, so that, depending on the context discussed in the preceding layer, applications adjust their behavior and adapt the services they provide to the user. In addition to the processing associated with services, the cloud is also used to store relevant information.

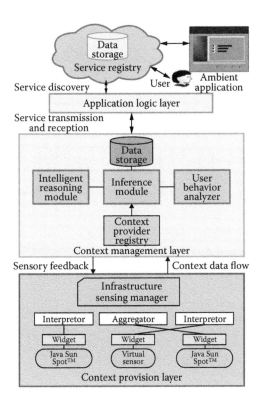

FIGURE 18.7
AMiCA architecture. (From Lee, K. et al., Proactive Context-Awareness in Ambient Assisted Living. Paper presented at the International Conference on Ageing, Disability and Independence, Newcastle, UK, 2010.)

Amigo

The Amigo project (AMIGO 2008), funded by the European Commission with the collaboration of 15 European companies and research institutes in different areas of knowledge, intends to support a networked home environment, focusing on aspects such as autonomy, loosely coupled components, and a heterogeneous structure. From a conceptual perspective, the Amigo project encompasses four key areas: such as personal computing, mobile computing, consumer electronics, and domotics.

Following a service-oriented paradigm, Amigo introduces a middleware layer, separating the platform layer (composed of the operating system and network modules) of the application layer. A middleware layer (Figure 18.8) encompasses several services that can be used by all other layers. Software components are divided into the following: base middleware, intelligent user services and legacy services (Janse et al. 2008).

The base middleware of Amigo is a flexible solution for the home network, integrating the most important technologies in terms of service platform, middleware protocols, programming paradigms, and security mechanisms (authentication and authorization of users and devices). The semantic technologies allow automated reasoning on the represented concepts by solving problems such as the heterogeneity of devices and services, research and service composition, context changes, and distribution of content.

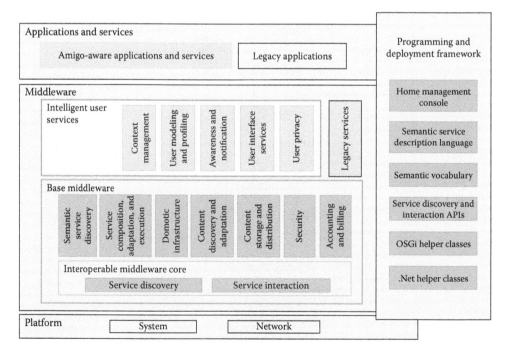

FIGURE 18.8

Amigo architecture. OSGi, open service gateway initiative. (With kind permission from Springer Science+ Business Media: *Amigo Architecture: Service Oriented Architecture for Intelligent Future In-Home Networks Constructing Ambient Intelligence*, vol. 11, 2008, pp. 371–378, Janse, M., Vink, P., and Georgantas, N.)

HERA

With a specific target audience of older people in early stages of Alzheimer's disease or with cardiovascular diseases or diabetes, the HERA project (Spanoudakis et al. 2010) aims to provide assistant services at reduced costs, improving users' lives at home and enhancing social interaction. The services provided here are grouped in three categories: cognitive enhancement services, specific residential services for patients, and residential services for older people in general. The challenges in developing the system are related to adaptability (to different users); heterogeneity (between different devices, solved with the implementation of an SOA); and simple, natural human–computer interaction.

Inspired by SOA, the overall architecture of the system identifies all the stakeholders in the project, among which we highlight the elderly (or patients) and health care providers (HERA Consortium 2010). Implicitly, Internet service providers (ISPs) and telecommunications operators are also presented. The main interface for users is a television, along with a set top box. Medical devices send their data via Bluetooth to the system so that doctors can access the clinical data of each user.

In more detail, the HERA architecture is shown in Figure 18.9. It is built according to three-tier architecture with Enterprise Java Beans (EJB) technology. The Apache server is used in conjunction with a MySQL database. At the intermediate layer, there are two groups of components, the first component relating to services and the second to the HERA system modules. The interfaces between components are based on web services and security and privacy technologies.

The services offered by the HERA platform include those of mental stimulation through specific games; asynchronous communication and information sharing between doctor and patient; monitoring of health conditions (weight, diabetes, blood pressure, etc.); alarm services (activities, medication, etc.); and nutritional counseling services.

MPOWER

The Middleware Platform for eMPOWERing cognitive disabled and elderly (MPOWER) project (SINTEF) is presented as an innovative middleware platform to support the rapid development of new services for the elderly or for people who have some type of cognitive impairment (Pitsillides et al. 2007). According to the authors, the goal of the project is to significantly improve its users' quality of life and adapt current technologies, such as those found in homes and smart sensor networks, to the specific needs of each. The platform focused its development on international standards, in order to simplify and accelerate the development of new services.

Figure 18.10 shows the architectural approach in technical terms. The platform is based on an SOA paradigm, using web services. From a global perspective, the three main categories for the interoperability of AAL services are the alarm and notification services (for sending messages), health services (export plans and medication schedules), and finally, voice and video communication services (Mikalsen et al. 2009).

The communication between different components is through hypertext transfer protocol (HTTP) or SOAP. To ensure high levels of modularity in its implementation, a UDDI service was added (OASIS 2004) as a broker, plus a message bus service inherent to the architecture.

From a detailed point of view, and with regard to development of the middleware itself, the services provided were organized according to five categories (Mikalsen et al. 2008):

- *Communication services*: services for communication of information of different kinds. They include alarm, external notification (email or short message service [SMS]),

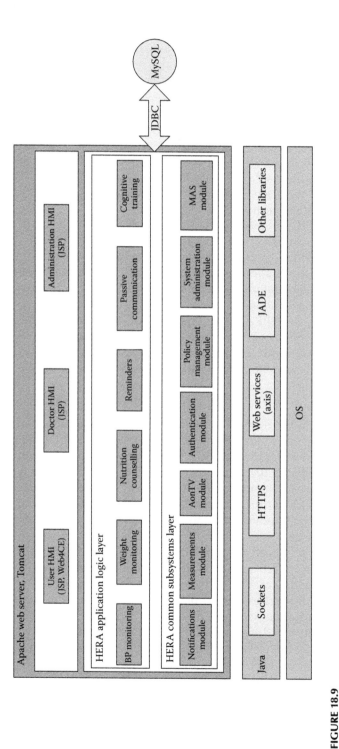

FIGURE 18.9
HERA server architecture. (From Spanoudakis, N. et al., A novel architecture and process for Ambient Assisted Living—the HERA approach. Paper presented at the 10th IEEE International Conference on Information Technology and Applications in Biomedicine [ITAB] Corfu, 2010.)

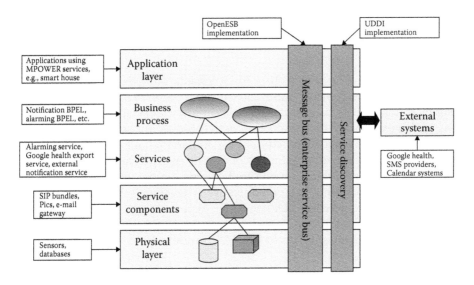

FIGURE 18.10
MPOWER SOA architecture and services. OpenESB, open enterprise service bus. (From Mikalsen, M. et al., Interoperability Services in the MPOWER Ambient Assisted Living Platform. Paper presented at the MIE. Retrieved from http://dblp.uni-trier.de/db/conf/mie/mie2009.html#MikalsenHFWW09, 2009.)

and Session Initiation Protocol (SIP) services for the management of external information.

- *Information services*: services oriented to scheduling, such as medication or alarm (event) services.

- *Management services*: services for the management of several types of users, for example, patients (addition, update, and search of patients).

- *Security services*: provide mechanisms for authentication, access control, and encryption as well as user management and auditing services.

- *Sensor services*: services for device configuration and obtaining information from them, such as temperature, location, doors, cameras, etc.

It is important to note that the architecture of this project is fairly complete. However, the complexity and the lower levels of heterogeneity in some decisions can also be an obstacle to its implementation.

Other Projects

Some other AAL reference projects are presented briefly below:

- Human Activity Recognition Engine (HARE)

    HARE aims to monitor the health status of people and their activities, through a heterogeneous sensor technology, processing activities in a cloud platform, increasing performance and reducing costs (Khattak et al. 2011). Initially, this system was developed for patients with Alzheimer's disease, to recognize a decrease in activity from analysis of data from several sensors, manipulated through ontologies to infer activities (feeding, falls, etc.), and make appropriate decisions according to information about the user profile.

- OASIS

  The goal of the open architecture for accessible services integration and standardisation (OASIS) project (OASIS 2008) is the creation of an open and innovative reference architecture based on ontologies and semantic services, which enables easy and inexpensive interconnection between existing services and those that will arise in the various areas required for an autonomous and independent lifestyle for the elderly. The target areas of OASIS are applications for independent living, including socializing, mobile applications, and applications for smart environments. With this aim, some modules were developed, highlighting the common ontological framework (COF) or OASIS hyperontology and also the reference architecture that uses the COF and support tools for the automatic linking of ontologies or emerging services to the OASIS architecture.

- openAAL

  The openAAL middleware platform represents a powerful and flexible open-source solution for AAL scenarios, allowing for easy deployment, configuration, and distribution of customized information technology (IT) services (Wolf et al. 2010). This platform provides generic services such as management contexts for abstraction and fusion of environmental data, system specification–based work flows, and semantic service research.

- PERSONA

  The perceptive spaces promoting independent aging (PERSONA) project aims to develop a scalable platform for the development of AAL services (Tazari et al. 2010). Its architecture, based on the Amigo platform, aims at easy, modular integration of components or services, emphasizing cost reduction, reliability, security, and adaptability to the requirements of each user or environment.

- SOPRANO

  Based on a combination of ontology techniques and service-oriented device architecture, the service-oriented programmable smart environments for older Europeans (SOPRANO) project aims to provide personalized IT services for the elderly or people with difficulty in maintaining a dignified, independent life (Wolf et al. 2008). The infrastructure consists of interfaces based on predefined contracts for each stakeholder (device vendors, developers, telecommunications engineers, or service providers) and is defined by ontologies. Ontologies act as mediators between the different components of the system, while the service-oriented infrastructure enables easy integration of new services or components.

- Universal Open Platform and Reference Specification for Ambient Assisted Living (universAAL)

  The universAAL project aims for the conception, design and implementation of new and innovative AAL services from a technical and economical point of view (universAAL 2010). Its main objective is the development of a complete set of interoperable components to form an environment for the development of open-source AAL applications. From a technological perspective, the universAAL platform consists of three essential service blocks: real-time support, development support, and community support.

Living Lab Ecosystem Conceptual Model

The concept of a living lab goes beyond a mere set of services or guidelines. It involves not only the inclusion of infrastructural aspects such as information and communication systems and peripheral devices but also development tools and specific methodologies for result analysis, specification, evaluation, or validation. Furthermore, for successful definition, the creation of a living lab ecosystem requires a constant collective effort—by stakeholders—to allow the R&D of new technologies and services. In our opinion, a living lab may be effectively divided into seven parts: (1) physical spaces, (2) physical infrastructure, (3) logical infrastructure, (4) development platform, (5) methodologies, (6) applications, and finally, (7) stakeholders.

Physical Spaces

A living lab must involve users in the innovation process from the early phases of research and idea generation until the later phases of development, implementation, and testing. Realistic scenarios must be provided specifically for older adults. This gives rise to the need to include a minimum set of environments or physical spaces: a laboratory apartment, a small family house, *real* apartments and/or family houses, and more standard laboratories.

To provide an accessible and easy-infrastructure *home*, a small apartment used for teaching gerontology courses at the University of Aveiro Health School was considered an essential physical space to include in the living lab. As partners in the project, the Centro de Medicina de Reabilitação da Região Centro–Rovisco Pais (CMRRP) has small houses used in the last stages of rehabilitation, and one, already with some domotics (Abreu et al. 2008) was also included.

As it is very important that researchers and students in health courses are also involved in the living lab, the living lab also includes two research labs as physical nodes, at the Institute of Electronic Engineering and Telematics of Aveiro (IEETA) in Aveiro and at the Microsoft Language Development Center (MLDC) in Porto Salvo.

Given the key aspects of service providers within the living lab, a more realistic point of view is provided by the inclusion of a social institution providing care to older adults (Santa Casa da Misericórdia de Oliveira do Bairro) and a rehabilitation center (CMRRP).

Physical Infrastructure

The living lab is composed of a complex network of devices or subsystems working together. The devices include the following: servers; personal computers (desktops, laptops); small portable computing devices (e.g., smartphones); sensors (on users and environment); video cameras; domestic appliances; input devices for interaction (e.g., Microsoft Kinect); actuators; and robots.

The creation and deployment of new, value-added services is enabled by networking technologies. Among those, next-generation network (NGN) technologies are considered essential because they provide the use of multiple broadband, QoS-enabled transport technologies (in which the underlying transport-related technologies are independent of service-related functions). NGN architectures also provide open interfaces and support for a wide spectrum of services, applications, and mechanisms based on service building blocks.

Logical Infrastructure

A common problem with AAL architectures is that different devices use different infrastructures and different protocols for communicating, resulting in interoperability issues. Given the heterogeneity inherent to LUL, NGN became our adopted solution due to its open interface support for a wide range of services, applications, and mechanisms based on service building blocks. NGN provides the bridge between them.

Figure 18.11 shows an overview of the logical connections enabled by the use of a broker, a diversity of services, and a monitor.

In order to ensure high interoperability and integration, all communications within the proposed architecture use both user datagram protocol (UDP) and transmission control protocol (TCP). Issues may rise with the use of UDP, given its unreliability, and some components may require high rate transmission capabilities without much attention to packet loss or traffic (real-time transfer protocol [RTP] video, for instance) (The Internet Society 1996). The choice of TCP (mainly via Internet Protocol) is obvious due to its well-known capabilities of overall packet delivery and error resistance.

Development Platform Architecture

The design and implementation of open distributed systems allowing the interaction of multiple, evolving heterogeneous devices is a difficult and complex task. Their development poses multiple challenges, such as the following: resource management, interoperability, synchronization, security, performance, scalability, and dependability.

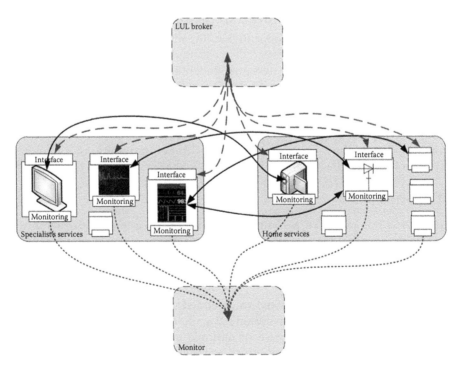

FIGURE 18.11
Communication between services, broker, and monitor.

The adopted development architecture is service based, and being the main focus of this chapter, it will be presented in section "LUL Architecture for New Service Development."

Methodologies

LUL, like all living labs, is not only about technologies. It is essentially an interactive environment to facilitate the research, development, integration, validation, and evaluation of adaptability and user monitoring technologies, new modes of interaction, and new services supported by NGN. In this sense, our living lab must propose and develop new methodologies with strong user involvement for the specification of new services, evaluation of these new services, and dissemination of knowledge.

Work on how to develop and evaluate new services is an important part of LUL. Regarding development, an iterative repetition of requirements, design, prototyping, and evaluation cycles has been applied.

In an LUL context, the services are tested involving potential end users in all development phases. This includes the conceptual design and, later, the prototypes, which allow for more realistic assessment, meeting the needs/preferences of users (Albers and Still 2010). This evaluation methodology presupposes a first phase of conceptual validation, followed by a prototype test and, finally, a pilot test. These phases are not isolated and are based on a spiral approach that follows the development progress from the beginning. The methodology should be flexible enough to allow moving forward, backward, and cross-wise between phases.

The first phase of evaluation aims to conceptually validate the interface and functionalities of the product or service. The prototype test intends to provide information about usability and user satisfaction for refinement of the requirements of the product or service. Finally, the pilot study tries to assess the significance of the product or service for its users, so that it can be integrated into their daily life.

The evaluation process involves techniques such as interviews, observation, system log recording, questionnaires, and recording of critical incidents (Bernsen and Dybkjaer 2009) to be used at different moments of data gathering.

Applications

The only way to evaluate/validate the various *components* resulting from the project is their use in practical services and applications. LUL identified three new applications as priorities: telerehabilitation (Teixeira et al. 2012), personal life assistant (Pires et al. 2011), and security at home. More information on the first will be presented in the sixth section of this chapter.

Stakeholders

As mentioned before, real users are essential within the living lab context. They are expected to be a source of ideas, to have a creative role in the development process, to help with their advice and concerns during the validation phase, as well to be diffusion agents.

In our case, users are not only the elderly end users but also health professionals (e.g., gerontologists), developers of new services, ICT developers, and institutional care providers.

LUL Architecture for New Service Development

In this section, we present the development architecture for LUL, based on an SOA paradigm (SOA). The choice of a *service architecture* comes from the need to obtain low rates of coupling between different components and ease their integration and deployment through simplified practices.

Low dependency between components becomes critical to ensure the autonomy of different functionalities with the lowest loss of service quality to the user. Due to the existing heterogeneity in technologies from different stakeholders, the architecture provides mechanisms for quick deployment via a set of support services aimed at application development.

One of the initial objectives of the project was to obtain efficient conditions for the creation of AAL business logics—by different stakeholders. Here, a major setback was due to the need to reimplement similar logics in each AAL project each time a new application was conceptualized. To some extent, this need leads to a waste of development time for simple recreation of common AAL capabilities. As such, LUL's architecture proposal has a strong focus on the conceptualization and development of *base* services that can reduce these limitations and allow expansion via future integration of *third-party* services.

Some of the previously described AAL projects included communication mechanisms inherent to the architecture. Although these mechanisms might provide higher security rates and robustness for the architectural option, these might also become limitative and problematic when introducing new business logics. As a solution, LUL's architecture adopts a simplified method related to how components communicate and are made available. According to SOA's paradigm, all modules are encapsulated as services, being accessed via web services. Security is obtained through the use of standards (such as SOAP) and additional authentication mechanisms (when necessary). Composition and orchestration are eased via service registry and integration of new logics sustained via several deployment locations and test environments.

LUL's architecture is represented in Figure 18.12. The architecture is composed of four layers: infrastructural, living lab services, common services, and applications.

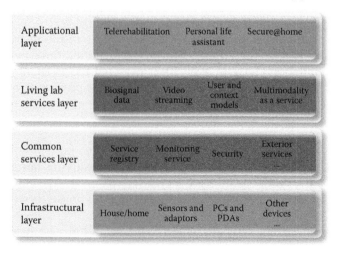

FIGURE 18.12
LUL development architecture overview.

Infrastructure Layer

The infrastructure involves the distributed lab physical nodes, particularly homes, and the entire set of devices at these different locations (sensors, adapters, mobile devices, set top boxes, desktop computers, etc.). As in most AAL architectures (e.g., see the work of Mikalsen et al. 2009), all are included in the *infrastructure layer*.

A common problem within several AAL scenarios concerns the constant add/remove operations of support devices. This raises two issues: the heterogeneity of communication technologies from each device and the high level of dependency between devices and software components.

While software dependency is natural, it can cause errors and lower rates of service quality. This dependency can be minimized, however, by introducing an intermediate mechanism between devices and software—middleware. By introducing middleware, it becomes the sole responsibility of the service to check the condition of the device as well as obtain *raw* data from it. The device's communication method (Wi-Fi, Bluetooth, ZigBee, among others) becomes invisible to the remaining services, with the middleware being the only *gateway* to the devices.

An issue with existing middleware solutions arises from their excessive complexity. In LUL's case, the middleware option is utilized in a minimized manner: each added device must be accessible via a specialized service—via a web service. As devices such as sensors might use a proprietary interface—common in commercial sensors—or contain no associated business logic, an adapter must be produced to provide communication with the device. This adapter must follow a *device-as-a-service* paradigm (de Deugd et al. 2006), offering its functionalities via a well-defined interface. In its design, the architecture's security and communication standards must be used in the implementation of the new service.

Common Services Layer

The *common services layer* provides services such as communication, security, monitoring, and user management. This layer is focused on all support services that are not directly associated with AAL or its application logics. By using this separation, a large set of services can be obtained through the inclusion of already-existing services created, for example, from previous international projects.

A serious issue with AAL architectures is their low reutilization rate. This problem is found not only with the architectures themselves but also with their associated services. Traditionally, a large set of AAL services is required to be rebuilt due to incompatibilities with the planned architecture. The living lab concept proposes a more open paradigm, in which already-existing services can easily be integrated as long as they provide their capabilities via web service technology. Above all, LUL's living lab aims to become a futuristic architecture where all who want to test their business logics in an AAL paradigm can do so without major technological constraints. The common service layer fulfills this objective.

In order to facilitate the search for services and their integration, any service within the architecture must advertise itself in the service registry. This service is critical to allow the system to offer orchestration and composition capabilities. Nevertheless, the purpose of the registry goes beyond that of a mere broker; it allows a service to inscribe itself and associate categories that describe its purpose and also to subscribe functional notifications of deployed services, such as changes in their status. With this subscription capability, services may be alerted, for example, to unavailability issues, which could result in system failure in the case of high dependencies.

Technologically, the registry runs at a central server serving all LUL nodes and functions like a WSDL (W3C 2001) repository. Given the SOA approach, the repository is implemented as a typical web service, accessible through SOAP (W3C 2007)—an XML format. As for registration, services rely on the WS-Notification specification (OASIS 2006), a common standard.

LUL Services Layer

The *LUL services layer* is composed of services developed to complement existing ones or to address areas not covered by existing AAL solutions. Examples are acquisition and data transmission by sensors, context and user information, robot control, and video streaming control, all developed in the LUL project. As such, it is in this layer that living lab associated services are placed and made available to the entire living lab ecosystem.

Some of LUL's base services were conceptualized and developed according to a *global* logic; that is, independently of the hardware used, services are able to *adapt* themselves and still propagate data. Two representative examples of this ideology are video streaming and the sensor and actuator services.

In order to keep the registry updated and functional, a monitoring service is also deployed in this layer, systematically querying services within the living lab ecosystem for *keep alive* information. This monitoring is essential in the case of errors or unavailability of a service, allowing the registry to notify the service's error. In addition, the monitoring service can evolve to be capable of composing QoS tests for registered services (such as latency and bandwidth) and be capable of using this information to compare similar services in order to recommend the most valuable and certifiable one.

More information on some of the services within this layer will be presented in section "LUL Services."

Application Layer

Finally, on top of the *architectural stack,* an *application layer* is included. In addition to their business logics, applications within this layer are distinguished by their interactive component. To help in this, applications make use of all inferior layers within the architecture. A representative example of this is the telerehabilitation application—presented in the section "Examples of Architecture Application."

LUL Services

In the previous section, two layers of services were introduced—one exclusively oriented to integrating specialized services to be developed as part of the LUL project. When implementing services, one of the first things that must be decided is where they will be deployed. Two possibilities arise: use of a central server accessible by all project nodes (scalable to a large increase in a more realistic AAL scenario) or use of a smaller home-based server. The need for both comes from the differences in the proposed services. While some are generic and must be readily available at a well-known address, others are more house dependent. Our option for LUL was to have a central server (named the LUL main server) where generic services are deployed and published, complemented by at least one server in each home (designated as *home gateway*).

Each home gateway should be placed near the senior, whether in their home, in a hospital ward, or a in a retirement home. The home environment is characterized by the presence of various sensors and actuators. The home gateway is responsible for all communication between the house and the outside world, i.e., between the LUL main server and living lab nodes. All local related problems are within the boundaries of this local server, reducing the complexity of its external communication.

Figure 18.13 shows integration of the different components or devices of the house, and the way they are made available for external access.

With the goal of providing an infrastructure to support the development, refinement, and testing of new services, the home gateway must fulfill some essential requirements at both the technical and user level, including the ability for automated installation or setup; remote maintenance; the possibility of start, stop, restart, update, or delete components without restarting the server; control of home devices; interoperability; security; scalability; monitoring; modularity; simplicity; and adaptability (to the user).

The approach to development of the living lab home gateway comprises the use of web services, benefiting from the advantages of SOA architectures.

During the development of the home gateway, some services were developed and added to the service layer. The services presented below are only a subset of all developed services, and they have been tested in a telerehabilitation scenario. In addition to all living lab services, additional services have been placed under home gateway *supervision*. Some examples include a robot, AdaptO (sound volume and font size adaption to the user) (Teixeira et al. 2011a), and personal life assistant (PLA) (audio and video conferences, among other functions).

In this section, we describe key services developed by the project, such as a video streaming service, a sensor and actuator service, and the application registry. The design and implementation of all LUL services must ensure that, regardless of the number, type, or complexity of the devices, the way the service communicates with others follows a specific, single protocol. This enables services to evolve and replace devices with others with better features without disrupting the outside communication layer.

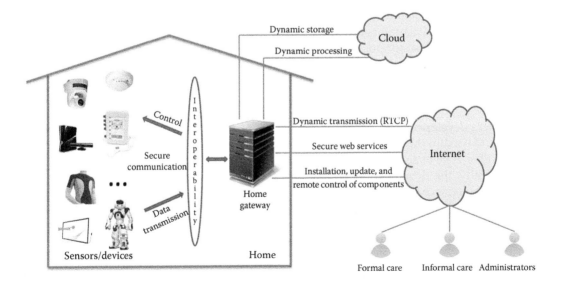

FIGURE 18.13
Living lab home gateway. RTCP, real time control protocol.

Application Registry

Many new services in AAL demand applications distributed over several locations. For example, the simple monitoring of an elderly person at home by means of video will require a part of the application to be at home and the other at the location of the professional in charge of the monitoring. It becomes necessary to create the means to deal with connectivity issues in such distributed applications. To accomplish a highly dynamic distributed architecture, a service must be provided for applications, allowing them to easily find, connect, and know the current status of others. This service is similar to the service registry integrating the common services layer, but, by serving as a registry for applications rather than services, it is a part of the LUL services layer.

Given the presented requirements, a new service for application registration was designed, implemented, and deployed in the LUL server. The service is closely related to a broker like the one used by the service registry. All applications register themselves at their startup in the registry; in addition, they must inform the registry of any status change. With this information, client applications can obtain the necessary information to connect and regain connectivity taking into consideration the status of their partners. In this way, in the case of a connection failure between two applications, the service can help to reestablish communication without the need for user interaction.

Given all the previous registration, scheduling, and connection information, the LUL server, through the monitor, scheduler, and broker modules, has detailed information about all the active sessions, as well as the status of all services that should be, but are not, involved in currently active sessions. Using such knowledge, the LUL server is able to automatically recover and reestablish abnormally terminated sessions and services.

Service for Sensors and Actuators

Sensor data and actuator control are fundamental for a typical AAL application. Information from sensors on user or environmental data is used by applications to process their business logics and to better adapt their user interfaces to match reality. In our architecture, devices and actuators are available through a specialized web service following a device-as-a-service paradigm. The first implementation of such a service was required for the retrieval of data gathered by one of the project's partners, Plux (2011). In this case, the service was required to retrieve data from specific sensors placed at home and make them available at both local and remote locations.

Due to the existence of several sensor types from different vendors, a generic sensor service was developed. This generic capability allows third-party devices to be easily integrated and used in the living lab ecosystem. Here, the Plux Bio Sensor was used, as could be any other type of sensor required in the future.

Technically, the developed service allows for real-time data to be available from the devices. The service itself is responsible for *grouping* the data, which can later be *consumed* by intermediate services. Each of these intermediate services is responsible for analysis and transformation of the acquired data according to their business logics.

Figure 18.14 represents how the service was deployed and subsequently used by a remote client application. Each generic sensor service has an interface, monitoring capabilities, and a set of devices. The service utilization process can be decomposed into parts: (1) service initialization—sensor service registers itself in the central service registry; (2) application authentication—each application that wants to obtain the service's data will ask the

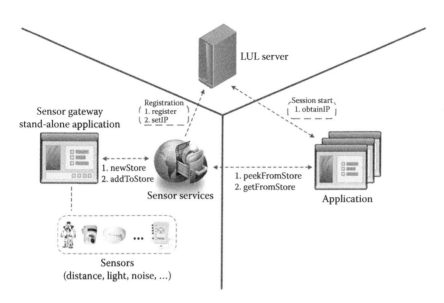

FIGURE 18.14
Deployment and use of the service for sensors.

application registry for information about it (such as location); and (3) data transmission—the application communicates with the sensor service, receiving all intended data.

Figure 18.14 shows an additional element—a stand-alone application. Some sensors require the use of an intermediate component that establishes direct communication with the device and then publishes the acquired *raw* data in the sensor service. This procedure is very common, especially with commercial sensors/actuators.

Video Streaming and Camera Control Services

Many potential applications in AAL require and can benefit from accessing images of a house and its inhabitants. Videoconferencing is the basis for many developments made in recent years in AAL projects (an example being the work of Peel et al. 2011). In some cases, it is also important to allow remote control of the camera, enabling the retrieval of images of a moving subject.

Since video transmission is not adequately addressed by the commonly used TCP protocol and poses real-time demands, the service must rely on protocols such as real time streaming protocol (RTSP) (The Internet Society 1998) to control the connection and RTP (The Internet Society 1996) for data transmission.

In the created service, actual transmission is not controlled due to possible delays in reception. However, to access the data, applications/services must get authorization from the service and, later, the actual feed link.

Similarly to other services, the video service has to register in the central server (via the application registry). To access the service, applications need first to question the central service, analyze the retrieved information, and then try to establish communication with the video service.

Figure 18.15 provides a generic view of the video service. Similarly to the service for sensors and actuators, the video service adopts a producer–consumer approach. The main

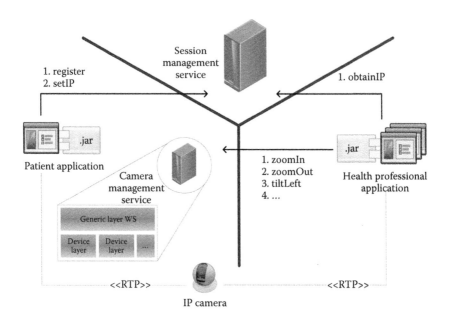

FIGURE 18.15
Video streaming and camera control service. WS, web services.

difference now is that the camera acts as an independent entity, providing video content without the need for a specialized application.

Data is only sent to an application via the initial connection. After the session is established, the client can directly use the service functionalities regarding camera control, such as pan, tilt, and zoom. Only one client at a time can control the camera. However, the video feed is accessible to many.

Other Services

Already existent but at an embryonic stage—minimal functionalities implemented—services for user modeling and profiling, context awareness, and multimodality were developed.

User modeling and profiling allow for methods such as tailoring information presentation to user and context, predicting the user's future behavior, helping the user to find relevant information, adapting interface features to the user and the context in which it is used, and indicating interface features and information presentation features for their adaptation to a multiuser environment. On the other hand, context awareness and notification provides the basic functionality required to develop applications allowing people and other applications to become aware of any significant change in context with minimal effort.

Multimodality—an interaction paradigm based on the use of several input/output options in a concurrent or redundant manner—is available on the platform via a specific algorithm called AdaptO (Teixeira et al. 2011a). AdaptO is based on output adaptation and possesses information on all available output methods by knowing their characteristics and current availability. Using context data such as distance to a screen or noise levels at a location, and user information such as vision or hearing disabilities, for instance, AdaptO establishes definitions of what modalities should be used or which are best suited at the time. When in execution, it provides applications with recommendations on how data should be made available to users upon request. AdaptO was successfully tested in LUL's telerehabilitation project as well as on a Microsoft PLA platform.

Examples of Architecture Application

This section presents an example of the use of the living lab and development architectures. This example is based on a new service to support remotely monitored rehabilitation sessions in elderly people's homes, called telerehabilitation (Teixeira et al. 2011a). For better understanding of the creational process, a guide explains how the LUL architecture was used in the development of this telerehabilitation service.

New Telerehabilitation Service for the Elderly

Telerehabilitation has the potential to facilitate access to rehabilitation services for clients who would otherwise be unable to access them for reasons such as distance from a health care facility, lack of trained clinicians in their geographic area, or mobility impairments (McCue et al. 2010). It allows the provision of rehabilitation services to remote and underserved populations, resulting in improved quality of life and prevention of secondary complications, decreasing the need and frequency of traveling to health care centers, and allowing health professionals to interact with clients and their families more often and follow up after discharge (Theodoros and Russell 2008).

At a technical level, a telerehabilitation service poses many demands—a distributed application with a high focus on components such as video, speech, user modeling, environment properties, and real-time communication.

Implementation

The first step in constructing the application to support such a new service is to be able to specify what its requirements are. Logically, given the goal of a telerehabilitation system, the first requirement is that the system will be used simultaneously at two different and possibly distant places: one being the health professional's location, the other, the elderly person's home. Communication between them is made available by the infrastructural layer of the development architecture and the bottom three parts of the LUL conceptual model (physical spaces, physical infrastructure, and logical infrastructure).

The second general requirement is related to support services. For a successful telerehabilitation session, information like sensor data, video, and feedback communication are critical for a health professional and must be made available. On the other hand, exercise information, instructions, and user adaptation become indispensable from a patient's perspective.

Most of these requirements are already met by the development architecture, particularly its LUL service layer. The developer must analyze what is available in the infrastructure and what services already exist. As such, the first step is to search through the architecture's service broker/registry. Using the results of the search, the developer finds the descriptions of services that might be of interest, for instance, video capture services on the applicational-services side and context/user services on the common-services side. An analysis of each of them is needed first, followed by the retrieval of their WSDL document—for client implementation. The developer then proceeds to integration of all of the functionalities within the application, including the necessary business logics. Finally, based on the home and hospital hardware, the application is deployed.

This is an example where it is inevitable to have a distributed logic within devices in the house and at the hospital (given the need for user interfaces), but other examples may involve exterior applicational deployment using only the infrastructure's available services.

Conclusion

This chapter presents both the LUL conceptual model and the architecture created for development of new AAL applications and services.

Following a service-oriented perspective, the architecture differs from others by assuming the need for certain services within AAL projects and presenting a new methodology for application development within AAL. Support services like user and context modeling, video streaming, or sensor information become fundamental to allow stakeholders to make use of AAL functionalities, with well-tested capabilities and without the need for repeated implementations. By separating different concepts into several layers and establishing a hierarchy between them, the occurrences of bottlenecks are reduced. Given SOA's standardization and the choice of Internet protocol (IP) as a communication technology, interoperability and integration issues are diminished, and scalability is assured for future expansion.

Test scenarios showed the value from both conceptual and service architectures. Additionally, the telerehabilitation service showed good usability rates and received good feedback from its users. Overall, with the conceptual and service architectures and consequent establishment of the living lab ecosystem, a step forward was taken to provide developers, researchers, and stakeholders with the means to create, test, and evaluate AAL logics in a simplified and integrated environment.

Future Work

To refine the proposed development architecture and its application to our LUL scenario, two areas appear to be most relevant: use and integration of cloud computing in our service-based architecture, and enhanced integration of our agent-based multimodal interaction support with the service-oriented view.

Use of cloud computing: Services and applications in use can be computer intensive, especially at the specialist site, when trying to analyze lengthy patient data records, or when processing complex information in real time. An approach to tackling this problem and alleviating the CPU load on the application site is to add a new element to the current architecture: the off-site processor. This off-site processor can be executed in a cloud computing environment, meaning that both peak and off-peak usage can be automatically handled by the cloud. The LUL server itself could also be on the cloud, benefiting from renewed scalability and availability. Integration of cloud computing in the proposed service development architecture should be based on the recent proposals of service-oriented cloud computing architectures (Tsai et al. 2010).

Service-oriented user interaction: An interesting area worth exploring is the service-oriented user interface (SOUI), a message-based architecture—meaning that everything in the user interface is controlled via messages. It enables control of both the appearance of the user interface and the interaction with services using a single messaging paradigm (Tsai et al. 2008).

Robot as a service: As LUL includes as one of its tasks the development of a service robot, the current trend toward robots as a service (Vasiliu et al. 2006; Matskin 2011) directly fits our architecture and should be explored.

References

Abreu, C., Fonseca, J. A., & Teixeira, A. (2008). Speech Enabled Interface to Home Automation for Disabled or Elderly People. Paper presented at the PROPOR 2008—Special Session. Retrieved from http://www.microsoft.com/portugal/mldc/news/propor2008MLDCSpecialSession/PapersPresentation.mspx (accessed January 18, 2012).

Aiello, M. (2006). The Role of Web Services at Home. Paper presented at the International Conference on Advanced International Conference on Telecommunications/Internet and Web Applications and Services. Retrieved from http://doi.ieeecomputersociety.org/10.1109/AICT-ICIW.2006.190 (accessed March 5, 2012).

Aiello, M., & Dustdar, S. (2008). Are Our Homes Ready for Services? A Domotic Infrastructure Based on the Web Service Stack. *Pervasive and Mobile Computing*, 4(4), 506–525.

Albers, M., & Still, B. (Eds.). (2010). *Usability of Complex Information Systems: Evaluation of User Interaction*. CRC Press, Boca Raton, FL.

AMIGO. (2008). Amigo—Ambient Intelligence for the Networked Home Environment. Retrieved from http://www.hitech-projects.com/euprojects/amigo/index.htm (accessed January 18, 2012).

Balzer, Y. (2004). Improve Your SOA Project Plans. Retrieved from http://www.ibm.com/developerworks/webservices/library/ws-improvesoa/ (accessed March 12, 2012).

Becker, M. (2008). Software Architecture Trends and Promising Technology for Ambient Assisted Living Systems. Paper presented at the Assisted Living Systems—Models, Architectures and Engineering Approaches. Retrieved from http://drops.dagstuhl.de/opus/volltexte/2008/1455 (accessed March 5, 2012).

Bernsen, N. O., & Dybkjaer, L. (2009). *Multimodal Usability*. Springer-Verlag, London.

de Deugd, S., Carroll, R., Kelly, K. E., Millett, B., & Ricker, J. (2006). SODA: Service-Oriented Device Architecture. *IEEE Pervasive Computing*, 5(3), 94–96.

Dohr, A., Drobics, M., Fugger, E., Prazak-Aram, B., & Schreier, G. (2010). Medication Management for Elderly People. Ehealth2010—Medical Informatics Meets Ehealth, 280.

Eriksson, L., Lindström, B., & Ekenberg, L. (2011). Patients' Experiences of Telerehabilitation at Home after Shoulder Joint Replacement. *Journal of Telemedicine and Telecare*, 17, 25–30.

Erl, T. (2008). What is SOA? An Introduction to Service-Oriented Computing. Retrieved from http://www.whatissoa.com/ (accessed January 18, 2012).

HERA Consortium. (2010). Deliverable D2.1: State-of-the-Art and Requirements Analysis. In Singular Logic SA (Ed.) (138 pp.).

Hsu, H. H., & Chen, C. C. (2010). RFID-based Human Behavior Modeling and Anomaly Detection for Elderly Care. *Mobile Information Systems*, 6(4), 341–354.

Huhns, M. N., & Singh, M. P. (2005). Service-Oriented Computing: Key Concepts and Principles. *Internet Computing*, 9(1), 75–81. doi: 10.1109/MIC.2005.21.

The Internet Society. (1996). RTP: A Transport Protocol for Real-Time Applications. Retrieved from http://www.ietf.org/rfc/rfc1889.txt (accessed January 18, 2012).

The Internet Society. (1998). Real Time Streaming Protocol (RTSP). Retrieved from http://www.ietf.org/rfc/rfc2326.txt (accessed January 18, 2012).

Janse, M., Vink, P., & Georgantas, N. (2008). *Amigo Architecture: Service Oriented Architecture for Intelligent Future In-Home Networks Constructing Ambient Intelligence* (Vol. 11, pp. 371–378). Springer, Berlin, Heidelberg.

Jara, A. J., Zamora-Izquierdo, M. A., & Gomez-Skarmeta, A. Y. (2009). An Ambient Assisted Living System for Telemedicine with Detection of Symptoms. *Bioinspired Applications in Artificial and Natural Computation*, Pt II, 5602, 75–84.

Khattak, A. M., Truc, P. T. H., Hung, L. X., Vinh, L. T., Dang, V.-H., Guan, D. et al. (2011). Towards Smart Homes Using Low Level Sensory Data. *Sensors*, 11(12), 11581–11604.

Kim, D., & Kim, D. (2006). An Intelligent Smart Home Control using Body Gestures. 2006 International Conference on Hybrid Information Technology, Vol. 2, Proceedings, 439–446.

Kung, A., & Jean-Bart, B. (2010). Making AAL Platforms a Reality. *Ambient Intelligence*, 6439, 187–196.

Lee, K., Lunney, T., Curran, K., & Santos, J. (2010). Proactive Context-Awareness in Ambient Assisted Living. Paper presented at the International Conference on Ageing, Disability and Independence, Newcastle, UK.

Loeser, C., Mueller, W., Berger, F., & Eikerling, H.-J. (2003). Peer-to-Peer Networks for Virtual Home Environments. Paper presented at the Proceedings of the 36th Annual Hawaii International Conference on System Sciences (HICSS'03)—Track 9, Vol. 9.

LUL Consortium. (2010). Living Usability Lab for Next Generation Networks. Retrieved from http://www.livinglab.pt (accessed January 18, 2012).

Matskin, M. (2011). Services, Clouds and Robots. Paper presented at the The Sixth International Conference on Internet and Web Applications and Services.

McCue, M., Fairman, A., & Pramuka, M. (2010). Enhancing Quality of Life through Telerehabilitation. *Physical Medicine and Rehabilitation Clinics of North America*, 21(1), 195–205.

Michelson, B. M. (2006). *Event-Driven Architecture Overview* (p. 8). Patricia Seybold Group, Boston.

Mikalsen, M., Walderhaug, S., & Stav, E. (2008). *MPOWER Project Deliverable: Overall Architecture*. SINTEF, Oslo, Norway.

Mikalsen, M., Hanke, S., Fuxreiter, T., Walderhaug, S., & Wienhofen, L. W. M. (2009). Interoperability Services in the MPOWER Ambient Assisted Living Platform. Paper presented at the MIE. Retrieved from http://dblp.uni-trier.de/db/conf/mie/mie2009.html#MikalsenHFWW09.

Mikulecky, P., Liskova, T., Cech, P., & Bures, V. (Eds.). (2008). Ambient Intelligence Perspectives. Selected Papers from the first International Ambient Intelligence Forum 2008, IOS Press.

OASIS. (2004). UDDI Spec Technical Committee Draft.

OASIS. (2006). OASIS Web Services Notification (WSN) TC. Retrieved from http://www.oasis-open.org/committees/tc_home.php?wg_abbrev=wsn (accessed January 18, 2012).

OASIS. (2008). OASIS—Project Presentation. Presentation. Retrieved from http://www.oasis-project.eu/index.php/lang-en/component/content/107?task=view&cat=21 (accessed January 18, 2012).

OASIS. (2011). Reference Architecture Foundation for Service Oriented Architecture Version 1.0. 120. Retrieved from http://docs.oasis-open.org/soa-rm/soa-ra/v1.0/soa-ra.pdf (accessed January 18, 2012).

Papazoglou, M. P., & van den Heuvel, W. J. (2007). Service Oriented Architectures: Approaches, Technologies and Research Issues. *VLDB Journal*, 16(3), 389–415.

Peel, N. M., Russell, T. G., & Gray, L. C. (2011). Feasibility of Using an In-home Video Conferencing System in Geriatric Rehabilitation. *Journal of Rehabilitation Medicine*, 43(4), 364–366.

Pires, C. G., Pinto, F. M., Rodrigues, E. M., & Dias, M. S. (2011). On the Benefits of Speech and Touch Interaction with Communication Services for Mobility Impaired Users. Paper presented at the 1st International Living Usability Lab Workshop on AAL Latest Solutions, Trends and Applications (part of BIOSTEC 2011).

Pitsillides, A., Themistokleous, E., Samaras, G., & Winnem, O. M. (2007). Overview of MPOWER: Middleware Platform for the Cognitively Impaired and Elderly. Paper presented at the IST-Africa 2007 Conference.

Plux. (2011). Plux Wireless Biosignals. Retrieved from http://www.plux.info/ (accessed January 18, 2012).

SINTEF. MPOWER. Retrieved from http://www.sintef.no/mpower (accessed January 5, 2012).

Sosinsky, B. (2011). *Cloud Computing Bible* (1st ed.). Wiley Publishing, Inc., Indianapolis, IN.

Spanoudakis, N., Grabner, B., Lymperopoulou, O., Moser-Siegmeth, V., Pantelopoulos, S., Sakka, P., & Moraitis, P. (2010). A Novel Architecture and Process for Ambient Assisted Living—The HERA approach. Paper presented at the 10th IEEE International Conference on Information Technology and Applications in Biomedicine (ITAB) Corfu.

Steg, H., Strese, H., Loroff, C., Hull, J., Schmidt, S. (2006). Ambient Assisted Living. Europe Is Facing a Demographic Challenge. Ambient Assisted Living Offers Solutions. European Overview Report, 1–85.

Subramanian, R., & Goodman, B. D. (2005). *Peer to Peer Computing: The Evolution of a Disruptive Technology*. Idea Group Publishing, Hershey, PA.

Sun, H., Florio, V. D., Gui, N., & Blondia, C. (2009). Promises and Challenges of Ambient Assisted Living Systems. Paper presented at the Sixth International Conference on Information Technology: New Generations (ITNG), Las Vegas, NV.

Tazari, M.-R., Furfari, F., Ramos, J.-P., & Ferro, E. (2010). The PERSONA Service Platform for AAL Spaces. In: *Handbook of Ambient Intelligence and Smart Environments* (pp. 1171–1199). Springer, New York.

Teixeira, A., Pereira, C., Oliveira e Silva, M., Pacheco, O., Neves, A., & Casimiro, J. (2011a). AdaptO—Adaptive Multimodal Output. Proceedings of the International Conference on Pervasive and Embedded Computing and Communication Systems (PECCS) 2011.

Teixeira, A., Rocha, N., Dias, M. S., Braga, D., Queirós, A., Pacheco, O. et al. (2011b). A New Living Lab for Usability Evaluation of ICT and Next Generation Networks for Elderly@Home. Paper presented at the 1st International Living Usability Lab Workshop on AAL Latest Solutions, Trends and Applications—AAL 2011 (Workshop of BIOSTEC 2011).

Teixeira, A., Pereira, C., Oliveira e Silva, M., Almeida, N., Sousa Pinto, J., Teixeira, C. et al. (2012). Health@Home Scenario: Creating a New Support System for Home Telerehabilitation. AAL 2012 (Workshop of BIOSTEC 2012).

Theodoros, D., & Russell, T. (2008). Telerehabilitation: Current Perspectives. *Studies in Health Technology and Informatics*, 131, 191–209.

Thies, G., & Vossen, G. (2008). Web-Oriented Architectures: On the Impact of Web 2.0 on Service-Oriented Architectures. Paper presented at the Asia-Pacific Services Computing Conference, 2008. APSCC '08. IEEE.

Tsai, W.-T., Huang, Q., Elston, J., & Chen, Y. (2008). Service-Oriented User Interface Modeling and Composition. Paper presented at the Proceedings of the 2008 IEEE International Conference on e-Business Engineering.

Tsai, W.-T., Sun, X., & Balasooriya, J. (2010). Service-Oriented Cloud Computing Architecture. Paper presented at the Seventh International Conference on Information Technology.

universAAL. (2010). UNIVERsal Open Platform and Reference Specification for Ambient Assisted Living. Brochure. Retrieved from http://universaal.org/index.php?option=com_content&view=category&layout=blog&id=8&Itemid=19 (accessed February 17, 2012).

Vasiliu, L., Sakpota, B., & Kim, H.-G. (2006). A Semantic Web Services Driven Application on Humanoid Robots. Retrieved from http://doi.ieeecomputersociety.org/10.1109/SEUS-WCCIA.2006.8 (accessed February 17, 2012).

W3C. (2001). Web Services Description Language (WSDL). Retrieved from http://www.w3.org/TR/wsdl (accessed February 17, 2012).

W3C. (2004). Web Services Architecture. Retrieved 17-02-2012, from http://www.w3.org/TR/ws-arch/#whatis (accessed February 17, 2012).

W3C. (2007). SOAP Specifications. Retrieved from http://www.w3.org/TR/soap/ (accessed February 17, 2012).

WHO. (2002). Active Ageing: A Policy Framework.

Wolf, P., Schmidt, A., & Klein, M. (2008). SOPRANO—An Extensible, Open AAL Platform for Elderly
    People Based on Semantical Contracts. Paper presented at the 3rd Workshop on Artificial
    Intelligence Techniques for Ambient Intelligence (AITAmI'08), 18th European Conference on
    Artificial Intelligence (ECAI 08), Patras, Greece. Retrieved from http://publications.andreas
    .schmidt.name/Wolf_Schmidt_Klein_AITAmI08_ECAI08_SOPRANO_AAL_Semantical
    _Contracts.pdf (accessed February 17, 2012).
Wolf, P., Schmidt, A., Otte, J. P., Klein, M., Rollwage, S., König-Ries, B. et al. (2010). openAAL—
    The Open Source Middleware for Ambient-Assisted Living (AAL). Paper presented at the
    AALIANCE Conference, Malaga, Spain. Retrieved from http://openaal.org/publications
    (accessed February 17, 2012).

19

Promoting Independent Living and Recreation in Life through Ambient Assisted Living Technology

Ângelo Costa, Juliana Teixeira, Nuno Santos, Ricardo Vardasca,
José Eduardo Fernandes, Ricardo J. Machado, Paulo Novais, and Ricardo Simoes

CONTENTS

ABSTRACT   The increase in life expectancy with a decrease in birth rates is contributing to the ageing of the European population. This phenomenon, coupled with greater awareness of the quality of life, the need to have cost-efficient assistive care, the intention of people to live independently in their homes, and the technological developments in recent decades, have contributed to the emergence of the concept of ambient assisted living (AAL). AAL solutions aim to provide healthy and safe ageing to users through promoting independence in performing daily activities and interacting with technology, taking into consideration the deterioration of the users' capabilities and the reduced costs of the solutions. In this chapter, AAL developments of monitoring activities of daily living (ADLs) and participation in a virtual community with the selected stakeholders are introduced, their roadmap with the expected technological developments are described, and the expected impact of these solutions on the end users of the developed solutions are discussed. This enables a real user guidance structure that represents the different needs and limitations of each user, presenting a highly structured project based on personas and possible solutions for them. The AAL4ALL Ambient Assisted Living for All (ALL4ALL) project is considered here as a case study to analyze and illustrate the ALL concepts discussed in this chapter.

KEY WORDS: *ambient assisted living, mobile architecture, AAL scenarios, AAL personas, functional profiles.*

Introduction

The increase in life expectancy at birth, the decrease in birth rates, and the growth of the older population (over 64) in Portugal, Europe, and the world contributed to an increase of the age dependency rate as seen in Figure 19.1. It can be seen that larger families are decreasing very fast while smaller families are increasing. This makes it very hard to renew the society's structure, leading to a population decrease. Figure 19.2 presents a comparison between people aged 0 to 19 years and people above 50 years in the different continents. This comparison can lead to the conclusion that the population is getting older. It is expected that by 2030, the number of elderly persons will greatly surpass that of the younger population in all continents. This ageing effect intensifies the demands for elderly

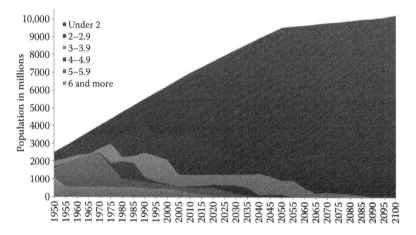

FIGURE 19.1
Children-per-family ratio of the world population. (From United Nations, Population estimates and projections section, 2012.)

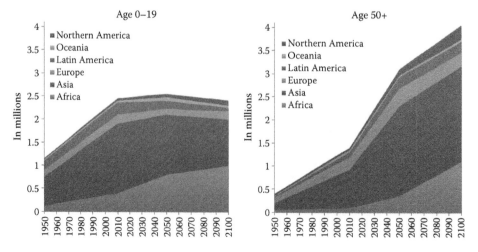

FIGURE 19.2
Population aged 0–19 and 50+ years. (From United Nations, Population estimates and projections section, 2012.)

care. In the worst-case scenario, the families' monthly income will not be sufficient to support an elderly person under their care. Current elderly care services are costly and will not be sufficient in the future to match needs [1,2]. Day care centers and nursing homes are expensive and do not have sufficient resources to attend to everyone in need. Furthermore, there are many people who are reluctant to leave their homes and go to an unknown environment, thinking that they will lose their independence and privacy.

Technology can be a real solution to this situation. By surrounding people with technological solutions that help them in their daily tasks while motoring them, a middle ground of compromise between independence and safety can be achieved.

The new eldercare demands, along with the evolution in technology usage, has created the required conditions for the development of information and communications technology (ICT) for independent living of the elderly. These ambient assisted living (AAL) solutions are intended to monitor and facilitate the health, safety, and well-being of individuals (handicapped and elder people) in specific scenarios, such as within their home, in mobility, in care centers, at work, and even during recreational activities. These solutions promote their independence, mobility, safety, and social contact through increased communication, inclusion, and participation by using ICT solutions [3].

ICT and web-based technologies offer new opportunities to create new living conditions and to facilitate social interaction and reduce limitations imposed by location and time, thus increasing personal control in daily life. AAL can, at best, be assumed as age-based assistance systems for a healthy and independent life that cater for the different abilities of their users. AAL comprises interoperable concepts, products, and services that combine new ICT and social environments with the aim to improve and increase the quality of life for people in all stages of the life cycle, incorporating intelligent systems of assistance for a better, healthier, and safer life in the preferred living environment; it also covers concepts, products, and services that interlink and improve new technologies and the social environment. Thus, it implies, not only challenges but also opportunities for citizens, the social and health care systems, as well as the industry and the European market [4]. Ambient intelligence represents an important role in AAL technologies, refers to electronic environments, and covers both the concept of ubiquitous computing and an intelligent social user interface.

Certainly, a good number of ideas have been tried out in many research projects and pilot experiments on ICT and ageing. Looking at some existing research projects, we can say that ICT solutions and their usage in AAL ecosystems have earned increased attention. The ePAL project [5] aims to explore innovative ways to best facilitate and support active ageing and ensure a balanced and inclusive postretirement lifestyle. A major hypothesis followed in ePAL is that ICT and, particularly, collaborative networks can provide an adequate framework for the implementation of effective support for active ageing. The SOPRANO project [6] aims to develop affordable, smart ICT-based assisted living services with interfaces that are easy to use for older people and familiar in their home environment. The universAAL project [7] will establish a store providing plug-and-play AAL applications and services that support multiple execution platforms and can be deployed to various devices and users. The PERSONA project [8] is working on a general-purpose technological platform for developing AAL services. Initial results include middleware that supports self-organization in an ad hoc manner and reference architecture for building AAL spaces. The conceptual architecture of PERSONA shows some of the platform components necessary for constructing AAL services. They are derived from a thorough analysis of different PERSONA scenarios. The CAALYX project [9] aims at increasing older people's autonomy and self-confidence by developing a wearable light device capable of measuring specific vital signs of the elderly, detecting falls, and communicating automatically in real time with the care provider in case of an emergency, wherever the elderly person happens to be, at home or outside. The CAALYX system's architecture is composed of three systems in cooperation: the roaming monitoring system, the home monitoring system, and the elderly care center.

The Ambient Assisted Living for All (AAL4ALL) project focuses on providing health care services and products to the elderly community; it implements the base structure of the foundations of the work presented. The objective is to present a roadmap and initial structures of an AAL project, focusing on the defined personas and a mobile solution to these personas. The current AAL projects lack a real user guidance structure, aiming at a broad area, whereas our opinion is that every user has different needs and limitations, meaning that the solutions should be personalized, solutions that will be presented in this chapter. The AAL4ALL project, similar to the Bridging Research in Ageing and ICT Development (BRAID) roadmap [10], adopts a holistic perspective of AAL concerning the adoption of life settings. These have been used to support the definition of scenarios and the respective sequence diagrams. Multiple viewpoints (like logical diagrams, sequence diagrams, or other artifacts) contribute to a better representation of the system and, as a consequence, to a better understanding of the system [11].

In this chapter, we intend to promote the use of AAL technology within *independent living* and *recreation in life* activities, with a focus on mobile and pervasive technologies. An analysis is conducted on existing technology for this domain and its applicability to the activities in question. We consider that this analysis must be conducted in the requirement phase of the project. We use sequence diagrams to represent the scenarios considered in both independent living and recreation in life, since they can be used to validate the elicited requirements in the analysis phase of system development. Additionally, we discuss technological issues and their relation to the presented scenarios, through profiling and framing techniques of the intended functionalities. The goal is to present a structure and development approach, demonstrating a new perspective on the problem and created from the start with the user in mind. Therefore, we present a design and plan that define, even before any development, the soft and hard requirements, based on questionnaires given to future users, which indicate their needs and the acceptance of technological solutions.

This chapter is structured as follows: the "AAL4ALL Project" section presents an introduction to the AAL4ALL project, discussing life settings, developments made, and scenarios. The "State of the Art" section presents ALL projects towards mobile implementation. The "Mobile Device Application Development of the AAL4ALL Architecture" section presents features for a mobile platform. The "Functional Profiles for Independent Living and Recreation in Life Scenarios" section discusses the profiling and framing techniques for independent living and recreation in life scenarios. Finally, the "Conclusions" section presents our conclusions and future work.

AAL4ALL Project

Although technologies for AAL are already available and often in use for different purposes, these *first offers* for primary and secondary end users are monolithic and incompatible and thus expensive and potentially unsustainable.

The AAL4ALL project brings together all relevant stakeholders, such as public institutions, industry, user organizations, and research and development institutions into the discussion and definition of the basic AAL services of general interest [12]. Analyzing already-existing standards and other international activities are key concepts of this project, which aims to capitalize on existing knowledge, avoiding redundant development, with a clear focus only on the missing pieces to achieve optimum solutions in this area.

Thus, the main objective of the AAL4ALL project is the development of a standard ecosystem of products and services for AAL, associated with a business model and validated through a large-scale trial [10,13–15].

Selected AAL Life Settings

The great challenges [16] established by the European Union (EU) commission for ageing societies and public health in the next 20 years are as follows:

- Modernizing European societies through creating better living conditions for people of all ages
- Enhancing the contribution of older people to the economy and society
- Strong expansion of needs for health and social care services
- Protection of the dignity of frail older people, who are often victims of neglect and abuse

Healthy ageing is defined as the process of optimizing opportunities for physical, social, and mental health to enable older people to take an active part in society without discrimination and to enjoy independence and good quality of life [17]. The EU commission strategy implies a rise in employability through the greater participation of older workers and the promotion of social inclusion, in particular, through the reduction of poverty.

It was suggested through the healthy ageing project [17] that the EU and the Member States have to do the following:

- Develop research to assess the effectiveness and the cost-effectiveness of health-promoting interventions and interventions for the prevention of disease or ill health throughout life and especially in later life.
- Strengthen research to find ways of motivating older people and changing their lifestyles, especially the *hard-to-reach* groups, paying special attention to environmental and cultural aspects.
- Strengthen research to develop indicators of healthy ageing and include data on the very old in health monitoring statistics and research.
- Disseminate research findings and promote their practical applications among all stakeholders.

Investing in healthy ageing [17] contributes to the labor supply, decreasing the likelihood of early retirement. The developments in technology influence all public domains and private life and how older people can cope with these developments. This population needs encouragement and time to become accustomed to the ever-changing world of technology.

The Lisbon Process [18] presented by the EU aims to promote active ageing by coordinating national policies, financial support, and the exchange of experience. Another report [19] from the EU Commission states that promoting *active ageing* results in longer working lives. Disease prevention is mentioned as an important measure for increasing productivity at work and reducing health care costs.

The focus of this research work within the scope of the AAL4ALL project is to address these challenges enunciated by the EU Commission guidelines developing the AAL area.

The BRAID project [10] aims to develop a comprehensive research and technological development (RTD) roadmap for active ageing by consolidating existing roadmaps and by describing and launching a stakeholder coordination and consultation mechanism; this project features key research challenges and produces a vision for a comprehensive approach in supporting the well-being and socioeconomic integration of increasing numbers of senior citizens in Europe, by approaching the ageing phenomenon and many of the resulting challenges through the development of a comprehensive roadmap for *ageing well*, which identifies advanced ICT-based approaches and mechanisms to support ageing of European citizens. This project has defined four main life settings: independent living, health and care in life, occupation in life, and recreation in life. Among these, the present research work focuses on two: independent living and recreation in life.

The standard AAL ecosystem, proposed by the AAL4ALL project, uses the description and characterization of the BRAID project as input to identify products, services, and business models. This ecosystem is built upon the concept of the availability of technology to the user in a form of set-and-forget. An easy setup and full integration of the devices are key requirements.

The target users for the AAL4ALL project include the elderly and those with disabilities, clearly with a high probability of poor technological knowledge. This results in reducing costs and minimizing problems for the user, thus providing a quality service with hassle-free operation.

The expected developments were designed having all of the described characteristics in mind, representing typical system users and devices, and providing a term of operation and development of future applications.

AAL Developments

The AAL4ALL project approached the AAL theme from a new point of view, not by adopting the standard forms that exist but by taking the current knowledge and creating new platforms, ontologies, and standards. These outcomes translate into a complex ambience of provided services, each having a different and crucial task. This implies connecting several appliances, sensors, and actuators present in the user's home, and coordinating them to follow rules created to better serve the user. Interfaces are also very important to the operation and user feedback to certain aspects; additionally, mobile monitoring and ubiquitous computing are important additions to provide pervasive monitoring and assistance.

Architecture and prototyping are considered the most important phases. They are the foundations of the project and must be carefully designed to ensure successful subsequent phases. Currently, there are several mangled projects that follow none of the specifications of other projects, thus creating badly stitched communication protocols and interfaces that rely on other interoperability bridging projects. In terms of creating solutions for the actors and concerning the development of solutions for mobile devices, specifications were made to achieve the proposed objectives.

In terms of technological solutions, the adoption of mobile devices opened a new gateway for providing and obtaining information. To develop the necessary conclusions in order to respond to the needs of the project, a roadmap was developed (Figure 19.3), leading to a specifications guide that serves as the foundation of the application and services

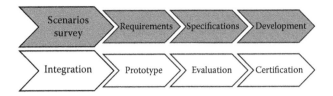

FIGURE 19.3
AAL4ALL project roadmap.

being developed in the mobile device. The roadmap is a strict composition of an over-all structure that defines the next steps of the project, providing the base guidelines for development.

Mobile devices are currently amazing pieces of technology, particularly considering their cost, not only packing processing capabilities that could outrun desktops made only 5 years ago but also bundled with several different communication systems and discrete sensors. Also, the availability of mobile devices and their operating systems provides the best solution for implementing pervasive communication services.

The mobile application proposed in this work is integrated in the resultant investigation scenarios: independent living and recreation in life.

Scenario Specification

In this section, we present scenarios regarding the independent living and recreation in life domains, by using specific sequence diagrams for elicitation purposes. Requirement elicitation is all about learning and understanding the needs of users and project stake-holders with the ultimate aim of communicating these needs to the system developers [20]. Stakeholders and developers have different points of view regarding requirements. Typically, for stakeholders, static requirement models are not enough, since stakeholders with non–computer science education are not able to discover all the interdependencies between the elicited requirements.

Thus, we adopt a requirement elicitation approach that starts by eliciting requirements based on the scenarios of the intended AAL domain. In this chapter, we considered the life settings as the starting point to define the scenarios (based on active ageing scenarios [21]) for the development of products and services within the AAL4ALL project. Among these, the present work focuses on the following two:

- *Independent living.* The individual should be safe and have all the care needed at home. Their activities should be managed, and they should have support for phys-ical mobility in terms of localization, positioning, and also mobility assistance.

- *Recreation in life.* The individual should be encouraged to socialize through real-world and virtual communities and in the management of social events. They should be requested to participate in entertainment activities, such as games, remote cultural activities, and remote recreation activities. They should engage in learning activities, experience exchange, and knowledge sharing.

These settings correspond to the main areas of life of a person in general and will need to be supported. The significance of defining these settings is that they comprehensively cover the main aspects related to active ageing and well-being of the elderly. The setup of the settings has resulted in the development of scenarios. These scenarios are built upon the concept of the availability of technology to the user in a form of set-and-forget. Easy setup and full integration of the devices are key requirements. The expected scenarios were designed to have all of the described characteristics in mind, represent typical system users and devices, and provide a term of operation and development of future applications.

The development of the scenarios intends to develop the assisted living environment in order to respond to the interactions between users and solutions and further the interactions of these solutions with the AAL4ALL platform. These solutions represent several technologies, such as medical technology, microsystems technology, ICT, and innovative services [13].

In terms of scenarios, a batch of them was developed, containing the resulting actors from the acquired data in order to respond to the most common requests of the user in general. The actors who are more related to the adopted technological solutions are those who are technologically resolute and aware, thus having medium to good knowledge of operating, for instance, mobile devices.

We now briefly describe the actors who participate in the scenarios available from the reports. Actor #1, Joana, is an elderly person who has a slight mobility problem but is very active, regularly goes to the theater, and possesses technical knowledge. The main interests concerning this actor are as follows:

- Have information about theatre shows
- Connect with friends from a virtual community
- Monitor health values
- Be accessible to family and have security systems for protection

With these interests and the knowledge about technology, Joana can work with the said technology to become more independent and active.

Our proposal leans towards the development of technological solutions for mobile devices. Mobile devices will be fully integrated into the concept of AAL and the operating system that controls the user's home. That means that the user has available at their fingertips an intuitive method to control their home and to connect with the rest of the world.

UML sequence diagrams have been constructed to capture the main AAL scenarios. Some approaches propose the usage of a stereotyped version of UML sequence diagrams to validate the elicited requirements in the analysis phase [22]. We can take into consideration that the scenarios expressed in the sequence diagrams are built using the candidate use cases in the form of activities that will be executed and must be computationally supported by the system to be implemented. These activities are placed in the sequence diagrams and associated with the corresponding actors [11]. Initially, in this project, it was necessary to establish the relationships between activities and actors. Interactions are used to define those relationships and can be represented in a UML sequence diagram. As an example for independent living and recreation in life, we consider two scenarios expressed in sequence diagrams: (1) *check health values* for independent living and (2) *participate in social community* for recreation in life.

In the scenario depicted in Figure 19.4, the user's health values (e.g., blood pressure, heart rate, etc.) are measured by using a device. Typically, the measurement device automatically submits the health values to be stored and accessed in the home or hospital.

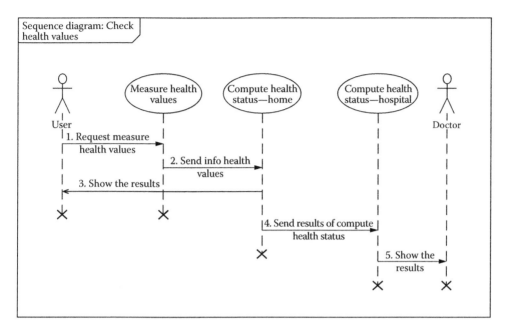

FIGURE 19.4
Check health values scenario.

Figure 19.5 depicts a scenario where the user can use a social network to participate in a social community. In this social community, the user can publish content (images, documents, presentations, videos, etc.).

There are already some approaches to this theme by other projects that can be integrated in an AAL concept. Taking cues from their development, we will present the advances in the development of an AAL mobile application.

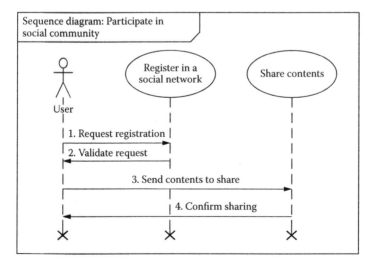

FIGURE 19.5
Participate in social community scenario.

State of the Art

The project presented relies on the concept of AAL being, in this case, implemented in mobile systems. As expected, due to the rise in this area in the last few years, there are already some projects that are being developed regarding the same concept and implementation strategy. There are some points in common but many more that are not, which will be presented next. The aim is to underline the benefits that our developments are implementing and differentiate them from the rest.

The Memory Aiding Prompting System (MAPS) project [22,23], developed at Colorado University, is a platform that supports people with cognitive disabilities, guiding them through daily tasks. This project has two technical aims: providing a remembering system and a social event sharing system.

The MAPS project works by using visual and audio signals, built from scripts, to guide the user on their daily schedule. This system works on both mobile devices and personal computers, the mobile version being very limited in comparison with the desktop version. The warning scripts are created by the caregivers, defining the appropriate way to notify the user of an impending task.

The work flow is established in the following way: The events/tasks are created on the desktop version, which also allows a user to share and store them; upon saving, the events are sent to the mobile version, which can only trigger the alarms to remind the user of the events/tasks. Wireless networks are used to upload the information to the mobile device. Moreover, the project relies on a third person to schedule and share events with the rest of the users.

MAPS is convenient in that it is easy to use and counts on the input of particular persons who know the user well. On the other hand, there are some problems: the mobile phone only acts as an alarm, only providing notifications to the user and not being a truly interactive system. The user cannot input the tasks themselves, thus always needing another person to help them. The system does not really create a community, being very limited in terms of user communication. Ultimately, it is just a suggestion system.

A community-oriented cognitive assistant was developed at the University of Rochester [24–26]. This project aimed to provide a platform used by various people (e.g., friends, family, caregivers) that connected all of them, allowing users to send their location so they can go to each other. It serves persons with cognitive disabilities, helping them to be located and receive attention from a caregiver, who is able to find the person and help them to safely get home or to other places. It relies on mobile phone GPS sensors and presents on the screen arrows pointing towards the direction the user has to go. This system can be controlled remotely, by a caregiver, sending the user to a safe place in case the user is lost or confused.

New advances in this project are at the personalization level, presenting algorithms to detect if a person who is interacting is a friend or a foe. The advances really impact the user's daily activities, thus expanding features that could integrate the mobility assistance.

The guiding system of this project is poor and does not have any type of interaction more than presenting the path to follow. It is not able to send the user's current location to other persons. This limits the assistance that the user could receive. For instance, if the caregiver wants to know where the user is, or if the user needs assistance, this cannot be done interactively or automatically. The caregiver or the user must phone the person to whom they want to relay the information, which develops a large entropy due to the fact that the caregiver must be allocated to counsel only one user, and this also can lead to much time being spent. Moreover, the user can only follow the path in the mobile device, being unable to change the route, and to change the list of routes, a technician is needed to create and upload the new data, making it very impractical.

The project Collaborative Memory Aids (CMA), developed by the University of Toronto, is a mobile device application that aims to help the user remember events [27]. It works only in mobile devices, thus being a direct interaction application. It uses adaptive interfaces that can be adjusted to each user and the creation of a community linked by events. The usability is a great component of the CMA. The operation process is done in the following way: The user (or other person) adds an event to the application scheduler, which is transmitted to a server that saves the events and the participants associated, setting an alarm in the mobile device of each participant.

Being easy to use, it was well accepted by the test subjects, but it fell short in terms of features. The users appreciated the fact that the interfaces are easy to learn and operate and that it connected automatically to their friends, scheduling all participants. However, these users had to do most of the tasks, adding, deleting, and editing, as it was not directly connected to a caregiver service provider. This led to a problem that was critical to the users, which was that if the users could not remember in the first place to schedule an event, how could the application remind them of it? This therefore somewhat defeated the whole purpose of the CMA project.

The presented projects brought about interesting points in their development that should serve as a basis for other projects' architecture and problems that should be addressed to not be repeated again. Next, we will present a preliminary architecture of an AAL platform that addresses the connection between the user and caregiver, to establish an environment of healthy cooperation between them.

Mobile Device Application Development of the AAL4ALL Architecture

From the projects presented, a mobile application can be structured that establishes a collaborative environment between the user and the caregiver. This application must follow the AAL4ALL architecture standard, meaning that it must follow the implemented integration systems. Therefore, it must be compliant with the communication norms that are provided by the communication node and the middleware standards.

Integration is crucial to a project with this dimension, as it has several different products and services from different providers. All the outcome products and services must obey the standards developed in this phase of development. Furthermore, a strict certification process will also result from this integration iteration, with the aim of verifying the product features and whether they stand up to the requirements of functionality and safety.

The mobile platform must be structured to comply with the platform communication nodes, thus being correctly integrated with the rest of the platform services.

Integration Features of AAL4ALL

The AAL4ALL ecosystem's architecture is extensible and scalable, requiring the core architecture to be just a backbone for the interoperability of members' components, offering basic services such as authentication, monitoring, and service discovery and subscription.

The mobile devices must then connect with the mobile gateway, ensuring the throughput of the data and the authentication of the information exchanged. The AAL4ALL project has great concern for information security and the privacy of the user, thus obligating the connecting services to use security safeguards.

The proposed AAL4ALL base architecture (Figure 19.6) consists of a mobile and home system gateway, AAL service providers, non-AAL-compliant/legacy services through adapters/gateways, and the core component AAL4ALL node. The AAL4ALL node is an interesting component to this mobile implementation. This is because of its ability to connect to the mobile devices and with web services such as Simple Object Access protocol (SOAP) and Representational State Transfer (Rest) [27–30].

In terms of development, the use of these technologies helps in terms of implementation and standardized communication systems, easing workload and decreasing time consumed.

Figure 19.7 presents how the mobile architecture will connect with the two domains. These domains consist of the system/device and mobile gateway. The system device

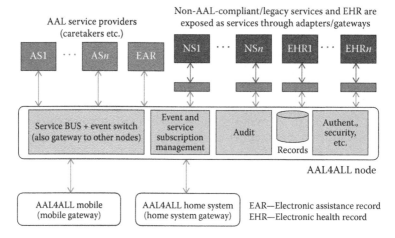

FIGURE 19.6
AAL4ALL system architecture.

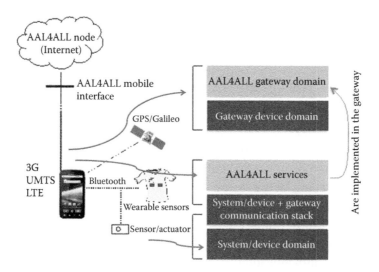

FIGURE 19.7
Mobile system components mapping to domains.

domain can be composed of wearable sensors or a GPS/Galileo service provider and will have connectivity with the gateway interface through a wireless sensor network (WSN); the mobile gateway domain is responsible for connecting to the AAL4ALL node and the Internet, providing the mobile AAL services.

The implementation of this integration system in a mobile application will be presented in the following section.

Mobile Device Application

In terms of development, AAL4ALL is, at this stage in the specification and definition of technological platforms, able to provide the required solutions for the presented personas. A significant part of the project will consist in the development of applications for mobile devices based on Android, to provide services at any location.

To operate in proper conditions, the mobile devices should have Internet connectivity available at all times. This allows the main features to operate correctly, by keeping information being sent and received. This means that the user can always be connected to their home, caregivers, and relatives. The application itself is divided into five major components:

1. Collecting local information and sending it to the central management: captures information directly from the sensors of the device and the interaction of the users with the mobile application.
2. Receiving information from the central management: provides the user with relevant information, which can be from the sensors or messages from other users. Due to the modular reception system, any information can be served to the user.
3. Providing interactive interfaces to display important information: the interfaces will be in compliance with standard regulations, directly accessed to be used by elderly persons.
4. Managing events: provides easy interaction with calendar and chat sessions with other users, rearranging the events if needed.
5. Providing localization and emergency services: access to the GPS built-in system and providing a *panic button* method to call for emergencies.

The application serves as a port to all the devices and services that the user subscribes to. It is able to receive communication, through the communication module and information from the sensors (whether home or body sensors), and display the information contained in it, using SOAP, OAUTH, and HTTPS protocols [30].

The connection with other persons can be established using chat or call sessions. Additionally, the system will provide a calendar management service that is able to receive incoming events or schedule new events using the JSON [30] data interchange format, containing all the important items about an event and other participants.

In terms of architecture, the whole system will rely on two platforms: the mobile and the home server. The home server establishes all the communications with the rest of the services available to the user, such as appliance control, in-home positioning system, advanced fall detection system, environment control, among others, using the available interfaces on the mobile to provide information about common house and user-related events.

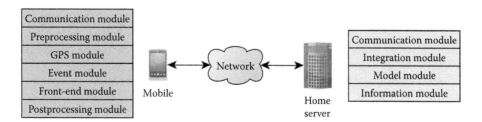

FIGURE 19.8
Mobile and home server modules.

Figure 19.8 represents all the modules needed to operate the system at this time. The separation of the modules provides a full separation, leading to easier upgrades and fail-proof operation. The mobile modules consist of the following:

- Communication module: establishes communication with the server, using secure protocols (OAUTH, HTTPS)
- Preprocessing module: processes incoming messages and separates them by module
- GPS module: retrieves user position and notifies the server
- Event module: gets events from an array of different calendar services and processes current and new events
- Front-end module: displays all the information, serving personalized interfaces; additionally provides a panic button to call relatives and send the user's current location
- Postprocessing module: packages all the information to respond to the server

The home server modules consist of the following:

- Communication module: establishes the communication with the mobile, using secure protocols (OAUTH, HTTPS)
- Integration module: provides the integration of the multiplicity of services and formats them into a universal standard
- Model module: per-service formatting standard service
- Information module: collects of user-readable information

Adaptive interfaces [31] will be available to provide information directly adjusted to the user's preferences and needs. This type of interface is commonly simple but informative, with the capability to be configured to display different types of information to adapt to people with different disabilities.

Due to the complexity of the AAL4ALL project, we presented only the services where the server has a direct impact on the mobile system. The collection of services greatly surpasses what is presented. This project is currently in development. As partnerships develop, the rest of the services of the mobile system following all these developments, leading to an exact integration with all systems. This therefore leaves only the following question: How does the mobile platform integrate with the presented scenarios?

Functional Profiles for Independent Living and Recreation in Life Scenarios

Technological and social developments, such as the Internet, wireless networks, and affordable communication and computing devices enriched with sensing capabilities, as well as other IT gadgets, contributed to the dissemination of computing. Embedding computing devices in objects or places for monitoring or control, along with mobile computing, enabled us to envision a *real* physical world enhanced with information and computing capabilities. These capabilities allow us to facilitate human life in its diverse facets (such as the personal or social), such as in AAL, or to improve businesses or other organizational processes. An AAL system aims to provide, through orchestration of cooperating pervasive devices and systems, a ubiquitous computing environment that allows a seamless and unobtrusive interaction when monitoring or assisting people in the realization of their activities.

The use of spontaneous cooperating smart objects, with access to online/Internet databases or services, offers great potential for applications [32]; it is not the enabling technology "[…] but the applications and the delivered services [that] will have a strong visible influence on our high-tech culture" [33]. Abowd et al. [34] believe that, to realize Weiser's vision [35] (a vision of ubiquitous/pervasive computing), beyond the understanding of the everyday practices of people and the augmentation of the world with heterogeneous interconnected devices, it is necessary to orchestrate these devices in order to provide for a holistic user experience.

With all the interconnected computing and other information-augmented objects, services are supported and deployed to enable higher-level applications that assist the user (either in a seamlessly or intensively interacting way). The pervasive information system (PIS) [36] inherent in these kinds of computation-enriched environments must be able to adapt to changes in the devices or in the structure of devices that compose the system. The design of the PIS must encompass an approach that recognizes those issues and that structures the needed concepts and adopts a proper strategy that allows fast development or integration of new or modified functionalities. These functionalities may correspond to new/changed system requirements, device capabilities, or device computational platform technology.

A PIS design takes into account relevant characteristics of PIS such as the following: (1) the elevated number of devices that can be involved; (2) the potential heterogeneity of the devices; (3) the pace of requirement changes due to technological or business innovations; and (4) the potential complexity of interactions among devices. Therefore, some issues that arise may influence the strategy taken in the approach to the design of PIS. Due to the complexity of PISs, software development for PIS can be facilitated by an approach that properly focuses the system, and the system development, with perspectives that help to abstract their relevant properties. Fernandes et al. [37] propose a development framework that encompasses concepts suitable for the model-driven development of PISs.

In this section, we relate the features presented in the previous section to the life settings considered in this chapter: independent living and recreation in life. In Figure 19.9, we apply computational entities to the scenario *check health values*. We are depicting the computational entities involved during the sequence flow (for instance, a measurement device, the home and hospital server, and the network). In the example, the measurement

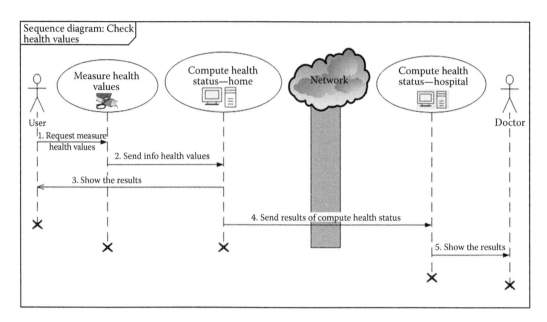

FIGURE 19.9
Check health values and computational entities.

device automatically sends the returned values to the home server. This information is available in the network. The hospital server can also access these health data in the same circumstances as the home server.

Figure 19.10 refers to the scenario shown in Figure 19.5. In this scenario, the user registers on a social network by using devices like smartphones, tablets, laptops, or the home server.

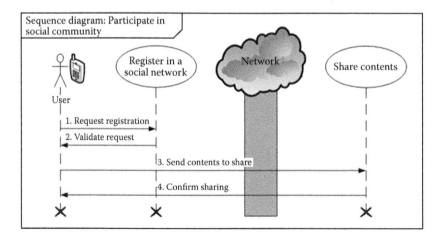

FIGURE 19.10
Participate in social community and computational entities.

The user is then capable of publishing content in the network, and the network allows access to the published content.

Our framework introduces and describes several concepts sustained on a few perspectives of relevance to the development structure, called dimensions (resources, functional, and abstraction); it also distinguishes two perspectives related to the development process: the global development process perspective and the elementary development processes perspective. Based on this development framework, profiling and framing structures [38] may be used as a way to effectively and consistently apply those concepts in PIS development projects independently of their size. These structures facilitate the definition of functional profiles, resource categories, and functional profile instances (concepts present in the development framework). Functional profiles define functionalities that are assigned to resource categories for their realization. The assignment of a functional profile to a specific resource category results in a functional profile instance, which will have a corresponding development structure that will be the subject of an elementary development process framed on a global development process.

Regarding the AAL4ALL project, Figure 19.11 illustrates the instantiation of the profiling and framing structure for AAL4ALL. The functional dimension axis (on the left of the figure) shows the functional profiles devised, and the resource dimension axis (at the top of the figure) shows the resource categories considered for the system. The plan formed by these axes shows the functional profile instances deemed relevant.

As seen in Figure 19.11, the profiling and framing of identified functionalities in the scenarios are structured in order to depict each of the functional profiles and their instances. The *health values retrieving* functional profile regards the reading and measurement of the user's health values (e.g., blood pressure, heart rate, etc.), by using a measurement device and storing the values in the server, without any data analysis or computation. Typically, measurement devices automatically send the returned values to another device (for instance, the home server). If these values are not automatically sent, alternatively, and hypothetically, values can be inserted directly by the home server, smartphone, tablet, or laptop. *Health data access* regards requesting and accessing the health data (measured in the previous functional profile) by using an information technology (IT) system. These data are stored and accessed in the home and hospital servers. *Home services orchestration* concerns the integration and orchestration of the services executed in the home environment. The home server is responsible for executing such a functional profile, since it is this device that is used as an integrator of the batch of installed and deployed devices in a user's homes (e.g., TV boxes, smartphones, laptops, tablets, sensors, etc.). *Platform service access* concerns providing access to the services available in the network. These services can be accessed by the user (via the home server) or a doctor or other medical service (via the hospital server). Alternatively, smartphones, tablets, and laptops can access the available services directly. *Contents publication* allows publication of content (images, documents, presentations, videos, etc.) in the network. Devices such as smartphones, tablets, laptops, or the home server can publish such content. *Publish contents availability assurance* regards the assurance of the availability of the published content (in the previous functional profile).

To attend to the profiling and framing structure for the AAL4ALL project and to the development framework for PIS, a development framework was established for this project (Figure 19.12). Figure 19.12 shows the framing of the development structures associated with the functional profile instances defined in the profiling and framing structure, as

526 *Ambient Assisted Living*

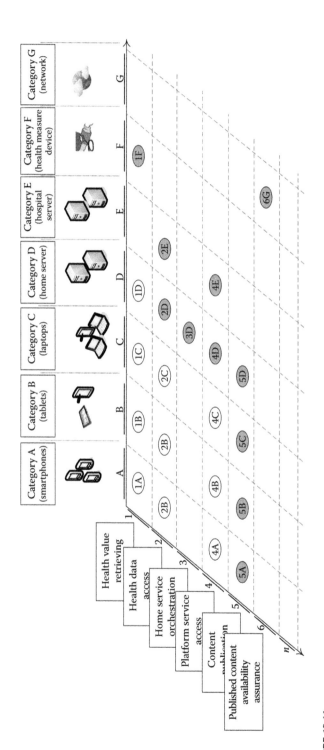

FIGURE 19.11
Profiling and framing structure for AAL4ALL.

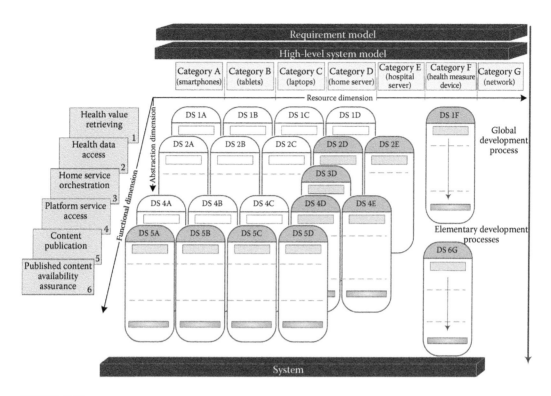

FIGURE 19.12
Development framework for PIS instantiated for AAL4ALL.

well as the corresponding elementary development processes that take place framed in a global development process.

The development structure instances identified in Figure 19.12 are composed of information regarding the development process for the functional profile. Development structures bring a first insight into how functional requirements and devices are organized. This representation serves as a starting point for identifying needs regarding functional modeling and the involved devices. In Figure 19.13, we depict the development structure associated with the functional profile instance 5A. In this functional profile instance, the *share contents* functionality regards a functional requirement that is defined in an early analysis phase. *Send contents* reflects the same functionality but in a lower abstraction level, by describing behavior at the system-level and independent from the adopted technology. The lower functionality within this development structure instance represents *send contents* with implementation requirements (i.e., nonfunctional requirements).

This framework ensures, then, the insertion of mobile devices in the ALL4ALL platform and full communication with the ALL4ALL node. At this stage, this is the most important step, as the certification and the pilot implementations are the next phases in the development roadmap of the AAL4ALL project.

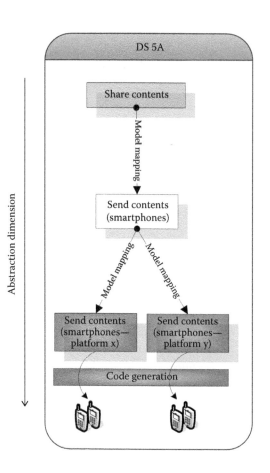

FIGURE 19.13
Content sharing.

Conclusions

This work presents the current development of an AAL4ALL consortium partner. Together with the current roadmap and the state of the art presented, the developments fall to the category of human interaction, where a user is represented in what is expected to be a normal everyday living situation. AAL4ALL aims at providing solutions in terms of AAL, by developing a platform from the bottom up, while taking advantage of the already-existing knowledge about AAL systems.

The current developments are presented in the form of requirements and specifications, constituting the base foundations of the project and a development in terms of architecture and conception. Due to the large participation of different contributors, such as universities and private companies, the expected results are a full-scale system with devices, such as sensors, actuators, and appliances, and large-scale services, such as electronic medical services and service call centers.

The presented scenario is a combination of other scenarios, in order to achieve a simple way to process and explain the complexity that every single scenario withstands. We use sequence diagrams to represent the scenarios and system requirements, thus contributing to a better representation and understanding of the AAL system. Our approach incorporates the mobile and home server modules in the sequence diagrams. Additionally, we defined a set of functional profiles that allow representation of the presented devices with the required functionalities for independent living and recreation in life scenarios. These functional profiles were identified through profiling and framing the functionality instances. Initial requirements for a solution domain are elicited through these functional profile instances and the presented development structures. The presented platform approaches a mobile solution that can handle the necessities of the user and the system. It implements a bidirectional communication solution that can be used to provide a simple way for the user to communicate, not only with persons but also with static computerized systems. It also supports assistance services such as localization and scheduling systems, and connection with body area networks, which can result in a sphere of communication and local processing, making available to users important information about their own status and to the silent monitoring systems complex information about the user's status in order to detect and act upon emergency situations.

In terms of next steps, the full development of the server and mobile platforms is expected, therefore consolidating results and validating the architecture and the framework. Due to the complexity and the branches that every deployment comprises, it is imperative to have a fully developed structure that conceptually validates the implementation. There is almost no margin for error, because upon deployment, the application is already in contact with the final users; therefore, any mistake could lead to serious consequences.

In summary, this system is expected to provide a safe and more secure life to the user by providing human and technological services, to keep users integrated in their communities and ensure a fulfilling ageing life.

Acknowledgments

This work is funded by national funds through the FCT—Foundation for Science and Technology, Lisbon, Portugal, through 3° Quadro Comunitário de Apoio, within projects PEst-C/CTM/LA0025/2011 and PEst-OE/EEI/UI0752/2011.

Project AAL4ALL is cofinanced by the European Community Fund FEDER through COMPETE—Programa Operacional Factores de Competitividade (POFC).

References

1. I. Martín, R. Neves, C. Pires, and J. Portugal, "Estatísticas de Equipamentos Sociais de Apoio à Terceira Idade em Portugal," 2006.
2. United Nations, "Population estimates and projections section," 2012. Available at http://esa.un.org/wpp/ppt/paa/PAA_2012_Heilig.pdf (accessed November 20, 2012).
3. R. Magjarevic, "Home care technologies for ambient assisted living," in *11th Mediterranean Conference on Medical and Biomedical Engineering and Computing 2007*, vol. 16, pp. 397–400, 2007.
4. M. Pieper, M. Antona, and U. Cortés, "Ambient assisted living," *ERCIM News*, pp. 18–64, 2011.
5. L. M. Camarinha-Matos, H. Afsarmanesh, A. del Cura, and J. Playfoot, "ePAL roadmap for active ageing—A collaborative networks approach to extending professional life," in *Proceedings of the 4th International ICST Conference on Pervasive Computing Technologies for Healthcare*, 2010.

6. SOPRANO Project, "Service-oriented programmable smart environments for older Europeans." http://cordis.europa.eu/project/rcn/80527_en.html (accessed December 15, 2011).

7. UniversALL Project, "Universal open platform and reference specification for ambient assisted living." Available at http://universaal.org/ (accessed December 15, 2011).

8. Persona Project, "Persona project." http://cordis.europa.eu/project/rcn/80532_en.html (accessed December 15, 2011).

9. A. Rocha, A. Martins, J. C. Freire, M. N. Kamel Boulos, M. E. Vicente, R. Feld, P. van de Ven, J. Nelson, A. Bourke, G. Olaighin, C. Sdogati, A. Jobes, L. Narvaiza, and A. Rodríguez-Molinero, "Innovations in health care services: The CAALYX system," *International Journal of Medical Informatics*, vol. 82, no. 11, pp. e307–e320, 2013. doi: 10.1016/j.ijmedinf.2011.03.003.

10. L. M. Camarinha-Matos, "BRAID's interim roadmap for ICT and ageing," 2010. Available at http://www.braidproject.eu/sites/default/files/BRAID-D6.1final.pdf (accessed November 20, 2012).

11. N. Ferreira, N. Santos, R. Machado, and D. Gašević, "Aligning domain-related models for creating context for software product design," *Software Quality. Increasing Value in Software and Systems Development Lecture Notes in Business Information Processing*, vol. 133, pp. 168–190, 2013.

12. K. Gaßner and M. Conrad, "ICT enabled independent living for elderly. A status-quo analysis on products and the research landscape in the field of ambient assisted living," 2010. Available at http://www.vdivde-it.de/publications/studies/ict-enabled-independent-living-for-elderly .-a-status-quo-analysis-on-products-and-the-research-landscape-in-the-field-of-ambient-assisted -living-aal-in-eu-27/at_download/pdf (accessed November 20, 2012).

13. R. Vardasca and R. Simoes, "Needs and opportunities in ambient assisted living in Portugal," in *2nd International Living Usability Lab Workshop on AAL Latest Solutions, Trends and Applications, AAL 2012, in Conjunction with BIOSTEC 2012*, pp. 100–108, 2012.

14. Â. Costa, J. C. Castillo, P. Novais, A. Fernández-Caballero, and R. Simoes, "Sensor-driven agenda for intelligent home care of the elderly," *Expert Systems with Applications*, vol. 39, no. 15, pp. 12192–12204, 2012.

15. A. Costa, P. Novais, J. M. Corchado, J. Neves, and Â. Costa, "Increased performance and better patient attendance in an hospital with the use of smart agendas," *Logic Journal of IGPL*, February 2011.

16. Commission of the European Communities, "Demography report 2008: Meeting social needs in an ageing society," 2008. Available at http://www.ec.europa.eu/social/BlobServlet?docId =2638&langId=en (accessed December 15, 2011).

17. BZgA and EuroHealthNet, "Healthy and active ageing," 2012. Available at http://www .healthyageing.eu/sites/www.healthyageing.eu/files/resources/Healthy%20and%20 Active%20Ageing.pdf (accessed November 20, 2012).

18. Swedish National Institute of Public Health, "Healthy ageing—A challenge for Europe," FHI, March 2007.

19. European Union, European Commission, Directorate-General for Employment, Social Affairs and Equal Opportunities, "Europe's demographic future: Facts and figures on challenges and opportunities," 2007. Available at http://www2.warwick.ac.uk/fac/soc/csgr/green/foresight /demography/2007_ec_europes_demographic_future_facts_and_figures_on_challenges_and _opportunities.pdf (accessed November 20, 2012).

20. D. Zowghi and C. Coulin, *Engineering and Managing Software Requirements*. Berlin/Heidelberg: Springer-Verlag, pp. 19–46, 2005.

21. L. M. Camarinha-Matos, J. Rosas, F. Ferrada, and A. I. Oliveira, "BRAID active ageing scenarios," 2011. Available at http://www.braidproject.eu/sites/default/files/Ageing_scenarios .pdf (accessed November 20, 2012).

22. R. J. Machado, K. B. Lassen, S. Oliveira, M. Couto, and P. Pinto, "Requirements validation: Execution of UML models with CPN tools," *International Journal on Software Tools for Technology Transfer*, vol. 9, no. 3–4, pp. 353–369, 2007.

23. S. Carmien, *Leveraging Skills into Independent Living- Distributed Cognition and Cognitive Disability*. Berlin: Springer, p. 256, 2007.

24. G. Fischer, E. Arias, S. Carmien, H. Eden, A. Kintsch, and J. F. Sullivan, "Supporting collaboration and distributed cognition in context-aware pervasive computing," in *Human Computer Interaction Consortium Winter Workshop (HCIC '04)*, 2004.
25. A. Sadilek, H. Kautz, and J. P. Bigham, "Finding your friends and following them to where you are," in *Proceedings of the Fifth ACM International Conference on Web Search and Data Mining— WSDM '12*, p. 723, 2012.
26. A. L. Liu, H. Hile, G. Borriello, H. Kautz, P. A. Brown, M. Harniss, and K. Johnson, "Evaluating a wayfinding system for individuals with cognitive impairment," in *CHI 2009*, 2009.
27. M. Wu, B. Richards, and R. Baecker, "Participatory Design of an Orientation Aid for Amnesics": "ACM Press," in *Proceedings of the SIGCHI Conference on Human Factors in Computing Systems— CHI '05*, vol. 1, New York: ACM, p. 511, 2004.
28. R. Englander, *Java and SOAP*, 1st ed., Vols. 11–12. Sebastopol, CA: O'Reilly Media, p. 288, 2002.
29. P. Adams, P. Easton, E. Johnson, R. Merrick, and M. Phillips, "SOAP over Java message service 1.0," W3C, 2011.
30. D. Crockford, "JSON: The fat-free alternative to XML," in *Proc of XML*, 2006.
31. J. A. Jorge, "Adaptive tools for the elderly," in *Proceedings of the 2001 EC/NSF Workshop on Universal Accessibility of Ubiquitous Computing Providing for the Elderly—WUAUC'01*, p. 66, 2001.
32. F. Mattern, "The vision and techical foundations of ubiquitous computing," *UPGRADE*, vol. 2, no. 5, pp. 3–5, 2001.
33. U. Hansmann, L. Merk, M. S. Nicklous, and T. Stober, *Pervasive Computing Handbook*, New York: Springer-Verlag, 2001.
34. G. D. Abowd, E. D. Mynatt, and T. Rodden, "The human experience of ubiquitous computing," *IEEE Pervasive Computing*, vol. 1, no. 1, pp. 48–57, 2002.
35. M. Weiser, "The computer for the 21st century," *Scientific American*, vol. 3, no. 3, pp. 94–104, 1991.
36. J. E. Fernandes, R. J. Machado, and J. Á. Carvalho, "Model-driven methodologies for pervasive information systems development," in *1st International Workshop on Model-Based Methodologies for Pervasive and Embedded Software—MOMPES'04*, pp. 15–23, 2004.
37. J. E. Fernandes, R. J. Machado, and J. Á. Carvalho, "Model-driven development for pervasive information systems," *Ubiquitous and Pervasive Computing: Concepts, Methodologies, Tools, and Applications*, pp. 408–438, 2010. doi: 10.4018/978-1-60566-960-1.ch028.
38. J. E. Fernandes, R. J. Machado, and J. Á. Carvalho, "Profiling and framing structures for pervasive information systems development," in *Virtual and Networked Organizations, Emergent Technologies and Tools Communications in Computer and Information Science*, pp. 283–293, 2012. doi:10.1007/978-3-642-31800-9_29.

Section V

AAL Research Topics

20

From Data to Knowledge: Towards Clinical Machine Learning Automation

Nuno Pombo, Kouamana Bousson, and Pedro Araújo

CONTENTS

ABSTRACT This chapter provides an overview of the machine learning (ML) concepts in the field of ambient assisted living (AAL). The ML techniques aim at structuring cognitive information stemming from raw data by means of a computer. Such data may be collected, for instance, by either patients or health care professionals (HCPs) during provided AAL services not only in the patient's home but also in medical and occupational environments; these data include, for example, activities and medication reminders, objective measurement of physiological parameters, feedback based on observed patterns, questionnaires, and scores. Both patients and HCPs are sources of raw clinical data that require computational processes that give rise to useful information capable of supporting clinical decision making. This chapter describes ML in terms of learning concepts emphasizing the follow approaches: supervised, unsupervised, semisupervised, and reinforcement learning. In addition, the principles of concept classification are explained, and the mathematical concepts of several methodologies are presented, such as neural networks, support vector machine, and fuzzy logic, among other techniques. Finally, an approach based on the fusion of several single methods is described for situations dealing with multiple learning models. The methods that are presented in this chapter were selected according to daily needs in medical data monitoring for the welfare of patients.

KEY WORDS: *machine learning, learning systems, classification, approximation functions, ambient assisted living.*

Introduction

Ambient assisted living (AAL) is a new paradigm in social computing that combines assisted living and ambient intelligence so as to provide care services not only in the patient's home, but also in medical and occupational environments. Patients should be asked to periodically interact with the system so as either to obtain health care information such as medication and clinical guidance or to keep their medical data up-to-date. AAL systems may include, for example, activities and medication reminders, objective measurement of physiological parameters, feedback based on observed patterns, questionnaires, and scores. On the one hand, patients are sources of health care raw data together with health care professionals (HCPs), which raises several challenges in terms of data acquisition and related to coordination regarding the collaboration between patients and medical professionals. On the other hand, AAL applications tend to be integrated into many other systems, which raises several concerns related to sensor technology, hardware, software, and communications. The main question arising from these scenarios is related to the management of data that are obtained, presented, and processed in the AAL systems. In other words, the AAL should be able to manage the collected data so as to produce meaningful and timely information with respect to medical practices. In line with this, machine learning (ML) methods may be used in knowledge refinement and discovery with the purpose of giving reliable explanations and support to HCPs and patients. Therefore, this chapter focuses on ML methods capable of producing information from rich sources of useful data and knowledge about the behavior and well-being of patients provided by AAL systems.

This chapter is organized as follows: The "Machine Learning" section describes the different ML approaches to knowledge acquisition by computers. Starting from the motivation for the use of function approximation, several techniques are illustrated and described. The section concludes with a description and examination of mathematical concepts that support reinforcement learning (RL). The "Classification" section describes the concept of classification and explains in detail several methodologies highlighting their mathematical explanation. Then, the "Approximator Fusion" section includes a description of its mathematical concepts. Finally, the last section concludes the chapter and summarizes the main points.

Machine Learning

For an ML system to be useful in solving medical diagnosis tasks, several features are desired: good performance, the ability to appropriately deal with missing and noisy data (uncertainty and errors in data), the transparency of diagnosis knowledge, the ability to explain decisions, and the ability of the algorithm to reduce the number of tests that are necessary to obtain reliable diagnosis (Kononenko 2001).

Data collected in AAL systems may include information used to send an alert about an emergency incident such as a fall or for unexpected behaviors such as deviation of a daily routine, reminders, and assistance in activities of daily living (ADLs), such as physical activities and taking medication. However, in medical practice, the acquisition of data from patients is often expensive and time consuming and may be cumbersome for the patients. Thus, it is desirable to make decisions based on a small amount of data that ideally may offer an accurate representation and explanation of the entire sample. It typically is expected that algorithms perform at least as well as the knowledge supported by human experts and/or databases. In addition, the algorithms must be able to explain decisions when faced with exceptional or new situations.

In line with this, the selection of estimators is applied to determine the appropriate subset of data using a function approximation ($y = f(x)$) drawn from giving a finite input–output scattered data set $(x_1, y_1),...,(x_m, y_m)$. Consider X and Y sets in space R^d and R, respectively. Assume that on the product $X \times Y$, Borel measure ρ is defined, which satisfies $\rho(X \times Y) = 1$ (Cucker and Smale 2002). Let g be any function defined on $X \times Y$, denoted by

$$E_\rho(g) = \int_{X \times Y} g(x,y)\,d\rho(x,y), \tag{20.1}$$

the expected value of the function g on $X \times Y$.

With the purpose of obtaining a function approximation, one of the following four approaches is used: supervised, semisupervised, and unsupervised learning, and RL.

Supervised Learning

Supervised learning assumes that the user knows beforehand the concepts, in other words, the classes and the instances of each class; that is, an exhaustive database built on external sources is available. The knowledge is obtained through a process or training that includes a data set called the training sample, which is structured according to the knowledge base supported by human experts, such as physicians in a medical context, and databases. As shown in Figure 20.1, this sample aims at tuning the system based on the minimization of the error signal determined by the differentiator, which represents the difference between the desired response (expected values) and the current response of the system (observed values). This produces an iterative learning process depending on the system environment.

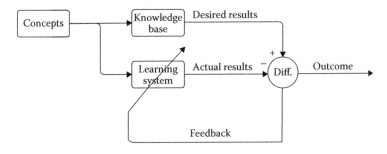

FIGURE 20.1
Supervised learning diagram.

The representative quantity of records in a training sample leads to a reduction of the discrepancy between observed and expected values and therefore results in a more accurate system. Supervised learning seeks to establish a relationship between dependent and independent variables so as to allow that one variable to be explained as a function of other variables.

Unsupervised Learning

Unsupervised learning assumes that the user is unaware of the classes due to the lack of sufficiently available information. Instead of supervised learning, which aims at establishing a relationship between dependent and independent variables, unsupervised learning treats all variables the same way so as to determine the different classes based on diverse features observed in the collection of unlabeled data that encompass the sample set. As shown in Figure 20.2, there is no feedback due to the fact that the unsupervised learning assumes that the learning system is reliable enough to produce accurate outcomes.

Semisupervised Learning

Semisupervised learning aims at propagating full labels to incompletely labeled data. Usually, the data set consists of a mixture of labeled data and unlabeled data. As shown in Figure 20.3, semisupervised learning combines the methodology of the supervised learning to process the labeled data with unsupervised learning to compute the unlabeled data (Singh et al. 2008). In fact, the outcome of the learning system that computes the labeled data represents an input of the unsupervised learning system, providing a complementary learning phase with the unlabeled data. Empirical results have shown that the use of unlabeled data can improve the performance of the classifier whereby semisupervised learning can considerably enhance the learning process.

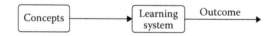

FIGURE 20.2
Unsupervised learning diagram.

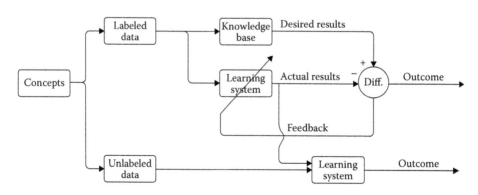

FIGURE 20.3
Semisupervised learning diagram.

Reinforcement Learning

RL is a paradigm of ML in which rewards and punishments guide the learning process. As shown in Figure 20.4, in RL, there is an agent (learner) that acts autonomously and receives a scalar reward signal that is used to evaluate the consequences of its actions.

The main goal of this agent is to find a policy, π, which is a mapping from states to actions, that maximizes the expected outcome (i.e., return) R_t defined by (Barreto and Anderson 2008)

$$R_t = r_{t+1} + \gamma r_{t+2} + \gamma^2 r_{t+3} + \ldots = \sum_{i=0}^{\infty} \gamma^i r_{t+i+1} \tag{20.2}$$

where $\gamma \in [0,1]$ is the discount factor. This parameter determines the relative importance of the individual rewards $r \in R$, which represent the quantification of the system outcome across time t. Thus, the agent selects an action $a \in A(s_t)$ as a function of the current state $s_t \in S$. S and $A(s_t)$ represent, respectively, the possible states of the system and the available actions in each one. Then, the reward r_{t+1} and a new state s_{t+1} is provided by the system as a response to an action a. Thus, the agent can learn and adapt continuously as a decision maker through interaction with the system while performing the required task and improving its behavior. This characteristic is useful for all dependent cases where a set of sufficiently large training data is difficult or impossible to obtain.

There are four elementary classes of techniques for maximizing the expected return as presented in Equation 20.2: dynamic programming, Monte Carlo algorithm, temporal-difference learning (TDL), and Q-learning.

Dynamic programming consists of a mathematical method that requires a complete and accurate model of the system. Consider a finite state space as the Bellman equation that yields a finite set of $|S|$ linear equations, which, using dynamic programming, is defined as follows:

$$V^*(s) = \max_{a \in A} \left(\sum_{s' \in S} P_{s,s'}^a \left(R_{s,s'}^a + \gamma V^*(s') \right) \right) \tag{20.3}$$

where s is the state, a the action, and γ the discount factor, the expected rewards $R_{s,s'}^a$ received at the transition from state s to state s' by executing actions a and transition probabilities P.

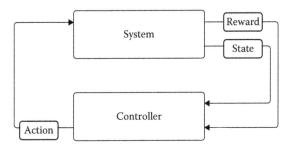

FIGURE 20.4
Reinforcement learning diagram.

Monte Carlo techniques do not use a model of the system, because they require only experience, in other words, based on sample sequences of states, actions, and rewards, or simulated interaction with the system. The value of state s_t is defined as the expected reward that is accrued from time t on; in other words, the expected value of p_t^τ that represents the reward that is accrued along trajectory $\tau = (s_t, s_{t+1}, s_{t+2}, \ldots)$,

$$V(s_t) = \sum_\tau P[\tau \mid s_t] \rho_t^\tau, \tag{20.4}$$

and given a policy π, the Monte Carlo policy evaluation generates state trajectories according to π and computes $V^\pi(s_t)$ as follows:

$$V^\pi(s_t) \leftarrow V^\pi(s_t) + \alpha_k \left[\rho_t^\tau - V^\pi(s_t) \right] \tag{20.5}$$

the parameter α_k being the learning rate at epoch k.

The TDL technique is flexible due to the fact that it does not require a model of the system and is defined by (Sutton and Barto 1998):

$$V(s) \leftarrow V(s) + \alpha[r_{t+1} + \gamma V(s_{t+1}) - V(s)] \tag{20.6}$$

where $V(s)$ is the value of state s, r_{t+1} is the reward received, α is the learning rate, γ is the discount factor, and s_{t+1} is the next state. In line with this, the value of a state is revised so as to match the value of the next state plus a reward signal. Thus, the last state equals the expected return.

Q-learning is one of the most popular methods in RL; it uses an off-policy technique so as to simplify the learning algorithm and facilitate convergence. Consider Q the action-value function:

$$Q(s,a) \leftarrow Q(s,a) + \alpha[r + \gamma \max_{a'} Q(s',a') - Q(s,a)] \tag{20.7}$$

where s is the state, a is the action, α is the learning rate, γ is the discount factor, r is the reward, and a' and s' are the next action and state, respectively.

Classification

The classification process varies according to the used learning methodology. When supervised learning is applied, the classification refers to the mapping of data items into one of the predefined classes. On the contrary, when unsupervised learning is utilized, the classification refers to the cluster analysis on the data set that offers a better understanding of the data set characteristics and provides a starting point for exploring further relationships.

Choosing the right classifier is a critical step in the knowledge acquiring process. A variety of techniques have been used in the classification of data sets, as described below.

Artificial Neural Networks

The artificial neural networks (ANNs) are composed of interconnected processing elements, called nodes (see Figure 20.5), that carry out the classification process, which was inspired by the way the brain recognizes patterns. Each element encompasses one or more inputs (signals) from other elements via the connections. These inputs represent propagation, either feedforward or backpropagation, of estimated weights through the nodes of the network so as to generate an output set where each component represents a particular classification for the input set. The net input of weighted signals received by a unit j is given by

$$\text{net}_j = w_0 + \sum_{i=1}^{n} w_i x_i \tag{20.8}$$

where w_0 is the biasing signal, w_i the weight on input connection ij, x_i the magnitude of signal on input connection ij, and n the number of input connections to node j.

The ANN can be either supervised or unsupervised learning. An ANN composed of a unique layer of nodes is called single-layer perceptron (SLP), whereas it is called multilayer perceptron (MLP) when it is composed of several layers, as presented in Figure 20.6.

The SLP is applied to learning from a batch of training, repeatedly, to find the accurate vector for the entire training set, whereas MLPs aim at the separation of input instances

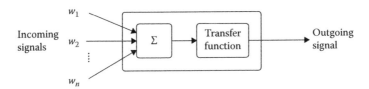

FIGURE 20.5
A single-network node.

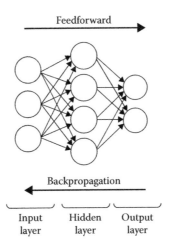

FIGURE 20.6
Illustration of an MLP.

into their appropriate categories. However, despite its robustness to noisy data and its ability to represent complex functions, its inability to explain decisions and the lack of transparency of data present an obstacle for its use in clinical settings such as AAL. Also, determining the adequate size of the hidden layer is sensitive to poor approximations caused by lack of neurons or overfitting from excessive nodes. A topology of SLN, called radial basis function neural network (RBFNN), is commonly used for solving machine learning problems that require short training time. Indeed, a RBFNN has only one hidden layer and the output of the network is a linear combination of the hidden nodes outputs (Li et al. 2008).

As depicted in Figure 20.7, a typical RBFNN structure encompasses an m-dimensional input vector x and an n-dimensional output vector $x \in R^m, y \in R^n, f{:}x \mapsto y$. There are several radial basis functions, such as the Gaussian function,

$$\phi_j(x) = \exp\left(-\frac{\|x - \mu_j\|^2}{\sigma_j^2}\right); \tag{20.9}$$

the multiquadrics function,

$$\phi_j(x) = \sqrt{x^2 + \sigma_j^2}; \tag{20.10}$$

and finally, the inverse multiquadrics function,

$$\phi_j(x) = \frac{1}{\sqrt{x^2 + \sigma_j^2}} \tag{20.11}$$

where $x = (x_1, x_2, \dots, x_m)^T$ is the input vector, μ_j is the center vector, and σ_j is the radius width of the jth hidden node. The output layer represents the outputs of the network, and each input node is a linear combination of the k radial basis functions of hidden nodes:

$$y_i = \sum_{j=1}^{k} w_{ji}\phi_j(x) \tag{20.12}$$

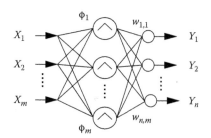

FIGURE 20.7
A standard RBFNN structure.

In addition, a statistical learning method called extreme learning machine (ELM) (Yoon et al. 2013) is also based on SLN topology. However, the ELM technique uses mathematical concepts to estimate the hidden output, avoiding the need to identify the best parameters with iterative tuning.

Giving a training set

$$N = \{(x_j, t_j) | x_j \in R^d, t_j \in R^m, j = 1,...,n\}, \tag{20.13}$$

the randomly generated input to hidden weights vectors is given by

$$w_i = (a_i, b_i), i = 1,...,l \tag{20.14}$$

where l is the number of hidden nodes.

$$\sum_{i=1}^{l} \beta_i g_i(w_i x_j + b_i) = t_j, j = 1,..., N \tag{20.15}$$

where $\beta = (\beta_{i1},...,\beta_{iN})$ is the output weight vector connecting the ith nodes and output nodes, and $W_i = (w_{i1},...,w_{in})$ is the output weight vector connecting the ith hidden node.

Then, the hidden layer output matrix H is given by

$$H(w_1,...,w_l, b_1,...,b_l x_1,...,x_n) = \begin{pmatrix} w_1 x_1 + b_1 & \cdots & w_l x_1 + b_l \\ \vdots & \ddots & \vdots \\ w_1 x_N + b_1 & \cdots & w_l x_N + b_l \end{pmatrix} \tag{20.16}$$

That is,

$$H\beta = T \tag{20.17}$$

$$\left\| H\hat{\beta} - T \right\| = \min_{\beta} \left\| H\beta - T \right\| \tag{20.18}$$

$$\bar{\beta} = H^+ T \tag{20.19}$$

where H^+ is the Moore–Penrose generalized inverse of the matrix.

Finally, a stochastic ANN based on MLPs, called Boltzmann machines (BMs) (Yaakob et al. 2011), was developed, aiming to represent a probability distribution of data that is obtained by changing recursively and gradually the network structure so as to achieve an optimal structure. Thus, probability rules are employed to update the state of nodes in the following manner:

$$P[V_i(t + 1)] = f(u_i(t)) \tag{20.20}$$

where $V_i(t + 1)$ is the output of node i, in the subsequent time iteration $t + 1$, f is the sigmoid function, and $u_i(t)$ is the total input to node i. $V_i(t + 1)$ is 1 with probability P and 0 with probability $1 - P$.

The total input to node i is given by

$$u_i(t) = \sum_{j=1}^{n} w_{ij} V_i(t) + \theta_i \qquad (20.21)$$

where w_{ij} is the weight between nodes i and j, θ_i is the threshold of node i, and V_i is the state of node i.

Self-Organizing Map

A different approach is verified by the self-organizing map (SOM), which is an unsupervised learning scheme that consists in positioning neurons in the network according to the input sample so as to reduce the dimension of data. The data vectors are projected onto positions on a two-dimensional grid, which consists of a set of $k \times k$ ordered nodes m_i, where $i = 1,\dots,k^2$ as presented in Figure 20.8. More similar models will be associated with nodes that are closer in the grid, whereas less similar models will be situated gradually farther away in the grid. There are two main approaches to achieve this purpose: a recursive stepwise approximation process and a batch-type process. On the one hand, the recursive approximation applies the input data one at a time in either periodic or random sequence, for as many steps as will be necessary until a stable state is reached.

Let the input data items constitute a sequence $\{x(t)\}$ of n-dimensional Euclidean vectors x and t the step sequence. Let $\{m_i(t)\}$ be another sequence of n-dimensional real vectors that represent the successively computed approximations of model m_i, where i is the spatial index of the grid node with which m_i is associated. Thus, the process converges and produces the desired ordered values for the models (Kohonen 2013):

$$m_i(t + 1) = m_i(t) + h_{c,i}(t)[x(t) - m_i(t)] \qquad (20.22)$$

where $h_{c,i}(t)$ is called the neighborhood function and c is the node index in the grid that represents the smallest Euclidean distance between $x(t)$ and $m_c(t)$, which is given by

$$c = \underset{i}{\mathrm{argmin}} \left\{ \| x(t) - m_i(t) \| \right\} \qquad (20.23)$$

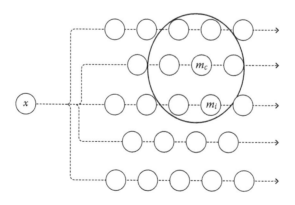

FIGURE 20.8
Illustration of an SOM structure. An input data item X is broadcast to a set of models m_i, of which m_c matches best with X. All models that belong to the neighborhood (larger circle) of m_c in the grid match better with X than with the rest.

These two equations represent a recursive step where first the input data item $x(t)$ selects the best matching model in the grid. The function $h_{c,i}(t)$ impels the modification rates at different nodes. A commonly used formula for this function is

$$h_{c,i}(t) = \alpha(t)\exp\left[-\frac{\text{sqdist}(c,i)}{2\sigma^2(t)}\right] \tag{20.24}$$

where $\alpha(t)$ and $\sigma(t)$ are a decreasing scalar function of t and $\text{sqdist}(c,i)$ is the square of the geometric distance between the nodes c and i in the grid, defined by

$$\text{sqdist}(c,i) = \text{distance}(m_c, m_i)^2 \tag{20.25}$$

The convergence of the process is given by

$$\forall i,\ E_t\{h_{c,i}(x(t) - m_i(t))\} = 0 \tag{20.26}$$

where E_t is the mathematical expectation value operator over t, whose state is denoted by

$$m_i^* = \frac{\sum_t h_{c,i}x(t)}{\sum_t h_{c,i}} \tag{20.27}$$

On the other hand, all of the input data are applied as one batch, and all of the models are updated in a single operation. With each node i, a model m_i and a list containing copies of certain input vectors $x(t)$ are associated. The initial values of m_i should be selected wisely. Usually, these values are selected as random vectors from the domain of the input vectors. A better selection in the case of the Euclidean metric is to assign to m_i values obtained from the two-dimensional hyperplane determined by the two largest principal components of x. Thus, consider the set of input data vectors defined by $\{x(t)\}$, where t is an index of a vector. Each $x(t)$ is compared with all of the models producing a sublist associated with the node that represents the model vector of best matches with $x(t)$ in the Euclidean metric.

Fuzzy Logic

Fuzzy logic represents a probabilistic logic model that uses reasoning to explain whether an event is about to happen (Dubois and Prade 2012; Zadeh 1965). A membership function (with values on a totally ordered set) is then interpreted as a possibility distribution π over S. Thus, the degree of possibility of an event A is

$$\Pi(A) = \max_{s\in A} \pi(S) \tag{20.28}$$

and the degree of necessity is given by

$$N(A) = \min_{s\notin A} v(\pi(s)) = v\left(\Pi(A^c)\right) \tag{20.29}$$

where v is the order-reversing map on L that yields a theory of epistemic uncertainty concerned with the handling of incomplete information, whereas $v(\Pi(A))$ is a degree of surprise if A occurs. This framework is often used in ML (Hall et al. 1992).

Support Vector Machine

The support vector machine (SVM) combines statistical methods and ML methods aiming to generate input–output mapping functions from a set of training data.

Consider the separable linear case in which two different classes are separated by the hyperplane:

$$f(x) = w^t x + b \tag{20.30}$$

The SVM finds the hyperplane that maximizes the separating margin between the two classes (Burges 1998). This hyperplane can be found by minimizing the cost function

$$\min J(w) = \frac{1}{2} w^t w = \frac{1}{2} \|w\|^2 \tag{20.31}$$

subject to the following separability constraints

$$w^t x_i + b \geq 1, \text{ for } y_i = 1 \text{ and } i = 1, 2, \ldots, l \tag{20.32}$$

or

$$w^t x_i + b \leq -1, \text{ for } y_i = -1 \text{ and } i = 1, 2, \ldots, l \tag{20.33}$$

Equivalently,

$$y_i(w^t x_i + b) \geq 1, \text{ where } i = 1, 2, \ldots, l \tag{20.34}$$

A slack variable can be introduced to relax the separability constraints:

$$y_i(w^t x_i + b) \geq 1 - \varepsilon_i; \text{ where } \varepsilon_i \geq 0 \text{ and } i = 1, 2, \ldots, l \tag{20.35}$$

Accordingly, the cost function in Equation 20.31 can be can be modified as follows:

$$J(w, \varepsilon) = \frac{1}{2} \|w\|^2 + c \sum_{i=1}^{l} \varepsilon_i \tag{20.36}$$

where c is a user-specified, positive, regularization parameter, and ε is a vector containing all the slack variables.

As depicted in Figure 20.9, the linear SVM only classifies two classes by means of a separating hyperplane, which is commonly insufficient when applied to medical decisions where several classes are usually needed. Therefore, nonlinear SVM is often used for complex real-world applications. Indeed, the nonlinear case occurs when the features in the sample space cannot be separated by mere hyperplanes.

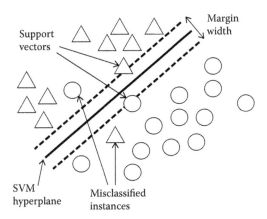

FIGURE 20.9
Illustration of a linear SVM decision function separating class +1 (circles) from class −1 (triangles).

Let us consider the input vector $x \in R^d$, which is transformed to a feature vector $\Phi(x)$ via a nonlinear map $\Phi: R^d \rightarrow R$. Then, the problem is solved by considering a kernel function $K: R^d \times R^d \rightarrow R$ defined as

$$K(x_i, x_j) = \Phi(x_i) \cdot \Phi(x_j) \tag{20.37}$$

where x_i and x_j represent any pair of input vectors.

Thus, the optimal separating contours are defined based on function f given by

$$f(x) = \sum_{k=1}^{l} \alpha_k y_k K(x_k, x) + \beta \tag{20.38}$$

where α_k and β are scalars and depend on x_k and y_k, $k = 1,..,l$.

The SVM provides good generalization capabilities; it is robust for high-dimensional data, is more suited to training, and performs better compared to traditional ANN. However, it is very sensitive to uncertainties, and a too-high-dimensional space may render the learning process too lengthy. The evaluation of function f may be cumbersome for some real-time applications. Therefore, a trade-off has to be found between the generalization characteristics of SVM and its sluggishness when faced with learning from large databases.

k-Nearest Neighbor

The *k*-nearest neighbor (*k*-NN) (Wang et al. 2013) classifier aims to evaluate the reduced feature vectors for the proposed two feature generation approaches. This algorithm presents low-computation-complexity methods for pattern recognition and is based on an intuitive concept that data points of the same class should be closer in the feature space.

Consider n training data defined by

$$\{(x_1, y_1),...,(x_n, y_n)\} \tag{20.39}$$

where (x_i, y_i) represents data pair i, in which x_i is the feature vector and y_i the corresponding target class. Thus, for a given data point x, the target class is determined as

$$y_p = 1 - NN(x) \tag{20.40}$$

where

$$p = \arg \min_i |x - x_i|^2 \tag{20.41}$$

k-Means Clustering

Cluster processing refers to partitioning the n samples into k groups or clusters based on some similarity metrics or on the combination of minimum intracluster and maximum intercluster distance (Chiang et al. 2011). Let $O = \{O_1, O_2,...,O_n\}$ be a set of n data samples, which are described by d features represented by a profile data matrix $O_{n \times d}$ composed by n row vectors, where each row vector has d dimensions. The ith row vector is defined by

$$O_i = \left\{ o_i^1, o_i^2, ..., o_i^d \right\} \tag{20.42}$$

where each element o_i^j is a scalar denoting the jth component of the corresponding data object. Thus, the aim of a clustering algorithm is to produce a partition of k groups or clusters $C = \{C_1, C_2,...,C_k\}$ where each one should contain at least one data object $C_i \neq \emptyset, \forall i \in \{1, 2,...,k\}$, different clusters should have no object in common, $C_i \cap C_j = \emptyset, \forall i \neq j$, and $i, j \in \{1, 2,...,k\}$, and the sum of objects in all clusters should be equal to the number of objects in the original data set $\bigcup_{i=1}^{k} C_i = O$. Then, one of the popular functions that is used to cluster the objects is the total mean square quantization error (MSE) (Jain et al. 1999), which is defined by

$$f(O,C) = \sum_{l=1}^{k} \sum_{O_i \in C_l} d(O_i, Z_l)^2 \tag{20.43}$$

where $d(O_i, Z_l)$ defines the dissimilarity between the object O_i and the centroid of cluster $C_l(Z_l)$, to be found by calculating the mean value of objects within a respective cluster. The Euclidean distance function is commonly used to determine the distance metrics between objects.

$$d(X_i, X_j) = \sqrt{\sum_{p=1}^{d} \left(x_i^p - x_j^p \right)^2} \tag{20.44}$$

It has been proven that despite performing well on small- to medium-sized data sets, traditional clustering algorithms fail to scale up well for large data sets, especially in terms of computation time (Vapnik 1995).

Linear Discriminant Analysis

Linear discriminant analysis (LDA) is a supervised dimension reduction used to transform one set of variables into another smaller set. Given m training data given by $\{x_1,...,x_m\}$

and L the number of classes, consider n_i the number of training samples in the ith class, where $i = 1,...,L$. The LDA aims to determine a transformation matrix W by maximizing the ratio $J(W)$:

$$J(W) = \frac{W^T S_B W}{W^T S_W W} \tag{20.45}$$

where the transformation matrix W is applied to maximize the ratio of $W^T S_W W$ and $W^T S_B W$, which represent the new within-class scatter and between-class scatter, respectively, in the new feature space. In other words,

$$S_W = \sum_{i=j}^{L} \sum_{j=1}^{n_i} \left(X_j^i - \mu_i \right)\left(X_j^i - \mu_i \right)^T \tag{20.46}$$

where X_j^i represents the jth sample of the ith class, and μ_i is the mean of class i.

The between-class scatter matrix is defined by

$$S_B = \sum_{i=1}^{L} n_i \left(\mu_i - \mu_{all} \right)\left(\mu_i - \mu_{all} \right)^T \tag{20.47}$$

where μ_{all} is the mean of all classes.

Then, a new feature vector y is obtained:

$$y = W^T x \tag{20.48}$$

Thus, the optimal W is computed as the solution of the following constrained quadratic minimization problem:

$$\underset{w}{\text{Min}}\left(-\frac{1}{2} W^T S_B W \right) \tag{20.49}$$

$$\text{subject to: } W^T S_W W = 1$$

By the Karush–Kuhn–Tucker (KKT) theorem (Boyd and Vandenberghe 2004), the solution of that minimization problem is

$$S_B W = \lambda S_W W \tag{20.50}$$

where λ is the Lagrange multiplier associated with the problem.

However, the LDA is based on a statistical model for feature extraction using a linear technique, which causes limitations in dealing with some features that have nonlinear relationships. Thus, some approaches are applied so as to overcome this problem, which are based on mapping the input data into an implicit feature space so as to allow their analysis, of these, kernel Fisher discriminant analysis is one of the most commonly used techniques (Liang and Shi 2004). Thus, consider the input space R^n mapped into an arbitrary dimensionality feature space F by a nonlinear mapping function ϕ:

$$\phi: R^n \rightarrow F, x \mapsto \phi(x) \tag{20.51}$$

The Fisher criterion function can be defined as

$$J_2(W) = \frac{W^T S_b^\phi W}{W^T S_t^\phi W} \tag{20.52}$$

where S_b^ϕ is the between-class scatter matrix and S_t^ϕ is the total population scatter matrix defined in the feature space F. These are defined by

$$S_b^\phi = \frac{1}{m} \sum_{i=1}^{L} l_i \left(m_i^\phi - m_0^\phi \right) \left(m_i^\phi - m_0^\phi \right)^T \tag{20.53}$$

$$S_t^\phi = \frac{1}{m} \sum_{i=1}^{m} \left(\phi(x_i) - m_0^\phi \right) \left(\phi(x_i) - m_0^\phi \right)^T \tag{20.54}$$

where m_i^ϕ is the mean vector of the mapped training samples in the ith class and m_0^ϕ is the mean vector of all mapped training samples.

Principal Component Analysis

Principal component analysis (PCA) (Chattopadhyay et al. 2013) is an unsupervised learning approach alternative to LDA for dimension reduction that is also widely used in data compression and statistical data analysis. PCA aims to find a subspace whose basis vector corresponds to the maximum-variance directions in the original space. In other words, PCA aims to reduce the original data set by identifying a small number of meaningful components. Let W represent the linear transformation mapping between the two space dimensions. The mean is defined by

$$\mu = \frac{1}{L} \sum_{i=1}^{L} x_i \tag{20.55}$$

where x_i are the vectors of the original feature space and L the number of classes.
The covariance matrix C is defined by

$$C = \frac{1}{L} \sum_{i=1}^{L} (x_i - \mu)(x_i - \mu)^T \tag{20.56}$$

Then, the eigenvalue associated with the eigenvector is defined by

$$\lambda_i e_i = C e_i \tag{20.57}$$

Sorting the eigenvalue λ_i and the corresponding eigenvectors in descending order and selecting the first g eigenvectors to compose W, we have

$$W = e^g_{i\ i=1} \tag{20.58}$$

Then, the PCA transformation is defined by

$$y_i = W^T x_i \tag{20.59}$$

Independent Component Analysis

Independent component analysis (ICA) (Comon 1994) is defined by

$$X = AS \tag{20.60}$$

where X is the random observed vector $\{X_1, X_2,...,X_m\}^T$ whose m elements are mixtures of m independent elements of a random vector $S = \{S_1, S_2,...,S_m\}^T$ and A represents an $m \times m$ mixing matrix. The main goal of ICA is to determine the unmixing matrix W that represents the inverse of A and thus to recover the hidden source using

$$S_k = A_k^{-1} X \tag{20.61}$$

where A_k^{-1} is the kth row of A^{-1}.

Assuming that data variables are linear or nonlinear mixtures of some latent variables, and the mixing system is also unknown, we can rewrite Equation 20.60 as follows:

$$X_i = a_{i1}S_1 + a_{i2}S_2 +...+ a_{in}S_n \quad i = 1, 2,...,n \tag{20.62}$$

Then, each S_i is statistically mutually independent, where each a_{ij} is the entry of the nonsingular matrix A. All random observed variables are defined by X_i, which is used to estimate the mixing coefficients a_{ij} and the independent components S_i.

There are several ways to measure independence, and each of them involves the use of different algorithms when it comes to performing an ICA, which results in slightly different unmixing matrices. These algorithms are divided into two main families: minimization of mutual information and maximization of non-Gaussianity.

The mutual information is composed for a pair of random variables and is defined by

$$I(X:Y) = H(X) - H(X|Y) \tag{20.63}$$

where $H(X)$ is the entropy of X and $H(X|Y)$ is the conditional entropy, which is defined as follows:

$$H(X|Y) = H(X,Y) - H(Y) \tag{20.64}$$

where $H(X,Y)$ is the joint entropy of X and Y and $H(Y)$ is the entropy of Y.

The entropy for a given variable is defined by (Shannon 1948)

$$H(X) = -\sum_x P(x)\log P(x) \tag{20.65}$$

$$H(Y) = -\sum_x P(y)\log P(y) \tag{20.66}$$

$$H(X,Y) = -\sum_{x,y} P(x,y)\log P(x,y) \tag{20.67}$$

where $P(x)$ is the probability that X is in the state x. Thus, entropy is a measure of uncertainty, of which the lower the value, the more information is represented about a given system.

A different method to estimate the ICA is focusing on non-Gaussianity; in other words, it is assumed that the data are not normally distributed. For this purpose, an approach called negentropy (reverse of entropy) is commonly used:

$$N(X) = H(X_{\text{Gaussian}}) - H(X) \tag{20.68}$$

where X is a non-Gaussian random vector, $H(X)$ is the entropy, and $H(X_{\text{Gaussian}})$ is the entropy of a Gaussian random vector whose covariance matrix is equal to that of X. However, due to the fact that the negentropy makes it difficult to compute Equation 20.68, a function approximation is frequently applied.

There are some differences between ICA and PCA; one of them lies in the fact that ICA finds a data set that is mutually independent, whereas PCA finds a data set that is mutually uncorrelated. In addition, ICA assumes that the data objects are statistically independent in the sense that the value of one gives no information about the values of the others.

Approximator Fusion

The learning outcome from each method described above may be limited not only by the approach itself but also by the pattern of the approximating function. For instance, in neural learning, the accuracy of the prediction is related to the number of hidden nodes and the output node function; in radial basis function learning, the number and the type of radial functions that are used influence the outcome of the learning process. To enable a learning outcome with higher generalization capabilities for a given application, several approximating functions stemming from different learning approaches may be combined in some way. Indeed, let $f_1,...,f_M$ be M independent approximating functions of a set $D = \{(x_1, y_1),...,(x_n, y_n)\}$ of scattered data. The problem of approximator fusion consists in finding a single approximating function f for the data set D and is defined as

$$f(x) = \sum_{j=1}^{M} \lambda_j f_j(x), \ (\lambda_j \geq 0, \ j = 1,..., M) \tag{20.69}$$

That problem summarizes to estimating the weight vector $\lambda = (\lambda_1, \ldots, \lambda_M)^T$ that minimizes the following cost functional:

$$J(\lambda) = \sum_{k=1}^{n} \left(y_k - \sum_{j=1}^{M} \lambda_j f_j(x_k) \right)^2 + \lambda^T W \lambda \qquad (20.70)$$

where W is a positive definite matrix. This is a regularized least-square problem that may be solved with well-known methods, described by Golub and Van Loan (1996).

The interest of approximator fusion lies in the high regularization power of the resultant approximating function; meanwhile, the fusion process may be time consuming since it requires the same set of data to be learnt using several different learning approaches and approximating functions. Here, too, a trade-off has to be found between the number of individual approximators to be used and the time that one has to invest in going through an approximator fusion process.

Conclusion

This chapter highlighted the importance of methodologies for obtaining knowledge starting from the collected data in the context of AAL and their capability to produce accurate and reliable outcomes for health care assistance professionals in clinical decision making. In line with this, an overview related to ML focused on complementary concepts such as learning, classification, and function approximation.

Four different ML methodologies were presented, supervised learning, unsupervised learning, semisupervised learning, and RL, as well specific unsupervised learning approaches such as LDA, PCA, and IDA. Finally, approximator fusion was explained, focusing on its capability to present more accurate outcomes obtained from the fusion of several sources compared with outcomes derived from the single usage of any other method.

The methods that are presented in this chapter are all suited for medical decision making involving various professionals and patients for high-quality and timely medical assistance.

Acknowledgments

The authors acknowledge the contribution of the Instituto de Telecomunicações, R&D Unit 50008, financed by the applicable financial framework (FCT/MEC through national funds and, when applicable, cofunded by FEDER–PT2020 partnership agreement). The authors also acknowledge the contribution of COST Action IC1303–AAPELE–Algorithms, Architectures and Platforms for Enhanced Living Environments.

References

Barreto, A.M.S., Anderson, C.W., 2008. Restricted gradient-descent algorithm for value-function approximation in reinforcement learning. *Artificial Intelligence* 172, 454–482.

Boyd, S., Vandenberghe, L., 2004. *Convex Optimization.* Cambridge University Press, New York.

Burges, C.J.C., 1998. A tutorial on support vector machines for pattern recognition. *Data Mining and Knowledge Discovery* 2, 121–167.

Chattopadhyay, A.K., Mondal, S., Chattopadhyay, T., 2013. Independent component analysis for the objective classification of globular clusters of the galaxy {NGC} 5128. *Computational Statistics & Data Analysis* 57, 17–32.

Chiang, M.-C., Tsai, C.-W., Yang, C.-S., 2011. A time-efficient pattern reduction algorithm for *k*-means clustering. *Information Sciences* 181, 716–731.

Comon, P., 1994. Independent component analysis: A new concept? *Signal Processing* 36, 287–314.

Cucker, F., Smale, S., 2002. On the mathematical foundations of learning. *Bulletin of the American Mathematical Society* 39, 1–49.

Dubois, D., Prade, H., 2012. Possibility theory, in: Meyers, R.A. (Ed.), *Computational Complexity.* Springer New York, pp. 2240–2252.

Golub, G.H., Van Loan, C.F., 1996. *Matrix Computations* (3rd ed.). Johns Hopkins University Press, Baltimore, MD.

Hall, L.O., Bensaid, A.M., Clarke, L.P., Velthuizen, R.P., Silbiger, M.S., Bezdek, J.C., 1992. A comparison of neural network and fuzzy clustering techniques in segmenting magnetic resonance images of the brain. *Neural Networks, IEEE Transactions on* 3, 672–682.

Jain, A.K., Murty, M.N., Flynn, P.J., 1999. Data clustering: A review. *ACM Computing Surveys* 31, 264–323.

Kohonen, T., 2013. Essentials of the self-organizing map. *Neural Networks* 37, 52–65.

Kononenko, I., 2001. Machine learning for medical diagnosis: History, state of the art and perspective. *Artificial Intelligence in Medicine* 23, 89–109.

Li, M., Tian, J., Chen, F., 2008. Improving multiclass pattern recognition with a co-evolutionary {RBFNN}. *Pattern Recognition Letters* 29, 392–406.

Liang, Z., Shi, P., 2004. An efficient and effective method to solve kernel Fisher discriminant analysis. *Neurocomputing* 61, 485–493.

Shannon, C.E., 1948. A mathematical theory of communication. *Bell System Technical Journal* 27.

Singh, A., Nowak, R.D., Zhu, X., 2008. Unlabeled data: Now it helps, now it doesn't, in: Koller, D., Schuurmans, D., Bengio, Y., Bottou, L. (Eds.), *NIPS.* Curran Associates, Inc., pp. 1513–1520.

Sutton, R.S., Barto, A.G., 1998. *Introduction to Reinforcement Learning* (1st ed.). MIT Press, Cambridge, MA.

Vapnik, V.N., 1995. *The Nature of Statistical Learning Theory.* Springer-Verlag New York, Inc., New York.

Wang, J.-S., Lin, C.-W., Yang, Y.-T.C., 2013. A k-nearest-neighbor classifier with heart rate variability feature-based transformation algorithm for driving stress recognition. *Neurocomputing* 116, 136–143.

Yaakob, S.B., Watada, J., Fulcher, J., 2011. Structural learning of the Boltzmann machine and its application to life cycle management. *Neurocomputing* 74, 2193–2200.

Yoon, H., Park, C.-S., Kim, J.S., Baek, J.-G., 2013. Algorithm learning based neural network integrating feature selection and classification. *Expert Systems with Applications* 40, 231–241.

Zadeh, L.A., 1965. Fuzzy sets. *Information and Control* 8, 338–353.

21

Soft Computing Drug Administration in the Ambient Assisted Living Environment

Filipe Quinaz, Paulo Fazendeiro, Miguel Castelo-Branco, and Pedro Araújo

CONTENTS

ABSTRACT   The central aim of this chapter is to present an overview of soft computing techniques designed for automatic drug infusion and modeling of patient response in the ambient assisted living environment. The advantages and limitations of automatic drug infusion systems are analyzed. In order to present the algorithms and concepts behind the patient response problem, across this chapter, special emphasis is given to the specific medical condition of hypertension. A brief description of the evolution of these systems, the identification of the most recent advances, and research trends are also provided. The specificities related to the implementation of medical systems in assisted living environments are analyzed, and possible solutions are suggested. The everyday usage of these systems in more familiar, nonhospital environments is discussed from an assisted living perspective.

KEY WORDS: *automatic drug administration, closed loop control, soft computing, neural networks, fuzzy logic.*

Introduction

With the constant evolution of computing technologies, the range of problems from the medical field that can be approached and effectively solved increases accordingly. The complexity inherent in medicine and its related areas of knowledge raises algorithmic construction difficulties, creating challenging problems, cf. Alexander (2010) and Eoyang (2007). There is a large range of solutions provided by computer technologies. These include management tools, patient identification, and communication methods, to mention just a few. While some of these systems are quite simple, applications for drug administration in AAL environments often require more sophisticated computer solutions due to their safety-critical nature and human-centric information processing requirements. These drug administration aiding systems range from simple reminders that are programmed to alert the patient of the need to administer the drug to complex systems that measure the patient's needs and administer the drug or advise the administrator accordingly (Medjahed et al. 2009; Suzuki and Nakauchi 2010; Yamamoto et al. 2010).

Drug administration is executed following a relatively broad protocol, cf. Webster et al. (2010) and Olasveengen et al. (2009). While there are drugs whose variations in dosage are tolerated, there are many drugs, such as insulin, whose precise administration is critical as it impacts patient safety and medical condition significantly (Dudde et al. 2006).

Additionally, patients tend to react differently to the same treatment, having great intra-patient and interpatient variability, due to their personal characteristics—these include the current clinical state, drug sensitivity, weight, and gender, among others.

The adaptation of the protocol to each individual is often a very challenging task even for health care professionals (Fazendeiro et al. 2007), where the administrator needs to analyze multiple sources of data in order to achieve the desired patient state. This situation is demanding and requires a great deal of attention and skill from the health care professionals in the treatment of their patients.

When talking about pharmacological intervention at home, in assisted living facilities or in a hospital environment, one of the most interesting and complex problems is the automatic administration of drugs. This chapter focuses on state-of-the-art and possible future solutions of soft computing techniques for the automatic drug administration problem in the assisted living environment. We start by describing the theoretical foundations behind the algorithms that allow the construction of these systems. In the development of this chapter, special emphasis is given to solutions for the concrete problem of arterial pressure control—an interesting problem that gives rise to a set of pertinent design issues common to many AAL setups due to the inherent complexity of the circulatory model and safety-critical nature of the treatment.

The work developed around the arterial pressure control problem can be extrapolated to other medical systems. Although most of the work available on this theme is focused on the hospital facet, it is expected that once these systems mature, they can be applied to assisted living facilities or home environments. The administration of insulin, a drug used by patients with diabetes, is an example of this change of technology environment (Campos-Delgado et al. 2006; Dudde et al. 2006). By analyzing professional hospital systems and algorithms, we can provide better insight into the current state of automatic drug administration, along with the current limitations, possible future developments, and applications.

Background

One of the major theoretical contributions that allowed automatic drug administration systems to be developed is control theory. Control theory is an interdisciplinary branch of engineering and mathematics, which studies the behavior of dynamic systems. In a very simple manner, when one or more output variables of a system need to follow a certain desired output value over time, a model-based controller manipulates the inputs to obtain the desired effect (Franklin et al. 1972; Sheppard 1980; Koivo 1981).

Control systems are ubiquitous in health care, ranging from simple controllers implemented only by hardware to more complex controllers implemented via hardware and/or software. Everyday examples of control systems include a boiler regulator for water temperature, the pressure controller of the cuff in an automatic arterial pressure meter, the humidity controller in dehumidifiers, or a pacemaker beat controller, just to mention a few (Lichtenstein 1984; Linkens 1994; Kami et al. 1996; Spratt 1997; Ritchart et al. 1998).

There are many important contributions of model-based controllers to the health care system, as can be seen from the applications found in the literature, cf. Carver and Scheier (1982). While the examples given above may not be strictly medical-related applications, they serve their purpose of illustrating some of the most basic characteristics of control systems. More complex controllers, related to automatic drug administration systems, provide an interesting application of these systems to medical problems.

The algorithms developed by using control theory techniques are model based. This means that they require one or several mathematical models that describe in a specific and well-defined form the problem to be approached.

From the beginning of scientific studies of the human body, researchers began to create mathematical models of the various body function systems. Nowadays, these mathematical models describe in a reasonably accurate form the way that our bodies operate (Montani and Vliet 2009). The pharmacological response can also be mathematically modeled, making it possible to be simulated through computerized means. Explicit knowledge about the various functional systems that constitute the human body has made it possible to address the challenge of automatic drug administration through the model-based solutions of control theory.

Most of the traditional controllers built to solve the hypertension problem are based on a mathematical model developed initially by Guyton et al. (1972). However, the linearity of the model prevents the accurate representation of nonlinear and time-varying features of the cardiovascular dynamics of the human body. Due to this characteristic, controller designs based purely on models, specially the optimal and adaptive ones, may not perform satisfactorily in practice. Modeling is generally difficult, and accurately modeling biological processes involving nonlinearity, time variance, and time delay is even more difficult due to the lack of information.

Such problems are common in the design of model-based controllers, and it is possible, through model-free, data-drive control systems, to increase the accuracy of the process models (Yardimci 2009). Therefore, the controller needs to have the ability to modify its behavior (adapt its parameters) in response to changes in the dynamics of the process and environment disturbances.

In addition to the precision and reliability required by these systems, there is also a need for high descriptive power in order to convey information about the behavior of the system and the actions being taken. Medical systems that offer a user interface and require an operator's interaction while functioning, as is the case for automatic drug administration applications, are examples of such critical applications. Due to their safety-critical nature, a mismatch between the designer's conceptual model and the user's mental model, or otherwise insufficient system feedback to allow the user to understand the current state of the system, can result in disastrous consequences (Palanque et al. 2007; Thimbleby 2007). This holds true when considering the assisted living application of these systems, where the user interface has to be well adapted to various types of users.

The latter developments of automatic drug infusion techniques in the medical field are characterized by the employment of some of the most advanced computer science technologies in order to solve the necessity for increased safety and accuracy through nonlinear controllers without prior process models. This has led to the emergence of data-driven methods applying artificial neural networks (ANNs) as a modeling tool and fuzzy logic as the control element (Ying and Sheppard 1994).

Fixed or adaptive fuzzy logic controllers (FLCs) can be used in response to both of these crucial system needs (accuracy and high descriptive power). Moreover, when the effective solution for the control problem requires the adaptation of the patient model, the hybridization of the FLC with ANNs results in a controller with self-learning ability. With this in mind, in this chapter, the reader will be presented with an overview of general fuzzy logic theory along with real-world, up-to-date automatic drug administration and patient response prediction systems.

Fuzzy Systems for Automatic Drug Administration

The successful synthesis of a fuzzy controller relies on the incorporation, under the form of linguistic IF-THEN rules, of the knowledge and experience about the processes being controlled. For this endeavor, a judicious choice of linguistic terms (fuzzy sets), inference engine (logical representation of fuzzy implication), and logical operators or connectives is a quintessential factors. In this sense, a fuzzy controller can be regarded as an expert system employing fuzzy logic for its reasoning.

Fuzzy controllers, being generally nonlinear, provide a practical means to solve nonlinear, time-variant, and time-delay control problems whether or not explicit mathematical models of the processes involved are available. The fact that medical professionals can manually and adequately control various complex human physiological variables involving nonlinearity, time variance, and time delay based on their knowledge and experience suggests the great potential of fuzzy controllers in biomedicine (Linkens 1994).

The first fuzzy mean arterial pressure (MAP) controller based on computer simulation (Slate et al. 1979) was constructed on a general-purpose fuzzy expert system shell. The fuzzy controller was improved to control MAP in pigs in the laboratory (Slate and Sheppard 1982) and MAP in postsurgical patients clinically (Ying et al. 1992).

Figure 21.1 illustrates the general structure of such controllers. Other researchers have conducted similar studies using simple fuzzy controllers (Isaka et al. 1988; Fukui and Masuzawa 1989; Ruiz et al. 1993).

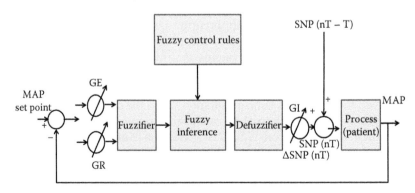

FIGURE 21.1
Block diagram of the fuzzy MAP controller. (From Ying, H., Sheppard, L.C., *Engineering in Medicine and Biology Magazine, IEEE*, vol. 13, no. 5, pp. 671–677, 1994. doi: 10.1109/51.334628.)

These controllers use two very simple calculations as inputs, the error and the rate of MAP. The error is measured as the difference between the desired and the obtained MAP in the previous instant. The rate of MAP identifies the change in MAP during the last interval.

The two inputs are scaled by input scalars, the error (GE) and the rate of MAP (GR), and then the scaled input is fuzzified and mapped to the *positive* and *negative* fuzzy sets, as shown in Figure 21.2.

L is an adjustable parameter of the controller. The output fuzzy sets describing the variation of sodium nitroprusside (SNP) dosage were three singleton fuzzy sets, *positive*, *zero*, and *negative*. A centroid defuzzifier was used to compute a crisp value for the variation of SNP dosage. The new SNP infusion rate was calculated based on the value of the current SNP dosage value, the variation of SNP dosage, the instant related to the variation calculation, and a configurable scalar.

Four fuzzy control rules were employed to relate linguistically the input fuzzy sets to the output fuzzy sets. These rules, though very simple, represented a rationally practical control strategy of human SNP infusion pump operators.

This controller is one of the simplest functional fuzzy controllers and was developed by adjusting different components of the controller, such as input and output fuzzy sets, and fuzzy control rules, using the trial-and-error method. Little effort was made to understand why and how the fuzzy controllers worked and what their explicit structures were in terms of classic control theory. While the black-box approach might be acceptable to some industries, such as consumer products, which could afford failure and/or expensive and exhaustive trails, it is not tolerable for control tasks directly involving human lives. In this light, this control mechanism was analytically converted to explicit control algorithms in terms of classic control theory. Such conversion enabled the authors to understand how the fuzzy controller operated and the role of different parameters in determining control performance. This understanding facilitated the design of the fuzzy MAP controller. Another important benefit was a dramatic reduction of the execution time of the fuzzy controller, which was initially based on a slow fuzzy expert system shell.

The system just described consists of the simplest hypertension controller. Based on this controller, other authors developed new methods and controllers.

Oshita et al. (1994) described a similar controller that administrates nicardipine instead of SNP. This variation involves different rules and has been tested in real patients, having achieved good results. The authors recommend the use of these kinds of controllers in medical procedures.

Other authors developed similar controllers based on the delivery of multiple drugs, where different and independent fuzzy controllers were used for each drug (Bauernschmitt

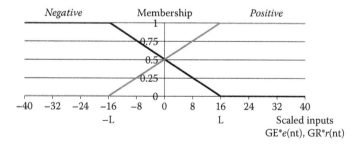

FIGURE 21.2

Fuzzy membership functions for MAP controller. (From Ying, H., Sheppard, L.C., *Engineering in Medicine and Biology Magazine, IEEE*, vol. 13, no. 5, pp. 671–677, 1994. doi: 10.1109/51.334628.)

et al. 2003). Tests were also conducted on humans with fairly good results. The authors noticed a need to increase the data artifact detection.

Artifacts occur quite frequently in any intensive care unit (ICU) due to manipulations in the patient or failure of sensors. Although the duration of drug application was too short to have hemodynamic consequences in the experiment, this activation has to be avoided in the clinical setup. Therefore, the integration of adequate artifact detection algorithms is necessary. Including more input and output variables, which was desirable, would lead to a huge increase in the number of rules. For these reasons, the authors described the need to develop a self-learning system taking into consideration important parameters like depth of narcosis and mechanical ventilation.

A similar but more recent approach was developed by Denai et al. (2007), where the rules used were altered. The testing was done with simulated data, having achieved good results. Keep in mind that the artifact problem described by Bauernschmitt et al. (2003) is nonexistent due to the simulator-generated data.

Another variation describes a similar controller based on three different models that are active depending on the clinical gravity of the situation of the patient (Held and Roy 2000). Only one of these three models is active at any given time. Two of these models are based on fuzzy controllers that use 36 rules to control 2 variables (cardiac output and MAP) with 2 different drugs. The drugs are also treated independently. This work is a fine tuning of the work done by the same authors in 1995 (Held and Roy 1995) and 1998 (Huang and Roy 1998). The system was tested on dogs.

Similar to the study developed by Held and Roy (2000), Sprunk et al. (2011) developed a three-model system to control the administration of four different drugs.

All of the approaches described above use the same basic concept of a fuzzy controller. Zheng et al. (2005) analyzed previous literature revealing that while past fuzzy controllers overcome some of the shortcomings inherent in the classical proportional integrative (PI) controller, no identification of the plant model is considered. Furthermore, the wide range of patient drug sensitivities to SNP is not considered. They developed a multiple-model adaptive control (MMAC) algorithm to identify the patient model and used a fuzzy control algorithm to design a controller bank. Thus, the proposed control method can provide satisfactory control performance and can handle changes in the system dynamics.

The MMAC procedure is based upon the assumption that the plant can be represented by one of a finite number of models and that for each such model, a controller can be designed a priori. All of these controllers together then constitute a controller bank. An adaptive mechanism is then needed for deciding which controller should be dominant for a given plant. One procedure for solving this problem is to form a weighted sum of all the controller outputs, where the weighting factors are determined by the relative residuals between the plant response and the model responses. These models are built upon the mathematical models using the recorded patient sensitivities and characteristics. The model bank consists of eight models with constant parameters characterizing the individual plant subspace.

To achieve desirable system performance and guarantee patient safety, the identification algorithm should converge quickly to the desired values and should react to time-varying plant characteristics, as well as ensure a reasonable rate of blood pressure change. Thus, the control output is computed as a weighted sum of controller bank signals.

The results of simulations indicate that the fuzzy controller–based MMAC algorithm can automatically control blood pressure over a fairly wide patient parameter envelope, even in the presence of much background noise.

Neuro-Fuzzy Systems for Automatic Drug Administration

ANNs, commonly called neural networks, are mathematical or computational models that are inspired by biological neural networks such as the brain (Yardimci 2009). The models most commonly used are far simpler than their biological counterparts. ANNs have become one of the most active research areas in recent years. Extracting explicit rules from data has the potential to allow applications to surpass the knowledge acquisition problem in artificial intelligence (Huang and Roy 1998).

These systems consist of interconnected layers of artificial neurons, and process information using a connectionist approach to computation. In most cases, an ANN is an adaptive system that changes its structure based on external or internal information that flows through the network during the learning phase. Modern neural networks are non-linear statistical data modeling tools and are usually used to model complex relationships between inputs and outputs or to find patterns in data.

Neural networks do not need to use complex mathematically explicit formulas or computer models. While neural networks can be used to solve complex problems, they have several disadvantages. According to Yardimci (2009), some of the characteristics that support the success of ANNs and distinguish them from the conventional computational techniques are as follows:

- The direct manner in which ANNs acquire information and knowledge about a given problem domain (learning interesting and possibly nonlinear relationships) through the *training* phase.
- Neural networks can work with continuous data that would be difficult to deal with by other means because of the form of the data or because there are so many variables.
- Neural network analysis can be conceived of as a black-box approach, and the user does not require sophisticated mathematical knowledge.
- The compact form in which the acquired information and knowledge is stored within the trained network and the ease with which it can be accessed and used.
- Neural network solutions can be robust even in the presence of *noise* in the input data.
- The high degree of accuracy reported when ANNs are used to generalize over a set of previously unseen data (not used in the *training* process) from the problem domain.

The most important shortcomings of ANNs are as follows:

- The data used to train neural networks should contain information, which, ideally, is spread evenly throughout the entire range of the system.
- There is limited theory to assist in the design of neural networks.
- There is no guarantee of finding an acceptable solution to a problem.
- There are limited opportunities to rationalize the solutions provided.

In the literature related to the control of hypertension, neural networks are mainly used as function approximators, but they can also be used as controllers for a given problem.

Figure 21.3 represents a common scenario where an unknown function describes an unknown system's dynamics. The objective is to adjust the parameters of the network so that it will produce the same response as the unknown function, if the same input is applied to both systems.

For hypertension control, the unknown function corresponds to the unknown circulatory system's dynamics for which control is attempted. With the approximation of this unknown function, the reaction of the patient to the administered drug can be calculated with increased precision.

Multilayer networks are universal approximators; however, they need to be trained in order to correctly predict the output of the unknown function. This is done by selecting the network parameters that will better approximate the desired value. One of the most common training procedures is called backpropagation (BP). In this method, a performance index is calculated. In general terms, this index represents the error in the output that is the difference between the output of the neural network and the desired output (output given by the unknown function).

The objective of the BP method of training is to minimize the error present in the output by correctly adjusting the network parameters. Each time the outputs are compared is called an epoch. The training is ended when the error is below a given threshold or when a given number of training epochs (or iterations) have ended. After the network has been trained, it is usually able to generalize the required outputs given different inputs. There are examples in the hypertension control literature that use ANNs (Polycarpou and Conway 1995; Chen et al. 1997).

The systems based on the usage of fuzzy logic together with neural networks (fuzzy neural networks) combine the humanlike reasoning of fuzzy systems with the learning and connectionist structure of neural networks (Negnevitsky 2005). The main strength of neuro-fuzzy systems is that they are universal approximators with the ability to elicit interpretable IF–THEN rules (Buckley and Hayashi 1995; Nauck and Kruse 1996).

Due to the fuzzy nature of the data present in fuzzy neural networks, the weight adjustment, training method, and activation functions are very different from a common neural network. A neuro-fuzzy system based on an underlying fuzzy system is trained by means of a data-driven learning method derived from neural network theory. There are many forms in which fuzzy logic theory can be used in neuro-fuzzy systems. Some of the more common applications use fuzzy logic as a means to input previous knowledge and information output.

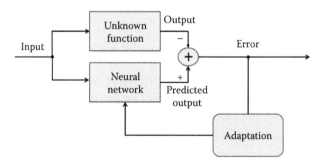

FIGURE 21.3
Neural network–based control system. (From Hagan, M., Demuth, H., Neural networks for control. *Proceedings of the American Control Conference*, 1999.)

In the case of blood pressure learning, the regularities of the network appear on hidden neurons. It is possible to extract rules or knowledge from these regularities. However, in many cases, there is no clear explanation of the relation between inputs and outputs, resulting in a black-box system.

Since the ANN structure is predetermined to learn only the relations between input and output characteristics of training data in medical diagnostic applications, the extraction of explicit rules from such a network structure is a difficult task. To avoid such a problem, Ichimura et al. (1997) proposed a method focusing on the cooperation of prior knowledge in the network formulation. The method enables the introduction of intermediate assumptions by medical experts into its network structure. The network structure is then trained on patient records. After the optimal network structure is achieved, the fuzzy rules are extracted from the network.

The network can converge into a suitable configuration based on the observation of training data and changing the connection weights accordingly.

After the network has reached a satisfactory set of results, the method proposed can give a clear explanation on the relation between inputs and outputs. To verify the method's effectiveness, the authors developed a model of the occurrence of hypertension and extracted fuzzy rules from the network. The obtained fuzzy rules were compared with prior knowledge.

Towell and Shavlik (1993) proposed a method of inserting knowledge into a neural network. The method is the specification of the seven-step rules to a network translation algorithm. This algorithm initially translates a set of rules into a neural network.

The first step of this algorithm transforms the set of rules into a format that clarifies its hierarchical structure and makes it possible to directly translate the rules into a neural network. If there is more than one rule for a consequence, then every rule for this consequence is rewritten as two rules. The second step establishes a mapping between a transformed set of rules, and a neural network using the map shown in Table 21.1.

Then, it creates networks that have a one-to-one correspondence with elements of the rule set. In the third step, the neurons in the network are numbered by their level. This number is a necessary precursor to several of the following steps. The fourth step adds hidden neurons to the network, thereby giving the network the ability to learn derived features not specified in the initial rule set but suggested by the expert. The fifth step adds neurons for known input features that are not referenced in the rules, because a set of rules that is not correct may not identify every input feature. In the sixth step, the algorithm adds links with zero weight to the network, even if the links are not specified by translation between all neurons in topologically contiguous levels. The final step is achieved by adding a small random number to each weight with the objective of perturbing all the weights in the network.

TABLE 21.1

Correspondence between Knowledge and Neural Network

Knowledge Bases	Neural Networks
Final conclusions	Output neurons
Facts	Input neurons
Intermediate conclusions	Hidden neurons
Dependencies	Weighted connections

Source: Towell, G. G. and I. W. Shavlik, *Machine Learning*, 13, 1993.

The neural network described above can only change the interconnection weights, and its structure has to remain fixed, limiting its adaptability. For such a problem, Ichimura et al. (1997) presented a structural learning method that aims at ameliorating the difficulties in a prior specification of network structure.

In a normal neural network's mechanism, the following behaviors may emerge during the learning phase: (1) a neural network does not have enough neurons, and then, the input weight vector will tend to fluctuate greatly even after a certain period of the learning process; and (2) the neural network is overspecified with nonfunctional or redundant neurons in the network.

In the first case, the network needs to generate new neurons, whereas in the second, it is necessary to delete the redundant neurons. Based on such behaviors, the criteria for the neuron generation/annihilation process is known, and the procedure of generating a new neuron and/or annihilating the specified neuron is done by the learning process of the neural network.

This algorithm was tested on real data, consisting of 16 input terms and 1 output term. There are two kinds of intermediate assumptions between the input terms and the output term. Ten terms are categorized into a biochemical test related to the measurement of blood pressure for the past 5 years; the remaining terms are *sex, age, obesity index,* gamma glutamyl transpeptidase *7-GTP,* and *volume of consuming alcohol.* One output term represents whether the patient has a hypertension attack, for the input record.

Using the standard BP learning, the network was trained for a real medical database consisting of 1024 patient records. In the referred test, the training set had 100 occurrence data records and 100 no-occurrence data records randomly sampled.

The developed system correctly diagnosed 95.0% of all patient records in the first instance. A neuron was found with large input weight vector variation in the second hidden layer related to blood pressure. According to the neuron generation algorithm, the neuron was split as its parent neuron's attributes were inherited. The network was trained again using the new network structure and correctly diagnosed 96.7% of all patient records. In the referred test, no redundant neuron was found.

After this step, extracting fuzzy rules from the network gives a clear explanation of the relation between inputs and outputs.

The number of weights in the neural network, and the weights between each neuron, has to be evaluated to quantify the degree of influence of input factors on output factors.

After this step, a set of fuzzy rules of the IF–THEN type is obtained. The method to extract fuzzy rules from the learned networks is further described in the work of Ichimura and Tazaki (1994) and Ichimura et al. (1995).

Case Study: The Self-Generating Fuzzy Neural Network Mean Arterial Pressure Controller

In this section, we describe a controller based on an adaptive nonlinear modeling technique: a self-generating fuzzy neural network (SGFNN) for modeling and controlling MAP via an SNP drug delivery system. The interested reader is referred to the original work of Fan and Joo (2010) for further details. This particular controller is the main focus of this section due to its ability to translate neural network learnt information into fuzzy logic rules. This is particularly important in the AAL environment, where descriptive power and adequate information transference are critical.

As mentioned before, there are mathematical models that aim to describe the pharmacokinetics of the human body. State-of-the-art blood pressure controllers incorporate this knowledge by associating these mathematical models with soft computing methodologies.

One of the most well-known mathematical models to describe the variation in blood pressure after SNP administration is shown as follows (Slate et al. 1979).

MAP is modeled by

$$MAP(t) = p_0 + \Delta p(t) + p_d(t) + n(t),$$

where p_0 is the initial blood pressure, $\Delta p(t)$ is the change in blood pressure due to SNP infusion, $p_d(t)$ is the change in blood pressure due to the rennin reflex, and $n(t)$ is modeled as the background noise.

The discrete-time deterministic model is given by

$$\Delta p(t) = \frac{q^{-d}(b_0 + b_m q^{-m})}{1 - a_1 q^{-1}} u(t),$$

where $\Delta p(t)$ is the change in blood pressure, $u(t)$ is the drug infusion rate, and $q^{(-1)}$ denotes a unit delay.

The pharmacokinetic/pharmacodynamic model parameters presented in Table 21.2 were deduced from medical studies done throughout the years according to the mathematical models referred to in the control theory literature. It is a table commonly used in practical applications.

The pharmacodynamic parameters d and m are associated with the initial transport delay and the recirculatory delay, respectively. a_1, b_0, and b_1 are the pharmacokinetic parameters modeling patient variability.

The SGFNN consists of a multilayer feedforward network based on ellipsoidal basis function (EBF) activation, identifying and executing a Takagi–Sugeno–Kang (TSK) fuzzy controller (Takagi and Sugeno 1985; Sugeno and Kang 1988).

Structure and parameter identification of the SGFNN can be done automatically and simultaneously. Structure learning is based on criteria of generating and pruning neurons. The Kalman filter (KF) algorithm (Lin and Lee 1996) has been used to adjust consequent parameters of the SGFNN. KF is a mathematical method that uses previous measurements to produce values that tend to be closer to the real values.

TABLE 21.2

Reference Values

Parameters	Minimum	Maximum	Nominal
a_0	0.606	0.779	0.741
b_0	0.053	3.547	0.187
b_1	0	1.418	0.075
d	2	5	3
m	4	10	6

Source: Fan, L. and Joo, E., An intelligent control approach for blood pressure system using self-generating fuzzy neural networks. Paper presented at the 11th International Conference on Control, Automation, Robotics and Vision, Singapore, 2010.

The main advantage of this methodology when compared to classical control theory methods is that it can model unknown nonlinearities of complex drug delivery systems and adapt to changes and uncertainties in these systems online.

It was previously pointed out that structure learning is based on the criteria of generating and pruning neurons. In other words, the output error of the SGFNN system with regard to the reference signal is an important criterion to determine whether a new rule should be recruited or not. The error is calculated based on the difference between the desired blood pressure and the blood pressure achieved in a given period of time. If the error is superior to a threshold, the creation of a new neuron is considered. The threshold is a value that decays over time, given an opportunity for the training of the network, allowing larger error values at the beginning.

The pruning strategy is based on the error reduction ratio (ERR) method (Chen et al. 1991). The ERR method is used to calculate the sensitivity and significance of fuzzy rules in order to check which rules would be deleted. When a rule has been generated, the allocation of its parameters is made for a Gaussian membership function, which includes centers and widths.

Once the premise parameters and structure of the SGFNN are determined, the KF algorithm is used to adjust the consequent parameters. In this context, the SGFNN is viewed as a modeling method. The information about a system's dynamics and mapping characteristics are stored in the network. The direct inverse control method is used to control blood pressure.

The direct inverse control method is based on the reference model of the system; neural networks or fuzzy neural networks are used to learn and approximate the inverse dynamics of the drug delivery system. Precise inverse dynamic calculations involve the knowledge of reactions yet to occur. This happens because the arterial pressure variations are calculated based on past administrations of the drug. When we invert the mathematical model, there are future values that are unknown. Due to the impossibility of measuring these kinds of events, soft computing methods are used, and the reference values are adopted. The resulting SGFNN can therefore be used to estimate the drug infusion rate given the desired blood pressure level $r(t)$.

The direct inverse control method is illustrated in Figure 21.4. When the SGFNN is used as a controller in a drug delivery system, the goal is to obtain appropriate control input $u(t)$ to make the output of system $y(t)$ approximate the desired blood pressure level $r(t)$. This

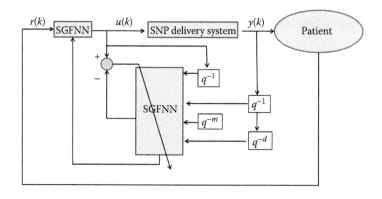

FIGURE 21.4
Direct inverse control method. (From Fan, L., Joo, E., An intelligent control approach for blood pressure system using self-generating fuzzy neural networks. Paper presented at the 11th International Conference Control, Automation, Robotics and Vision, Singapore, 2010.)

system consists of two stages: the learning stage and the application stage. In the learning stage, the SGFNN is used to identify the inverse dynamics of the drug delivery system. In the application stage, the SGFNN is viewed as a controller to generate the control input.

According to Fan and Joo (2010), the proposed SGFNN can learn from the training data without any prior knowledge of the drug delivery system. Simulation studies demonstrate the effectiveness of the proposed SGFNN algorithm to model and control the drug delivery system even in the presence of noise.

Final Remarks

Assisted living systems must combine the characteristics of output comprehensibility and increased input simplicity with robust error detection, high accuracy, and recovery capabilities in order to be usable by nonmedical professionals.

The systems described in this chapter are valid solutions for automatic drug administration, many of them tested in professional medical care environments. Although most of the work available on this theme is focused on the hospital environment, once the systems mature, they can be applied to assisted living facilities or even to the patient's homes. The administration of insulin, a drug used by patients with diabetes, is an example of this change of paradigm. Despite the practical adhesion to some of these systems, key issues still exist in pursuing the design of more robust and clinically safe controllers. Determination of an appropriate underlying process model is a difficult issue for biomedical control in general but essential for stability and convergence of the controller.

The controllers present in the literature rely on the minimization of the error between the desired reference level (blood pressure or neuromuscular relaxation, for instance) and the actual achieved value. If a readmission event occurs, the patient will be submitted to the standard controller. This implies that a new learning phase will be created for that particular patient, discarding the information gathered in the previous clinical admissions. Methods for explicitly increasing the knowledge about a patient are not easily found in the literature. The creation of a holistic health model for each patient that could be used in future interventions is an interesting research problem.

Current mathematical reference models are inherently empirical (see, for example, the hypertension model of Montani and Vliet), promoting controllers based on soft computing methodologies as a very interesting tool to model new concepts or adjust previous ones regarding the precise definition of the system. Data gathered from the patient may be analyzed in order to create soft comprehensible models for presently unmodeled physiological behaviors or to enhance the precision inherent to currently defined models.

Health care professionals do possess a general patient vision, evaluating several key biometric values in order to assess the stability of the patient. This allows the detection of anomalies in the treatment or in the patient's condition. This capability enables the professionals to react to the actual patient response and adapt the therapeutic action. The integration of complementary models (e.g., circulatory system's model) with the pharmacodynamic model of a given drug may be a way of decreasing the limitation of these systems, accompanied by the increase in stability and reliability. While hypertension control is based on the circulatory system, it would be interesting if controllers processed more information than just that directly related to arterial pressure in order to verify the overall patient response.

Most of the systems currently found in the literature were built, tuned, and tested using medical simulators. While some authors state that their team built the simulator, others do not mention the source. This may lead to different results and, therefore, to a mismatch between the capabilities of the systems and their evaluation. Also, this characteristic makes it very hard to compare the various algorithms and their real performance, advantages, and drawbacks. One of the possible solutions for this problem could be the possibility for readers and researchers to have access to the same simulators. The development of a de facto standard open-source simulator (or even a commercial one) seems to be an endeavor that would be worth pursuing.

As for the teams and researchers whose algorithms and systems were tested on real patients or that used patient data, it would be recommended, in order to better understand their work, that those particular data are also made available to the scientific community. Humans have very high intrapatient and interpatient variability in terms of their biological systems. Having different data sets chosen to train, test, and evaluate the algorithms and systems may lead to a large fluctuation of results. Having a good understanding of other authors' work would also be very useful when additional patient information is gathered. This information should be data set related and completely anonymous. This need is due to the fact that a patient biological system's response to treatment strongly varies depending on other pathologies or characteristics, such as drug sensitivity, patient weight, or age.

Fuzzy logic–based controllers have been proven to be a viable solution for the closed-loop automatic medical drug administration problem. While maintaining the accuracy and reliability that is critical for medical controllers, they provide the ability to input patient information and output a system's results in a more human-friendly manner. They provide a natural language interface, allowing users to better assess the system's execution model, increasing the descriptive power of automatic drug administration technologies. This increase in the interface's descriptive capabilities is especially relevant when considering the assisted living application of these technologies. This relevancy is due to the existence of highly heterogeneous groups of medical system users. While technology interfacing is a very common problem for developers, it is usually very challenging to perfect. Medical systems require an interface that is informative and conveys the data in a precise form often required by trained professionals.

By analyzing professional hospital systems and algorithms, this chapter intends to provide a better insight into the current state of automatic drug administration, along with the current limitations, possible future developments, and applications that enable the deployment of such systems in a less constrained AAL environment.

References

Alexander, C. (2010). *Complexity & Medicine: The Elephant in the Waiting Room*. Nottingham, UK: Nottingham University Press.

Bauernschmitt, R., Hoerer, J., Schirmbeck, E.U., Keil, H., Schrott, G., Knoll, A., Lange, R. (2003). Fuzzy-logic based automatic control of hemodynamics. *Computers in Cardiology, 2003*, pp. 773–776, September 21–24. doi: 10.1109/CIC.2003.1291271.

Buckley, J., Hayashi, Y. (1995). Neural networks for fuzzy systems. *Fuzzy Sets and Systems*, vol. 71, pp. 265–276.

Campos-Delgado, D.U., Hernandez-Ordonez, M., Femat, R., Gordillo-Moscoso, A. (2006). Fuzzy-based controller for glucose regulation in type-1 diabetic patients by subcutaneous route. *IEEE Transactions on Biomedical Engineering*, vol. 53, no. 11, pp. 2201–2210. doi: 10.1109/TBME.2006.879461.

Carver, C., Scheier, M. (1982). Control theory: A useful conceptual framework for personality–social, clinical, and health psychology. *Psychological Bulletin*, vol. 92, no. 1, pp. 111–135.

Chen, C., Lin, W., Kuo, T., Wang, C. (1997). Adaptive control of arterial blood pressure with a learning controller based on multilayer neural networks. *IEEE Transactions on Biomedical Engineering*, vol. 44, no. 7, pp. 601–609.

Chen, S., Cowan, C., Grant, P. (1991). Orthogonal least squares learning algorithm for radial basis function network. *IEEE Transactions on Neural Networks*, vol. 2, pp. 302–309.

Denai, M., Mahfouf, M., Ross, J. (2007). A fuzzy decision support system for therapy administration in cardiovascular intensive care patients. *IEEE International Fuzzy Systems Conference, 2007. FUZZ-IEEE 2007*, pp. 1–6, July 23–26. doi: 10.1109/FUZZY.2007.4295361.

Dudde, R., Vering, T., Piechotta, G., Hintsche, R. (2006). Computer-aided continuous drug infusion: Setup and test of a mobile closed-loop system for the continuous automated infusion of insulin. *IEEE Transactions on Information Technology in Biomedicine*, vol. 10, no. 2, pp. 395–402. doi: 10.1109/TITB.2006.864477.

Eoyang, G. (2007). Human systems dynamics: Complexity-based approach to a complex evaluation. In B. Williams and I. Imam (Eds.), *Systems Concepts in Evaluation an Expert Anthology*. Point Reyes, CA: EdgePress, pp. 123–140.

Fan, L., Joo, E. (2010). An intelligent control approach for blood pressure system using self-generating fuzzy neural networks. Paper presented at the 11th International Conference Control, Automation, Robotics and Vision, Singapore.

Fazendeiro, P., Valente de Oliveira, J., Pedrycz, W. (2007). A multi-objective design of a patient and anaesthetist-friendly neuromuscular blockade controller. *IEEE Transactions on Biomedical Engineering*, vol. 54. no. 9, pp. 1667–1678.

Franklin, G.F., Powell, J.D., Emani-Naeini, A. (1972). *Feedback Control of Dynamic Systems*. Boston: Addison-Wesley.

Fukui, Y., Masuzawa, T. (1989). Development of fuzzy blood pressure control system. *Iyodenshi-To-Seitai-Kogaku*, vol. 27, pp. 79–85.

Guyton, A., Coleman, T., Granger, H. (1972). Circulation: Overall regulation. *Annual Review of Physiology*, vol. 34, pp. 13–44.

Hagan, M., Demuth, H. (1999). Neural networks for control. *Proceedings of the American Control Conference*.

Held, C.M., Roy, R.J. (1995). Multiple drug hemodynamic control by means of a supervisory-fuzzy rule-based adaptive control system: Validation on a model. *IEEE Transactions on Biomedical Engineering*, vol. 42, no. 4, pp. 371–385. doi: 10.1109/10.376130.

Held, C.M., Roy, R.J. (2000). Hemodynamic management of congestive heart failure by means of a multiple mode rule-based control system using fuzzy logic. *IEEE Transactions on Biomedical Engineering*, vol. 47, no. 1, pp. 115–123.

Huang, J.W., Roy, R.J. (1998). Multiple-drug hemodynamic control using fuzzy decision theory. *IEEE Transactions on Biomedical Engineering*, vol. 45, no. 2, pp. 213–228. doi: 10.1109/10.661269.

Ichimura, T., Tazaki, E. (1994). Learning and extracting method for fuzzy rules using neural networks with modified structure level adaptation. *Proc. of the 2nd European Congress on Fuzzy and Intelligent Technologies (EUFIT'94)*, vol. 3, pp. 1237–1241.

Ichimura, T., Tazaki, E., Yoshida, K. (1995). Extraction of fuzzy rules using neural networks with structure level adaptation—Verification of the diagnosis of hepatobiliary disorders. *International Journal of Biomedical Computing*, vol. 40, no. 2, pp. 139–146.

Ichimura, T., Ooba, K., Tazaki, E., Takahashi, H., Yoshida, K. (1997). Knowledge based approach to structure level adaptation of neural networks. *1997 IEEE International Conference on Systems, Man, and Cybernetics. Computational Cybernetics and Simulation*, vol. 1, pp. 548–553, October 12–15. doi: 10.1109/ICSMC.1997.625809.

Isaka, S., Sebald, A.V., Smith, N.T., Quinn, M. (1988). A fuzzy blood pressure controller. *Proc. IEEE Tenth Ann. EMBS Conf.*, New Orleans, LA, pp. 1410–1411.

Kami, K., Adachi, H., Umeyama, K., Kosaka, Y., Yamaguchi, S., Fuse, E., Sato, M., Nakamura, M., Tanaka, Y., Fukaya, T., Matsuno, K., Suzuki, K. (1996). Endoscope system with automatic control according to movement of an operator. US Patent 5558619.

Koivo, A. (1981). Microprocessor-based controller for pharmacodynamical application. *IEEE Transactions on Automatic Control*, vol. AC-26, no. 5, pp. 1208–1213.

Lichtenstein, E. (1984). Computer-control medical care system. US Patent 4,464,172.

Lin, C.T., Lee, C.S. (1996). *Neural Fuzzy Systems: A Neuro-Fuzzy Synergism to Intelligent Systems*. Upper Saddle River, NJ: Prentice Hall.

Linkens, D.A. (1994). *Intelligent Control in Biomedicine*. London: Taylor & Francis.

Medjahed, H., Istrate, D., Boudy, J., Dorizzi, B. (2009). Human activities of daily living recognition using fuzzy logic for elderly home monitoring. *IEEE International Conference on Fuzzy Systems, 2009. FUZZ-IEEE 2009*, pp. 2001–2006, August 20–24. doi: 10.1109/FUZZY.2009.5277257.

Montani, J.P., Vliet, B.N.V. (2009). Understanding the contribution of Guyton's large circulatory model to long-term control of arterial pressure. *Experimental Physiology*, vol. 94, pp. 382–388.

Nauck, D., Kruse, R. (1996). Neuro-fuzzy classification with NEFCLASS. In P. Kleinschmidt, A. Bachem, U. Derigs, D. Fischer, U. Leopold-Wildburger and R. Möhring (Eds.), *Operations Research Proceedings*. Berlin: Springer, pp. 294–299.

Negnevitsky, M. (2005). *Artificial Intelligence, A Guide to Intelligent Systems*, Second edition. England: Pearson Education Limited.

Olasveengen, M., Sunde, K., Brunborg, C., Thowsen, J., Steen, P., Wik, L. (2009). Intravenous drug administration during out-of-hospital cardiac arrest. A randomized trial. *The Journal of American Medical Association—JAMA*, vol. 302, no. 20, pp. 2222–2229.

Oshita, S., Nakakimura, K., Sakabe, T. (1994). Hypertension control during anesthesia. Fuzzy logic regulation of nicardipine infusion. *Engineering in Medicine and Biology Magazine, IEEE*, vol. 13, no. 5, pp. 667–670.

Palanque, P., Basnyat, S., Navarre, D. (2007). Improving interactive systems usability using formal description techniques: Application to healthcare. In *HCI and Usability for Medicine and Health Care*, vol. 4799 of *Lecture Notes in Computer Science*. Berlin: Springer, pp. 21–40.

Polycarpou, M., Conway, J. (1995). Modeling and control of drug delivery systems using adaptive neural control methods. *Proceedings of the American Control Conference*, vol. 1, pp. 781–785.

Ritchart, M., Burbank, H. (1998). Control system and method for automated biopsy device. US Patent 5,769,086.

Ruiz, R., Borches, D., Gonzalez, A., Corral, J. (1993). A new sodium-nitroprusside-infusion controller for the regulation of arterial blood pressure. *Biomedical Instrumentation & Technology*, vol. 27, pp. 244–251.

Sheppard, L. (1980). Computer control of the infusion of vasoactive drugs. *Annals of Biomedical Engineering*, vol. 8, pp. 431–444. Springer Netherlands.

Slate, J., Sheppard, L.C. (1982). Automatic control of blood pressure by drug infusion. *IEE Proceedings, Part A*, vol. 129, no. 9, pp. 639–645.

Slate, J., Sheppard, L.C., Rideout, V.C., Blackstone, E.H. (1979). A model for design of a blood pressure controller for hypertensive patients. *5th IFAC Symp. Identification Syst. Parameter Estimation*, Darmstadt, F. R. Germany, September 24–28.

Spratt, R. (1997). Automatic X-ray exposure control system and method of use. US Patent 5,617,462.

Sprunk, N., Mendoza, G.A., Knoll, A., Schreiber, U., Eichhorn, S., Horer, J., Bauernschmitt, R. (2011). Hemodynamic regulation using fuzzy logic. *2011 Eighth International Conference on Fuzzy Systems and Knowledge Discovery (FSKD)*, vol. 1, pp. 515–519, July 26–28. doi: 10.1109/FSKD .2011.6019570.

Sugeno, M., Kang, G. (1988). Structure identification of fuzzy model. *Fuzzy Sets and Systems*, vol. 28, pp. 15–33.

Suzuki, T., Nakauchi, Y. (2010). Interactive medicine case system for elderly recipient. *2010 3rd IEEE RAS and EMBS International Conference on Biomedical Robotics and Biomechatronics (BioRob)*, pp. 253–258, September 26–29. doi: 10.1109/BIOROB.2010.5627737.

Takagi, T., Sugeno, M. (1985). Fuzzy identification of systems and its applications to modeling and control. *IEEE Transactions on Systems, Man, and Cybernetics*, vol. 15, pp. 116–132.

Thimbleby, H. (2007). User-centered methods are insufficient for safety critical systems. In *HCI and Usability for Medicine and Health Care*, vol. 4799 of *Lecture Notes in Computer Science*. Berlin: Springer, pp. 1–20.

Towell, G.G., Shavlik, W. (1993). Extracting refined rules from knowledge-based neural networks. *Machine Learning*, vol. 13, pp. 71–101.

Webster, C., Larsson, L., Frampton, C., Weller, J., McKenzie, A., Cumin, D., Merry, A. (2010). Clinical assessment of a new anaesthetic drug administration system: A prospective, controlled, longitudinal incident monitoring study. *Anaesthesia*, vol. 65, no. 5, pp. 490–499.

Yamamoto, Y., Huang, R., Ma, J. (2010). Medicine management and medicine taking assistance system for supporting elderly care at home. *2010 2nd International Symposium on Aware Computing (ISAC)*, pp. 31–37, November 1–4. doi: 10.1109/ISAC.2010.5670451.

Yardimci, A. (2009). Soft computing in medicine. *Applied Soft Computing*, vol. 9, pp. 1029–1043. Amsterdam, The Netherlands: Elsevier Science Publishers B. V.

Ying, H., Sheppard, L.C. (1994). Regulating mean arterial pressure in postsurgical cardiac patients. A fuzzy logic system to control administration of sodium nitroprusside. *Engineering in Medicine and Biology Magazine, IEEE*, vol. 13, no. 5, pp. 671–677. doi: 10.1109/51.334628.

Ying, H., McEachem, M., Eddleman, D.W., Sheppard, L.C. (1992). Fuzzy control of mean arterial pressure in postsurgical patients with sodium nitroprusside infusion. *IEEE Transactions on Biomedical Engineering*, vol. 39, pp. 1060–1070.

Zheng, H., Zhu, K.Y., Zhang, D.G. (2005). Design of an adaptive drug delivery control system. *International Conference on Control and Automation, 2005. ICCA '05*, vol. 2, pp. 846–851, June 26–29. doi: 10.1109/ICCA.2005.1528240.

22

Semantic Framework for Context-Aware Monitoring of Ambient Assisted Living Ecosystems

Lyazid Sabri, Abdelghani Chibani, Yacine Amirat,
Gian Piero Zarri, and Patrick Gatellier

CONTENTS

ABSTRACT The Web of Objects is a new emerging concept that represents a new way of organizing physical or abstract objects—or things—delivering a high level of services that can be discovered, composed, executed, and monitored. Building an ambient assisted living (AAL) ecosystem, according to this vision, is of great interest since it consists of multiple heterogeneous objects that need to be semantically and automatically interoperable. In this chapter, a new semantic framework for monitoring AAL heterogeneous ecosystems is presented. This framework deals with context awareness and closed-world assumption (CWA) based semantic reasoning for designing management rules and ontologies. It preserves, on one hand, the structural expressiveness provided by ontologies, through compatibility with the World Wide Web Consortium (W3C) recommendations and, on the other hand, it takes advantage of the full benefit of the production rule reasoning. It is capable of dynamically detecting real-world objects and capturing their contexts, in order to identify the specific changes that are happening in the environment, to infer the current situation and to react accordingly. Context management is designed by combining the micro-concept ontology language into a set rules and queries using the SEMbySEM business rule language. These rules allow us to express high-level reasoning over context events, sent from the façade layer of the Framework architecture, while the queries allow us to generate high-level monitoring views, concerning manageable objects status and context, as well as their measures and produced activities. Conversely, the monitoring rules can trigger control actions that are translated, by the façade, into concrete operations on the targeted manageable object. In order to validate the proposed framework, a scenario dedicated to the safety of elderly people in smart homes is proposed and implemented hereby.

KEY WORDS: *semantic reasoning, closed world assumption, ontologies, context awareness, web of objects, ambient assisted living.*

Introduction

The latest advances in consumer electronics miniaturization, embedded systems, and wireless networking technologies are transforming our living and working environments into complex and pervasive ecosystems. These ecosystems—such as, interactive smart home or building automation systems—aim to protect, assist, and satisfy the daily life needs of *ordinary* people any time and anywhere. We call such ecosystems ambient assisted living (AAL) environments [1–3]. For example, integration of miniature and wearable health monitoring devices within home automation and communication infrastructures will make the health monitoring process smart, and wearable monitoring devices will become an important instrument for the prolongation of life. Other devices such as smartphones or TVs can deliver vital information as reminders to take medications or to provide early detection of behavioral changes (fall, heart attack, etc.) as an adequate measure of an emergency situation [1,4–6].

The emergence of new challenging domains in the *Internet of the future* mode—where we talk about the "Web of Objects" (WoO)—emphasizes even more the interest in building an AAL environment. WoO depicts, in fact, the future Internet as being a collection of objects—or things—delivering high-level services that could be discovered, composed, executed, and monitored [7,8]. The WoO enlarges the universe of current devices that are part of the Internet to cover *objects* that can correspond to both physical (like everyday domestic devices, sensors, actuators, plants, or machines) and abstract (web services, multimedia content providers, directories, mashups) ones. According to the WoO vision, an AAL ecosystem consists of a high amount of heterogeneous entities that have mutual interactions, such as switching a light on, sitting on a chair, opening the door, moving, etc. Some of these interactions may be related to complex and dynamic behaviors such as cooking, sleeping, etc. From a management perspective, all these objects must be capable of capturing *events* and their context, a condition that is necessary, on the one hand, to get the full understanding of the environment and citizens' situation and, on the other hand, to react to the identified ones.

However, the complexity of such ecosystems is very high, and important challenges must be addressed in order to implement efficient management systems on both small- and large-scale levels. The most important challenges are as follows: context awareness, semantic interoperability of knowledge and services, and the integration of autonomic computing capabilities such as reactive reasoning and self-* features [9–11].

Addressing these challenges needs multiview management frameworks with semantic knowledge representation and reasoning capabilities. These kinds of frameworks should be capable of providing a rich and semantic description of the interacting objects with respect to both their *static* (physical) context characteristics and their dynamic behaviors or situations [9]. From a concrete point of view, the objects (devices/sensors/actuators) that interact in an AAL environment need to be made semantically and automatically interoperable. Any management system will be, then, capable of dynamically detecting these objects and capturing their contexts in order to identify the changes occuring in the environment, infer the current situation, and react accordingly.

The recent progress in the field of pervasive computing, thanks to the semantic web and service-oriented computing (SOC), have resulted in some interesting context awareness frameworks [12–17]. Indeed, a context awareness framework provides representation and reasoning functionalities that allow a software entity to capture its context and self-adapt its behavior to the changes occurring in the context over time. In general, context is considered as an interpretation of the environment from the observation of a set of interrelated physical objects. The most popular definition of context is that given in Ref. [18]: Context is any information that can be used to characterize the situation of an entity (e.g., a person, place, etc.) that is considered relevant to the interaction between a user and an application. Information such as location, identity, time, and activity are considered as the primary context types for characterizing the situation of an entity. *Situation* is defined in Ref. [19] as an external semantic interpretation of context. The meaningful interpretation of context is done from the application or system observer point of view, rather than from sensors or context itself. In AAL, the concepts of context and situation awareness are useful, on the one hand, to get a better understanding of living persons and the activities of their surrounding objects and, on the other hand, to adapt the behavior of the AAL system by applying actions on the environment actuators. Symbolic reasoning on context using ontologies constitutes the most adopted approach for AAL and pervasive computing [12,20]. This kind of reasoning is generally used to transform raw data captured independently from real-world sensors into meaningful interpretations of context. Situation reasoning is based on the interpretation of context captures according to space and time. For example, Wang et al. [21] designed a context awareness framework based on the combination of ontologies with Horn-like rules for the inference of specific contexts in the physical environment such as the bedroom, kitchen, etc.

The main contribution of our research work consists of designing a new semantic framework to build monitoring systems, tailored to ambient intelligence (AmI) requirements. This framework is the result of the research activities that were undertaken with partners in the context of the European project SEMbySEM [22–24]. The latter aimed, in fact, at the construction of a common software framework allowing different domain administrators to easily set up and handle different *real-world* heterogeneous entities, called *manageable objects* (MOs). An MO corresponds to a physical or abstract object disseminated in the real world, which can deliver a service, i.e., acting as an information provider, or on which control can be applied. It is characterized by specific identities and a set of attributes/properties. The SEMbySEM monitoring system allows domain experts to easily set up and reuse monitoring rules and handle different monitoring views coping with different levels of perception of AAL in the real world.

More precisely, the framework deals with context awareness and closed-world assumption (CWA) semantic reasoning over heterogeneous ecosystems by preserving the structural expressiveness provided by ontologies and the compatibility with the WoO vision through the compliancy with the recommendations of both the W3C and the open standards for global information society Organization for the Advancement of Structured Information Standards (OASIS). The latter specify how semantic knowledge and web services can be shared over the future Internet. In addition, the proposed framework exploits in full all the possible benefits of production rule reasoning for managing an infrastructure composed of connected things.

In this chapter, we present a detailed description of the architecture of our framework and the ontology management techniques that are used to build up the *reasoning on context* procedures according to the closed-world reasoning paradigm. We claim that our semantic-based architecture approach provides (1) standardized and reliable mechanisms for developing dynamic and context-aware monitoring views that can give rise to a high level of semantic representation of the situations occurring in the AAL environment, and (2) the possibility of a seamless integration of the real-world MOs' descriptions and of their communication technologies according to a common semantic model. The semantic model is specified using the *micro-concept* (μ-concept) ontology language and is interoperable with Resource Description Framework Schema (RDFS) and Web Ontology Language (OWL) 2 [25]. A μ-concept is a binary concept that describes the structure and interactions of an atomic or composite MO. The monitoring activities are then implemented by combining these μ-concepts and their properties into a set of production rules and queries using the SEMbySEM *μ-concept rule language*. The production rules are used for reasoning over the events sent from the MOs while the queries allow us to infer knowledge to be used to generate the monitoring views that concern MOs status and context as well as their measures and produced activities.

For the validation of the proposed framework, a concrete scenario dedicated to the monitoring of elderly people in smart homes has been proposed and implemented.

The chapter is organized as follows: The section "AmI Context Events Management Using Rules and Ontologies" presents the main challenges regarding the management of AAL ecosystems and the combination of ontologies with *production rules* as suitable solution to address them. Then, in the section "CWA-Based Semantic," a CWA-based semantic model is proposed to describe semantically manageable objects' structure and context (status, behaviors) of an AAL ecosystem according to the CWA, and make semantic reasoning on context through the SEMbySEM Business Rule Language. The section "SEMbySEM Framework Architecture" presents the multi-layered architecture of the proposed framework for the monitoring of AAL environments, and the section "Elderly Safety Monitoring Scenario" details the implementation of an AAL scenario dedicated to safety monitoring of elderly people. The "Conclusion" summarizes the contributions of this research work and gives an outlook on the ongoing works.

AmI Context Events Management Using Rules and Ontologies

The management of AAL ecosystems needs to take on some challenges concerning the integration into an industrial and ubiquitous monitoring system of principles such as management model maintenance; extensibility and scalability; and also persistency, privacy, and security. The appropriate instrument to address these challenges according to the CWA is the combination of ontologies with *production rules*—i.e., formal abstractions of management policies and practices that are directly executable on a machine making use of a rule engine [26,27].

Production Rules

In general, the technical solutions used to implement management rules range from the so-called sequential algorithms to production rules pertaining to a logic programming context and making use (normally) of the *Rete* algorithm. A management system based on production rules relies on a rule engine (or *inference engine*) for unifying the antecedent of the rules with information included in the *working memory* where the *facts* corresponding to the targeted application are collected. If the unification is successful, the corresponding rule *fires*, and new knowledge is derived by executing the operations proper to the *action* part (the consequent) of the rule [28]. It is possible that the production of this new knowledge leads to some changes in the working memory: in the next cycle of operations performed by the inference engine, other rules can then be fired, producing new knowledge and inducing new changes in the working memory, etc. Firing rules are based on the powerful pattern-matching mechanism proper to the Rete algorithm, which is designed to minimize the evaluation of repetitive tests across many objects/attributes and many rules during the consecutive operation cycles: An in-depth description of this algorithm based on a concrete example can be found in Ref. [29].

Semantic Web Ontologies

Independent from the technical issues about the design of context-aware monitoring systems, a fundamental problem to be solved consists in the choice of the sort of *formal vocabulary* to be used to write rules that react to various events. Given the increasing use of *ontologies* as a way of *cleverly* structuring a terminological domain making use of *hierarchical* (IsA) and *property/value* relationships, utilizing a vocabulary of concepts/instances in order to describe *rules* represents a very popular approach. The most popular language in the domain of semantic knowledge modeling, making use of ontologies, is OWL [30]. OWL is a semantic mark-up language for publishing and sharing ontologies using Resource Description Framework (RDF) extensions; see Figure 22.1. The first version, OWL 1, consists of three specific sublanguages characterized respectively by an increasing level of complexity and expressiveness, OWL Lite, OWL Description Logics (DL), and OWL Full [31]. The new release OWL 2 (see Ref. [32]) extends the *standard* version, OWL 1, with a small set of features, e.g., a sort of meta-modeling device called *punning* that relaxes the mandatory disjointedness of vocabularies in OWL DL when it is possible to disambiguate the exact meaning of a name (e.g., a name like *Person* can

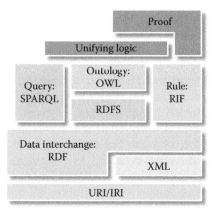

FIGURE 22.1
Representation and reasoning languages of the semantic web stack from W3C. IRI, internationalized resource identifier; SPARQL, SPARQL Protocol and RDF Query Language; URI, uniform resource identifier.

be used as a class, an individual, or a property). Specific working groups are actively working to promote the *core rule language* Rule Interchange Format (RIF), Datalog based, to allow rules to be translated between different rule languages and then used across different rule systems; see http://www.w3.org/TR/rif-core/. A specific *dialect* of RIF, the Production Rules Interchange Format (RIF-PRD), can be used for allowing easy interchange between different production rule languages; see http://www.w3.org/2005/rules/wiki/PRD [33].

In spite of the positive contribution supplied by OWL 1 and its successor OWL 2, for example, for describing context through a semantic representation and incorporating tools for querying and reasoning to simplify context management and interpretation, OWL suffers from three conceptual and practical issues that can be summarized as follows.

The first issue concerns the sort of knowledge representation proper to OWL. OWL is, in fact, a *binary* language, which means that properties in OWL are strictly limited to expressing a binary relationship linking two individuals or an individual and a value. This is a real issue when we have to deal with situations requiring the description of relatively complex events, like those that can involve complex manageable things, in order to take into account the context of these events and to efficiently manage any sort of *dynamic* and *real-time* information; see Refs. [33] and [34].

The second issue concerns the lack of support of CWA reasoning. In fact, both OWL 1 and OWL 2 follow an *open-world assumption (OWA)* paradigm, while in systems management, we need to follow the *CWA* like in active databases [29,35,36]. OWA does not make any hypothesis about the truth or falsity of a fact unless it can be proven. Thus, if truth or falsity of some fact is unknown, nothing can be inferred about it, and both scenarios must be considered [26,27,37]. This apparent flexibility implies logical inconsistencies that are conflicting with management system requirements. For example, we cannot assume in OWL the uniqueness of concept names, i.e., two different instances can refer to the same object. On the contrary, a semantic reasoning system based on the CWA like the system we have proposed in the SEMbySEM project assumes that every fact that cannot be proved as true is implicitly assumed to be false. This requires that the existing facts are assumed to be complete or that common-sense conclusions can be drawn from existing evidence under incomplete information [38]. The CWA renders inference nonmonotonic: The presence of new evidence can invalidate previously drawn conclusions, while the name of the concepts must be unique to avoid any possible contradiction. Chen et al. [39] proposed a reasoning approach for context awareness for AmI spaces based on the combination of F-logic rules [40] with Standard Ontology for Ubiquitous and Pervasive Applications (SOUPA) ontology [39]. F-logic is a rule-based language that integrates the concepts of deductive databases with object-oriented programming such as classes, objects, and types.

The third issue concerns the fact that OWL relies on a limited reasoning paradigm, i.e., *inference by inheritance*. This means that all the OWL-based so-called reasoners like KAON, Pellet, Racer, Fact++, or Hoolet are, in practice, more useful in solving the most common classification (*subsumption*) problems than in executing real reasoning operations where new knowledge must be produced from existing [25,39,41]. In addition, the lack of *native* support for variables in OWL makes the building up of *real* ontology inference engines practically impossible within the strict limits of this language. To deal with this situation, OWL-compatible rule languages like RuleML, TRIPLE, and Semantic Web Rule Language (SWRL)—all based, roughly, on extensions of the inferential properties of Horn clauses and Datalog to deal with OWL-like data structures—have been proposed. Nevertheless, they appear to be, at least for the time being, quite limited with respect to the range of their possible applications and particularly complicated to use in practice. Let us consider, for example, SWRL, which, until recently, was considered a sort of *standard* in the W3C rule domain [42].

This rule language *augments* OWL by allowing a user to create *if/then* rules written in terms of OWL classes, properties, and individuals. By using OWA, SWRL does not support *negation by failure* (NAF), as well as classical negation, disjunctions, and nonmonotonicity; being based on a combination of OWL Lite and OWL DL sublanguages, it cannot support OWL Full and RDF/RDFS. Moreover, being more *expressive* than OWL DL, SWRL is not *decidable*; more precisely, it is *semidecidable*. As a consequence, SWRL rules are often written in a decidable subset of SWRL called *DL-Safe SWRL*. One of the consequences of this restriction is that DL-Safe SWRL variables can only be bound to known individuals in an OWL ontology. This is too restrictive for many applications where variables must also be bound (i.e., when a specific instance is unknown) to the general concept *subsuming* this instance. The *normal* strategy for executing the SWRL rules is then to make use of *external* rule engines like Jess, a reimplementation in Java of CLIPS, an *old* Rete-based and LISP-oriented rule engine. Building context-aware ambient intelligent environment by using semantic web rules (see Ref. [42]) leads, in several cases, to complex rule bases that are closely related to the requirements of specific application fields and are therefore difficult to maintain, evolve, and reuse.

CWA-Based Semantic Model

The semantic model proposed in SEMbySEM project provides representation capabilities to describe semantically manageable objects' structure and context (status, behaviors) according to the CWA [43,44]. This model also provides the capability to ground the reasoning in any possible production rules engine existing in the market without losing the semantic properties of the reasoning.

The semantic model refers to the μ-concepts that compose the AAL ontology, their relationships, the consistency rules, etc. The resulting μ-ontology (1) describes ubiquitous sensors and actuators disseminated in the AAL environment; (2) defines their characteristics, e.g., by declaring the control operation allowed on them and the way they can be used for reasoning purposes; and (3) defines groups of objects sharing common characteristics concerning, e.g., information they can provide, actions that can be applied on them, etc.

μ-Concept Language

The μ-concept language consists of the following conceptual components: concept, property, instance, and action [45]. A coherent knowledge base (KB) using the μ-concept model can be represented in Equation 22.1 as a n-uplet:

$$\sum_{\mu CM} = \langle C, P, I^P, A^I \rangle \tag{22.1}$$

where C is a μ-concept and P is the set of its properties $I^P : P \cap C = \{\}$.

The main similarity of μ-concept with OWL and RDF lies in the way of defining relations that are represented independently from the concepts and may then symbolize a relation with any kind of μ-concept. On the other hand, multilingual support makes μ-concept ontologies readable in several languages. For instance, a set of attributes is given to define a label and a description in a particular language for each element of the model. Listing 1 shows an example of the μ-concept *Room* and its multilingual names defined in the μ-concept native representation.

```
<smc:Concept smc:ID = "LighSpot">
<smc:Label xml:lang = "en">LightSpot</smc:Label>
  <smc:Label xml:lang = "fr">Lumière</smc:Label>
  <smc:Description xml:lang = "en">The semantic description of
    lightspot device</smc:Description>
</smc:Concept>
```

LISTING 1
The μ-concept *Room* in SEMbySEM format.

Listings 2a and 2b show the concept *Room* and its properties declared respectively in RDF and the μ-concept native representation.

```
<smc:Concept rdf:ID = "Room">
<rdfs:subClassOf rdf:resource = "#Location">
<smc:restriction>
  <smc:PropertyRestriction>
  <smc:onProperty rdf:resource = "#Temperature"/>
  <smc:default rdf:datatype = "&xsd;integer">17
    </smc:default>
  </smc:PropertyRestriction>
</smc:restriction>
    </smc:Concept>
```

LISTING 2a
The μ-concept *Room* with property in RDF format.

```
<smc:Concept smc:ID = "Room">
  <smc:Inherits smc:Reference = "Location"/>
</smc:Concept>
<smc:Property smc:ID = "Temperature">
<smc:Default smc:LiteralType = "Integer">17</smc:Default>
</smc:Property>
```

LISTING 2b
Room μ-concept with property in SEMbySEM format.

An instance *I*, associated to a concrete MO, is described using a single concept; *I* can have any number of P values of the same property. Two different instances cannot refer to the same object (the name of the instance must be unique to avoid any possible contradiction). The property value of a concept instance can be declared in the μ-concept native representation as a literal inside the instance declaration, and it can be declared as a constant; see Listings 3a and 3b.

```
<smc:Instance smc:ID = "BedRoom1" smc:Concept = "Room">
  <smc:Description xml:lang = "en">Alice Bedroom</smc:Description>
  <smc:PropertyValue smc:Property = "PersonPresent" smc:LiteralType =
   "String">Alice</smc:PropertyValue>
</smc:Instance>
```

LISTING 3a
μ-concept instance in RDF format.

```
<smc:Instance smc:ID = "BedRoom1" smc:Concept = "Room">
  <smc:Description xml:lang = "en">Alice Bedroom
    </smc:Description>
  <smc:PropertyValue smc:Property = "PersonPresent"
    smc:Constant = "true" smc:LiteralType = "String">Alice
  </smc:PropertyValue>
</smc:Instance>
```

LISTING 3b
μ-concept instance in SEMbySEM format.

The main differences with OWL concern the fact that every μ-concept is used to describe the aim of MOs and can then define *actions* that each instance (or concrete MO) depending on this μ-concept will be able to execute [33,43]. For instance, in Equation 22.1, A^I is a concept that represents the actions that I, as an instance of μC, can carry out. The A^I semantic description differs from a μ-concept only in the way that inverse-functional and inverse properties must not be used to describe an action concept.

The action concept description may also include restrictions on properties that are separated in two parts: The first one concerns properties specifying the restrictions when the action is launched (input restrictions), while the second one is related to the restrictions when the action is complete (output and effect restrictions). These restrictions behave exactly like property restrictions declared in μ-concept, overriding the default property behavior on its domain; see Listing 4.

```
<smc:Action rdf:ID = "switchOff">
  <smc:actionDomain rdf:resource = "#LighSpot"/>
  <rdfs:Label xml:lang = "fr">Eteindre</rdfs:Label>
  <rdfs:Label xml:lang = "en">SwitchOff</rdfs:Label>
  <smc:Property rdf:ID = "InRoom" smc:Input = "true">
    <MinCardinality>1</MinCardinality>
  </smc:Property>
  <smc:Property rdf:ID = "ReasonMessage">
    </rdfs:domain rdf:resource = "#switchOff">
    </rdfs:range rdf:dataType = "&xsd;string">
  </smc:Property>
</smc:Action>
```

LISTING 4
Action description in μ-concept ontology language.

In addition, the action concept is characterized by a set of special properties: *Agent, Object, Source, Beneficiary, Modality, Topic, and Context*; possible extensions concern more general properties like *Cause, Goal, Coordination, Alternative*, etc. [33,46]. All these properties are optional, with the exception of *ActionAgent*, whose presence is mandatory in the definition of each of the actions associated with the model and in the description of the corresponding instances. The possibility of defining this sort of action implies that the μ-concept model can be considered free from any constraints of the *binary* method of OWL or description logics to describe relations among μ-concepts. We can consider that the μ-concept is closer to conceptual models in the entity/relationship style [33].

SEMbySEM Business Rule Language

The SEMbySEM *business* rule language allows users to set up monitoring rules following the standard *if/then* production rule format (if *condition* then *consequence*) [26]. The *condition* pattern is characterized by a set of μ-concepts or variables that can be bound to a μ-concept with the possibility to put a single constraint or a set of constraints. The μ-concept format is characterized by the syntax of Equation 22.2:

$$C\left(\sum_{0}^{n} S\right) <=>$$

$$\sum_{\mu CM} = \langle C, P, I^P, A^I \rangle \tag{22.2}$$

In Equation 22.2, C can be a *concept* in the current ontology and corresponds then to a *class* in the standard W3C languages, or to a *variable* that can be bound to a class. An instance referenced by a variable will then have a class type. S may represent either a single constraint or a set of constraints to satisfy in order to match variables and concept instances. A rule expressed without restrictions allows us to match every instance of a given concept. All the types of variables declared in Equation 22.2 will be automatically deduced from the corresponding matched elements. Note that the results of the evaluation of Equation 22.2 may be linked to a variable V, which can be accessed directly within the current rule when included in the action part. Thus, we can rewrite Equation 22.2 as follows:

$$V := C\left(\sum_{0}^{n} S\right) \tag{22.3}$$

The *action* pattern (*consequent*) represents operations to perform on instances when a rule is triggered. These operations, O, are the standard ones: create or remove instances in/from the knowledge base, update property values or global variables, etc. The most important among them corresponds to a *do* action on an instance J. All these operations follow the schema represented by Equation 22.4.

$$O\left(\sum_{I}^{n} J\right) \tag{22.4}$$

Multivalued (multicardinality) properties can be associated with actions and can then be considered as another way of getting rid of the *binary* limitations associated with W3C languages. Note also, in this context, the introduction of the key word *one*—to be used with multivalued properties only—in order to select one value from all those corresponding to multi-instance matching.

Apart from the possibility of defining and executing complex actions on the MOs, other features of the μ-concept rule language that are missing in the W3C languages concern the possibility of defining inequality constraints on the properties, and properties calculated as a combination of other ones. For instance, the following rule, in Listing 5, allows the triggering of an event each time a person enters an area covered by a radio-frequency identification (RFID) reader.

```
import ontology "./AmI.smc";
rule "Rule1"
conditions
    ?w := Person(?tPos := locatedAt,
               ?curLM := one (hasRFIDTag)) ;    Predicates
    ?lm := RFIDTag(?lPos := locatedAt,
                    isnot(?curLM) ) ;
    ?tPos( ?x1 := position) ;

actions
    Geofencing_Notification ?notif :=
        createInstance(Geofencing_Notification);
    ?notif->locatedAt:= ?lm;                    Actions
end
```

LISTING 5
SEMbySEM business rule example.

Due to space limitations, we do not introduce here the complete μ-concept rule language grammar; see a fragment of this grammar in Table 22.1 for more details. Equation 22.5 illustrates the syntax of variables where the name of a variable is then composed of alphanumerical characters or underscores, starting with a "?". The first character after the "?" must be a letter or an underscore.

$$<\text{Variable Name}> :: = \text{'?'}[a\text{-}zA\text{-}Z\_][a\text{-}zA\text{-}Z0\text{-}9\_\$]* \tag{22.5}$$

TABLE 22.1

Part of the μ-Concept Rule Language Grammar

```
RULES → e | RULE RULES
RULE → rule " Name " BODY RULES
BODY → ATTRIBUTES BODY | when LHS then RHS end
LHS → VAR Concept (EXPRESSIONS) FROM
FROM → e | from Variable | LHS
VAR → e | $Variable :
ATTRIBUTES → e | ATTRIBUTE Value ; ATTRIBUTES
ATTRIBUTE → no-loop | salience | ...
EXPRESSIONS → e | CONSTRAINT EXPRESSION
EXPRESSION → e | , EXPRESSIONS
CONSTRAINT → VAR Property RESTRICTION | eval
                                    (EXPRESSION_BOOLEAN)
RESTRICTION → e | OPERATOR Value1
OPERATOR  → < | > | <= | >= | == | != | contain | not contain |
Value → Value | Variable
Value → real | date | string | boolean
Variable → Identifier
Name → string
```

SEMbySEM Framework Architecture

Monitoring of AAL environments using the SEMbySEM framework can be designed according to a layered and loosely coupled architectural model that allows a clear separation between the management and visualization of monitoring views and the reasoning process based on the real-world model and MOs. The SEMbySEM architecture, illustrated in Figure 22.2, is structured in three main layers: (1) the visualization layer that presents personalized views of the monitoring information to the end user, (2) the reasoning core layer that handles monitoring operations and reasoning, and (3) the façade layer for interaction with the real-world MOs [33,47]. The communication module is a transversal technical layer that enables some types of asynchronous communications between the layers.

Visualization Layer

This layer allows the generation of customized views representing specific information about MOs. Users and stakeholders interact with MOs through the views by sending queries, actions, or visualizing information corresponding to μ-concept instances updated in real time [47]. It exchanges semantic data with the core layer by forwarding μ-concept actions and receiving notifications coming from the MOs. The action queries that are handled respectively by the visualization and the core can be ordered directly by the end user or preregistered queries in the working memory of the reasoning module, during run-time.

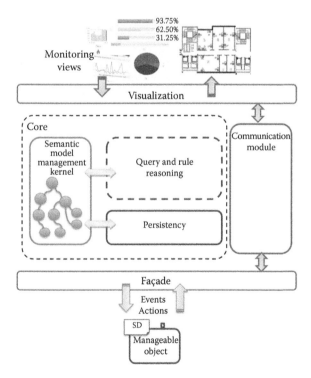

FIGURE 22.2
SEMbySEM framework architecture. SD, semantic description.

The visualization layer is designed to generate web-based views [47,48]. It includes two main modules: the *Visu-Core Communication* module and the visualization engine. The *Visu-Core Communication* layer allows message-based bidirectional communication with the core layer using two main functionalities: management of μ-concept instances and properties, and sending actions corresponding to the μ-concept instance description given in the monitoring view. The management of μ-concept instances includes the update, deletion, and storing of the μ-concept instance data currently used by end users. This visualization engine module allows the generation and delivery of the view graphical interface to an end user's web browser according to a predefined graphical user interface (GUI) model of the view. This engine updates the view content by dynamically pulling or pushing data or widgets to the GUI web browser.

SEMbySEM Reasoning Core Layer

The core layer architecture consists of specific modules that encapsulate the semantic model management, the monitoring and reasoning operations, the persistency of context knowledge, and the communication aspects (see Figure 22.3).

The main modules of the core are described as follows.

Kernel Module

This module provides a set of technical functionalities that are necessary to manage the content of the knowledge base, its consistency regarding the μ-concept ontology, and the reasoning operations that are handled by the rules and query modules. These functionalities are grouped into the following submodules:

- *Semantic model*: This module checks the setup of μ-concept instances and constraints, updates the model according to the messages it receives, and sends notifications to the visualization layer each time the semantic model is updated. This includes the following operations: (1) read the semantic model definition (ontologies, μ-concepts, properties, actions, etc.); (2) read the μ-concept instances and their property values; (3) modify μ-concept instance property values; (4) create or delete μ-concept instances; and (5) register the modifications on the semantic model.

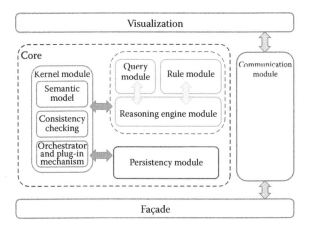

FIGURE 22.3
The core layer internal architecture.

- *Consistency checking*: This module checks for the consistency of the semantic representation according to a set of predefined constraints (defined in the semantic model). The checking is done for each modification of the model to ensure that the model's instance values are always consistent regarding their corresponding μ-concepts and properties definitions.
- *Orchestrator*: This module acts as a scheduler for processing the core's modules. This scheduling is specified by system designers at design time. The order of execution is optimized in such a way that only the modules executing read operations on the semantic model are handled simultaneously while the modules that modify the semantic model have to be executed in an exclusive way.
- *Plug-in support and kernel messaging service*: The core also provides an interface for plug-in support to publish some specific synchronous services to other modules, get some specific services from other modules, and read/process their messages according to the registered semantic model modifications or from other services' events. It also allows the sending of services' events. The kernel messaging service allows the core plug-in modules to send and receive synchronous messages to/from each other. Each plug-in module has a message queue. The queue processing method automatically calls the right callback of a module, depending on message type. However, because modules treat their messages according to their own internal logic, the messaging service can be viewed also as asynchronous and thread safe. Sometimes, callback methods may block messages in case of concurrent access but only for the time to post a set of messages. The plug-in modules that are external to the core cannot directly access the internal messaging service method and may use instead the asynchronous communication module service, also used by the façade.

Query, Rule, and Reasoning Modules

The rule module is responsible for loading and wrapping the registered SEMbySEM rules into a target format accepted by the reasoning engine, such as Drools [49]. The query module handles the queries coming from the visualization layer, making use of the rule wrapping process implemented in the reasoning engine module. The latter interoperates with any possible sort of Rete-based production rule systems. It corresponds to the core reasoning logic used within the whole SEMbySEM framework. It has also its own working memory that is populated with μ-concept Java objects of the MOs' description ontology and their corresponding semantic rules and queries. The reasoning engine module is driven by the orchestrator and does not need to work synchronously each time a modification is performed in the semantic model. This implies that the reasoning engine must notify the kernel only when the reasoning starts or stops. The rule engine must also notify the kernel wherever there are any changes in the working memory; it will react by firing the rules and updating the semantic model if some modules ask to alter this model. It handles, on one side, the static input data composed of μ-concept definitions and management rules that are loaded at core start-up. On the side, it handles the dynamic input data composed of modified μ-concept instances provided by MOs through the façade layer. Moreover, it provides dynamic output data corresponding to new context inferences and action triggering. These output data are handled by the kernel as an update operation of the semantic model; see Figure 22.4.

Jess and Drools are the most widely used open-source reasoning engines based on the Rete algorithm. We have chosen to integrate the first release of the SEMbySEM framework

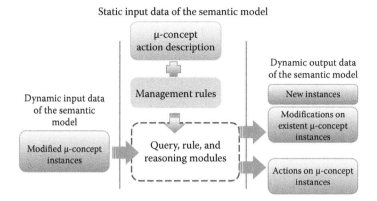

FIGURE 22.4
Reasoning process.

software using the Drools engine execution environment. This choice is motivated by the fact that Drools is an enhanced and optimized implementation of the Rete algorithm for object-oriented Java systems. Compared to Jess, Drools is a procedural language that provides some additional possibilities for the management of functions. Unlike semantic web, writing rules in Drools format is very close to production rules, at the difference of tools such as Jena 2 or Bossam. Despite having integrated forward-chaining mechanisms based the Rete algorithm, Jena and Bossam are fundamentally semantic web oriented and suitable for OWA reasoning. Moreover, they suffer from the same type of limitation already evoked with respect to SWRL in the section "Production Rules"—e.g., restrictions on the use of RDFS, OWL, etc.

The persistency module allows for restoring of the semantic model and rule engine working memory in case of a breakdown.

Façade Layer

This layer, also called the *real-world communication façade*, provides an abstraction of the real world and therefore hides the heterogeneity and complexity of the data formats and the communication technologies used by the MOs. The most basic functional requirement of the façade is to recognize and handle the protocols needed to allow the communication between MOs in a given place with a monitoring system core. An MO is an abstraction computed from a number of atomic objects. In the case where the MO is directly associated with a single atomic object, the façade must compute the MO attributes from the values returned by the façade and must translate the methods called on the MO into actions that must be executed by the associated atomic object. In the other cases, an MO must be built from a number of atomic objects. An MO, for example, may be represented in the façade as a composite object, hierarchical or not, whose leaves are atomic objects.

For better manageability of AmI environments, the core and the façade should be fully distributed and not necessarily deployed in the same network area. For instance, a typical monitoring system of an AmI environment can be composed of one core and multiple façades. The core is not aware of the network location of the deployed façades. The MOs are registered to one single façade and must have unique identifiers, in order to be recognized independently from the devices on which they are mapped. They can be deployed on different façades and can move between façades and reconfigure dynamically. Communication protocols that can be used in the interaction with the MOs range from raw protocols on serial or peer-to-peer (P2P) connections to standard protocols such as SNMP, HTTP, Simple Object Access protocol (SOAP), representational state transfer (REST), universal plug and play (UPnP), Java remote method invocation (Java RMI), devices profile for web services (DPWS), etc. In this context, it is too difficult to build a generic architecture that provides homogeneous access functionalities that support these protocols and data encoding of any manufacturer device.

SEMbySEM provides two integration models of the façade. In the first one, the façade is composed of atomic MOs, where each MO is mapped to one single device that uses a single communication protocol for events or actions. In the second model, the façade allows the creation of the abstraction of a monitoring subsystem using the Service Abstract Machine (SAM) middleware [47,50,51]. The latter provides a homogeneous representation for high-level object management. It provides features for composite entities, dynamic façade discovery, and distributed MOs. The SAM physical layer is made of service frameworks that manage services and/or devices that communicate using a number of protocols. The current version of the SAM middleware offers an abstraction of Open Service Gateway initiative (OSGi), UPnP, DPWS, SNMP, and SOAP web services. Using the SAM middleware, the monitoring subsystem is considered a complex MO that provides high-level events corresponding to atomic μ-concepts. In this context, the processing is hidden for the core and done inside the MO. Note that it is possible to instantiate several façades according to the two models that can coexist in the same AmI monitoring system.

The façade architecture, depicted in Figure 22.4, proposes three bootstrap modes for the integration of MOs. In the first one, an MO can be any software component, including legacy systems that implement one of the communication protocols supported by façade communication layer to communicate captured context data in raw format. In this mode, the façade executes all the transformations from the raw data format into the μ-concept format and provides also the attribute information requested to identify the corresponding μ-concept definitions and properties. This bootstrap is useful when a sensor network with poor computing capabilities is used. The main limitation concerns the update of the façade every time a new data format is needed to handle the changes in MOs. In the second bootstrap mode, the MOs communicate with the façade using the standard façade message. In this case, the façade executes only the transformation of the message attribute values into μ-concept instance values that should be managed by the core. In the third bootstrap mode, the façade and the MO communicate using a μ-concept–compliant message format. The façade acts therefore only as a message router between MOs and the core. This bootstrap is supported in the current version of the SEMbySEM framework using the SAM middleware. However, supporting a new device technology in the third bootstrap requires a lot of development effort compared to the first and second bootstraps.

The detailed architecture corresponding to the three bootstraps, depicted in Figure 22.5, is composed of the following modules:

- *MO Service Registry*: This administration module is a directory that stores an MO's relevant information, such as its associated μ-concepts and communication details, either on the event or the action side when actions are supported.

- *Façade End Points*: Event Source and Action Destination modules are used as end points of the façade to communicate with the MOs using the corresponding protocols such as SOAP, HTTP, SNMP, etc. The Event Source end point handles event reception for an identified source of information and feeds the Event Controller with event content according to one of the integration modes of MOs within the façade (legacy, façade message [to be standardized], or even μ-concept message). A

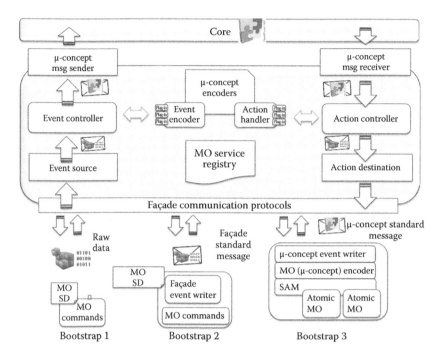

FIGURE 22.5
The façade architecture. SD, semantic description.

filter can be used to control the messages handled by the Event Source. The Action Destination end point allows the sending of action requests to an identified MO. The communication protocol and end point data mapping should be set up during the design stage according to the supported protocol stack of the façade and message encoders, respectively.

- *Event and Action Controllers*: There are two modules that handle, respectively, action and event message transformation operations. The Event Controller module handles the transformation of façade message content into a μ-concept message. It can also handle the registration of MOs (their associated service description) in the MO Service Registry. The Action Controller handles μ-concept messages containing μ-concept action, converts them into the right (expected) format of the identified Action Destination via the Action Handler, and sends them to the identified Action Destination.

- *μ-concept message Senders/Receivers*: These two modules allow independent management of μ-concept message exchange with the core. In the case of an incoming action message from the core, this message is provided to the Action Controller that will handle its transformation. On the other hand, the Event Controller module is invoked to route the transformed μ-concept message to the core layer.

- *MO encoders*: These are plug-ins that are used to manage, on the one hand, action messages that should be handled by the MOs and, on the other hand, context event data that are sent by the MOs. Two types of encoders are considered: the Action Encoder, also called Action Handler, converts a μ-concept message into the expected format of an identified Action Destination of an MO, while the MO Event Encoder transforms context events data into μ-concept messages.

Façade Message Standard

The façade message standard (FMS) is used as an open message-formatting tool for all contents that can be exchanged between the façade and MOs [47,48]. It does not address any specific application or telecommunication method. Based on an XML schema (see Listing 6), FMS can be used within the most well-known application communication protocols such as SOAP, SNMP, or HTTP. This ensures the interoperability of the façade with all kinds of MOs, even complex or atomic ones. In addition, FMS has a simple and portable structure that can be handled by any type of computing device that supports a basic XML processing stack and does not imply either an important footprint or an overhead of monitoring data processing. This way of encoding remains sufficiently abstract to be adaptable to other coding schemes. In addition, the FMS allows multiuse encoding, where one message schema can support multiple message types, such as getting information, update, order action, cancellation, acknowledgement, and error messages.

```
<?xml version = "1.0" encoding = "UTF-8"?>
...
<element name = "identifier" type = "string"/>
<element name = "sender" type = "string"/>
<element name = "sent" type = "dateTime"/>
<element name = "msgType">
...
  <simpleType>
  <restriction base = "string">
  <enumeration value = "Action"/>
  <enumeration value = "Info"/>
  <enumeration value = "Ack"/>
  <element name = "address">
   ...
  <complexType>
  <sequence>
  <element name = "url" type = "anyURI" maxOccurs = "1" minOccurs = "1"/>
  <element name = "protocol" type = "string" maxOccurs = "1"
    minOccurs = "0"/>
  </sequence>
  </complexType>
...
</element>
...
```

LISTING 6
A partial presentation of the XML schema used to create a μ-concept message.

The standard façade message of the SEMbySEM framework consists of the following mandatory segments:

- *Message*: The *message* segment provides basic information about the current message. It includes the following information: message purpose, message source, as well as a unique identifier for the current message and links to other related messages. The message segment may be used alone for message acknowledgements, cancellations, or other system functions. Most message segments include at least one content segment.

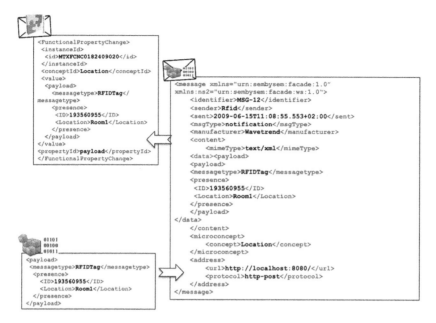

FIGURE 22.6
Context event encoding using the façade standard message.

- *Content*: The *content* segment not only hosts the exchanged data but also provides additional information related to the data type.
- *μ-concepts*: The *μ-concept* segment provides additional information about the semantic concept associated with the message sender.
- *Address*: The *address* segment provides additional information related to the way to communicate with the message sender.

To understand how the façade works, let us consider the simple case of tracking a person's position at home using RFID. According to the first bootstrap mode, an MO is implemented to send an event to the façade if an RFID tag is detected in the reader's coverage area. The event is represented (see Figure 22.6), using two XML tags; the ID XML tag corresponds to the detected RFID tag's unique sequential number, and the location XML tag corresponds to the place where the reader is installed. The context event message is transformed by the façade layer into a μ-concept message and then forwarded to the core layer. The latter updates the semantic model with an instance of the new position.

Elderly Safety Monitoring Scenario

This scenario aims at building a health monitoring system for improving the safety of elderly persons living alone in their own homes even when their conditions worsen and the home cannot support their safety. The main requirement of our monitoring system is its capability to detect any injury that can be caused by an abnormal situation: falls, cardiovascular attacks, respiratory crisis, gas propagation, fire, nonauthorized intrusion into the home, etc. In addition, the system should be able to reason on the given emergency and the events appropriate to its related context to avoid triggering a wrong alarm if there is no emergency situation. The reaction to an emergency from a monitoring perspective consists of providing a system endowed with monitoring rules that allow the triggering of some actions, such as closing the gas jet valves, switching on lights, sending alert messages, etc.

The scenario begins with an elderly person, Mary, who was hospitalized 1 week ago due to pacemaker failure. She had been allowed to return home; a monitoring system has been installed in her house and connected to the hospital in order to allow her physician to be aware day by day about her vital signals and follow the effect of the ordered therapy program. As Mary is living alone, the monitoring system allows a continuous remote surveillance of her activity to ensure her safety. In the following, we make use of the following storyboard to describe a typical emergency situation.

Emergency Situation Monitoring

After leaving her bedroom, Mary goes to Kitchen to prepare her meal. At t0, she turns on the cooker to prepare her meal. Then, she returns to the bedroom and switches on the TV. Ten minutes later, she feels unwell and decides to have a short sleeping period, but she forgets to switch off the stove. The consequence is that all the temperature sensors, located in the kitchen and near the cooker, give notification that the temperature values are higher than the normal range. In this case, the monitoring system should automatically switch off all the kitchen devices and notify Mary through one of the speakers nearest to her. Let us assume now that the RFID location system detects the presence of Mary in the bedroom, but the camera, sound, and motion sensors installed in the ceiling of the bedroom do not detect any activity of the elderly. Moreover, the vital sensors indicate that her blood pressure is out of the normal range. Considering that all these events occur in the same period, the monitoring system will conclude that Mary's vital status is abnormal and will trigger an emergency alert.

Scenario Requirements

The following general requirements are taken into account when designing the monitoring rules and MOs to meet the scenario storyboard described:

- The RFID MO must send Mary a presence notification to the core each time the RFID active reader detects Mary's RFID tag.
- The motion-detection MO must listen 180 s before sending a notification to the core that no movement has been detected.
- The sound-detection MO must listen 60 s before sending a notification to the core that no sound has been detected.
- If the stove is on for a period higher than 10 min, its corresponding MO must notify the core that the stove is still on and must turn off the stove for safety.
- The vital-signals MO must send a notification of abnormal vital status to the core each time the blood pressure value exceeds the systolic threshold of 180 mm Hg or the diastolic threshold of 110 mm Hg.
- The core layer must send a turnoff action message to all the MOs if the stove is on for a period that exceeds 10 min and if the kitchen temperature is higher than 42°C and Mary is not present in the kitchen.

- The core should check for the presence of Mary in the bedroom before triggering any action in this area.
- If an emergency situation is inferred, the core layer must trigger an action corresponding to an emergency alert message. The messaging MO sends this message to the hospital and acknowledgment requests to Mary's relatives.

Semantic Model

The ontology-based semantic model of our scenario is depicted in Figure 22.7. It is composed of μ-concepts describing the ambient environment context and a set of rules that instantiate new context events and actions to react in response to specific context events. This model has been built up using the rule editor and ontology editor developed within the consortium SEMbySEM [33].

The μ-concepts that are taken into account for the emergency case are presented in the following using uppercase letters.

- PERSON: This μ-concept is a superconcept that describes Mary's identity and context. It has two properties, hasID and hasPersonalContext specifying, respectively, the RFID tag serial number used to identify the person in the AAL space and the details of the context of the inferred situation.
- SITUATION: This μ-concept is a superconcept that describes any situation in the ambient environment. The subconcept EMERGENCY describes an emergency situation that can occur for a person.
- PERSONAL_CONTEXT: This μ-concept is a superconcept that describes context information attributes such as vital signals provided by the MO using physical sensors. It has a single functional property that is used to log the time stamps of context captures. The Boolean properties isSleeping and fixedOnSite are used in conjunction with a third property, locatedAt, as fact-events within the monitoring rules to infer the personal context. The property locatedAt describes precisely the location in which a person with a specific ID is located. The range values of the locatAt property are all the instance of the μ-concept LOCATION or its subconcepts BED and ROOM.

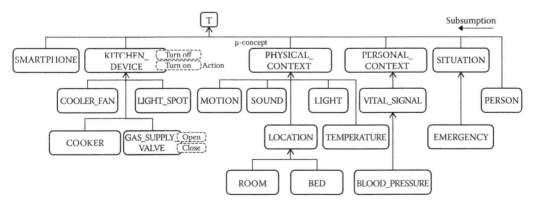

FIGURE 22.7
Partial schema of the scenario μ-concept ontology.

- VITAL_SIGNAL: This is a subconcept of PERSONAL_CONTEXT that describes the vital signal status. The AbNormalVitalSignal property, a Boolean data type, corresponds to an event triggered by a manageable objet if some abnormal values of vital signals are detected. BLOOD_PRESSURE is a subconcept of VITAL_SIGNAL.
- PHYSICAL_CONTEXT: This μ-concept is a superconcept that describes any context information provided by an MO corresponding to a physical sensor in the environment. It has a single functional property used to log the time stamps of context captures.
- LOCATION is a subconcept of PHYSICAL_CONTEXT that describes any location in the home. It consists of two subconcepts: ROOM and BED.
- LIGHT: This is a subconcept of PHYSICAL_CONTEXT that describes the ambient light status. It consists of two properties: LightOnDetected and LightOffDetected. The Boolean property LightOnDetected corresponds to an event triggered when the light is switched, on while the Boolean property LightOffDetected corresponds to an event that is triggered when the light is switched off.
- MOTION: This is a subconcept of PHYSICAL_CONTEXT that describes a motion detected by a motion sensor. It has a single property, MotionDetected, with Boolean range.
- SOUND: This is a subconcept of PHYSICAL_CONTEXT. It has a single property, soundDetected, that corresponds to an event flag indicating that an ambient sound is detected.
- KITCHEN_DEVICE: This superconcept describes all the MOs allowing execution of an action in the kitchen. The main subconcepts that are considered in the scenario are COOLER_FAN, COOKER, LIGHT_SPOT, and GAS_SUPPLY_VALVE.

The main actions considered in this scenario are the following:

- TurnOn and TurnOff: These two actions are executed on the instances of the μ-concept KITCHN_DEVICE or its subconcepts. The instances correspond to the physical device present in the kitchen.
- Open and Close: These two actions are executed on the instances of the μ-concept GAS_SUPPLY_VALVE.
- Send: This action is executed on the instances of the μ-concept MESSAGE. In the scenario, the façade translates this action into a *send message* command that is executed using an MO corresponding to an e-mail or short message service (SMS).

Monitoring Rules

In this section, we describe some monitoring rules written in the SEMbySEM rule language. As previously mentioned, the inference of an emergency situation needs several contexts; for instance, Mary is sleeping in the bedroom, no sound is detected, and her vital signals are out of range. Rule #2 depicted in Listing 7 allows inference of the context *Mary is sleeping.* The condition part of this rule requires the evaluation of the properties FixedOnSite and SoundDetected using rule #1. This rule allows the inference that no sound is detected and that Mary, who is located in the bedroom, is fixed on site. The condition part of rule #1 refers to the μ-concepts position, person, and sound, while the consequence includes a special predicate to update the semantic model with new instances.

```
import ontology "./Aml.smc";

Rule "Rule #1"
priority = 2;
declare noMotionDetected
@role (event)

Conditions
    ?v_person:=PERSON (?v_person:=all(hasID)),
            exists (one in ?v_person (hasID=="MaryRFID");
    ?v_context:=exists (PERSONAL_CONTEXT
            (locatedAt (BEDROOM),
            locatedAt (BED));

Actions
    POSTURE posture_event:=createInstance (POSTURE)

    ?posture_event->FixedOnSite(BED));
    ?posture_event->timestamp:=datetime("now");

End
```

```
import ontology "./Aml.smc";

Rule "Rule #2"
priority = 3;
declare noMotionDetected
@role (event)

Conditions
    ?v_person:=PERSON (?v_person:=all(hasID)),
            exists (one in ?v_person (hasID=="MaryRFID");
    ?v_context:=exists (POSTURE (FixedOnSite(BED)),
                SOUND (SoundDetected(false)),
                MOTION (MotionDetected(false),
                timestamp=datetime("now"));

Actions
    Update (SoundDetected:=false);
    Update (MotionDetected:=false);
    Update (timestamp:=datetime("now"));

    PERSONAL_CONTEXT v_person_context_event:=
            createInstance (PERSONAL_CONTEXT);

    ?v_person_context_event->IsSleeping(true);
    ?v_person_context_event->timestamp:=datetime("now");

End
```

LISTING 7
SEMbySEM business rules #1 and #2.

As it is depicted in Listing 8, Rule #3 is responsible for turning off the cooker when Mary is sleeping in the bedroom. Rule #4 detects when Mary is in an emergency situation through the conjunction of four contexts: sleeping, abnormal vital status, no sound detected after the speaker warning, and kitchen temperature is out of range.

```
import ontology "./AmI.smc";

Rule "Rule #3"
priority = 3;
declare noMotionDetected
@role (event)

Conditions
    ?v_person:=PERSON (?v_person:=all(hasID)),
        exists (one in ?v_person (hasID=="MaryRFID");
    ?v_context:=exists (COOKER(isRunning(true)),
        PERSONAL_CONTEXT (IsSleeping(true),
        timestamp==datetime("now");

Actions
    createAction(KITCHEN_DEVICE(?turnOff));
    'KITCHEN_DEVICE/TurnOff' ?turnOffAction:=
    createAction('KITCHEN_DEVICE/TurnOff');
    ?turnOffAction->Reason:='ActionReason/SafetyProcedure';
    execute(?turnOffAction);
End
```

LISTING 8
SEMbySEM business rule #3.

Rule #4, depicted in Listing 9, allows the inference of an emergency situation and triggers actions on MOs to ensure the safety of Mary, for instance, turning off the cooker (turnoff), closing the gas supply valve, switching lights on/off, and sending an alarm message. Note that the μ-concepts EMERGENCY and MESSAGE have similar roles but are managed differently in the semantic model. The μ-concept EMERGENCY is used for the visualization of the situation in the monitoring view, while the action MESSAGE is used to trigger a command for sending a message through the façade.

```
import ontology "./AmI.smc";

Rule "Rule #4"
priority = 1;
declare noMotionDetected
@role (event)

Conditions
        ?v_person:=PERSON (?v_person:=all(hasID)), exists (one in ?v_person
                   (hasID=="MaryRFID");

        ?v_context:=exists (TEMPERATURE(Degree("HIGH")), PERSONAL_CONTEXT
                      (IsSleeping(true), timestamp==datetime("now"), ?v_kitchen_device:=
                      COOKER(isRunning(true)), VITAL_SIGNAL(AbnormalVitalSignal(true),
                      ?v_home_device:=GAS_SUPLLY_VALVE);

Actions
        EMERGENCY v_situation:=createInstance (EMERGENCY);
        ?v_person -> currentSituation (?v_situation);

        'KITCHEN_DEVICE/TurnOff' ?turnOffAction:=createAction(?v_kitchen_device,
                                    'KITCHEN_DEVICE/TurnOff');

        ?turnOffAction->Reason:='ActionReason/SafetyProcedure';
        execute(?turnOffAction);

        'KITCHEN_DEVICE/GAS_SUPPLY/Close' ?closeAction:=createAction(?v_home_device,
                                       'GAS_SUPPLY/Close');
        ?closeAction->Reason:='ActionReason/Emergency';

        execute(?closeAction);

        'MESSAGE/Send' ?sendMessage:=createAction(?v_home_device, 'MESSAGE/Send');
        ?sendMessage->Reason:='ActionReason/EmergencyAlert';

        execute(?sendMessage);
End
```

LISTING 9
SEMbySEM business rule #4.

Façade of the AmI Infrastructure

The AmI infrastructure (see Figure 22.8) consists of the following sensors:

- The MEMSIC Imote2 sensors provide the current climate in a specific place, such as temperature, light, pressure, etc.
- The Wavetrend L-RX400 RFID readers are used to identify and locate physical objects equipped with TG1800 active tags.
- The MEMSIC Cricket infrastructure is a grid of motes that provides the current location of physical objects in an indoor space.

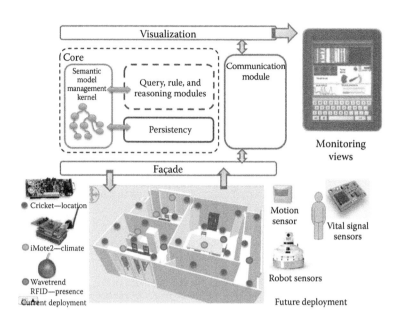

FIGURE 22.8
The architecture of the AmI infrastructure.

For practical issues, sensors providing blood pressure signals are simulated using Java threads. In future deployment, we plan to integrate MOs that interface with motion sensors, the Pekee II mobile robot components, and an SpO_2 sensor based on a Corscience ChipOx connected to an Atmel board.

The pragmatic approach for the implementation of the SEMbySEM façade prototype was the use of a Java service bus. The latter facilitates the registration and communication with the MOs that can be built by a third party or delivered by the manufacturers as out-of-the-box components. For this purpose, the current SEMbySEM façade is implemented using the open-source service bus Apache ServiceMix. The latter allows interoperation with software components in an event-driven way and the seamless discovery, registration, and replacement of MOs disseminated in the network. In addition, it is based on ActiveMQ, a publish-subscribe message-oriented middleware that provides reliable and flexible asynchronous message passing based on the Java Messaging Service (JMS) specification [48]. This middleware provides easy management of both internal and external events corresponding to the communication with the sensors and actuators. Note that external events concern all the events triggered by the MOs, while internal events concern the messages exchanged between the façade modules and the core.

We have taken into account a simplified but realistic integration hypothesis to integrate the MOs of the AmI infrastructure according to the first bootstrap mode; see the subsection "Façade Layer." In this mode, a sensor or an actuator is mapped onto a single MO. This choice is motivated by the fact that we are dealing only with atomic MOs located in a common network area and that the processing of the context data requires only a single instance of the reasoning core.

SEMbySEM at Run-Time

The reasoning core starts by loading the μ-concept ontology in the kernel working memory. This will dynamically generate *Java bean* objects in the working memory of the reasoning engine module that correspond to the AmI ontology instances matching with the μ-concepts description. The main operations on μ-concepts that are performed for monitoring issues concern: (1) the capturing of context events coming from the façade layer and (2) the inference of the corresponding reactive actions to be executed on the MOs, such as switching on the light or turning off the cooker.

When a context event occurs in the real world, the corresponding MO detects this event and encodes it into a façade message according to the second bootstrap. The façade transforms this message into a μ-concept message using the corresponding μ-concept and properties described in the ontology. The message is sent to the core to update the semantic model. When the core communication module receives the message, the orchestrator in the kernel module starts the rule engine to update the working memory with new instances corresponding to the new context event.

In the case where the instances created by the core match with some action-triggering rules, the core creates an instance of the μ-concept *action* for each action predicate in the consequence part of the rule. For instance, in the rules given in Listing 8, the instance of cooker turnoff will be wrapped into a μ-concept message that will be processed by the façade. When the façade receives the message, it encodes it into a façade message (see Listing 10) and sends it to the MO that handles the cooker device.

```
<smc:Action smc:ID = "TurnOff">
    <smc:Domain smc:Reference = "Cooker"/>
    <smc:Property smc:ID = "ReasonMessage" smc:Range = "String"/>
</smc:Action>
```

LISTING 10
Representation of cooker turnoff action in a μ-concept message format.

To update the monitoring view with new context information, the visualization layer sends a μ-concept query to the core. The query module maps this query with one of the Drools queries registered in the working memory. The orchestrator triggers the rule engine to notify the visualization layer of the query execution results. Note that the query registration in the current release of the framework is done at core bootstrap time.

Conclusion

In this chapter, we presented a new semantic framework to build monitoring systems, tailored to the requirements of AAL environments. This framework aims, in fact, at the construction of a common software framework allowing different domain experts to easily manage real-world heterogeneous—physical or abstract—entities, called manageable objects. The proposed framework deals with context awareness and CWA semantic reasoning over heterogeneous ecosystems such as AAL, by preserving, on the one hand, the structural expressiveness provided by ontologies and the compatibility with the WoO vision through compliance with the W3C and OASIS recommendations for knowledge and service sharing over the future Internet and, on the other hand, by exploiting in full all the possible benefits of production rule reasoning. The proposed semantic-based architecture approach provides: (1) standardized and reliable mechanisms for developing dynamic and context-aware monitoring views that can give rise to a high level of semantic representation of the situations occurring in AAL environments, and (2) the possibility of a seamless integration of the real-world MOs' descriptions and of their communication technologies according to a common semantic model. The semantic model is specified using the μ-concept ontology language and is interoperable with RDFS and OWL 2. Through the implementation of an AAL scenario dedicated to safety monitoring of elderly people, we have shown how to exploit the framework to build a semantic model for monitoring the targeted application, i.e., the μ-concepts describing the ambient environment context and the set of rules that instantiate new context events and actions to react in response to specific context events. The ongoing work concerns the exploitation of the proposed framework in scenarios involving composite intelligent objects such as a companion robot.

References

1. G. Van den Broek, F. Cavallo, C. Wehrmann, *AALIANCE Ambient Assisted Living Roadmap*, IOS Press, 2010.
2. E. Zelkha, B. Epstein, From devices to 'ambient intelligence': The transformation of consumer electronics. Presentation at the Digital Living Room Conference, 1998.
3. M. Bielikova, T. Krajcovic, Ambient intelligence within a home environment. *ERCIM News*, No. 47, 2001.
4. P. Wolf, A. Schmidt, M. Klein, SOPRANO: An extensible, open AAL platform for elderly people based on semantic contracts. *Proceedings of the 3rd Workshop on Artificial Intelligence Techniques for Ambient Intelligence (AITAmI '08)*, colocated with the 18th European Conf on Artificial Intelligence (ECAI 08), Patras, Greece, July 21–24, 2008.
5. K. Ducatel, M. Bogdanowicz, F. Scapolo, J. Leijten, J. C. Burgelman, Scenarios for ambient intelligence in 2010. Final Report of the IST Advisory Group (ISTAG), 2001. Available at ftp://ftp.cordis.lu/pub/ist/docs/istagscenarios2010.pdf.
6. S. Helal, W. Mann, H. El-Zabadani, J. King, Y. Kaddoura, E. Jansen, The gator tech smart house: A programmable pervasive space. *Computer Journal*, 38(3), 50–60, 2005.
7. M. Winkler, J. Cardoso, G. Scheithauer, Challenges of business service monitoring in the internet of services. *iiWAS '08: Proceedings of the 10th International Conference on Information Integration and Web-based Applications & Services*, pp. 613–616, 2008.
8. N. Ibrahim, F. Le Mouël, A survey on service composition middleware in pervasive environments. *International Journal of Computer Science Issues, IJCSI*, 1(1–12), 2001.
9. P. Roeder, M. Mosmondor, R. Obermaisser, H. Boos, UniversAAL Project of the 7th Framework Program, D6.1. A Training Plan and Training Material, 2010. Available at http://www.universaal.org/ (accessed June 6, 2010).
10. E. Niemelä, J. Latvakoski, Survey of requirements and solutions for ubiquitous software. *Proceedings of the 3rd International Conference on Mobile and Ubiquitous Multimédia MUM '04*, pp. 71–78, 2004.
11. J. A. Kientz, R. G. Hayes, L. T. Westeyn, T. Starner, G. D. Abowd, Ubiquitous computing and autism: Assisting caregivers of children with special needs. *Ubiquitous Computing, IEEE Publication*, 6(1), 28–35, 2007.

12. J. Schaefer, A middleware for self-organising distributed ambient assisted living applications. *Proceeding of ECEASST 27*, 2010.
13. B. Schilit, N. Adams, R. Want, Context-aware computing applications. *Proceedings of the Workshop on Mobile Computing Systems and Applications*, IEEE Computer Society Press, Los Alamitos, CA, pp. 85–90, 1994.
14. M. Baldauf, S. Dustdar, F. Rosenberg, A survey on context-aware systems. *International Journal of Ad Hoc and Ubiquitous Computing*, 2(4), 263–277, 2004. Inderscience Publishers.
15. C. Bettini, O. Brdiczka, K. Henricksen, J. Indulska, D. Nicklas, A. Ranganathan, D. Riboni, A survey of context modelling and reasoning techniques. *Pervasive and Mobile Computing*, 6(2), 161–180, 2010.
16. S. W. Loke, Representing and reasoning with situations for context-aware pervasive computing: A logic programming perspective. *The Knowledge Engineering Review*, 19, 213–223, 2004.
17. T. Gu, H. Pung, D. Zhang, A service oriented middleware for building context-aware services. *Journal Network Computing Applications*, 28(1), 1–18, 2005.
18. A. K. Dey, Understanding and using context. *Personal and Ubiquitous Computing*, 5(1), 4–7, 2001.
19. J. Coutaz, J. Crowley, S. Dobson, D. Garlan, Context is key. *Communications of the ACM*, 48(3), 49–53, 2005.
20. D. Riboni, C. Bettini, OWL 2 modeling and reasoning with complex human activities. *Journal Pervasive and Mobile Computing*, 7(3), 379–395, 2011. Elsevier Science.
21. X. H. Wang, D. Q. Zhang, T. Gu, H. K. Pung, Ontology based context modeling and reasoning using OWL. *Proceedings of Pervasive Computing and Communications Workshops*, pp. 18–22, 2004.
22. ITEA, SEMbySEM. 2010. Available at https://itea3.org/project/sembysem.html (accessed June 6, 2010).
23. G. P. Zarri, L. Sabri, A. Chibani, Y. Amirat, Semantic-based industrial engineering: Problems and solutions. *Complex, Intelligent and Software Intensive Systems (CISIS), 2010 International Conference*, pp. 1022–1102, 2010.
24. L. Sabri, A. Chibani, J. Beck, G. P. Zarri, Y. Amirat, J. S. Brunner, P. Gatellier, An editor for micro-concept rules design. *Proceedings of the 3rd International RuleML2009 Challenge (CEUR-WS)*, 2009. Available at http://ceur-ws.org/Vol-549/paper8.pdf (accessed November 6, 2009).
25. F. Baader, D. Calvanese, D. McGuinness, D. Nardi, P. Patel-Schneider, *The Description Logic Handbook: Theory, Implementation, and Applications*. Cambridge University Press, New York, 2003.
26. C. V. Damasio, A. Analyti, G. Antoniou, G. Wagner, Supporting open and closed world reasoning on the Web. *Principles and Practice of Semantic Web Reasoning*, 4187(506779), 149, 2006. Springer.
27. I. Horrocks, P. F. Patel-Schneider, H. Boley, S. Tabet, B. Grosof, M. Dean, SWRL: A semantic web rule language combining OWL and RuleML. W3C Member Submission, 2004. Available at http://www.daml.org/2004/11/fol/rules-all (accessed July 10, 2010).
28. C. L. Forgy, RETE: A fast algorithm for the many pattern/many object match problem. *Artificial Intelligence*, 19(1), 17–37, 1982.
29. E. Bertino, B. Catania, G. P. Zarri, *Intelligent Database Systems*. Addison-Wesley and ACM Press, London, 2001.
30. I. Horrocks, P. F. Patel-Schneider, Knowledge representation and reasoning on the Semantic Web: OWL, Chapter 9. In *Handbook of Semantic Web Technologies*, J. Domingue, D. Fensel, and J. A. Hendler, eds., pp. 365–368. Springer Edition, 2010.
31. S. Bechhofer, F. van Harmelen, J. Hendler, I. Horrocks, D. L. McGuinness, P. F. Patel-Schneider, OWL Web Ontology Language Reference—W3C Recommendation, 2004. Available at http://www.w3.org/TR/2004/REC-owl-ref-20040210/ (accessed September 3, 2010).
32. OWL 2 Web Ontology Language, W3C Recommendation, 2012. Available at http://www.w3.org/TR/2012/REC-owl2-overview-20121211/ (accessed September 7, 2012).
33. L. Sabri, A. Chibani, Y. Amirat, G. P. Zarri, Semantic reasoning framework to supervise and manage contexts and objects in pervasive computing environments. *IEEE Workshops of International Conference on Advanced Information Networking and Applications, AINA 2011*, Biopolis, Singapore, pp. 47–52, March 22–25, 2011.

34. J. Beck, L. Sabri, G. P. Zarri, Business rules languages. SEMbySEM Project Deliverable D3.2, 2009. Available at http://ubiquitous-intelligence.eu/contact (accessed June 7, 2011).

35. G. Wagner, A. Giurca, I.-M. Diaconescu, G. Antoniou, A. Analyti, C. V. Damasio, Reasoning on the Web with open and closed predicates. *Proceedings of the 3rd International Workshop on Applications of Logic Programming to the (Semantic) Web and Web Services (ALPSWS2008). CEUR Workshop Proceedings,* 2008.

36. E. Thomas, J. Z. Pan, Y. Ren, E. Thomas, J. Z. Pan, Y. Ren, TrOWL: Tractable OWL 2 reasoning infrastructure. *The Semantic Web: Research and Applications, Lecture Notes in Computer Science,* vol. 6089, pp. 431–435, 2010.

37. Y. Ren, J. Z. Pan, Y. Zhao, Closed world reasoning for OWL2 with NBox*. *Journal of Tsinghua Science and Technology,* 15(6), 692–701, 2010.

38. G. Meditskos, N. Bassiliades, DLE Jena: A practical forward-chaining OWL 2 RL reasoner combining Jena and Pellet. *Journal of Web Semantics, Elsevier,* 8(1), 89–94, 2010.

39. H. Chen, T. Finin, A. Joshi, The SOUPA ontology for pervasive computing. In *Ontologies for Agents: Theory and Experiences, Software Agent Technologies Series.* V. Tamma, S. Cranefield, T. Finin and S. Willmott (Eds), Springer, 2005, pp. 233–256.

40. M. Kifer, G. Lausen, J. Wu, Logical foundations of object-oriented and framebased languages. *Journal of ACM,* 42, 741–843, 1995.

41. J. Tao, E. Sirin, J. Bao, D. L. McGuinness, Integrity constraints in OWL. *Proceedings of the 24th AAAI Conference on Artificial Intelligence (AAAI-10),* Atlanta, GA, July 11–15, 2010.

42. J. S. Brunner, J. Beck, Micro-concept: Model reference. SEMbySEM Project Deliverable D2.3, working draft version 1.4, 2009. Available at http://www.sembysem.org (accessed April 12, 2009).

43. D. Bonino, E. Castellina, F. Corno, DOG: An ontology-powered OSGi domotic gateway. *Proceedings 20th IEEE International Conference on Tools with Artificial Intelligence, ICTAI '08,* vol. 1, pp. 157–160, 2008.

44. M. Knorr, J. J. Alferes, P. Hitzler, Towards tractable local closed world reasoning for the Semantic Web. *Proceedings of the 13th Portuguese Conference on Artificial Intelligence EPI,* Springer, 2007.

45. Y. Ren, J. Z. Pan, Y. Zhao, Closed world reasoning for OWL2 with negation as failure. *Chinese Semantic Web Symposium, CSWS2010,* 2010.

46. G. P. Zarri, Using rules in the Narrative Knowledge Representation Language (NKRL) environment. In *Handbook of Research on Emerging Rule-Based Languages and Technologies: Open Solutions and Approaches-volume 1,* A. Giurca, D. Gasevic, K. Taveter (Eds), IGI Global, 2009, pp. 50–75.

47. J. Estublier, SEMbySEM global architecture. SEMbySEM Project Deliverable D3.1, 2010. Available at http://www.sembysem.org (accessed April 9, 2009).

48. C. E. Laporte, SemBySem technical specifications. SEMbySEM Project Deliverable D3.2, 2010. Available at http://www.sembysem.org (accessed April, 9, 2009).

49. Drools, Business rules engine. Available at http://www.jboss.org/drools/drools-fusion.html (accessed July 12, 2012).

50. J. Estublier, I. Dieng, E. Simon, D. Moreno, Opportunistic computing experience with the SAM platform. *ACM Proceedings of the 2nd International Workshop on Principles of Engineering Service-Oriented Systems (PESOS),* pp. 1–7, 2010.

51. L. Baresi, E. Di Nitto, C. Ghezzi, Towards open-world software: Issues and challenges. *30th Annual IEEE/NASA Software Engineering Workshop SEW-30 (SEW '06),* pp. 249–252, 2006.

23

Collaborative Ecosystem Architecture for Ambient Assisted Living

Luis M. Camarinha-Matos, João Rosas, Ana Inês Oliveira, and Filipa Ferrada

CONTENTS

ABSTRACT A conceptual architecture is introduced to guide the development of a collaborative ecosystem of care services supporting active ageing. A holistic perspective of ambient assisted living (AAL), focusing on the elderly and considering four important life settings, is adopted: (1) independent living, (2) health and care in life, (3) occupation in life, and (4) recreation in life. In order to provide a better understanding and interrelate concepts, a three-layered model is adopted: infrastructure layer, care and assistance service layer, and AAL ecosystem layer. The notion of integrated care services, which are to be provided by multiple stakeholders through well-elaborated collaboration mechanisms, is explored. In this context, the architecture explores the paradigm of collaborative networks. The proposed conceptual framework is aligned with the recommendations of the European bridging research in ageing and ICT development (BRAID) roadmap on information and communication technology (ICT) and ageing.

KEY WORDS: *care ecosystem, elderly care services, AAL architecture, collaborative networks.*

Introduction

Decreasing birth rates and increasing life expectancy observed in most developed countries, which is leading to a rapid increase in the percentage of the aged population, raises tough challenges to our society. Additionally, migratory patterns within Europe have resulted in movement (of largely young people) from rural to urban areas and to more affluent Member States. This movement has resulted in a reduction in traditional extended family structures and community cohesion, and has been associated with a growth in the perception of isolation and loneliness, especially amongst older people. In this context, there is an urgent need to find effective and affordable solutions to provide care and assistance to the elderly.

Information and communication technologies (ICTs), particularly high-speed pervasive broadband connectivity, intelligent robotics, sensing, natural user–machine interfaces, cloud computing, and web-based technologies, offer new opportunities to provide care and assistance, as well as new ways of working; facilitate social interaction; and reduce limitations imposed by location and time. Many research projects and pilot experiments have focused on ICT and ageing (see, for instance, Refs. [1–4]).

But many good ideas and promising pilot cases fail to scale because the adopted approaches have been excessively technocentric. A purely technology-centered approach, without consideration of the socio-organizational aspects is likely to add only marginal value, not being accepted by users or not finding a sustainable business approach for wider deployment. Therefore, while designing a new conceptual architecture for ICT and ageing, it is fundamental to also address the need for organizational and cultural change.

On the other hand, the frequent association of senior citizens with a dependent stage of life no longer matches reality. The adoption of the concept of *active ageing* provides a more appropriate understanding of the later phases of life [5]. Furthermore, the notion of *productive ageing* [6] has opened new perspectives for a change in the way society often perceives older people. Thus, supporting the active ageing process is about creating not only an environment exclusively focused on providing health care and assistance but, rather, a more comprehensive one, in which the elderly citizens do not feel excluded, and have a chance to use their knowledge and expertise in a fruitful way, by making a valued contribution to the communities in which they live [7–9]. Indeed, some seniors will require additional support and care, for which ICT can be used to support innovation and effective service development. But it is also necessary to temper the *tsunami* discourse on ageing by challenging stereotypical notions of seniors as a homogenous group of vulnerable people. The aim should be to enable all citizens to live independently and be active in society, increasing efficiency of care systems and promoting a dynamic and flourishing ICT and ageing industry. Seniors are a diverse group with much to contribute to society, and the role of ICT should also be focused on value creation, extending working life, and user-generated knowledge.

In order for ICT to achieve its full potential as a vehicle to support the agenda of ageing well and enable citizens to age with dignity, it needs to be underpinned and governed by supportive organizational structures and robust regulatory frameworks.

Aiming at providing a contribution to the ICT and ageing area, the Portuguese Ambient Assisted Living for All (AAL4ALL) project is focused on the development of an ecosystem of products and services for ambient assisted living (AAL), complemented with an adequate business model for this ecosystem. The AAL4ALL consortium involves 32 partners from industry, service providers, and academia, associated with the Health Cluster Portugal.

The underlying assumption in this project is that the creation of effective support environments for ageing citizens requires the involvement and effective coordination of multiple stakeholders, from diverse sectors and distinct backgrounds. Hence, before addressing specific (technical) implementation approaches and technologies, it is important to consolidate concepts in order to mobilize and align all the needed stakeholders. As such, one of the initial results of the project was the establishment of a conceptual architecture for AAL, which is summarized in this chapter. The aim is not simply to support the development of (complex) technological artifacts, but rather, to conceive systems to support the formation and operation of sustainable AAL ecosystems.

Trends and Challenges in Elderly Care Services

Although substantial research has been carried out in this area, past developments in elderly care services as well as current market offers are still characterized by some fragmentation. The focus has been predominately put on the development of isolated services—e.g., monitoring of some health-related parameter, fall detection, agenda reminder, alarm button, etc.—each one typically provided by a single organization and often showing an excessive technocentric flavor. A current trend is to move from fragmented services to progressively more *integrated care services* [9,10], which are likely to be provided by multiple stakeholders through well-elaborated collaboration mechanisms. Furthermore, the importance of the role of communities and other forms of collaborative networks involving all stakeholders, operating as an ecosystem, is being recognized.

At this point, we should note that a term frequently causing misunderstandings is the concept of *service*, which is used with different meanings by different communities. Therefore, we distinguish two types of services:

- *Software services*: basically software functionalities that are (remotely) accessible or callable (e.g., web services). This concept corresponds to the view of service typically adopted by ICT experts.
- *Care and assistance services*: correspond to the services provided to the end users (senior citizens, in this case). This notion is equivalent to what is usually called *business services*. A care and assistance service may involve a number of software services and human intervention. The actual structure of such a service also depends on the interaction between the provider and the user, and may ultimately (and dynamically) vary according to the flow of that interaction.

Associated with the notion of service—either software service or care and assistance service—there is the notion of a *service provider*. Since a provider might offer more than one service, it is convenient to introduce the concept of *service entity*—an encapsulation of the various services provided by the same entity, in other words, a representation of a service provider [9,10]. For instance, a device used in AAL can be represented (modeled) as a service entity that provides several software services (the software functionalities of the device). Similarly, a care institution can be represented by a service entity encapsulating all care and assistance services provided by that institution.

On the other hand, developments in this area should not be exclusively focused on ICT (and related technologies, e.g., sensors, intelligent home appliances, service robotics) but need to also consider the design and launching of adequate policy actions in order to guarantee the success of any such developments. Complementarily, training actions, not only for the senior citizens but also for all the other stakeholders, are a condition for success.

This trend was clearly confirmed by the BRAID roadmapping project [11,12]. This European initiative went through an extensive consultation of stakeholders in the AAL area towards identifying the most relevant research actions in this sector for the next decade. Unlike previous initiatives, BRAID attempted to develop a holistic perspective of the area. ICT and ageing indeed represents a complex area that can be analyzed from multiple perspectives and requires the contribution of multiple disciplines. As such four perspectives or *life settings* were considered particularly relevant and selected as the basis for focused consideration in the various phases of the roadmapping process:

- *Independent living*: how technology can assist in normal daily life activities, e.g., tasks at home, mobility, safety, agenda management (memory help), etc.
- *Health and care in life*: how technology can assist in health monitoring, disease prevention, and compensation for disabilities.
- *Occupation in life*: how technology can support the continuation of professional activities along the ageing process.
- *Recreation in life*: how technology can facilitate socialization and participation in leisure activities.

The identified strategic actions are briefly described in Tables 23.1 to 23.4. As they result from a large-scale consultation of relevant stakeholders across Europe, we think they will

TABLE 23.1

Strategic Actions for Support in Independent Living

Research Actions for Independent Living
<ul><li>*Establish collaborative environments*: Design and develop novel and effective collaborative environments, according to a design-for-all perspective, combining social networking and collaborative networks of care provision stakeholders to facilitate support, companionship, and community participation with trust establishment.</li><li>*Extend capabilities*: Investigate, develop, and integrate intelligent functionalities to compensate for diminishing cognitive and physical capabilities and to design and develop intelligent, user-centered, context-aware, and self-adapting tools for personal assistance in planning and performing daily activities and facilitating societal participation.</li><li>*Assist mobility*: Integrate and customize methods and tools to assist mobility, including services for localization, trip planning, navigation, orientation in complex environments, driving assistance, and intermodal transportation, focusing on elderly needs with special relevance on adequate and adaptable user interfaces, taking into account the built environment and issues of trust and safety.</li><li>*Monitor well-being*: Design, develop, and integrate open, affordable, and scalable sensor network environments, both home centered and human centered, with intelligent monitoring, including new levels of security, safety, unintrusiveness, and privacy towards supporting better caring services.</li><li>*Build supportive environments*: Design, develop, and validate prevention and interventions based on responsive situational awareness, considering different contexts (e.g., at home, at work, outside), while trying to avoid creating dependency.</li><li>*Align independent and sustainable living*: Explore the alignment of ICT for independent living with smart grid and sustainable development technologies, including interoperability concerns, with the aid of users and relevant stakeholders.</li><li>*Assess impacts*: Promote integrative studies on the sociological, economic, ethical, and quality-of-life impacts of introducing services and technologies for independent living.</li><li>*Elicit needs of focus groups*: Comprehensively characterize different focus groups and their needs, as well as facilitators, obstacles, and acceptability potential.</li></ul>

be important drivers of the next developments in AAL care service provision. In total, about 150 stakeholders, representing both technological and socio-organizational areas, contributed to the roadmap through a number of consensus building events organized in different regions of Europe.

When asked to prioritize the identified actions, participants in the roadmapping process clearly emphasized actions such as the following:

- Establishing collaborative environments for independent living
- Establishing health care ecosystems
- Building collaboration platforms and systems for occupation in life
- Building participatory communities for recreation in life
- Etc.

These priorities confirm the mentioned trend towards integrated services provided through collaborative ecosystems. Figure 23.1 shows these findings of BRAID. Each square represents one (needed) research and development (R & D) action; the area of the squares

TABLE 23.2

Strategic Actions for Support in Health and Care in Life

Research Actions for Health and Care in Life
• *Establish health care ecosystem*: Define new organizational and business models, driven by affordability concerns, and develop support tools for the establishment of collaborative health care ecosystems involving families, health care providers, social security, and regulatory authorities, forming the backbone for the emergence of new services for healthy living support, integrating formal and informal care.
• *Develop health monitoring systems*: Design, develop, and integrate affordable sensorial systems for health condition monitoring, combined with intelligent diagnosis functionalities, understanding of the environment, and other context factors, that are easily adaptable to the needs of each senior individual and considering acceptability issues.
• *Establish safe infrastructure*: Develop a safe and adaptable infrastructure, aligned with relevant standards in e-health, to support the provision of consumer-driven health care services, including prevention and healthy lifestyle assistance.
• *Design integrated assistive services*: Create a multistakeholder framework for the emergence of integrated information-based assistive health care services, with particular emphasis on user-centered design, quality of service (QoS), and recipient's quality of life.
• *Develop intervention tools*: Design, develop, and assess advanced devices, intelligent robots, and intelligent tools to support home and health care institution–based interventions and associated support systems, like prevention systems, which are self-adapting to the cognitive, emotional, and physical status of the senior and respect the established safety and ethical principles.
• *Introduce ICT-based innovative therapeutic approaches*: Explore ICT to create novel therapeutic environments, support palliative care and cognitive and mental well-being, and promote healthy lifestyles. Issues like interoperability and affordability should be considered.
• *Raise ICT awareness and skills in health and care*: Launch actions and develop mechanisms to increase the potential of ICT support for *healthy living environments* and to form a consensus on values, ethical principles, rights, safety, and privacy issues, as well as a better understanding of the consequences of a shift towards getting health services at home.
• *Develop regulatory framework*: Promote studies to elaborate, assess, and regulate new organizational forms, legal structures, and protocols for health care provision to the ageing population from a multisectoral collaboration perspective.
• *Establish organizational and business models*: Identify critical elements in ICT-based support services for healthy living, taking into account all the potential actors and stakeholders, and promote the design of sustainable business models.

TABLE 23.3

Strategic Actions for Support in Occupation in Life

Research Actions for Occupation in Life
• *Build collaboration platforms and systems*: Design and develop open ICT collaboration platforms, support, and systems aimed at facilitating value creation, addressing the specific needs of communities of senior professionals, and that promote intergenerational interaction and socialization, which are enhanced by affective computing, context awareness, and trust establishment.
• *Leverage legacy*: Develop environments that empower and enable seniors to create a legacy capitalizing on their invaluable and transferable personal/professional knowledge and experience.
• *Create adaptive solutions and services*: Develop and integrate self-adaptive and configurable technology solutions and services in ICT environments, applying principles of e-accessibility, design for all, and usability in order to facilitate technology acceptance and enable customization for/by seniors.
• *Create a model framework*: Develop approaches, models, and reasoning methods related to older people's occupation life cycle and their participation in the economic system, including value systems, behaviors, and issues of physical, cultural, and emotional health.
• *Create trusted knowledge networks*: Create a trusted knowledge network that provides an integrative framework to enable seniors within their occupation in life, whether professional or voluntary.
• *Weave online and off-line collaboration*: Develop an integrative framework for identity management that effectively and seamlessly joins online and off-line collaboration for seniors, to create invaluable connections between virtual and real-world aspects of their occupation in life, as in the case of keeping links with former employers.
• *Guide career transition*: Define new lifelong training programs and realistic practices that prepare senior knowledge holders and guide them in the successful transition from full employment to occupation in life.
• *Improve working practices*: Investigate new models of working practices and related reward and taxation models for seniors, taking account of work–life balance, ageing well, and gender, and promote the findings to positively influence societal perception of older workers, also considering existing standards.
• *Enhance policy and legislation*: Identify and assess current national and European policy, legislation, and incentives relevant to active participation of seniors in the socioeconomic system and recommend new approaches that lower barriers and promote and support active ageing according to cultural issues. Evaluation of the impact on society from older peoples' engagement should be considered.

is proportional to the number of votes given by participating stakeholders. In addition to the technology-oriented development actions, BRAID also identified the need to develop, at the same time, a number of policy-related actions (dashed boxes in Figure 23.1).

AAL4ALL Care Ecosystem Conceptual Architecture

AAL4ALL takes into account the findings and recommendations of the BRAID roadmap, while adapting them to a national context [13]. As an important element to facilitate the creation of synergies among stakeholders, a conceptual architecture was designed. This architecture aims at structuring the developments for AAL by defining a unified terminology and describing the functionality and roles of components.

A *services ecosystem* model is considered in which the basic idea is to have an environment that facilitates rapid composition of (eventually multistakeholder) services, forming integrated care and assistance services (implicitly calling for a collaborative consortia formation). This requires that services and their providers be prepared to collaborate with each other. While designing this architecture, a sociotechnical approach was followed,

TABLE 23.4

Strategic Actions for Support in Recreation in Life

Research Actions for Recreation in Life
• *Build participatory communities*: Design, develop, and implement local and regional participatory communities that combine online and off-line participation through social networking, intergenerational interaction, volunteering, and local government involvement, focusing on participatory recreational life and well-being.
• *Build novel interfaces*: Develop novel human–machine interfaces with high quality of usability and applying design for all principles, oriented towards seniors' active engagement in recreational activities, considering their cognitive and physical capabilities, and including augmented reality, affective computing, companion artifacts, pervasiveness, multimodal interfaces, etc.
• *Build recreational platforms, solutions, and services*: Design and develop open, secure, interoperable, flexible, accessible, customizable, and affordable ICT recreational platforms, solutions, and services for senior citizens.
• *Find new recreational channels*: Elaborate innovation portfolio of new ICT-supported recreational activities for seniors, exploring telepresence, augmented reality and immersive technologies, remote participation in cultural events, collaborative gaming, intelligent urban environments, etc. All these should consider cultural aspects.
• *Create and promote gaming*: Design, develop, and promote novel physical, recreational, and cognitive games for seniors, serious games dynamically responsive to users' physiological and affective state, and integrated physical–cognitive gaming, with a holistic focus on recreation, well-being, socialization, and intergenerational collaboration.
• *Train for digital lifestyle*: Create and deploy training programs and mechanisms oriented to help senior citizens enter and explore new lifestyles in the digital age, with particular attention to rural areas.
• *Assess recreation impact*: Promote multidisciplinary studies on the impact of physical and cognitive recreational activities for seniors, in either urban or rural contexts.
• *Promote studies on recreation*: Promote studies on all aspects of ICT-enabled/induced social innovation oriented to participatory involvement of the elderly in recreational, cultural, and social life. One challenging result is the creation of taxonomies for understanding the activities that are important for the well-being of elderly persons.

since socio-organizational aspects are vital to realize the potential benefits of technology in support of the ageing population. Similar to a virtual organization breeding environment (VBE), we can consider in this environment the existence of supporting entities that take care of issues such as QoS, billing, etc.

In order to facilitate understanding and better interrelate the involved concepts, a three-layered model is adopted for the AAL4ALL conceptual architecture, as illustrated in Figure 23.2. Each layer is focused on specific aspects of the intended AAL environment, and a logical hierarchical structure is established among these layers.

The lowest level—the *support infrastructure*—represents a facilitator (providing support) for the development and delivery of care and assistance services. Such infrastructure should provide, among other functionalities, channels and mechanisms for safe communications and information sharing and exchange among the members of a given AAL ecosystem. As a *support* component, the infrastructure is neutral regarding any specific set of care and assistance services or any specific organizational model of the ecosystem. The infrastructure comprises two sublayers (Figure 23.3): (1) local infrastructure, corresponding to the support infrastructure located in a specific *location* (e.g., user's home, care center), and (2) global infrastructure, supporting the network of *spaces* (or local environments) *inhabited* by the various stakeholders. This division is justified by both the different technical specificities of each sublayer and (possibly) different business models associated with each one.

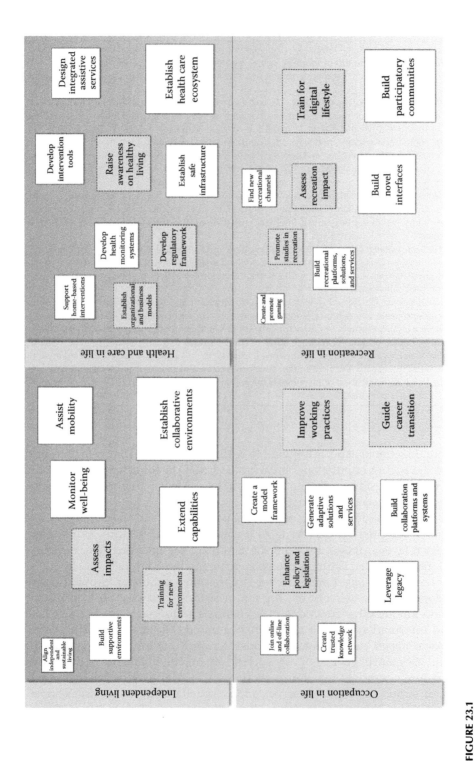

FIGURE 23.1
Prioritization of research actions in BRAID roadmap.

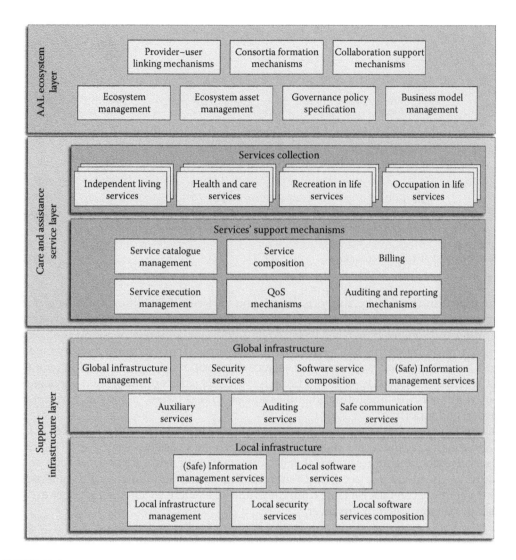

FIGURE 23.2
AAL4ALL conceptual architecture.

The local infrastructure provides support for the user care services in one's current location. It should allow the installation of sensors and actuators through adequate network standards. Examples of local infrastructure are the senior's home, senior hotels, care centers, senior in movement outside, and intelligent built environments.

The local infrastructure supports critical services, processes, and data, requiring high-level security. It will manage multiple networked sensors and actuators of several kinds, including implantable/wearable devices, as well as automation and robotic mechanisms. All these devices are modeled/wrapped as software service entities. In this sense, the local (physical) infrastructure is transformed into a software services ecosystem (which is distinct from the concept of an AAL ecosystem). Main functional blocks at this level include the following: (1) local infrastructure management, (2) local security services, (3) local software service composition, (4) safe information management services, and (5) local software services.

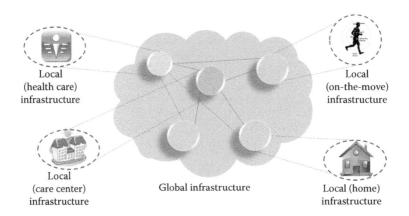

FIGURE 23.3
Scope of local and global infrastructures.

The global infrastructure supports interaction between the entities/nodes engaged in care provision. It supports multinode services, distributed processes, and software service invocation and composition. It can be based on a dedicated portal or on a cloud computing approach. Main functional blocks include the following: (1) global infrastructure management, (2) security services, (3) software service composition, (4) safe information management services at a global level, (5) auditing services, (6) safe communication services, and (7) auxiliary services (including identification of critical issues, assessing performance, statistics, and reporting).

The intermediate layer—*care and assistance services*—provides functionalities for managing and making available an open collection of care and assistance services. The notion of *open* collection of services means that it is dynamic in the sense that services can be easily introduced, edited, replaced, and removed. Functionalities allowing the construction of new and more complex services from the available elementary (atomic) services are also possible and envisioned in this layer.

In AAL4ALL, a number of demonstrative services are being developed, addressing relevant needs as identified through scenario analysis, complemented with requirements derived from an extensive set of questionnaires used to identify user needs.

This layer is logically split into two sublayers: service collection and service support mechanisms. The higher level represents the open care and assistance service collection. To facilitate the organization and management of the collection, care and assistance services are divided into four groups according to the four life settings: *independent living, health and care in life, occupation in life,* and *recreation in life.*

The lower-level layer comprises a set of support mechanisms for the management of services. Main functional elements include the following: (1) service catalog management, (2) service composition mechanisms, (3) billing, (4) service execution management, (5) QoS mechanisms, and (6) auditing and reporting mechanisms.

The top layer of the architecture—*AAL ecosystem*—provides organization, governance, and collaboration support for the multiple AAL stakeholders from a sociotechnical perspective.

An AAL ecosystem can involve, in addition to senior citizens, a combination of formal care and informal care networks, as illustrated in Figure 23.4.

The purposes of the AAL ecosystem can only be achieved if adequate functionalities for modeling and management are provided. Such functionalities should then give support

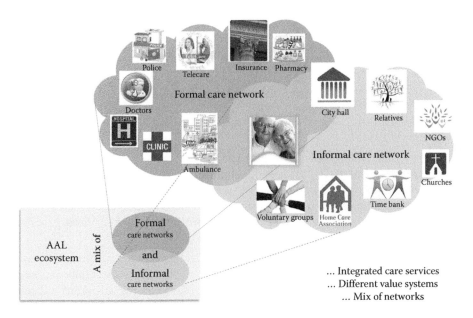

FIGURE 23.4
Example of AAL ecosystem–combining formal and informal care networks.

to organize and structure dynamic organizations, define and enforce governance policies; define profiles, roles, and business models; launch collaborative processes; and support links between providers and clients/users. The main functional elements of this layer include the following:

1. *Ecosystem management*: to provide effective management of the AAL ecosystem in terms of service providers, users, regulators, and support entities. Functionalities for membership and role management, profile and competency management (providers), user profile management, other stakeholder management, and management of interaction with external entities. It also includes a model of the organizational structure.

2. *Asset management*: to provide mechanisms that allow the management of all AAL ecosystem assets: products, services, shared knowledge, etc. It includes modeling of assets and their ownership and access rights and mechanisms for sharing of assets, as well as market gap analysis.

3. *Governance policy specification*: to provide mechanisms that allow the specification of the governance policies of the AAL ecosystem, including collaboration agreements. It includes a definition of governance policies through instantiation of templates, rules/clauses, etc., as well as a definition of rights and duties and identification of performance indicators.

4. *Business model management*: to provide means for identification, characterization, and management of specific business models adopted by the AAL ecosystem and its members. Such mechanisms include the specification of the business models, contracting, accounting services, specific business plans, support mechanisms, etc. Associated with the business models, value systems are also modeled. Models for assignment of responsibilities/liabilities and benefit distribution are included.

This element also includes the definition of service packages tailored to each user/class of users.

5. *Provider–user linking mechanisms*: to provide mechanisms to support links between AAL services or product providers and end users of the AAL ecosystem. In other words, offering mechanisms to promote usage of the care and assistance services offered by the AAL ecosystem. A variety of mechanisms can be considered in each ecosystem, including the following: e-marketplace, brokerage, dissemination and marketing, etc.

6. *Consortia formation mechanisms*: to provide mechanisms that allow (rapid) consortia formation among AAL providers, including external entities if needed, in order to deliver integrated services. It also includes consortia formation mechanisms in response to emergency situations and selection criteria specific to each ecosystem and involving elements such as stakeholders' profiles/offered services, past record of QoS, availability, collaboration readiness, costs, etc.

7. *Collaboration support mechanisms*: to provide mechanisms to support cooperation and/or collaboration among the AAL ecosystem members. A collaboration platform allowing multiple collaboration processes, involving different subsets of stakeholders. Therefore, different virtual collaboration spaces should be allowed.

Care and Assistance Services

As mentioned, the potential value of an AAL conceptual architecture depends on its capability to support scalable development and delivery of care and assistance services to the users. These services must be useful in a context of an aged, but more active, population and thus not only cover health care but also help in maintaining an active social and professional life.

Considering the four life settings mentioned, a set of examples of care and assistance services can be exemplified as follows.

Independent Living

This life setting is about the very basic needs of a person in everyday life activities that are easily taken for granted. Examples of aspects of independent living include the following:

- Access to relatives, caregivers, and the community
- Daily life activities, such as housekeeping, buying food, and personal hygiene care, among others
- Mobility and transport
- Privacy, security, and safety and a suitable environment

It should also be noted that *independent* living by no means advocates being isolated. However, an ageing citizen should, as much as possible, be supported in living

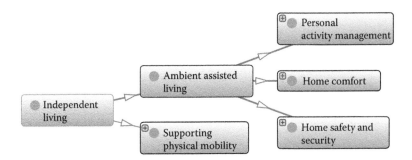

FIGURE 23.5
Example services in the dimension of independent living.

independently and autonomously, in order to have the choice of how much to depend on others.

As illustrated in Figure 23.5, the AAL dimension includes services that provide support for people to remain in their home environment, enhancing the quality of their daily life. Looking further into this dimension, we can consider several services:

- *Personal activity management*: services for monitoring of meals, dietary help, Internet shopping, agenda reminding, reminders to take pills, bill payment reminders, meal and dieting advisor, etc.
- *Home comfort*: services such as assistance in operation of smart appliances, light control, temperature control, and blind controlling, which can be configurable and adaptable to each person living at home, contribute to providing comfortable homes.
- *Home safety and security*: services consisting of proactive environmental sensors and assistive technology and contact with friends and family, including giving reassurance.

Supporting physical mobility includes localization/positioning assistance, which corresponds to services that provide the positioning and localization of people both indoors and outdoors. Questions such as *where am I?*, *what is near me?*, and *which way to go?* are answered. It also includes mobility and transportation services, which correspond to services that give support to mobility through offering transportation assistance for driving, parking, and trip planning and also support in the public transportation network.

Health and Care in Life

This life setting deals not only with a healthy lifestyle but also with care for physical and mental well-being, e.g., promoting exercise and preventing sickness as well as interventions related to health issues. The activities of concern are very individualized for every ageing citizen. Example areas include the following:

- Self-management (e.g., exercise, nutrition)
- Engagement with primary care (e.g., caregivers, pharmacist)
- Engagement with acute care (e.g., emergency admission, stay in hospital)

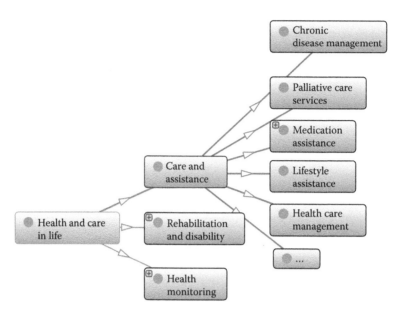

FIGURE 23.6
Example services for health and care in life.

As illustrated in Figure 23.6, this class of services includes the care and assistance services, which support daily activity according to personal health conditions and provide assistance in situations of illness, injury, or other unhealthy events. It includes, for instance, the following services:

- *Medication assistance*: support for remembering and/or dispensing, e.g., prescription and medication reminding
- *Lifestyle assistance*: services that help in maintaining a healthy lifestyle
- *Chronic disease management*: services that provide assistance in cases of diagnosed chronic diseases
- *Palliative care*: support in palliative care
- *Personal health care management*: services that support diverse care assistance, for instance, a user checking their health record updates or engaging in video conferencing for interaction with a physician for a checkup

Health and care in life also includes rehabilitation and disability compensation services to support people's rehabilitation of functional limitations and disability compensation. These services include rehabilitation, i.e., assistance services aiming to improve and recover lost functions after an illness or injury event, which might have caused functional limitations. It also includes neurocognitive compensation, which corresponds to assistance services provided in case of neurocognitive disabilities, e.g., helping with disorientation in the case of people with Alzheimer, providing cognitive reinforcement, and performing behavior monitoring for detecting potential harmful behavior.

Lastly, this dimension also includes health monitoring, which corresponds to services aimed at monitoring people's health condition to look for anomalies or out-of-pattern behaviors. Health monitoring can be either at home or outdoors.

Occupation in Life

Occupation in life addresses how technology can support the continuation of professional activities either with a salary or on a voluntary basis. Similar to the other life settings, occupation in life can look very different for each individual, depending on the background work structure, sector, individual goals, capabilities, flexibility, opportunities, and functional ability. Some examples of cases to be considered under this life setting include the following:

- Adaptation of working conditions
- Mentoring/coaching/consulting
- Teamwork
- Intergenerational teamwork
- Leaving a legacy

As illustrated in Figure 23.7, *extending professional life* corresponds to technological services for facilitation of an active professional life after retirement and staying in touch with ongoing and new developments in the expertise area. It includes the following example services:

- *Working in professional communities*: services that allow the creation and maintenance of professional communities that enable senior professionals to remain professionally active.
- *Keeping links with former employers*: services that allow senior professionals to maintain links with former employers so that knowledge and experience can continue to be used.
- *Freelancing and entrepreneurship*: services that allow senior professionals to perform professional activities on a freelancing basis and promote entrepreneurship activities.

The *workplace enhancement services* correspond to services and technology support to enhance seniors' workplace and working conditions, adjusted to people's needs as they get older.

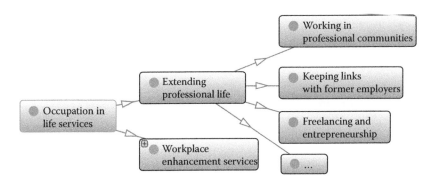

FIGURE 23.7
Example services for occupation in life.

Recreation in Life

This includes a wide range of activities where technology can be applied, for example,

- Crafts and hobbies
- Sports and physical activity
- Entertainment, taking part in cultural life, and playing games
- Family interaction and socializing
- Travel and leisure
- Political engagement
- Spiritual and faith groups
- Lifelong learning and passing on personal wisdom

As illustrated in Figure 23.8, recreation in life includes entertainment, which corresponds to services for people's amusement and distraction with the aim to promote leisure, socialization, and cultural activities. Related services include the following examples:

- *Gaming*: services for brain stimulation games and online entertainment games (e.g., bingo, cards)
- *Cultural activities*: services of online reading and storytelling, and remote attendance at concerts, cinema, theatre, etc.
- *Recreation activities*: services representing specialized and remote sports centers (attending classes from home), sports, etc.

Learning services help promote and provide learning, training, and education for people. It includes remote learning, which corresponds to services for remote access to libraries, painting, the Internet, etc. It also includes services for experience exchange and knowledge sharing, which relate to services for remote teaching/consulting (highlight intergenerational relationships and skills sharing).

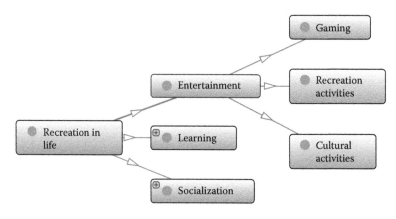

FIGURE 23.8
Examples of recreation in life services.

Lastly, socialization includes services that give support to social networking and community building with the aim of keeping people engaged in society. It corresponds to *social events management*, which refers to services that help the elderly engage in outdoor activities and volunteering activities, time banks, etc. It also includes participation in virtual communities and specialized social networks.

Many of these services clearly benefit from a collaborative multistakeholder approach. In fact, the development of high-quality and sustainable support services for ageing well requires a stronger engagement and collaborative effort among all relevant stakeholders, including local communities, which is reflected in the notion of a care ecosystem.

Implementation Aspects

Implementation architectures. As mentioned, the purpose of the AAL4ALL conceptual architecture is to provide a kind of reference framework for the various stakeholders in the sector [13]. Particular implementations will require the derivation/instantiation of implementation architectures that detail the intended systems and give guidance on how to implement them. In order to validate the conceptual framework, which was already the result of wide consultation among stakeholders, AAL4ALL engaged in implementing a number of pilot cases (large-scale trials), covering an extensive set of scenarios.

The feasibility of sustainable AAL ecosystems supported by an environment developed according to the concepts of the proposed architecture depends on the elaboration of appropriate business models that go hand in hand with the techno-organizational developments. Therefore, a number of critical questions related to the business models need to be addressed: Who pays for/owns the infrastructure? Which business model for implementations based on cloud computing should be used? Which service billing criteria should be used? Which value systems and benefit distribution model should be used? Etc.

AAL ecosystem: regional or national? One of the characteristics of the Internet and computer networks in general is that it allows some independence from geographical barriers. This characteristic allows remote delivery of care and assistance services, which could suggest the possibility of building an AAL ecosystem at a national (if not European) level. On the other hand, we cannot ignore the reality of existing organizational structures—many entities operate on a regional/local basis, e.g., care centers, health care centers, city hall related entities, etc. Furthermore, the importance of local communities in the process of supporting social inclusion of senior citizens is well recognized. Therefore, it seems more realistic to focus on regional/local AAL ecosystems. Even within one (small) geographical area, we might foresee the emergence of different AAL ecosystems based on different criteria (e.g., culture, interests, economic level).

Certainly, there are major stakeholders (e.g., infrastructure operators, special service providers, insurance companies, etc.) that operate at a national (or international) level. But this fact is not an obstacle for a model based on local ecosystems, since such stakeholders might participate in several local ecosystems.

It should be noted that the notion of local ecosystem, although appearing to be associated with a community present in a given geographical area, is not strictly bounded by geographical borders. For instance, relatives of senior citizens might be living in different geographical regions and still be part (mostly through remote access) of a local ecosystem where their senior relatives live.

Nevertheless, although AAL4ALL can foresee a future scenario in which care and assistance to elderly is provided through a multiplicity of local ecosystems, there are clear advantages, from the perspective of economy of scale, in all these local ecosystems being built following a common conceptual architecture (a kind of reference architecture at a national level). Some form of *federation* of those *ecosystems* would also be useful to allow more affordable access to some specific services (e.g., very specialized health care services) and also to guarantee continuity of services when users travel from one region to another (a kind of *roaming* between ecosystems).

Smart (energy) grid infrastructures. The so-called smart grid represents a move from a centralized, energy producer–controlled network to one less centralized and more consumer interactive. Initially, it corresponds to an overlay of the energy distribution grid with an information and metering system. At the current stage, most efforts in this area are very focused on infrastructure aspects [14,15]. Current pilot implementations offer both a bidirectional energy and information infrastructure, which opens new opportunities for the development of intelligent home automation and supervision systems. Besides the possibility of implementing energy optimization, these infrastructures allow for remote operation of home appliances, home security and surveillance, etc. However, establishing a truly smart grid that is economically viable and sustainable requires the participation of a large number of stakeholders, including producers, transmission and distribution operators, regulators, policymakers, consumers, and providers of novel services. The development of home-centered assistance services for the elderly on top of this infrastructure is a natural possibility, which calls for synergies between the two areas. Thus, the next challenge in smart grids is to adopt organizational models and governance structures and develop advanced tools to support collaboration among these players, which provides an opportunity for AAL service providers.

Intelligent transport infrastructures. Current development trends towards intelligent transport systems are leading to the progressive introduction of new technologies based on electronics, sensorial systems, and communication and information technologies. For instance, new road management policies, based on new user-paying models, and increasing concerns about traffic safety establish requirements for a new family of emergent business services. A promising strategy to promote sustainable and safe mobility aims at offering new comprehensive service contracts integrating multiple possibilities of access to public transport systems, parking areas, subscription to innovative insurance policies, etc.

The next challenge in this area is the development of a collaborative eco-driving environment, focused on effective support of integrated services targeting transportation energy efficiency, cost saving, and improvement of safety in mobility across Europe. There is enormous potential for reducing accidents, optimizing mobility time, and improving energy efficiency. This requires enabling the vehicles and road infrastructures with a new generation of intelligent transportation systems. Furthermore, achieving such infrastructure on a large scale needs the currently fragmented scenarios of multiple stakeholders acting independently (and even in competition) to disappear and be replaced with a collaborative context promoting integrated services and service innovation.

The underlying assumption is that new business models and novel business entities will progressively emerge in the transportation domain. In the future eco-driving environment, integrated transportation service providers will act as either service brokers or integrators directly interacting with the end users, providing them with a range of integrated services. The actual service providers and their transactions will become invisible for the individual drivers. Through a single contract, the driver is released from the burdensome details of dealing with separate business entities and, additionally, gains an advantage in reduced cost via subscribing to several services at once. The actual composition of elemental services into more complex (integrated) service packs is built dynamically and depends only on the subscription options taken by each driver. For instance, one customer might be interested in the service for optimal routing and optimal parking, as well as navigational information. Such services are likely to involve a number of different actors, such as road and highway operators, city traffic controllers, parking lot and gas station owners, payment clearance operators, etc., for which significant interoperability is required.

Some successful *specialized* examples have already started to emerge on the market although still with much of an ad hoc nature. Take, for instance, the case of Via Verde in Portugal. This integrated service offer extends the traditional electronic tolling service of motorways by covering parking services, gas station payments, food at drive-in restaurants, etc. The growing success of this initiative clearly shows the potential for integrated transportation-related services, supported by a collaborative network of service providers.

This general context needs to be taken into account by AAL developments, particularly in areas concerning the development of mobility services for the elderly. On one hand, business models for service packaging being adopted in this sector may inspire solutions for the elderly care sector; on the other hand, mobility services for the elderly need to cope with the trends in intelligent urban transportation infrastructures and smart cities.

Cyber physical systems (CPSs). The developments in CPSs and the Internet of Things (IoT) can have a considerable impact on AAL developments.

CPSs are engineered systems that are built from and depend upon the synergy of computational and physical components [16]. IoT is an integrated part of future Internet and could be defined as a dynamic global network infrastructure with self-configuring capabilities based on standard and interoperable communication protocols where physical and virtual *things* have identities, physical attributes, and virtual personalities and use intelligent interfaces, and are seamlessly integrated into the information network [17]. A thing in this context could be defined as a real/physical or digital/virtual entity that exists and moves in space and time and is capable of being identified. Things are commonly identified by assigned identification numbers, names, and/or location addresses.

Examples of applications of CPS for independent living include the following:

- Detecting the activities of daily living using wearable and ambient sensors, monitoring social interactions using wearable and ambient sensors, monitoring chronic disease using wearable vital signs sensors and body sensors.
- Things can learn regular routines and raise alerts or send out notifications in anomalous situations.

Examples in health care include the following:

- Measurement and monitoring methods of vital functions (temperature, blood pressure, heart rate, cholesterol levels, blood glucose, etc).
- Implantable wireless identifiable devices could be used to store health records that could save a patient's life in emergency situations.
- Edible, biodegradable chips could be introduced into the body and used for guided action.

Applications in intelligent buildings, which might also support AAL, include the following:

- Smart metering for measuring energy consumption and transmitting this information to the energy provider electronically.
- Sensors for temperature and humidity provide the necessary data to automatically adjust the comfort level and to optimize the use of energy for heating or cooling (ubiquitous sensor networks).
- Monitoring and reacting to human activity, such that exceptional situations could be detected and people can be assisted in everyday activities, e.g., supporting the elderly.
- Home automation, operation of home appliances.
- Security.

Conclusions

The combination of ICT with new collaborative organizational structures represents a promising contribution to face the challenges of providing care and assistance services to a rapidly growing percentage of the aged population. In this direction, many efforts have been carried out during the last decade, but most of them were focused on the development of single, nonintegrated services. Current trends point to the need for more integrated services, which are likely to result from contributions of various stakeholders. In fact, demographic pressure, economics, and technology, individually and collectively, are spawning rapid changes in service delivery and care provision across a range of sectors including health, employment, and welfare.

In this context, the AAL4ALL project has developed a conceptual architecture to support an ecosystem of integrated (collaborative) services. The architecture follows a holistic sociotechnical approach, which is reflected in the ecosystem notion, in opposition to more traditional technocentric solutions. This proposal is aimed at acting as a facilitator for the necessary *convergence* of stakeholders and effective support for their collaboration. Having a technology-independent conceptual architecture facilitates evolution and coping with emerging technologies. The set of technology/service developers that adhere to a common conceptual architecture can more easily collaborate in specific ecosystems (shorter adaptation time), which represents a competitive advantage in comparison with outsiders.

In terms of implementation, any technological development in AAL needs to also take into account and establish links with other areas such as smart grids, intelligent (urban) transportation systems, smart cities, and CPSs in order to ensure sustainable solutions.

Acknowledgments

This work was funded in part by the project AAL4ALL (QREN 13852), cofinanced by the European Community Fund through COMPETE—Programa Operacional Factores de Competitividade. Partial support was also obtained from the European Commission through the BRAID project (FP7 program). The authors also thank the contributions from their partners in these projects.

References

1. Aguilar, J. M.; Cantos, J.; Exposito, G.; Gómez, P. (2004). The improvement of the quality of life for elderly and relatives through two tele-assistance services: The TeleCARE approach. In *Proceedings of TELECARE 2004 Workshop—Tele-Care and Collaborative Virtual Communities*, Porto, Portugal, INSTICC Press, pp. 73–85.

2. Camarinha-Matos, L. M.; Rosas, J.; Oliveira, A. (2004). A mobile agents platform for telecare and teleassistance. In *Proceedings of TELECARE 2004—Int. Workshop on Tele-Care and Collaborative Virtual Communities in Elderly Care*, Porto, Portugal, INSTICC Press, pp. 37–48.

3. Costa, R.; Novais, P.; Costa, A.; Neves, J. (2009). Memory support in ambient assisted living. In *Leveraging Knowledge for Innovation in Collaborative Networks*, IFIP AICT 307, Springer, pp. 745–752.

4. Vontas, A.; Protogeros, N.; Moumtzi, V. (2009). Practices and services for enabling the independent living of elderly population. In *Leveraging Knowledge for Innovation in Collaborative Networks*, IFIP AICT 307, Heidelberg, Springer, pp. 753–758.

5. USDHHS (1997). Active aging: A shift in the paradigm—Denver Summit of Eight (Industrial Countries), May 1997, U.S. Department of Health and Human Services. Available at http://aspe.hhs.gov/daltcp/reports/actaging.pdf (accessed March 15, 2013).

6. Garlick, S.; Soar, J. (2007). Human capital, innovation and the productive ageing: Growth and senior aged health in the regional community through engaged higher education. In *Annual AUCEA Conference*, Alice Springs, Australia, July 2–4.

7. Llmarinen, J. (2006). Aging and work life balance in the EU, June 6.

8. HSBC Insurance (2007). The future of retirement—The new old age, May 2007. Available at www.hsbc.com/1/PA_1_1_S5/content/assets/retirement/gender_perspective_eurasia _africa_1.pdf (accessed March 15, 2013).

9. Franco, R.; Bas, A.; Prats, G.; Varela, R. (2009). Supporting structural and functional collaborative networked organizations modeling with service entities. In *Leveraging Knowledge for Innovation in Collaborative Networks*, IFIP AICT 307, Heidelberg, Springer, pp. 547–554.

10. Cardoso, T.; Camarinha-Matos, L. M. (2011). Pro-activity in collaborative service ecosystems. In *Adaptation and Value Creating Collaborative Networks*, IFIP AICT 362/2011, Springer, pp. 377–387.

11. Camarinha-Matos, L. M.; Afsarmanesh, H. (2011). Collaborative ecosystems in ageing support. In *Adaptation and Value Creating Collaborative Networks*, IFIP AICT 362/2011, Springer, pp. 177–188.

12. Camarinha-Matos, L. M.; Ferrada, F.; Oliveira, A. I.; Rosas, J. (2011). Consolidated roadmap for ICT and ageing. Deliverable D6.21, BRAID project, October 2011. Available at http://www .braidproject.eu/ (accessed November 6, 2014).

13. Camarinha-Matos, L. M.; Rosas, J.; Oliveira, A.; Ferrada, F. (2012). A Collaborative service ecosystem for ambient assisted living. In *Collaborative Networks in the Internet of Services*, IFIP AICT Series 380/2012, Springer, pp. 117–127.

14. Breuer, W.; Povh, D.; Retzmann, D.; Urbanke, C.; Weinhold, M. (2007). Prospects of smart grid technologies for a sustainable and secure power supply. In *20th World Energy Congress*, Rome, Italy, November 11–15.

15. Kok, J. K.; Warmer, C. J.; Karnouskos, S.; Nestle, D.; Dimeas, A.; Weidlich, A.; Strauss, P.; Buchholz, B.; Drenkard, S.; Hatziargyriou, N.; Lioliou, V. (2009). Smart houses for a smart grid. In *20th International Conference on Electricity Distribution*, Prague, Czech Republic, June 8–11.

16. NSF (2010). Cyber physical systems. Available at http://www.nsf.gov/funding/pgm_summ .jsp?pims_id=503286 (accessed November 6, 2014).

17. Sundmaeker, H.; Guillemin, P.; Friess, P.; Woelfflé, S. (Eds.) (2010). Vision and challenges for realising the internet of things. CERP-IoT, European Commission.

24

Social Ambient Intelligence for Assisted Living: Social Context, Networking, and Privacy

Antonio Sapuppo and Boon-Chong Seet

CONTENTS

ABSTRACT Ambient intelligence (AmI) is a key enabling technology of Ambient Assisted Living (AAL) systems. One of the specified objectives of AAL is to improve social interaction and minimize isolation of individuals with their communities. This calls for the design of AAL systems with the primary goal of assisting people in their interaction with others in their daily environments. In addition, whether or not an AAL system is intended for promoting social interaction, it must intelligently and naturally support its human users, who by nature are social beings. This necessitates the need for social context awareness by these systems to adapt and respond to the changing social context of the users. In this chapter, we first discuss the emerging concept of social ambient intelligence (socAmI). We then review the underlying methods and technologies to address three important challenges of socAmI: the acquisition of social context, enhancing ubiquitous social networking, and privacy protection.

KEY WORDS: *social ambient intelligence, assisted living, social context, social networking, privacy.*

Introduction

Ambient intelligence (AmI) is an emerging technological paradigm that takes a human-centric view of the applications of technology. AmI envisions a future where everyday objects and living spaces will be augmented with unobtrusive networked sensing devices, creating a smart environment that is sensitive and responsive to the needs of its inhabitants in order to support and enhance their well-being, productivity, and lifestyle (Aarts and Encarnacao 2006). AmI technologies have been applied across the different domains of lifestyle, with a majority of applications focused on health care (Cornejo 2010; Riva and Gramatica 2003; Seet and Casar 2007) and education (Li et al. 2009; Olsevicova and Mikulecky 2008). Recently, AmI has also been applied as a persuasive technology to encourage people to make behavioral changes by delivering persuasive content tailored to the users at the right time at the right place (Kaptein et al. 2010).

Ambient assisted living (AAL) is a concept to enhance people's quality of living, in particular, the elderly and the disabled, by supporting their everyday activities at home, at work, and in the community through AmI technologies (Nehmer et al. 2006). One of the specified objectives of AAL is to improve social interaction and minimize isolation of individuals from their communities (AALIANCE 2011). This is important as research has shown that social connectedness plays an important role in the physical and mental well-being of an individual (Cohen 2004; Rook et al. 2007; Seeman 1996). Social connectedness refers to the sense of belonging and relatedness with others, which could be supported by social care assistive systems enabled through socially aware AmI. This calls for the design of AAL systems with the primary goal of assisting people in their interaction with others in their daily environments, for example, systems that inform users of the presence, activities, and other social contexts of the people in their communities with the aim of reinforcing their existing social relationships or even creating new social networks.

Whether or not an AAL system is intended for promoting social interaction or for assisting other activities of daily living (ADLs), it must intelligently and naturally support its human users, who, by nature, are social beings. As human behavior, preferences and needs can be influenced by the social environment, which varies in time and space, this necessitates the need for social context awareness by these systems to adapt and respond to the changing social contexts of the users. Thus, social ambient intelligence (socAmI), which can be seen as an evolution of AmI where a social dimension has been added to the technology's awareness of humans (Youngblood et al. 2005), is the foundation for realizing socially aware systems for assisted living.

The remaining structure of the chapter is organized as follows. The second section on "Social Ambient Intelligence" reviews the concepts of socAmI with a view on enabling the development of AAL systems for social care support. The third through fifth sections—"Acquisition of Social Context," "Ubiquitous Social Networking," and "Privacy Designs and Models"—discuss the respective underlying technologies for acquiring users' social context, enhancing social networking between inhabitants, and addressing related privacy issues, in socAmI environments. Finally, this chapter ends with the "Conclusion."

Social Ambient Intelligence

SocAmI has been studied in institutional (Boella et al. 2008), work (Rocker 2009), and social (Erl 2005; Hasswa and Hassanein 2010) environments as well as in assisting individual living and health support for elderly users (Cornejo 2010; Rocker et al. 2010), while aiming at enriching users' social lives and improving their communication possibilities. In particular, the target of socAmI environments is to anticipate upcoming circumstances (Joly et al. 2009) in order to enhance people's lives by supporting social actions that the users are currently engaged in.

SocAmI environments are based on context-awareness research, which enables creation of systems that provide information or services based on their relevance, evaluated according to the acquired context. In particular, any information that is used to characterize the situation of an entity (e.g., person, place or object) can be defined as context (Dey and Abowd 2000). In order to achieve more reliable and truly context-aware smart spaces, both environmental and social contexts must be considered. While the environmental context comprises physical characteristics of the surroundings, such as temperature, lights, sounds, etc., the social context refers to the information about inhabitants of the socAmI, for example, users' identities, types of social relationships, social interactions, and user preferences (Hasswa and Hassanein 2010).

In order to obtain environmental context information, sensor networks have been deployed in socAmI environments. However, these sensors are incapable of gathering users' social context information due to their limited resources, such as restricted energy, networking, and storage capabilities (Liu and Das 2006). Notably, to overcome these limitations, recent research explores the usage of mobile phones as social sensors (Eagle 2011). Mobile phones are already equipped with GPS, an accelerometer, and other sensing components, enabling acquisition of environmental context information (Breslin et al. 2009; Musolesi et al. 2008). Moreover, they are also ideally suited to provide an insight into social behavior patterns because they can be seen as wearable and inconspicuous sensors, constantly carrying users' personal information (Breslin et al. 2009). Finally, they are also considered to be gateways to social networks, which are significant sources of users' social context such as a user's preferences, list of friends, etc. (Breslin et al. 2009; Eagle 2011).

The vast amount of social context information, acquired by using mobiles as social sensors, enables more personalized applications, where inhabitants of socAmI environments are the primary targets of sensing. Thus, we can consider these smart spaces to be based on people-centric sensing approaches (Campbell et al. 2008; Lu et al. 2009; Murty et al. 2008). Specifically, those environments consist mainly of intangible social components, such as user preferences, identities, and relationships between the users, rather than just machines and devices. This collection of information provides a crucial foundation for ubiquitous services to better empower people in their social conduct and enhance their sense of social connectedness. However, in order to enable those services, it is necessary to address the following mutually dependent technological and psychological challenges (Streitz and Nixon 2005).

1. *Social context*: the socAmI environments must be capable of acquiring users' social context. Further, an evaluation of the obtained social context must be carried out to elaborate its significance and relevancy, which is conducive to learning users' behavioral and social patterns for personalizing social networking services.

2. *Social networking*: the socAmI environments must be capable of enhancing ubiquitous social networking between its participants. In particular, those services have to be applied not only among acquaintances but also between strangers with interpersonal affinities. Hence, it would lead to highlighting relevant social paths between users in the physical world that would otherwise remain hidden.

3. *Privacy*: the socAmI must be capable of providing a secure and safe exchange and dissemination of participants' personal information. This challenge arises due to the fact that the foundation of ubiquitous social networking is based on automated sharing of participants' personal information, which can provoke potential privacy threats. If not addressed responsibly, these threats could motivate users to withhold their personal information due to mistrust in socAmI environments (Abowd and Mynatt 2000; Bohn et al. 2005).

In the following sections, we are going to discuss these socAmI challenges and present potential solutions.

Acquisition of Social Context

The social context of inhabitants of socAmI environments, shown in Figure 24.1, can be acquired by using different technologies. First, we are going to discuss previous works that investigated acquisition of users' identities and understanding types of relationships between the users. Then, we will look into other studies, which focus on detection of users' social activities. Finally, we will explore research that integrated online social networks in socAmI environments to retrieve users' profiles (e.g., list of friends, preferences, etc.) as another source of social context.

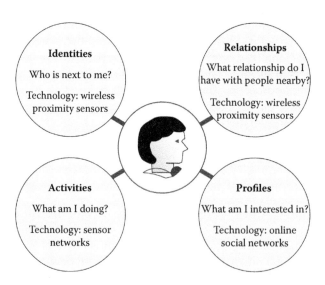

FIGURE 24.1
Social context of the user.

Users' Identities and Types of Relationships

In regard to the acquisition of users' identities and social context in terms of types of relationships, mobile phones have been exploited as social proximity sensors because of their wireless capabilities. Among the wireless technologies available, Bluetooth was usually preferred due to its common adoption in mobile phones and characteristics such as device and service discoveries. In this case, the acquisition range of social context depends on the power classes of the Bluetooth radio. Obviously, a more powerful radio implies larger power consumption. Thus, mobile phones are typically equipped with class 2 Bluetooth radios, which provide a range of up to 10 m for use as social proximity sensors.

Bluetooth-enabled mobile phones were used as social proximity sensors by Lawrence et al. (2006) in their research on the subject of familiar strangers. Two people are classified as familiar strangers if they encounter each other regularly without interacting or forming an explicit relationship of a social nature (Milgram 1977). The challenge of the authors was to identify the social groups among familiar strangers. They defined those groups as copresence communities, i.e., groups of individuals who regularly share a particular location at the same time. Members of copresence communities are not required to have any social interactions, but due to repeated collocations of individuals, they were expected to have common interests in the functioning of the local area (e.g., punctuality of a bus among the people who tend to take the same bus). Thus, the authors implemented an ambient information dissemination environment (AIDE), which is able to acquire and exploit relevant social context. AIDE detects mobile devices, identifies users and the community to which they belong, and automatically disseminates contents in the background, based on the preferences specified by the users.

Acquisition and applications of the social context of users' identities in socAmI environments were further explored by Perkio et al. (2006). The main objective of their research was to predict users' locations by monitoring their Bluetooth neighborhoods in a work environment. The socAmI environments were equipped with several passive Bluetooth beacons. The purpose of the beacons was to scan the surroundings and detect Bluetooth-enabled mobile phones, carried by users as wearable sensors. The collected data were stored in a back-end server and subsequently used as input data for training naive Bayes models (Lewis 1998) in order to predict inhabitants' location in the socAmI environments. Test results showed that they were able to reach an average prediction accuracy of 94.8% in their office environment, using a time-dependent dynamic model.

Similar methodology and objectives have been employed by Eagle and Pentland (2006). However, in contrast to the previously discussed project, the authors focused on investigation of social relationships among the inhabitants of socAmI environments, in addition to predicting users' locations. Specifically, three locations were considered: work, home, and elsewhere. Moreover, the Bluetooth neighborhood of the users was not only investigated by using passive Bluetooth beacons. Mobile phones were also scanning, detecting, and identifying other users in opportunistic meetings, thus providing more complete information about the users' Bluetooth surroundings. Apart from data related to Bluetooth neighborhoods, the collected information further included call logs, cell tower IDs, application usage, and phone status to be used in order to provide insight into both the individuals and their communities. Thus, the acquired data were applied not only to predict user locations but also to anticipate the probability of user meetings and define types of relationships between the socAmI inhabitants. The authors employed a hidden Markov model (Eddy 1996), which was trained for 1 month and afterwards resulted in accuracy greater than 95% in anticipating users' locations. Bayes rules were used to predict the probability of user encounters with an accuracy of 90%. And finally, the social proximity context information was used in order to investigate types of relationships between users. Particularly, the nature of the relationships between the participants of socAmI was deduced by combining users' proximity information with temporal and spatial information. Specifically, it was expected that being near someone in a canteen at 3 pm implies a different relationship than being detected in the proximity downtown on a late weekend night. Based on these assumptions, the authors trained a Gaussian mixture model (Duda et al. 2001), which achieved a prediction accuracy of over 90%.

Users' Activities

Identifying users and predicting their locations and types of participants' relations were not the only challenges addressed in socAmI. In addition, Cook et al. (2010) further explored the social context by attempting to detect users' social activities. They collected social context data of two inhabitants by using in-house sensor networks and stored them in an Structured Query Language (SQL) database. In order to recognize the activities that occurred in the socAmI environments, they applied hidden Markov (Eddy 1996) and naive Bayesian classifier (Han and Kamber 2006) statistical models. The former model achieved an average activity recognition accuracy of 90%, while the latter one obtained an accuracy level of 49%; thus, the hidden Markov model can be assumed to be a more effective approach for this type of classification problem. However, it must be noted that attempting to recognize social activities between more than just two users would result in a significant increase of complexity of the system.

Detecting users' activities was also the objective of the CenceMe project (Miluzzo et al. 2008). However, the authors used a methodology different from Cook et al. (2010) to acquire users' social context. They exclusively relied on sensing components of mobile phones to anticipate current activities of participants of socAmI. Particularly, CenceMe uses the following sensing components of smartphones:

- Accelerometers to predict the current condition of users (e.g., sitting, standing, walking, etc.)
- A microphone to recognize quiet or noise environments and conversation between people
- Bluetooth as a social proximity sensor to classify the neighborhood members (e.g., friends, strangers, etc.)
- GPS to identify the current position of the user and mobility patterns such as traveling in a vehicle or not, being stationary, walking, running, etc.

Therefore, the CenceMe mobile application is capable of recognizing the current users' activities by utilizing the combination of these data acquired from the mobile sensing components. For example, by combining the current location of the user, information from the proximity sensor (e.g., coworkers in the neighborhood) as well as information from the accelerometers (e.g., sitting) and microphone (e.g., talking), it can be inferred that the user is participating in a business meeting.

User Online Profiles

As previously discussed, sensor networks have the possibility to acquire social context such as users' identities, relationships, and current activities within the smart spaces. However, they do not develop awareness of users' interests and preferences, which would present much added value for socAmI. Indisputably, online social networks are a vast source of users' personal information. Thus, by integrating online social networks into sensor networks, socAmI environments can become more accurate context-aware smart spaces, and consequently, more advanced solutions can be provided (Breslin et al. 2009; Hasswa and Hassanein 2010).

The integration of online social networks and sensor network technologies could be accomplished by modeling them through semantic web technologies. Subsequently, it would be possible to develop a unified layer of social context on top of existing applications. This approach has also been discussed by Joly et al. (2009) and Breslin et al. (2009).

Miluzzo et al. (2008) investigated the acquisition of social context through online social networking sites, in addition to the prediction of users' activities, discussed in the section "Users' Activities." In particular, CenceMe retrieves the user's list of friends from social networking sites, such as Facebook and MySpace, to update them about their current activities. Thus, CenceMe presents new opportunities to keep friends close by providing constantly accessible information about users' locations and activities.

Another approach, which exploits data from online social networking sites, is the Astra project (Mavrommati and Calemis 2008). Astra is based on service-oriented architecture principles (Erl 2005), which enable effective service delivery in dynamic environments. In particular, Astra has the purpose of accommodating users' wishes through available network technologies. A model to manage the users' information and preferences was implemented, based on the concepts of Nimbus and Focus (Calemis et al. 2010). While Nimbus represents the information that the user would like to share, Focus represents the set of information that the user is interested in receiving. Thus, a customized response to each user's preferences can be created by exploiting the social context gathered from smart objects and sensors in the user's surroundings. According to users' preferences, automatic updates about the users' availability for interaction (e.g., going for a walk or a phone conversation) can be delivered to the community of users (e.g., friends, family members, etc.).

Ubiquitous Social Networking

As noted in the previous section, some studies have already acquired and applied social context from online social networks in order to enhance ubiquitous social networking services. Specifically, Astra and CenceMe focused on keeping friends and family members close by giving updates about their current activities, locations, availability, etc. However, these approaches cannot be identified as *networking*, due to their principal focus on existing acquaintances. In fact, *networking* has been previously defined as relationship initiation, often between strangers (Boyd and Ellison 2008). It leads to new opportunities to leverage interpersonal affinities for personal benefits between people who do not know each other but probably should. Thus, socAmI must be capable of promoting sociability not only among friends but between strangers as well.

Hasswa and Hassanein (2010) promoted social networking among socAmI participants with similar interests. The authors utilized mobile devices both as wearable sensors and as gateways to social networks in order to obtain a more detailed social and environmental context. The proposed architecture comprised Internet access points in order to enable the socAmI environments, as shown in Figure 24.2a. When mobile phones connect to the smart space dedicated access point, users give permissions to retrieve their social context,

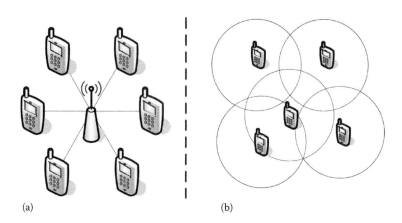

(a)   (b)

FIGURE 24.2
(a) Centralized and (b) decentralized social networking architectures.

stored in online social networks. Consequently, users' preferences, interests, personal data, and list of friends become available for that specific socAmI environment, which, in turn, develops a complete and deep understanding of the users in the surroundings and thus is able to provide personalized services to its inhabitants. For example, socAmI smart space is capable of classifying users within the environment into different groups based on relationships and similar interests. Consequently, it is able to promote networking (e.g., exchange public, private, and group messages, pictures, etc.) among the identified groups.

However, the work by Hasswa and Hassanein (2010) is based on an architecture that exclusively relies on a central unit, as shown in Figure 24.2a. In this case, the socAmI environment is limited to a physical location, and the offered services are restricted to a certain network (Schollmeier 2001). However, the elevated mobility of mobile phone users could potentially enable unrestrained sensing coverage of socAmI environments (Campbell et al. 2008), which would inspire new system architectures. Consequently, we further investigate ubiquitous social networking that is established during purely ad hoc meetings, as shown in Figure 24.2b. This solution leads towards sociable opportunistic networks, where nodes are wirelessly interconnected and have the possibility to identify each other (Heinemann 2007). Thus, sociable opportunistic networks contribute to addressing sociability issues by enabling dynamic and mobile socAmI environments, applied in the everyday physical world. As a result, the value of social networking is significantly enhanced, and benefits are available immediately upon demand.

The MIT Serendipity project (Eagle and Pentland 2005) was the pioneer of sociable opportunistic networks. The software architecture of Serendipity is shown in Figure 24.3. When Serendipity users randomly meet, they exchange Bluetooth identification. This information is sent to a central server, which contains all the Serendipity users' profiles along with their matchmaking preferences. The server evaluates similarities between encountering users, and if the similarity score identifies a mutual match, the server notifies both users about their presence and the related affinities.

Another sociable opportunistic networking approach is the MobiSoc (Gupta et al. 2009) application. When MobiSoc peers meet, the application captures and manages the social context of physical communities such as social profiles and people-to-people and people-to-place affinities. Further, MobiSoc exploits learning algorithms to notify users about relevant matches according to their preferences.

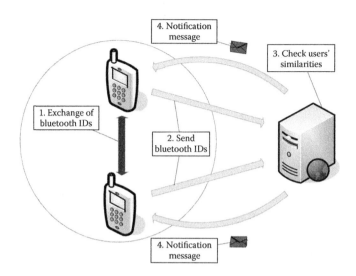

FIGURE 24.3
Centralized solution for ad hoc socAmI environments.

However, even if relying on opportunistic meetings, the previously discussed solutions still comprise interactions between the nodes and a central server, as shown in Figure 24.3. Recently, those centralized solutions were replaced with new decentralized approaches, which exploit dynamic mobile connectivity in terms of peer-to-peer communications. In fact, peer-to-peer solutions are considered to be more suitable for socAmI environments, due to the fact that inhabitants engage in opportunistic ad hoc social interactions (Toninelli et al. 2010).

Figure 24.4 shows an example of peer-to-peer communication (Schollmeier 2001) on mobile phones, using the Bluetooth technology. Each node of the peer-to-peer network can simultaneously play two different roles: server and client. The task of the server is to publish a service and accept concurrent connections, whereas the task of the client is to search and connect to services in order to exchange data. One of the well-known implementations of decentralized architecture was the Nokia Sensor (Persson and Jung 2005), which relies exclusively on opportunistic connections between devices nearby. Using the Bluetooth technology, similarly to Figure 24.4, Nokia Sensor users are able to discover each

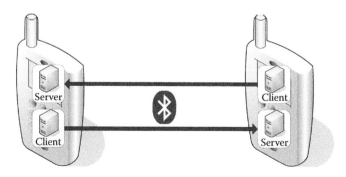

FIGURE 24.4
Decentralized solution for ad hoc socAmI environments.

other within a short communication range and exchange users' contents, stored in the local memory of their mobile phones (e.g., profiles, pictures, etc.). Other works that have also investigated decentralized sociable opportunistic networks aimed at analyzing users' personal social networks (Nicolai et al. 2006), displaying users' encounters (Kostakos and O'Neill 2008), and disseminating contexts such as messages (Pietilainen et al. 2009).

Among those decentralized sociable opportunistic networks, Sapuppo and Sørensen (2011) presented an approach called local social networks, which aims at providing ubiquitous social networking services while preserving users' privacy. A local social network has been introduced as a distributed network architecture where nodes are linked to online social networking profiles and wirelessly interconnected to exchange personalized contents. As shown in Figure 24.5, a local social network is based on an integration of online social networks and opportunistic networks. Thus, a local social network node behaves as both an online social network node and an opportunistic network node at the same time.

The first prototype of local social networks is called Spiderweb (Sapuppo 2010), which was implemented in Java 2 Micro Edition for Symbian OS (de Jode 2004). In order to evaluate users' acceptance of local social networks, the Spiderweb services were tested according to the Technology Acceptance Model (Davis 1989) by investigating the perceived ease of use and usefulness of the application. Both tests returned satisfactory results, with users finding Spiderweb to be an interesting and innovative application, which is also very easy to use. The majority of the respondents claimed that they would be potential users of those ubiquitous social networking services. In particular, they emphasized and appreciated the fact that social networking was no longer in front of a stationary PC, but these technologies were disappearing in the background.

Additionally, in order to address potential privacy threats in local social networks, a privacy model called Diverged Personalities was proposed (Sapuppo 2010). This model is based on the following assumption: the sensitivity of the users' personal information varies depending on activities and interactions in which the user is involved. Specifically, the proposed privacy model suggests representing the user with different personalities in different circumstances. Thus, the personality of a user would be composed of a user's personal information that is relevant, though not sensitive, in those specific circumstances. We will further investigate privacy in socAmI environments in the next section.

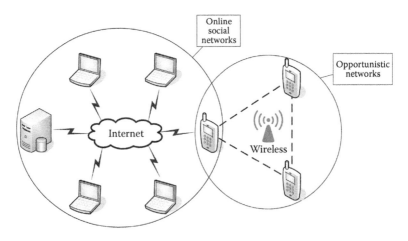

FIGURE 24.5
Local social network architecture.

Privacy Designs and Models

Even when ubiquitous computing (ubicomp) was just a vision (Weiser 1995), privacy threats were already identified as the greatest barrier to long-term success (Bünnig 2009a; Hong et al. 2004). Nowadays, sensors are capable of not only acquiring environmental data but obtaining users' personal information as well. Thus, the technological development is moving towards a people-centric era, where humans are the main focus of sensing. In people-centric sensing, users are parts of mobile sensor networks, where mobile devices are conceptually tied to individuals. Consequently, new challenges arise for privacy of ubicomp, which specifically include safe collecting, storing, processing, and disseminating of users' personal information, related to daily users' activities (Johnson et al. 2007).

Fundamentally, privacy is not considered anymore as having "the right to be left alone" (Brandeis and Warren 1890), but it is now understood as having "the right to select what personal information about me is to be disclosed and to whom" (Westin 1967). Therefore, the main challenge of ubicomp is shifting from hiding personal data to ensuring successful management of disclosure of users' personal information. Particularly, socAmI environments must ensure individuals' awareness of when/what information is collected and data management afterwards (e.g., stored, encrypted, combined with other information, etc.). Moreover, the methods and purposes of applying the collected data must be not only transparent but also, most importantly, endorsable by the users (Bellotti and Sellen 1993; Motahari et al. 2007). Consequently, socAmI environments must be designed to provide possibilities for their inhabitants to enforce their own preferences for the acquisition, management, and dissemination of their personal information.

Privacy Design Guidelines

In the following, we are focusing on the design guidelines for socAmI environments, which do not aim to ensure total security but instead target prevention of accidental data disclosure, where personal information is unintentionally revealed, even if not inquired. Initially, we review previous works that provide design solutions for trustable and feasible AmI-based applications, including AAL systems, by drawing on the legal privacy framework and management of personal data to be shared with other individuals. Further, we discuss existing privacy models that contribute to ubiquitous social networking targets.

Legal Regulations

The design of socAmI environments has achieved significant progress in recent years, and simultaneously, the privacy concerns have been discussed in the legal as well as academic worlds. The legal regulations draw the primary framework for privacy preservation in ubicomp. However, when interpreting them, usability and applicability must also be considered. Although the legal world calls for total privacy and preservation, the essence of sociability and networking demands disclosure of relevant information. Thus, improper application of legal regulations could result in threats to the success of socAmI environments, as the user could be overwhelmed by unnecessary privacy protection measures.

Both regional and international legal frameworks have been adopted by researchers as reference guidelines to develop methodologies for privacy protection. This includes the

US Privacy Act of 1974 and Directive 2002/58/EC (2002) adopted by the European Union (EU), which concerns the processing of personal data and protecting their privacy in the electronic communications sector. The US Privacy Act of 1974 is based on fair information practices and is among the earliest guidelines that indisputably influenced all subsequent data protection legislation, based on information practices (Langheinrich 2001). The principle of fair information practices is summarized in the following:

- *Collection limitation*: the collection of data should be limited and obtained by lawful and fair means with the knowledge or consent of the data subject.
- *Use limitation*: prior to data collection, the purpose should be specified, and the subsequent use of these data should be limited to those purposes.
- *Data quality*: the data should be accurate, complete, up to date, and relevant to the main purposes of their use.
- *Reasonable security*: the data should be protected from risks such as loss, unauthorized access, destruction, use, modification, or disclosure of data, through implementing appropriate security safeguards.
- *Openness and transparency*: there should be openness about the existence, nature, purpose, and location of the collected data.
- *Individual participation*: the data subject should have the right to challenge the data and, if the challenge is successful, to have the data erased, rectified, completed, or amended.
- *Accountability*: the data controllers should be accountable for complying with measures, which give effect to these principles.

Later, in 1995, the EU Directive was enacted, and it provided two additional relevant aspects: (1) limit data transfers to non-EU countries that present an inadequate level of privacy protection and (2) introduce the notion of explicit consent, which refers to the process of obtaining personal data only after unambiguous consent from the interested party (Langheinrich 2001).

These legislation privacy laws were subsequently adapted to the design of ubicomp by Langheinrich (2001), who identified several main areas of innovation and system design for data protection in ubicomp: notifying the user appropriately; taking into account the user's choice and seeking consent; enforcing limitation of scope within the concepts of proximity and locality; enabling anonymity and pseudonymity when necessary; and providing adequate security and appropriate data access.

In the context of information and communication technologies (ICTs), le Metayer (2010) also discusses and advocates the adoption of the *privacy by design* approach. This refers to treating the privacy issue not as an afterthought but as a first-class requirement from the beginning of the system's design phase. An example of adopting such an approach is an agent-based architecture proposed for enhancing privacy protection in AmI (PRIAM 2007). The key feature of this architecture is the use of privacy agents, which are software components installed on devices in the proximity of or on the data subject. The privacy agents manage the personal data according to the wishes of the subject, expressed in a restricted natural language devised for privacy policies. In the domain of ambient assisted living, privacy by design has also been viewed as a more effective solution for privacy protection over one that is based on the data subject's freely given and informed consent (Rost 2010).

Personal Privacy

The legal regulations, outlined in the previous section, define the principles for designing trustable socAmI environments. In this section, we focus on personal privacy, which is related to the management of personal data to be shared with other individuals (Lederer et al. 2004). This concept cannot be seen as a static notion, where users set rules and enforce them, but rather, it should be considered a dynamic process, representing continuous negotiation and management of the boundaries that shape personal data disclosure (Altman 1975, 1977; Palen and Dourish 2003).

Lederer et al. (2004) discussed the crucial importance of empowering the inhabitants of socAmI environments to make conscious personal data disclosure decisions. They proposed relevant privacy guidelines that focused on both enabling users to understand the impact of data disclosure on personal privacy as well as allowing them to perform natural social actions. These privacy guidelines depict five pitfalls to be avoided in the design of privacy management systems for ubicomp environments. Ubicomp privacy management systems should not obscure the potential (pitfall 1) and actual (pitfall 2) information flows. For instance, the individuals should be informed of who the recipient is and what information is disclosed, as well as about the privacy implications of their data disclosure, e.g., how the information is shared, the presence of third-party observers, etc. Moreover, designers of privacy models for ubicomp environments should not emphasize configuration over action (pitfall 3). In fact, ubicomp should allow users to manage privacy as a natural consequence of their normal engagement with the environment. Ubicomp should also not lack coarse-grained control (pitfall 4), but a binary choice for halting and resuming data disclosure should always be provided. Finally, ubicomp should not inhibit established practice (pitfall 5). For example, the design of ubicomp should give the opportunity for users to transfer established social practice, such as ambiguous information and plausible deniability, to emerging technologies.

Privacy Models

In this section, we present existing privacy models that attempt to incorporate the legal and data disclosure challenges. Particularly, the suitable privacy models for socAmI environments should follow the legal requirements, while still facilitating data disclosure and as well replicating the natural data privacy handling of the individuals.

A privacy protection model, which followed the outlined legal regulations of personal data privacy, was implemented by Yee (2010). In particular, the author provided a solution where socAmI environments are owned by an entity, which sets a framework of information policies, established according to the legal requirements. Moreover, each user is given an opportunity to personalize their privacy policy, by specifying what they are interested in sharing (observe) and under what terms. Thus, before any actual interaction with the socAmI environment, the user is asked to present their own set of information policies to be verified by the socAmI entity. If the policy is found to be compatible, the user is permitted to interact with the environment; otherwise, a negotiation is attempted.

Indisputably, while primarily addressing personal data privacy in terms of legal regulations, Yee's (2010) model requires more attention to the dynamic nature of personal data disclosure. Other privacy protection solutions (Jendricke et al. 2002; Kapadia et al. 2007; Myles et al. 2003) presented more extensive considerations of personal data disclosure by incorporating possibilities for dynamic sharing choices. Specifically, these models were implemented by enabling users to share varying personal data subsets, depending on the location of the inquiry.

However, Sadeh et al. (2009) proved that socAmI inhabitants encountered difficulties while selecting their privacy preferences according to the single *location* factor. Lederer et al. (2003a) conducted a survey that investigated the important determinants for data disclosure decisions. In particular, the research was focused on the inquirer and the current situation parameters. The inquirer is considered to be the individual that the user is interacting with, and the situation is defined according to the circumstances at that time. The authors determined the identity of the inquirer to be the most important value for influencing the users' privacy choices, followed by the situation as a parameter of secondary significance. Consequently, in the following, we present three different privacy models: Faces, Diverged Personalities, and Disclosure Decision Model, for managing dynamic data disclosure based on the inquirer and circumstances (e.g., location, time, current activity) as determinants.

Faces

The management of data disclosure in socAmI environments was first implemented in a privacy model called Faces (Lederer et al. 2003b). This privacy model was inspired by the work of Goffman (1978), who observed that an individual is inclined to present themselves to a certain audience by undertaking a particular role or face and that they will attempt to maintain that chosen face throughout the time. The authors implemented Faces according to the results of the privacy survey, previously introduced, which identified that the inquirer and the current situation present major influence over users' preferences of data disclosure. Thus, they designed the software prototype Faces to allow the user to decide *who* can access *what* and *when*. Faces supports four predefined levels of privacy protection, ranging from *undisclosed*, which denotes absolute confidentiality, to *precise*, which allows openness of the entirety of a user's personal information. The process of the Faces privacy model is shown in Figure 24.6.

As the first step, prior to any actual disclosure, users set the privacy rules through a desktop application, by creating a 3-tuple of inquirers, situations, and faces (Figure 24.6a). Afterwards, when the user meets one of the predefined circumstances, the Faces repository, where all the predefined preferences are stored, is queried. Based on the input of

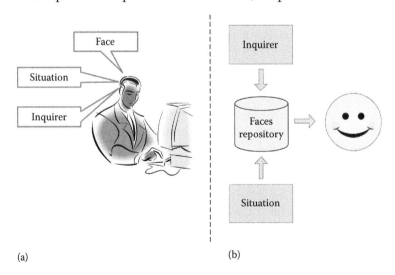

(a)   (b)

FIGURE 24.6
Faces privacy model process. (a) Manual configuration of the faces privacy model and (b) retrieval of user's data disclosure decisions based on the inquirer and situation parameters.

the current situation and inquirer, the repository returns the corresponding face to be presented for the inquirer (Figure 24.6b). Additionally, in case of unknown inquirers or situations, a default face is returned.

Faces was tested by first users, who indicated that the predefined privacy preferences were not an accurate solution for guiding data disclosure in socAmI environments. Specifically, the users encountered difficulties in predicting their own data disclosure preferences precisely, as sometimes, they wished to adjust their decisions while meeting the actual circumstances. Even more importantly, some of the users were not able to remember their predefined preferences, which further highlights the complexity of the privacy model. Thus, the test results imply that the Faces privacy model would permit invasion of privacy, in case the actual/real preferences did not meet the rules predefined by the user. Consequently, due to the encountered issues, Lederer et al. (2004) upgraded the Faces concept into the Precision Dial model.

In comparison to Faces, Precision Dial removed the preconfigured privacy preferences and added quick manual selection of one of the four privacy protection levels, introduced in the Faces privacy model. Thus, while encountering different circumstances, the user has the opportunity to manually adjust his/her precision privacy settings when needed. However, the usability of the model was not taken into consideration, and despite achieving the primary goal of dynamic privacy management, the model required too much of the users' attention in order to enable ad hoc data disclosure preferences. These issues are being addressed through the privacy models presented in the following.

Disclosure Decision Model

The privacy models discussed in the previous section present crucial disadvantages. Faces, as well as the other solutions (Jendricke et al. 2002; Kapadia et al. 2007; Myles et al. 2003), do not take into account the dynamic nature of data privacy, as they rely on preconfigured static privacy preferences. Precision Dial attempted to overcome these disadvantages by providing the opportunity for users to adjust their ad hoc data disclosure decisions. Despite achieving the goal of enabling ad hoc privacy control, Precision Dial might demand a considerable amount of users' attention and intervention, in case users continuously need to adjust their precision settings. Moreover, Precision Dial is based on four predefined levels of data disclosure, which limits the range of disclosure to a finite number of preference levels. Undeniably, such a solution does not entirely correspond to the nature of natural privacy handling, where no fixed number exists for data disclosure levels.

To address these limitations, Bünnig (2009b) suggested a privacy model called the Disclosure Decision Model (DDM), which focuses on relieving the users from frequent data disclosure decisions. Specifically, DDM can be considered an agent that manages information disclosure on behalf of the user through the process shown in Figure 24.7.

The first step of the DDM model is taken by the users, who manually set disclosure rules that are generalized privacy protection guidelines for particular circumstances. These rules are the primary determinant for the data disclosure decisions (step 2). However, if the general predetermined rules do not directly apply for a particular situation, the knowledge of DDM is taken into consideration for that particular disclosure choice (step 3). In case of a user's disagreement with the automated disclosure decision of a specific data set, the design allows a manual veto possibility, which highlights a wrong disclosure choice made by DDM (step 4). Consequently, the DDM sends to the user a rule template, which enables the user to manually deal with the current circumstances (step 5). Afterwards, the fulfilled rule template will be added to the existing set of rules, thus enabling a continuous DDM learning mechanism.

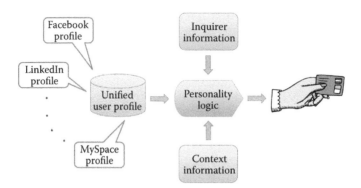

FIGURE 24.7
Disclosure Decision Model process.

In order to investigate different data mining algorithms to be applied for developing DDM, the authors asked test users to set their hypothetical privacy protection guidelines for socAmI. Subsequently, a socAmI environment was implemented and used as a test environment for simulating potential service providers requesting users' personal information (Bünnig and Cap 2009). Among data mining algorithms tested, such as rule learner, decision tree, s-nearest neighbor, support vector machine (SVM), and naive Bayes classifier, test results have indicated that naive Bayes classifier was the most suitable algorithm, as it presented the highest results, with an approximate accuracy of 95%, and potential for further increasing performance.

Diverged Personalities

Sapuppo and Sørensen (2011) introduced a privacy model, called Diverged Personalities (DiP), which attempts to address the same issues identified in the Faces and Precision Dial privacy mechanisms. DiP was originally designed for the local social network environments, as discussed in the fourth section. According to the DiP privacy model, the unified user profile is diverged into different users' personalities to be presented under different circumstances, in order to gain interpersonal benefits while facilitating safe communication in local social networks. The most suitable personality for each circumstance is generated by the process shown in Figure 24.8.

The central component of DiP is the Personality Logic. The Personality Logic receives as input the unified user profile, which is composed of a collection of a user's online profiles, stored in online social network sites. Moreover, the Personality Logic also processes the inquirer's social information (e.g., stranger, coworker, familiar stranger, friend, etc.) and environmental information (e.g., current activity, location, time, etc.). Based on these inputs, algorithms automatically provide the best personality to be shared, which can be compared to a business card that people often exchange for interpersonal benefits. When selecting the best personality to be disclosed, the Personality Logic takes into account both previous data disclosure decisions and influential factors, already identified to influence users' data disclosure decisions in previous investigations. For instance, we refer to the following influential factors, already identified to impact users' personal data disclosure decisions in ubiquitous social networking: identity of the inquirer (Davis and Gutwin 2004; Lederer et al. 2003a; Weise et al. 2011), current environment (Sapuppo 2013), activity (Jones et al. 2004; Sapuppo 2012, 2013; Sapuppo and Seet 2012), mood (Consolvo et al. 2005; Sapuppo 2013), location familiarity (Sapuppo 2012, 2013; Sapuppo and Seet 2012), purpose

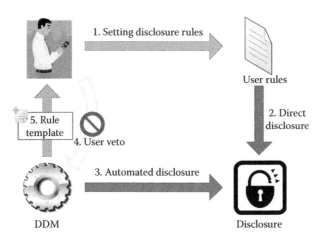

FIGURE 24.8
Diverged Personalities privacy model.

of disclosure (Consolvo et al. 2005; Sapuppo 2012, 2013), and number of previous meetings and mutual friends with the inquirer (Sapuppo 2012, 2013).

In conclusion, Sapuppo (2013) conducted quantitative research for investigating the relationship between these influential factors and ad hoc data disclosure decisions. The participants' ad hoc data disclosure decisions were collected by exploiting a ubiquitous social networking prototype. The collected data, i.e., at least 1650 data disclosure decisions per each participant, were analyzed by applying the binary logistic regression statistical model. Thus, we were capable of simulating the DiP privacy model and presenting the results about the overall proportion of cases that the binary logistic regression statistical model classified correctly. The achieved overall success of prediction is approximately 90%, with a peak accuracy of 93% and a potential for further increasing performance.

Despite the good prediction results achieved by the DDM and DiP privacy models, it was recommended that these ad hoc privacy control mechanisms limit their autonomy by providing only suggested data disclosure choices and obtaining a user's approval before any actual disclosure, in case of inquiry for highly sensitive data to be disclosed (Bünnig 2009a; Sapuppo 2013).

Conclusion

In this chapter, we have shown the need for social context awareness in AAL systems, for which socAmI is an important enabling technology. As socAmI is still a relatively new and evolving field, there is a need for the research community to understand the challenges in the development of socAmI environments. We have identified three important challenges, which are the acquisition of social context, enhancing ubiquitous social networking, and privacy protection. Thus, we have reviewed methods and technologies to acquire the social context of socAmI environment inhabitants, such as users' identities and relationships, users' activities, as well as personal users' information from online social networks. In addition, we presented architectures and technologies for enhancing social networking not only among acquaintances but also between strangers with matching interests. Finally, we identified privacy as the main threat to long-term success of socAmI, arising due to its principal goal of promoting sociability, which requires disclosure of users' personal information. Therefore, we first investigated socAmI design principles based on legal data privacy protection requirements as well as possibilities to conduct socially meaningful actions in those environments. Afterwards, we reviewed and evaluated diverse privacy protection models, focusing on ubiquitous social networking in socAmI environments. We concluded that privacy models that apply preconfigured data disclosure decisions are not suitable for representing the dynamic natural privacy handling of the users. Consequently, for socAmI environments, we recognized predominantly automated ad hoc privacy management as the most feasible privacy model, as long as highly sensitive personal information is not a part of the disclosed data set. As future work, we recommend further focus on the above three challenges with careful consideration of the aims and characteristics of the assisted living environment.

We recommend further research on acquisition of detailed social and additional environmental context for helping privacy management systems to better understand and consequently evaluate current users' circumstances. For example, we refer to the prediction of detailed social activities in highly complex situations, such as collaborative actions within groups of two or more participants.

Moreover, we suggest that designers carefully evaluate advantages and disadvantages of different software architectures, i.e., centralized and decentralized, when designing privacy protection models for ubiquitous social networking, by taking into consideration privacy guidelines and principles, reviewed in this chapter. For instance, a pure peer-to-peer approach might present advantages that would motivate users to disclose their personal information, as disclosure of personal data would only occur between end users by exactly replicating an exchange of paper business cards. However, when in close proximity, users can wirelessly exchange their personal profiles, but they cannot thereafter modify them, which might be considered a crucial disadvantage of this software architecture. On the contrary, a centralized architecture might be ideal for enabling users to modify their personal data, even after actual disclosure. In fact, the third-party entities might store users' personal data disclosure decisions to be accessed, updated, or even removed at any time. However, this kind of solution would certainly require embracing disclosure to third-party components.

Finally, following the significant results achieved by statistical models for predicting users' personal information disclosure decisions, we recommend further focus on automation of data disclosure choices. We also strongly encourage further research on updating the current design guidelines, proposed by Lederer et al. (2004). In fact, while these guidelines indisputably contribute to the target of helping designers to enable informed management of users' personal privacy in socAmI environments, they fail to enable the ease of maximizing users' potential networking possibilities while preserving their personal privacy. Consequently, there exists a need to identify other guidelines for enabling the design of more trustable and functional ubiquitous social networking services that would motivate users to share their personal data in such environments.

References

AALIANCE. 2011. Ambient assisted living roadmap. Available at http://www.aaliance.eu/public /documents/aaliance-roadmap/aaliance-aal-roadmap.pdf (accessed May 15, 2011).

Aarts, E., and Encarnacao, J. 2006. *True Visions: The Emergence of Ambient Intelligence*. Berlin: Springer.

Abowd, G. D., and Mynatt, E. D. 2000. Charting past, present, and future research in ubiquitous computing. *ACM Transactions on Computer-Human Interaction*, 7(1):29–58.

Altman, I. 1975. *The Environment and Social Behavior: Privacy, Personal Space, Territory, and Crowding.* Monterey, CA: Brooks/Cole Publishing.

Altman, I. 1977. Privacy regulation: Culturally universal or culturally specific? *Journal of Social Issues*, 33(3):66–84.

Bellotti, V., and Sellen, A. 1993. Design for privacy in ubiquitous computing environments. *Proceedings of the Third European Conference on Computer-Supported Cooperative Work*, September 1993, Milano, Italy.

Boella, G., van der Torre, L., and Villata, S. 2008. Institutional social networks for ambient intelligence. *Proceedings of the Society for the Study of Artificial Intelligence and the Simulation of Behaviour Convention: Communication, Interaction and Social Intelligence*, April 2008, Aberdeen, Scotland.

Bohn, J. et al. 2005. Social, economic, and ethical implications of ambient intelligence and ubiquitous computing. In *Ambient Intelligence*, eds. W. Weber J. M. Rabaey, and E. Aarts, 5–29. Berlin: Springer.

Boyd, D. M., and Ellison, N. B. 2008. Social network sites: Definition, history, and scholarship. *Journal of Computer Mediated Communication*, 13(1):210–230.

Brandeis, L. D., and Warren, S. D. 1890. The right to privacy. *Harvard Law Review*, 4(5):193–220.

Breslin, J. G. et al. 2009. Integrating social networks and sensor networks. *Proceedings of the W3C Workshop on the Future of Social Networking*, January 2009, Barcelona, Spain.

Bünnig, C. 2009a. Simulation and analysis of ad hoc privacy control in smart environments. *Proceedings of the International Conference on Intelligent Interactive Assistance and Mobile Multimedia Computing*, November 2009, Rostock-Warnemünde, Germany.

Bünnig, C. 2009b. Smart privacy management in ubiquitous computing environments. *Proceedings of the Symposium on Human Interface*, July 2009, San Diego, CA.

Bünnig, C., and Cap, C. H. 2009. Ad hoc privacy management in ubiquitous computing environments. *Proceedings of the Second International Conference on Advances in Human-Oriented and Personalized Mechanisms, Technologies, and Services*, September 2009, Porto, Portugal.

Calemis, I. et al. 2010. Astra: An awareness connectivity platform for designing pervasive awareness applications. In *Innovations and Advances in Computer Sciences and Engineering*, ed. T. Sobh, 185–190. Netherlands: Springer.

Campbell, A. T. et al. 2008. The rise of people-centric sensing. *IEEE Internet Computing Magazine*, 12(4):12–21.

Cohen, S. 2004. Social relationships and health. *American Psychologist*, 59:676–684.

Consolvo, S. et al. 2005. Location disclosure to social relations: Why, when & what people want to share. *Proceedings of the SIGCHI Conference on Human Factors in Computing Systems*, 81–90, ACM.

Cook, D. J. et al. 2010. Detection of social interaction in smart spaces. *Cybernetics and Systems*, 41(2):90–104.

Cornejo, R. 2010. Integrating older adults into social networking sites through ambient intelligence. *Proceedings of the 16th ACM International Conference on Supporting Group Work*, November 2010, Sanibel Island, FL.

Davis, F. D. 1989. Perceived usefulness, perceived ease of use, and user acceptance of information technology. *MIS Quarterly*, 13(3):319–340.

Davis, S., and Gutwin, C. 2004. Using relationship to control disclosure in awareness servers. *Canadian Human-Computer Communication Society*, 145–152.

de Jode, M. 2004. *Programming Java 2 Micro Edition on Symbian OS: A Developer's Guide to MIDP 2.0.* West Sussex, UK: John Wiley & Sons Ltd.

Dey, A. K., and Abowd, G. D. 2000. Towards a better understanding of context and context-awareness. *Proceedings of the CHI Workshop on: The What, Who, Where, When, and How of Context-Awareness*, April 2000, Hagel, The Netherlands.

Directive 2002/58/EC. 2002. Directive 2002/58/EC of the European Parliament and of the Council on the processing of personal data and the protection of privacy in the electronic communications sector.

Duda, R. O., Hart, P. E., and Stork, D. G. 2001. *Pattern Classification*. New York: John Wiley and Sons.

Eagle, N. 2011. Mobile phones as social sensors. In *The Handbook of Emergent Technologies in Social Research*, ed. S. N. Hesse-Biber, 492–521. New York: Oxford University Press.

Eagle, N., and Pentland, A. 2005. Social serendipity: Mobilizing social software. *IEEE Pervasive Computing Magazine*, 4(2):28–34.

Eagle, N., and Pentland, A. 2006. Reality mining: Sensing complex social systems. *Personal and Ubiquitous Computing*, 10(4):255–268.

Eddy, S. R. 1996. Hidden markov models. *Current Opinion in Structural Biology*, 6(3):361–365.

Erl, T. 2005. *Service-Oriented Architecture: Concepts, Technology, and Design*. Upper Saddle River, NJ: Prentice Hall PTR.

Goffman, E. 1978. *The Presentation of Self in Everyday Life*. Harmondsworth: Penguin.

Gupta, A., Kalra, A., Boston, D., and Borcea, C. 2009. Mobisoc: A middleware for mobile social computing applications. *Mobile Networks and Applications*, 14(1):35–52.

Han, J., and Kamber, M. 2006. Bayesian classification. *Data Mining: Concepts and Techniques*, 310–317. San Francisco, CA: Elsevier.

Hasswa, A., and Hassanein, H. 2010. Using heterogeneous and social contexts to create a smart space architecture. *Proceedings of the IEEE Symposium on Computers and Communications*, June 2010, Riccione, Italy.

Heinemann, A. 2007. *Collaboration in Opportunistic Networks: Rethinking Mobile Ad-Hoc Communication*. Saarbrücken, Germany: VDM Verlag.

Hong, J. I., Ng, J. D., Lederer, S., and Landay, J. A. 2004. Privacy risk models for designing privacy-sensitive ubiquitous computing systems. *Proceedings of the 5th Conference on Designing Interactive Systems: Processes, Practices, Methods, and Techniques*, August 2004, Cambridge, MA.

Jendricke, U., Kreutzer, M., and Zugenmaier, A. 2002. Pervasive privacy with identity management. *Proceedings of the Workshop on Security in Ubiquitous Computing*, September 2002, Göteborg, Sweden.

Johnson, P. et al. 2007. People-centric urban sensing: Security challenges for the new paradigm. Technical Report TR2007-586. Hanover, NH: Dartmouth College.

Joly, A., Maret, P., and Bataille, F. 2009. Leveraging semantic technologies towards social ambient intelligence. In *Ubiquitous and Pervasive Computing: Concepts, Methodologies, Tools, and Applications*, ed. J. Symonds, 1643–1668. Hershey, PA: IGI Global.

Jones, Q. et al. 2004. Putting systems into place: A qualitative study of design requirements for location-aware community systems. *Proceedings of the 2004 ACM Conference on Computer Supported Cooperative Work*, 202–211.

Kapadia, A., Henderson, T., Fielding, J., and Kotz, D. 2007. Virtual walls: Protecting digital privacy in pervasive environments. *Proceedings of the 5th International Conference on Pervasive Computing*, May 2007, Toronto, Canada.

Kaptein, M. C., Markopoulos, P., de Ruyter, B., and Aarts, E. 2010. Persuasion in ambient intelligence. *Journal of Ambient Intelligence and Humanized Computing*, 1(1):43–56.

Kostakos, V., and O'Neill, E. 2008. Cityware: Urban computing to bridge online and real-world social networks. In *Handbook of Research on Urban Informatics: The Practice and Promise of the Real-Time City*, ed. M. Foth, 195–204. Hershey, PA: IGI Global.

Langheinrich, M. 2001. Privacy by design—principles of privacy-aware ubiquitous systems. *Ubicomp 2001: Ubiquitous Computing*, 273–291, Springer.

Lawrence, J., Payne, T. R., and Roure, D. D. 2006. Co-presence communities: Using pervasive computing to support weak social networks. *Proceedings of the 15th IEEE International Workshops on Enabling Technologies: Infrastructure for Collaborative Enterprises*, June 2006, Manchester, UK.

Le Metayer, D. 2010. Privacy by design. In *Data Protection in a Profiled World*, ed. S. Gutwirth, 323–334. Netherlands: Springer.

Lederer, S., Mankoff, J., and Dey, A. K. 2003a. Who wants to know what when? Privacy preference determinants in ubiquitous computing. *Proceedings of the CHI Conference on Human Factors in Computing Systems*, April 2003, Fort Lauderdale, FL.

Lederer, S., Mankoff, J., Dey, A. K., and Beckmann, C. 2003b. Managing personal information disclosure in ubiquitous computing environments. Technical Report UCB/CSD-03-1257. Berkeley, CA: EECS Department, University of California.

Lederer, S., Hong, J. I., Dey, A. K., and Landay, J. A. 2004. Personal privacy through understanding and action: Five pitfalls for designers. *Personal and Ubiquitous Computing*, 8(6):440–454.

Lewis, D. 1998. Naive (Bayes) at forty: The independence assumption in information retrieval. *Proceedings of the 10th European Conference on Machine Learning*, April 1998, Chemnitz, Germany.

Li, X., Feng, L., Zhou, L., and Shi, Y. 2009. Learning in an ambient intelligent world: Enabling technologies and practices. *IEEE Transactions on Knowledge and Data Engineering*, 21(6):910–924.

Liu, Y., and Das, S. K. 2006. Information-intensive wireless sensor networks: Potential and challenges. *IEEE Communications Magazine*, 44(11):142–147.

Lu, H. et al. 2009. Soundsense: Scalable sound sensing for people-centric applications on mobile phones. *Proceedings of the 7th International Conference on Mobile Systems, Applications, and Services*, June 2009, Kraków, Poland.

Mavrommati, I., and Calemis, I. 2008. Astra awareness connectivity platform based on service oriented concepts. *Proceedings of Workshop on Architectures and Platforms on AmI*, November 2008, Nuremberg, Germany.

Milgram, S. 1977. The familiar stranger: An aspect of urban anonymity. In *The Individual in a Social World: Essays and Experiments*, eds. J. Sabini, and M. Silver, 68–71. New York: McGraw-Hill.

Miluzzo, E. et al. 2008. Sensing meets mobile social networks: The design, implementation and evaluation of the Cenceme application. *Proceedings of the 6th ACM Conference on Embedded Network Sensor Systems*, November 2008, Raleigh, NC.

Motahari, S., Manikopoulos, C., Hiltz, R., and Jones, Q. 2007. Seven privacy worries in ubiquitous social computing. *Proceedings of the 3rd Symposium on Usable Privacy and Security*, July 2007, Pittsburgh, PA.

Murty, R. et al. 2008. Citysense: A vision for an urban-scale wireless networking testbed. *Proceedings of the IEEE International Conference on Technologies for Homeland Security*, May 2008, Waltham, MA.

Musolesi, M. et al. 2008. The second life of a sensor: Integrating real-world experience in virtual worlds using mobile phones. *Proceedings of the 5th ACM Workshop on Embedded Networked Sensors*, June 2008, Charlottesville, VA.

Myles, G., Friday, A., and Davies, N. 2003. Preserving privacy in environments with location-based applications. *IEEE Pervasive Computing*, 2(1):56–64.

Nehmer, J., Becker, M., Karshmer, A., and Lamm, R. 2006. Living assistance systems: An ambient intelligence approach. *Proceedings of the 28th International Conference on Software Engineering*, May 2006, Shanghai, China.

Nicolai, T., Yoneki, E., Behrens, N., and Kenn, H. 2006. Exploring social context with the wireless rope. *Proceedings of the OTM Workshop on Mobile and Networking Technologies for Social Applications*, October 2006, Montpellier, France.

Olsevicova, K., and Mikulecky, P. 2008. Learning management systems as an ambient intelligence playground. *International Journal of Web Based Communities*, 4(3):348–358.

Palen, L., and Dourish, P. 2003. Unpacking privacy for networked world. *Proceedings of the SIGCHI Conference on Human Factors in Computing Systems*, 129–136, ACM.

Perkio, J. et al. 2006. Utilizing rich Bluetooth environments for identity prediction and exploring social networks as techniques for ubiquitous computing. *Proceedings of IEEE/WIC/ACM International Conference on Web Intelligence*, December 2006, Hong Kong, China.

Persson, P., and Jung, Y. 2005. Nokia sensor: From research to product. *Proceedings of the Conference on Designing for User eXperience*, November 2005, San Francisco, CA.

Pietilainen, A. K. et al. 2009. Mobiclique: Middleware for mobile social networking. *Proceedings of the 2nd ACM Workshop on Online Social Networks*, August 2009, Barcelona, Spain.

PRIAM. 2007. PRIAM: Privacy issues and ambient intelligence. INRIA. Available at http://priam.citi.insa-lyon.fr (assessed May 15, 2011).

Riva, G., and Gramatica, F. 2003. From stethoscope to ambient intelligence: The evolution of health-care. *International Journal of Healthcare Technology and Management*, 5(3):268–283.

Rocker, C. 2009. Acceptance of future workplace systems: How the social situation influences the usage intention of ambient intelligence technologies in work environments. *Proceedings of the 9th International Conference on Work with Computer Systems*, August 2009, Beijing, China.

Rocker, C. et al. 2010. Towards adaptive interfaces for supporting elderly users in technology-enhanced home environments. *Proceedings of the 18th Biennial Conference of the International Communications Society: Culture, Communication and the Cutting Edge of Technology*, June 2010, Tokyo, Japan.

Rook, K. S. et al. 2007. Optimizing social relationships as a resource for health and well-being in later life. In *Handbook of Health Psychology and Aging*, eds. C. M. Aldwin, C. L. Park, and A. Spiro, 267–285. New York: The Guilford Press.

Rost, M. 2010. Privacy protection in AAL systems. European Privacy Seal. Available at https://www.european-privacy-seal.eu/results/fact-sheets/Privacy Protection-in-AAL-20101022-en.pdf (assessed May 15, 2011).

Sadeh, N. et al. 2009. Understanding and capturing people's privacy policies in a mobile social networking application. *Personal and Ubiquitous Computing*, 13(6):401–412.

Sapuppo, A. 2010. Spiderweb: A social mobile network. *Proceedings of the 12th European Wireless Conference*, April 2010, Luca, Italy.

Sapuppo, A. 2012. Privacy analysis in mobile social networks: The influential factors for disclosure of personal data. *International Journal of Wireless and Mobile Computing*, 5(4):315–326.

Sapuppo, A. 2013. The influential factors for the variation of data sensitivity in ubiquitous social networking. *International Journal of Wireless and Mobile Computing*, 6(2):115–130.

Sapuppo, A., and Seet, B.-C. 2012. An empirical investigation of disclosure of personal information in ubiquitous social computing. *International Journal of Computer Theory and Engineering*, 4(3):373–378.

Sapuppo, A., and Sørensen, L. T. 2011. Local social networks. *Proceedings of the International Conference on Telecommunication Technology and Applications*, May 2011, Sydney, Australia.

Schollmeier, R. 2001. A definition of peer-to-peer networking for the classification of peer-to-peer architectures and applications. *Proceedings of the First IEEE International Conference on Peer-to-Peer Computing*, August 2001, Linkoping, Sweden.

Seeman, T. E. 1996. Social ties and health: The benefits of social integration. *Annals of Epidemiology*, 6(5):442–451.

Seet, B.-C., and Casar, J. R. 2007. Physical object search and reminding in ambient intelligent spaces. *Proceedings of Conference of the Spanish Association for Artificial Intelligence*, November 2007, Salamanca, Spain.

Streitz, N., and Nixon, P. 2005. The disappearing computer. *Communications of the ACM*, 48(3):32–35.

Toninelli, A. et al. 2010. Middleware support for mobile social ecosystems. *Proceedings of the IEEE 34th Annual Computer Software and Applications Conference Workshops*, July 2010, Seoul, Korea.

Weise, J. et al. 2011. Are you close with me? Are you nearby? Investigating social groups, closeness and willingness to share. *Proceedings of the 13th International Conference in Ubiquitous Computing*.

Weiser, M. 1995. The computer for the 21st century. *Scientific American*, 272(3):78–89.

Westin, A. F. 1967. *Privacy and Freedom*. New York: Atheneum Press.

Yee, G. 2010. Using privacy policies to protect privacy in Ubicomp. *Proceedings of the 19th IEEE International Conference on Advanced Information Networking and Applications*, April 2010, Perth, Australia.

Youngblood, M., Cook, D. J., and Holder, L. B. 2005. Seamlessly engineering a smart environment. *Proceedings of the IEEE International Conference on Systems, Man and Cybernetics*, October 2005, Hawaii.

25

WeCare: Cooperating with Older People in the Design and Evaluation of Online Social Networking Services

Marc Steen, Mari Ervasti, Marja Harjumaa, Sarah Bourke,
Victor Hernandez, Marlou Min, and Sharon Prins

CONTENTS

ABSTRACT   The WeCare project focused on improving older people's well-being by enabling them to engage in online social networking and thus promoting social interaction and participation. Participation in social networks, both online and *in real life*, is intended to help them to stay in touch with family and friends and to meet new people. The project involved industry partners, care or service providers, and research institutes from four countries: Finland, Spain, Ireland, and the Netherlands. For each country, a human-centered design approach was followed, in which an online social networking service was developed through codesign and evaluated in older people's daily lives through user trials, both in close cooperation with different groups of users. Four different services were developed in order to match different user groups' needs and usage contexts. More specifically, the codesign process and user trials involved older people (*primary users*) and people in their social networks and professional caregivers (*secondary users*). In this chapter, we discuss the codesign process, which involved interviews and creative workshops, and the user trials, which involved observations, interviews, and surveys. Based on our findings in the WeCare project, we articulated recommendations for the development and implementation of social networking services for older people.

KEY WORDS: *older people, social networking, well-being, codesign, user trials, recommendations.*

Introduction

People, especially in more developed countries, get older than ever before. This, however, does not always mean that expectations for a happy life improve as well. For example, loneliness seems to increase and many people live alone. New information and communication technology (ICT) possibilities may offer opportunities to combat loneliness and hence improve the number of *quality-adjusted life years* of older people. A longitudinal study on loneliness and contact with friends, by Holmén and Furukawa (2002), shows a downward trend of *contact with friends* and *perceived health* as people age. Moreover, social interaction is assumed to positively affect health (Seeman 1996; Helliwell and Putnam 2004; Golden et al. 2009).

The goal of the WeCare project was to enable older people to participate in social networking, both online and face-to-face, in order to empower them to improve their well-being. The working hypothesis was that participation of older people in social networks, both online and *in real life*, helps them to stay in touch with family and friends, and to come in contact with new people, and thereby enables them to improve their well-being. The aim was to encourage older people to participate in social networks and to continue to participate in these when they age. If they are active in social networks before ill health or other problems arise, they can help each other. This approach will improve older people's autonomy so that they can live at home longer, which enhances their quality of life. Furthermore, the people who provide family care or informal care can share tasks among each other or have peer support, which prevents them from *burning out*. As a result of these two developments, the demand for professional care and social services will decrease.

The WeCare Project

Four online social networking services were developed, evaluated, and implemented in the WeCare project. The services are tailor-made for the four different contexts in Finland, Spain, Ireland, and the Netherlands, in close cooperation with older people and organizations that represent older people.

The WeCare services offer communication, coordination, and information applications, which older people can use together with family and friends, and with people in their neighborhoods, for example, based on shared interests or shared activities. The services include easy-to-use applications for social communication, such as video communication or discussion forums, and applications to coordinate social activities, such as shared calendars and ways to request or offer support. In the development of these applications, special care is given to ease of use and privacy. The project views ICT as a means toward an end: to empower people to live more happily.

In each country, a codesign process was organized in close cooperation with users and user organizations, and different services were developed for different contexts, target groups, and goals. Moreover, pilot projects and user trials were organized in each country to evaluate the services, including the underlying technologies and business models.

In each of the four participating countries, an organization that represented older people participated in the project:

- *Finland*: Caritas-Säätiö, a provider of care services
- *Spain*: FASS, which later merged into ASSDA, a provider of care services
- *Ireland*: the Irish Farmers Association (IFA)
- *The Netherlands*: ANBO, an older people's organization, and HWW, a provider of care services

The WeCare project was organized as *open innovation*, as *multidisciplinary teamwork*, and as an *iterative process*. The term *open innovation* (Chesbrough 2003) refers to organizing innovation processes in ways that enable the sharing of ideas and knowledge between organizations. The WeCare project is an example of open innovation because diverse project partners cooperated in it: technology- and application-oriented industry partners Videra (Finland), Skytek (Ireland), Ericsson, and Simac/ShareCare (the Netherlands); care and service providers Caritas-Säätiö (Finland) and ASSDA (Spain); user organizations the IFA and ANBO (the Netherlands); and research organizations VTT (Finland), I2BC (Spain), and TNO (the Netherlands).

Furthermore, the project was based on *multidisciplinary teamwork* in that people from different disciplines and with different perspectives cooperated in the project (e.g., technology, social science, design). The project was organized in four work packages (WPs) that cooperated closely with each other: user involvement and codesign (WP1); technology development (WP2); prototyping and piloting (WP3); and the development of business models (WP4).

Moreover, the project was organized as an *iterative process*, with iterations of research, design, and evaluation, which enabled project team members to better understand users' practices, needs, and preferences, and to explore, develop, and evaluate solutions. These iterations facilitated trying out and learning, especially by organizing codesign processes and user trial pilots in close cooperation with prospective users.

This chapter's goal is to share our experiences and findings. Below, we will discuss the ways in which project team members cooperated with older people during the design and evaluation of a series of online social networking services. The goal of these discussions is to better understand how to organize such cooperation in such ways that both the users—in our cases, older people—and the project team members can benefit from these interactions.

In the section "Codesign," we will discuss the codesign process and its results, and in the section "User Trials," the user trials and their findings will be discussed. This chapter closes by articulating a range of practical recommendations for the development and implementation of social networking services for older people (in the section "Recommendations").

More information about the WeCare project can be found at the website http://www .wecare-project.eu.

Codesign

The involvement of potential users during research and design was critical to the success of the project. The project followed a human-centered design (HCD) approach, which can be characterized using four principles (ISO 1999): (1) involving prospective users in research, design, and evaluation in order to better understand their experiences, needs, and preferences; (2) finding an appropriate allocation of functions between users and technology; (3) organizing productive iterations of research, design, and evaluation; and (4) organizing multidisciplinary teamwork throughout the project.

HCD aims to promote cooperation with users or customers during research, design, and evaluation activities, with the goal to jointly develop innovations that better match people's needs and preferences. In HCD, *users* are not seen as passive recipients but as active participants and creative contributors to research and design activities (Steen 2011, 2012, 2013).

In order to profit optimally from users' knowledge and ideas, the older people that participated in the WeCare project were treated as *experts of their experience* (Sleeswijk-Visser et al. 2005); they participated on the basis of being experts on their own daily life experiences and their knowledge about their practical needs and preferences. The project team members aimed to develop the WeCare services *together with* them, rather than *for* them. (In the Finnish user trial, several older people were unable to participate in the HCD activities themselves due to their physical challenges; in those cases, their nurses represented them in order to also represent their user requirements.)

Below, we discuss the codesign activities in the four countries: their contexts, target groups, and goals, as well as their user involvement activities and the services that were developed.

Finland

In Finland, the team members followed an iterative process in which interviews and workshops were organized by Caritas-Säätiö and VTT. Care personnel at Caritas were actively involved, also as a way to represent those older people that were unable to effectively participate in interviews or workshops.

The Finnish pilot was organized in cooperation with end-user organization Caritas, technology provider Videra, and research organization VTT. The study aimed at designing both a service and a product, and thus, the users were involved in the process in several phases.

The pilot environment in Finland was provided by Caritas: a not-for-profit organization that provides assisted living and rehabilitation services. The service offerings of Caritas cover a range of services for older or disabled people. In this study, the focus was on *rehabilitation service*. Rehabilitation is seen as a core enabler for tackling problems related to loneliness and isolation, as it can address problems from physical mobility to cognitive and psychological issues. Currently, the care service concept is based purely on face-to-face meeting and other arranged activities that require physical meetings. Caritas wishes to expand this service concept with virtual connection between the participants of the rehabilitation, their caretakers, close ones, and the professional contacts provided by Caritas and other interest groups. The goal is to expand the existing service concept to better address the long-term needs of the users and better integrate the rehabilitation service with the everyday lives of the users.

The starting point for the service development in Finland is the Videra Caring TV, which allows both the sender and the recipient to see and hear each other simultaneously via a two-way video link. The system is especially designed for older users, and it can be used for communicating, for example, with health care professionals or social workers. The goal is to provide different digital services for older people with the help of this technology and to support their independent living. Videra Caring TV also allows older people to communicate with each other and to participate in diverse interactive programs, such as exercise classes, interactive conversations, expert lectures, and other health-promoting services. Videra Caring TV allows older people to stay in touch with their children who may live far away. Family members can have Caring TV installed on, for example, a laptop computer.

The customers of rehabilitation services are a challenging user group regarding technology design and adoption. They are usually aged, handicapped, or ill people, whose abilities have been reduced, and they normally receive care from their informal caregivers, i.e., their family members or other intimate persons. However, sometimes they receive care temporarily at the rehabilitation services. Many of them have little or no experience with computers, and they may have difficulties in imagining how such a technology could help them or how they could use it themselves. It is assumed that besides the customers of rehabilitation services, their relatives and the personnel of Caritas will also be using the service.

Since the project followed an HCD approach, the project team members did not make a detailed design at the start of the project. However, they did have ideas for what the service would look like, how it would work, and how it would help older people to evolve their social lives. The service and its functionalities evolved in an iterative process of design, evaluation, and development.

The personnel and customers of Caritas have been in a strategic position in the design, and the personnel of the technology provider and researchers have provided their experience and knowledge as well, aiming to realize all requirements put by the participants. Requirements were formulated through an extensive series of interviews and workshops.

The basis for the service has been the Videra Caring TV video communication system, which was needed to optimally match with the existing services of Caritas (see Figure 25.1).

There was intensive cooperation between project team members (both researchers and developers) and users (both older people and nurses). In the course of the project, there were five interviews and twelve meetings, and two user studies. This was done in an iterative process. In a first iteration, the one-to-one video chat feature was evaluated in the context of the respite care service. The goal was to evaluate whether video communication during respite care would alleviate the separation anxiety that was experienced sometimes by the informal caregiver, sometimes the person in need for care, and sometimes by both of them.

The evaluation showed that the WeCare service was very easy to use, both for the frail and older users. However, challenges were identified in integrating the service into the care processes. A second iteration extended the video communication feature of the WeCare service by broadcasting functionality. The broadcasting functionality extends Caritas group activities by broadcasting the event through video to those users who are at home or at another facility of Caritas.

The HCD activities had the following effects, in chronological order, on the process of idea generation and service development:

- Understanding respite care and older people, e.g., their characteristics and limitations
- Understanding the role of technology in practice, e.g., its possibilities and limitations

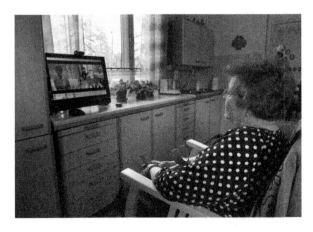

FIGURE 25.1
A participant in the Finnish user trial using the WeCare service of Caritas-Säätiö.

- List of functionalities that would be needed, e.g., to call other people and to follow broadcasts
- Understanding nurses that work in respite care, e.g., their attitudes toward technology
- Understanding of needs and ideas development, e.g., no need for phone book, need for content developed by Caritas, need for training of nurses, customers, and relatives, and communication with them about the service
- Changing the setting: from using the service in respite care (which proved to be too challenging for service adoption) to using the service at home (with broadcasts to people's homes)
- Ideas for the user interface design, e.g., phone book and feedback, and the idea to personalize the user interface for each individual user, and other ideas, e.g., for user-generated content and integration with occupational therapy

The main findings of HCD and effects on idea generation and service development were the following:

- User requirements and specifications for the service based on interactions with older people, nurses, and other staff
- The decision to focus no longer on usage in the context of respite care, but on usage in the context of people's homes
- Knowledge about which functionalities are or are not needed, and knowledge about which user interface design solutions will or will not work

Spain

The HCD process in Spain involved two user trials: iVillage and iOrganization. In the iVillage concept, a local community can share local information fostering social interaction among them. In the iOrganization concept, the social networking service is integrated into a care service that is targeted to older people. Both concepts have been explored.

The Institute of Innovation for Human Well-being (i2BC) organized an iVillage pilot in Lebrija (a medium-size town near Seville), with the support of the town hall and other local organizations. Traditionally, the main economic activities in Lebrija have been related to the agricultural sector and the construction sector—however, both sectors will probably not have enough capacity to support Lebrija's economy. Additionally, Lebrija is facing the consequences of a social and economic crisis, which, together with the demographic changes related to the aging of the population, leads to an increase in the unemployment rate, as well as early retired elderly adults. The end users of the WeCare service in Lebrija will be elderly adults, of ages ranging from 55 to 65 years old, with no relevant health problems. In this context, the goal of WeCare in Lebrija is to promote active aging by improving social participation and allowing elderly people to be active members in their communities—not only passive subjects or beneficiaries but also productive members. Prevention is also another benefit, since users can obtain more benefit from it, when they will need to be cared for later on.

The Andalusian Foundation for Social Services (FASS, which later merged into ASSDA) organized an iOrganization pilot in Malaga and Seville. FASS/ASSDA is the provider of the Andalusian Telecare Service, a system of customized attention, providing immediate response to emergency situations or insecurity, loneliness, and isolation, based on new communication technologies. This system also enables users to be reached by phone. The participants' profiles of this pilot correspond to people who are over 65 years old. They are also users of the Andalusian Telecare Service, and many of them are currently suffering from dependency, loneliness, and social isolation. The goals of the iOrganization pilot are twofold: to introduce users to the world of new technologies, which will not only provide possibilities to enhance their quality of life but can also provide a means of personal fulfillment, and to test the feasibility of introducing an ambient assisted living service like WeCare in an organization like the FASS.

The iVillage (Lebrija) and iOrganization (Málaga and Seville) user trials did follow a relatively traditional approach of not only bringing users to the laboratory and asking them what they needed but also moving researchers to the real contexts, where they can observe the older people and these people's daily lives' contexts. In Lebrija, a two-day event was organized, including general participatory talks in which citizens discussed their social status, daily life problems, and (nontechnological) needs in the areas of education, health, or well-being. Next, several associations and citizens were recruited to participate in the project, and a collaborative atmosphere was created to discover their problems and needs. A similar session was organized by FASS, inviting some of their users for breakfast. During this session, a WeCare demo was presented and discussed, and a first group of users was recruited for the user trial.

The needs and preferences of older people were investigated by means of interviews, by focus groups, by direct observation of participants' daily lives, and via desk research. The information collected was used together with service requirements to articulate user requirements and to define the components to be included in the WeCare service. These requirements include information about what kind of applications they need and would like to use in order to promote their social lives by participating in community activities and fostering the exchange of cultural experiences and hobbies. Furthermore, participants in the user trials received an initial training session to learn the basic functionalities. During this session, some initial comments and difficulties are collected in order to improve the WeCare service in future design iterations.

The WeCare system used for the pilots in Spain (iVillage and iOrganization) is an Internet portal that includes several components: profile management, news, events' calendar, neighbors, and medical reminder. Using these different applications, people can share and comment on user-generated content, organize events, match other users with similar interests, or use reminders to recall medication schedule.

The HCD process in Spain involved 25 interviews with citizens in Lebrija, 3 codesign sessions with FASS/ASSDA clients/users and stakeholders, and 3 project meetings and weekly meetings with software developers.

The basis for the service has been the combination of components that were developed in cooperation among Ericsson, Skytek, and Simac/ShareCare, and the integration of the new service into the existing telecare services of FASS/ASSDA (see Figure 25.2).

The main contributions of HCD to idea generation and service development were the following:

- Prioritizing different functionalities, e.g., news, events, and reminder modules were found more relevant than forum and chat.

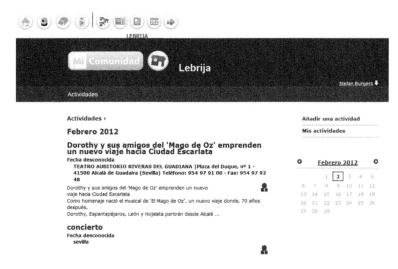

FIGURE 25.2
Screenshot of the Spanish version of the WeCare service, deployed by ASSDA.

- User requirements, focusing on the ease of use of the platform and its different functionalities.
- Additional requirements for further improving some of the functionalities, e.g., *closed* and *open* groups, links between events and reminders, and reminder used more generically (rather than only for medicines).

Ireland

In Ireland, the WeCare service is targeted at Irish farmers over 55 years of age in order to ascertain whether this system can help to combat loneliness and isolation in older Irish people. At present, in Ireland there are 130,000 Irish farmers receiving the single farm payment. There are 65,000 farmers on the combined Early Retirement Scheme and the Rural Environmental Protection Scheme (REPS). The IFA has over 21,250 members aged over 65 who live in rural isolated locations all over Ireland. The IFA has a website called iFarm.ie, which is actively used by the younger farming community but not by the older farming community. Furthermore, the iFarm system provides a means for the IFA to communicate with their members and for the members to request information from the IFA, but it does not focus on the social interaction of the members with each other or with the provision of support services such as social care.

The IFA wished to address the issue of rural isolation among older farmers using WeCare 2.0 in conjunction with iFarm. The IFA saw this as an opportunity to encourage older, less computer-literate farmers to use technology as a means of communication and as part of their daily activities and also as part of a larger farming community. The IFA wanted to offer WeCare 2.0 to the entire farming community, enabling farmers both young and old to develop a *buddy system* where tips, advice, and help can be exchanged. Home computers will be used to test the system in people's homes during these trials. In addition, the system was tested on Android portable devices and on iPads. The trials were organized in Co Kilkenny and Co Louth, both of which are involved in a government initiative called *Age Friendly Counties*. The objective of this program is to increase the participation of older people in the social, economic, and cultural life of the community for everyone's benefit and to improve the health and well-being of older people in the county.

Initially, development officers of the IFA in each county profiled members aged over 55 years who were active participants in the IFA and who might be interested in being participants in the project and trials. The development officers made a list of potential participants in each county and approached them with the idea. Once they received positive feedback, they sent the results to the customer services department in the IFA Head Office. IFA customer services then further interviewed each potential participant and asked them whether they currently use a computer or laptop, whether they have an Internet connection, whether they use a mobile phone, and whether they would like to participate in the trial. If the response to these questions was positive, then the participant was invited to join a focus group, in which they viewed and evaluated the WeCare service. They were very positive about the system, especially about the social networking applications. They found the system easy to use on an iPad and on an Android smartphone. The majority of farmers who came to the focus group decided to participate in the trials. Some farmers decided not to proceed because of hardware or Internet connection issues. Ten older Irish farmers from Co Kilkenny and Co Louth made up the initial trial test group.

The HCD process in Ireland was relatively focused, and relatively fast, and was based upon a close cooperation between Skytek and the IFA. Potential users were recruited among farmers. They were interviewed and then invited to participate in a focus group to evaluate the WeCare service. Many of them participated in user trials, in which they practically used and evaluated the WeCare service. HCD has helped to practically and quickly evaluate project team members' ideas and to practically and quickly modify and improve the service.

The basis for service development has been the combination and integration of several relevant components into an easy-to-use *portal* that offers general communication (VoIP phone), general information (sports, news), relevant information for farmers (weather and markets), and an application for farmers (in cooperation with Agfood, i.e., for payments and applications). Furthermore, the service has been made available on mobile devices and tablet computers (see Figure 25.3).

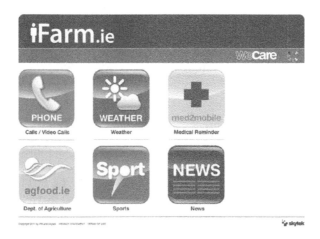

FIGURE 25.3
Screenshot of the Irish version of the WeCare service, suitable for tablet computers.

The Netherlands

In the Netherlands, the WeCare service was piloted among older people living independently in their own home in Escamp, a part of the city of The Hague. Escamp consists of several neighborhoods. The housing and population of Escamp are diverse and range from apartment buildings and houses built before World War II, which are typically owned by housing corporations and which house relatively many older people and relatively many people from an ethnic minority background, to modern houses and apartment buildings, which are typically owned by younger people and young families. Escamp has 113,000 inhabitants (The Hague, 500,000 total). The primary user group is defined as independently living older people, and the secondary user group is defined as these older people's family members, friends, and informal caregivers.

ANBO and TNO interviewed 28 older people and their informal caregivers to better understand their situation, and their needs and wishes regarding a service like WeCare. Four of them participated in codesign sessions in which they spoke about their needs and preferences and actively contributed to the articulation of user requirements for the WeCare service.

A group of ten people participated in the user trial. These people were recruited and invited by a local chapter of ANBO, in close cooperation with HWW, an organization that provides formal care at people's homes. HWW was interested in experimenting with ICT services as possible supplements to their current services. In several cases, the older person was supported by their children and/or informal caregivers to use the WeCare service. Some older people also received formal care from HWW, in which case these formal caregivers were also involved in the pilot. People's experiences were evaluated during the pilot, involving both the older people themselves (primary target group) and their family members, friends, and/or formal caregivers (secondary target group).

The service development process started with project team members' ideas on a service that would help older people to communicate with others, in social networks, both online and *in real life*. These ideas were based on earlier and similar research projects, and were further developed, evaluated, and modified in an iterative process, in close cooperation with several older people: First, several older people (*expert users*) were interviewed. Next several other older people (*expert users*) participated in a creative workshop, in which we jointly further developed and modified these ideas (see Figure 25.4).

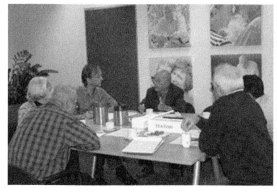
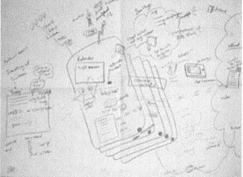

FIGURE 25.4
Creative session with older people, in the Netherlands, in cooperation with ANBO.

The findings from interviews and workshop were the basis for the user requirements and the user interface design, which were discussed in a series of six project team meetings. In these meetings, the project team members that had been involved in the interviews and creative workshop represented older people and their needs and preferences (*user advocates*). The HCD activities were especially valuable for choosing and further developing the key functionalities, for articulating user requirements (which were also used for the Spanish version of the WeCare service), for developing ideas for the user interface design, and for improving the usability of the service (see Figure 25.5).

Discussion and Conclusions

It is interesting to see that the HCD process was organized differently in the different countries. These differences were anticipated because the contexts are different in the different countries:

- In Finland, the WeCare service was developed in close cooperation between care provider Caritas-Säätiö, technology provider Videra, and research organization VTT. The service was based on a video communication system, which was integrated into existing care services, through an iterative, hands-on process in close cooperation with Caritas personnel. HCD helped to articulate user requirements and specifications for the service, to make the decision to switch focus in the context of usage (from respite care to people's homes), and to develop and fine-tune easy-to-use functionalities and user interface design solutions.

- In Spain, the WeCare service was developed in cooperation with research organization i2BC, care service provider FASS/ASSDA, and technology-oriented

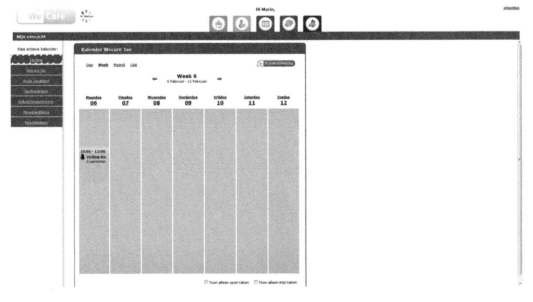

FIGURE 25.5
Screenshot of the Dutch version of the WeCare service, with shared online calendars.

project partners Ericsson, Skytek, and Simac/ShareCare. Groups of citizens were interviewed, codesign sessions with FASS/ASSDA clients and stakeholders were organized, and the service was developed iteratively, through weekly meetings with software developers. The service was integrated into the current services of FASS/ASSDA. HCD helped to prioritize different functionalities, to focus on ease of use of the service, and to further improve several functionalities.

- In Ireland, the WeCare service was developed in a relatively focused and fast process through close cooperation between technology developer Skytek and users'/farmers' organization IFA. Potential users were recruited and interviewed. Several participated in a focus group and then in user trials. The basis of the service has been the combination and integration of several components into an easy-to-use *portal*. This *portal* has also been made available on mobile devices, such as tablet computers. HCD helped to practically and quickly evaluate and modify project team members' initial ideas and improve the service.

- In the Netherlands, the service development process started with project team members' ideas. These ideas were further developed, evaluated, and modified iteratively, involving interviews and a creative workshop with older people—and a series of project team meetings, in which older people's perspectives were represented by project team members. HCD helped to better understand older people and their needs and preferences, to develop user requirements and user interface design solutions, and to provide input to the service development process on older people's needs and preferences on a continuous basis.

One may note that in all cases, older people were actually involved in the process. One may also note that in all cases, other people—not only older people—helped to represent older people or contributed in other ways to the service development process:

- In Finland, Caritas personnel, especially nurses, represented several older people who were unable to participate and provided input for integrating WeCare into existing services.

- In Spain, people within FASS/ASSDA also had a stake and an important say in the process of service development and in integrating the service into the existing services.

- In Ireland, people from the IFA represented users' perspectives and contributed to the organizing of the user trials and service development.

- In the Netherlands, people from research organization TNO and user organization ANBO (who had been involved in interviews and workshops with older people), represented older people during the development of user requirements and user interface solutions.

Involvement of not only the *users* but also of other people that represent *users* is in line with an HCD approach. In the ISO 13407 standard for HCD (ISO 1999), it is advised to organize multidisciplinary teamwork that includes a *variety of skills* and *range of personnel*: users, and also, for example, application domain specialists, systems engineers and programmers, marketers and salespersons, user interface designers, human–computer interaction specialists, trainers, and support personnel.

Furthermore, one may note that in all cases, there were already ideas for the service to be developed and ideas to further develop systems or applications that were already available:

- In Finland, the idea was to use the Videra video communication system and to modify it so that it matches the Caritas services.
- In Spain, the idea was to choose several relevant modules from the current services of Simac/ShareCare (*Care Site* and *Neighbourhood Site*; partly after service development process in the Netherlands, chronologically).
- In Ireland, the idea was to combine and cleverly integrate several relevant components into an easy-to-use *portal*, specifically for farmers.
- In the Netherlands, the idea was to further develop and modify several relevant modules from the current services of Simac/ShareCare (*Care Site* and *Neighbourhood Site*) (so that Spain could choose from these modules, after service development in the Netherlands).

Again, there is nothing inherently good or bad with starting with an idea in HCD. The advantage of starting with an idea is that the project can have more focus. A risk of starting with an idea is that *users* have less influence on the idea generation process and can *only* contribute to service development: to the modification and further improvement of ideas into services. *Only* is between quotes because this is indeed not a small contribution. However, this risk has been mitigated by carefully examining the initial ideas and assumptions at the start of the process, both by conducting desk research and by conducting interviews, observations, and workshops with older people, in order to evaluate and validate these initial ideas and assumptions. Moreover, and probably most importantly, this risk was mitigated by fostering an open attitude among project team members toward older people throughout the entire HCD process, which allowed for learning and for adopting and modifying their ideas and assumptions, e.g., the decision, in Finland, to focus the project on another context of usage, based on interactions with users.

In summary, the HCD processes have been organized appropriately and differently in the different countries and have resulted in different, relevant, and easy-to-use services. The services that were developed optimally match the different contexts (e.g., iOrganization, iVillage) and the needs and preferences of the different types of older people (e.g., frail clients of care services or independently living farmers).

We found that following an HCD approach, e.g., by organizing interviews or workshops, was especially helpful and had added value for the following purposes:

- Understanding users' contexts, needs, and preferences, as a basis for joint idea generation and for screening of ideas
- Steering service development, e.g., making the decision to focus on another context of usage, based upon knowledge about people's needs
- Prioritizing and choosing between different functionalities, based on knowledge about which functionalities are or are not needed by users
- Choosing between and further developing user interface design solutions, based on knowledge about which will or will not work for users
- Further detailing and improving functionalities and user interface solutions, based upon user input and feedback

User Trials

In order to validate the WeCare services in actual use, and to evaluate the benefits and challenges related to the service, field trials were organized. Both quantitative and qualitative data were gathered in the evaluation, and various methods were used, including interviews, questionnaires, user observation, and collection of system log data. Some key figures of the user trials are summarized in Table 25.1.

A common evaluation framework was developed in order to monitor and evaluate each pilot site outcome and impact. In each trial, the following issues were measured:

1. Well-being and loneliness
2. User experience
3. Expectations (before user trials)
4. Perceived value (after user trials)
5. Expected value versus perceived value
6. Usability and accessibility (during and after user trials)
7. Social networks (before and after user trials)
8. Usage information

The findings related to aforementioned research topics are discussed next, also per country, for each of the four countries.

Well-Being and Loneliness

The WeCare project has aimed to improve the quality of life and well-being of older people, preventing them from suffering loneliness and isolation by using an Internet service that reinforces their social networks. In this sense, some relationships are assumed between users' experience with the technology and improvements in users' daily life. The hypothesis is that the use of the WeCare Internet service will reduce loneliness feelings and isolation of older users that subsequently will impact positively on perceived quality of life and well-being.

The experiences of well-being and loneliness were measured using a questionnaire before and after the trial. For the measurement and analysis of well-being data in WeCare, we adopted the well-being module from the European Social Survey (ESS). ESS has collected a vast amount of well-being data over Europe (Huppert et al. 2009). For the WeCare project, the phrasing of some of the questions was changed, questions were omitted,

TABLE 25.1

Key Figures of User Trials

Country	Schedule	Number of Users	Average Age
Finland	April 2011–Jan 2012	13 (9 older people, 4 relatives)	72 (81 among older users)
Ireland	April–May 2011	10	65
The Netherlands	Sept 2011–Jan 2012	9	75
Spain	Sept–Oct 2011	19 (10 older people, 9 mediators)	48 (58 among older users)

questions were added, and the order of the questions was changed. In addition, questions related to loneliness were added.

Loneliness can be considered as the perceived isolation of a certain person. Feeling loneliness is not equal to being alone, but includes feelings of isolation, disconnectedness, and not belonging. For its measurement in WeCare, the Three-Item Loneliness Scale, a short questionnaire constructed and validated by Hughes et al. (2004), was adopted.

However, because the trial exposures of all test subjects were not equal, and also the data were collected a bit differently in different counties (users were not able to fill in questionnaires by themselves, but the questions were asked as interview questions), data could not be used for proper statistical analysis. Also, because the number of users was relatively small, no significant results were found.

User Experience

In this study, an evaluation framework was defined in order to guide the data collection of the researchers. Our criteria were that the framework should be easy to comprehend and adopt by all researchers and it should apply to all research activities, including user studies and field trials. Our goal was not to build a comprehensive research framework but to select a group of parameters that would match with our practical need to solve the research question. The goal of this study was to understand the users' interaction with the technology using a holistic user experience approach.

Finland

The experiences of the home users were quite positive. The touch screen device was easy to adopt and use, the basic functionalities of one-to-one communication and broadcasting services for people at home provided value for the users, there were not any major obstacles that would have hindered technology use, and the technology had a positive influence on the social relationships of the participants. Two functionalities were most valued by the home users: (1) one-to-one communication with the families and relatives, and (2) service broadcasts. In one-to-one communication, participants valued the video image, which provided added value compared to other communication methods. Group communication functionality was barely used. However, it was observed that people used the WeCare technology for group communication; they joined the broadcast a while before the actual show started, and thus they had some time to share their thoughts. This was found to be meaningful for them.

Ireland

During the trial, participants found the WeCare service very useful, with some users establishing an increased interest in technology as a result of the service. Following the user trial, all participants felt that the WeCare service was beneficial, particularly in a rural context and that the service fulfilled or even exceeded their expectations. Overall, the users were impressed by the reliable and real-time information that the service was capable of providing, with the weather and news applications proving especially helpful. Some participants experienced Internet connectivity issues, which also affected connectivity to Skype, occasionally. Although all modules were used by the trial participants, the news, weather, and Skype components were most popular. The weather feature was particularly effective for forecasting and planning farming activities days in advance. The news component was popular among the participants who wished to be updated with real-time information during *out-of-coverage* times of the day, and the Skype feature was popular among the majority of trial participants, particularly those with family and friends living abroad.

The Netherlands

The users were generally optimistic on the ease of use of the service. They understood the main features and enjoyed trying them out. Their motivation for testing the service came from extrinsic motivators. They enjoyed testing the service because they felt it important having been chosen to test a product especially designed for older people. But they did not feel like the service was designed for them. In retrospect, the most liked part of the service was the contact list. Several people used it to call or email friends and family. In the beginning, people expected much of the forum functionality. They hoped to share hobbies and discussions there. But there was little activity in posting on the forum, due to the relatively small user group, which had not enough *critical mass*, which made it a relatively dull part of the site. When asked why they did not use the forum, they explained that they felt no use in typing messages to people they did not know or had seen only once. But they did regret there was no activity there. So they would have liked an active forum, but they found it hard to initiate activity and participate themselves.

Spain

The two most used features of the WeCare service were the news and events components. Participants claimed that the most appreciated functionalities of the service were those allowing them to be updated and in touch with their communities. It is important to notice that the WeCare system was perceived by participants not as a personal communication tool (e.g., between me and other or others) but as a tool for communication within a community (e.g., between me and the whole community). In this sense, the service was more easily adopted by those participants with an existing active role in the community, which encouraged others to be also active members.

Expectations (before User Trials)

We define *expected value* as the expectations that the user has regarding the technology or the service before usage. The user might not be able to describe the expectations, but probably they have a problem or a need that they think that the service is suitable for.

Finland

In Finland, home users were mainly expecting to receive a novel communication channel that they would be able to use despite their various functional limitations—a channel that would also entail a visual connection: "It would feel nice if I would be able to learn to use this." They also expected the service to bring emotional value for them: "This would provide a nice pastime"; "This cheers up an old person"; "You now get revived when you start using this (the service) from the morning." Home users were also expecting the service to bring stimulation and epistemic value by giving an older person a chance to learn new skills. People were also expecting the service to bring the value of belonging: "Could this somehow bring us closer?"; "It's could be good to know what is happening (in close ones' lives)." They also expected the service to bring safety value in terms of increased feeling of security and freedom from fear: "You will see if the things are alright on the other side." One user also proposed that the home care could utilize the system for providing their services, and they could, for example, call and "give directions for taking the right medicine from looking at the medicine package." Informal caregivers experienced that the service would be especially valuable and useful for their spouses, the persons they are caring for: "My spouse will get the connection; hopefully they will find new friends with whom they will be able to make a connection."

Ireland

Before the trial commenced, the Irish participants were looking forward to using the WeCare service. Many saw it as an opportunity to improve their Internet and computer literacy skills and also as a way of advancing their communication ability through the use of Skype. Some of the users had family and friends living abroad and considered the Skype feature as a valuable aspect of the service. In particular, the farmers were eager to engage with the weather and also the market application, as these were considered by them as the most important and relevant features regarding their occupation.

The Netherlands

At the start of the trial, we asked the participants in the Netherlands what they expected of the WeCare service. Below we summarize some of the expectations of the users:

- An easy medium to contact all relatives.
- The calendar gives my daughter and sons the ability to look where I am, so they don't come to visit me in vain.
- A nice start page on the Internet.
- A good way to get to know more people in the neighborhood.
- A nice way to find people to do some activity with, e.g., walking, cycling, card games.
- A medium to keep family and friends updated on my activities, traveling, going out.
- It is a nice way to get more used to Internet and computers in general.
- "I like to know what's new on the market."

Spain

In order to identify the users' expectations regarding the service, two sessions were organized with the older users and the mediators. Some of the expectations were as follows:

- Services for the Lebrija community
- Support network for informal caregivers, in order to cope with their social isolation
- Added value in comparison with generic social networking services (e.g., additional services specialized in health, quality of life, active aging, and so on)

- A network for exchanging and sharing resources (e.g., assistive technologies or wheel chairs)
- News service intended for the Lebrija community
- A medium to distribute health and social support to the community beyond personal assistance
- A way to give value to the "life experience" of older people (e.g., a retired teacher telling their experiences and giving advice on how to face retirement)

Perceived Value (after User Trials)

We define "perceived value" as something that is composed of the perceived, subjective experience of the user in interaction with the service and technology (Isomursu et al. 2010). The value is not determined by the functionalities of the service but instead by the advantage that the user gets by using the service and the positive consequences and impact related to the user's own meaningful goals in life. Value is a result of a process where the service provider and the end user work together (value co-creation). The perceived value was studied by interviewing the user and observing what the service does for the end user, and how the user is able to use the service for the goals that they find important, and evaluating how likely the user would like to buy and use the service outside the pilot.

Finland

The home users reported that they were very satisfied and pleased with the service. Users especially experienced added value through the visual communication. Especially in the case of two families, the service also brought value to the informal caregivers in the form of providing value for their spouses, the persons they were caring for: "When I have gone away (when she is, e.g., doing home chores, or when her spouse is at temporal care) it has provided pleasure (for her spouse)." Service usage also provided the value of freedom for the informal caregivers. The service seemed to also bring safety value: "We have discussed issues related to medication and also other important things." People also experienced that through the chair exercises provided through the service broadcasts, they were now exercising more than they would without the device: "Considering the exercises, this device has been useful for us"; "We wouldn't have exercised this much (without the device)"; and "If you exercise by yourself, it remains short. It is good that there is this separate time reserved for exercising."

For the caregivers, it was rewarding to learn to use the service and to teach others to use it. The person who was mostly in charge of the project reported that it had been easy to introduce the service to others and show them how to use it. Interviewees also valued the possibility to present the service for students and other people who were visiting the care facilities, because it gave a modern impression of their organization.

Although the nurses evaluated that more people participate in live activities than in video broadcasts, it was found that sometimes, when there had been only a couple of people present on site, chair exercises or other activities would have been cancelled without the participation of home users and people at the other care facilities.

The song performer, who sent the music broadcasts in addition to his "normal" job, got many benefits from the service. Before the project, he used to visit other care facilities 4 days a week, but after he started to use the service, he was able to cut the visits to one. Because traveling between the care facilities is time consuming, he said that he saves approximately 5 or 6 hours a week for his *normal* care job. He said that he has adopted the service as an integral part of his job and he finds it to be a good tool. The service has also had indirect consequences for his life, because now he can cycle to work most of the week instead of driving a car, which he previously needed for driving between the care facilities.

The service had an effect on the social relationships of the nurses. The interviewees in the distant facilities said that they had experienced feeling a bit isolated from the main facility, and one of the benefits of the service has been the possibility to be in contact with the main facility and thus feel more connected. One interviewee also experienced that during the project, she has been in cooperation with the caregivers of the main facility and the project has brought caregivers from different facilities together.

Ireland

Following the completion of the trial, the majority of the participants felt that the WeCare service was of great use to them. When the users were asked if they felt they needed a service like WeCare, the response was notably positive all round. The IMI result for value and usefulness scored highly among the participants. The score of 5.6 out of 7 indicates that, generally, participants found the WeCare service to be a valuable and useful activity.

For the most part, the participants felt it was practical to have the six chosen features available on one screen. They found this to be convenient and useful, particularly for users with little previous technology experience. One participant, who was using the WeCare service from his home PC, commented that it would be more useful to him if the service was available on his mobile phone, as he has recently purchased an Android phone.

When the participants were asked if the service provided a new benefit or advantage to them, the response was, generally speaking, a positive one. Seven of the participants commented that following the trial, they were now less dependent on others and more independent and confident in relation to technology. The WeCare service allowed some of the users to finally understand and realize the benefits of technology.

The Netherlands

During the exit interviews, participants expressed their perceived value, which sometimes varied from their expected value. Most relevant aspects were as follows:

- There weren't enough participants for active discussions on the forum, so you don't get in touch with other people.
- The other participants weren't as active as I am, so I didn't find myself buddies to go out with. I only got reactions like "I can't cycle anymore, hope you find someone else."
- I would have liked to find more information on the site, like actual newsfeeds.
- I would have liked to play games together with other participants.
- I would have liked to upload more photos.
- Nobody reacts on the forum, so it is a bit dull.
- I had expected to do more with it, but it's easier to pick up the phone and call.
- I liked it because it gave me more confidence to use the Internet.
- I liked trying out the service and helping other people by testing it.

- In my opinion it looks a bit like a dating website, and that's something I don't want.
- It turned out that my children don't look at my service, so there's no use in filling out the calendar.

Spain

During the exit interview, participants expressed their perceived value in the following ways:

- The user trial period has been very limited, and it was not possible to post enough contents or to organize enough events for community building.
- Due to iterative designs, there were errors and changes in the design at the beginning of the pilot that produced some disorientation. Because of this, they cannot figure out the real value of the platform because they have not interacted with a finalized product but with prototypes.
- Positively, they see the system as potentially helpful for the Lebrija community, especially for those people that need it most (e.g., people with limited social networks).
- They have seen value in the user involvement itself, assessing their participation as 7 in a scale of 10. Important points have been the communication with the project team and other participants.
- The main value was found in meeting with people with similar difficulties of life circumstances, in the empowerment of the community, and as a channel to meet new people and being active.

Expected Value versus Perceived Value

It can be concluded that in Finland and Ireland, users' expectations were mostly met, whereas in the Netherlands and Spain, technology did not fully meet users' needs. The findings show that the WeCare services engaged people with new activities, gave confidence, and provided variety in their lives. It also provided a possibility to meet people in a similar life situation and increased the amount of social relationships.

However, in the Netherlands, some of the more experienced computer users stated that WeCare did not provide enough value compared to existing technologies and services: it is possible to find the same information elsewhere, it is easier to pick up the phone, or it is easier to use a normal calendar than starting up the computer. People also got confused with private calendar vs. neighborhood calendar, and some stated that it is no use to fill out the calendar if the social network did not look at the service.

In Finland, the problem was that people turned off their computers and thus others could not always reach the person on the other end spontaneously. In Ireland, a couple of users missed online help features and they had difficulties with Internet connections. Some people in the Netherlands also had difficulties to write or remember their usernames and passwords, which strongly influenced their user experience. In the first user trial in Spain, the technology was not ready for piloting and there were errors and changes that influenced users.

There were also findings related to the user trial itself. Because a limited group of people used WeCare for a limited time period, social media features, such as forums and public calendars, were lacking content. Because there were not that many participants, people had difficulties to make new friends: "The others couldn't ride a bike anymore." In the

Netherlands, some had false expectations: they hoped to be provided with a new computer, for example. In Finland and in the Netherlands, some people quit the pilot because of health problems. In the Netherlands, delays on the pilot had a negative influence on the motivation of the users, although they were informed as soon as possible. Also, just using WeCare and participating in codesign sessions, interviews, and group situations engaged people in new activities and made them learn new things.

Usability and Accessibility (during and after User Trials)

Usability was very relevant for this project, and usability studies at the beginning of the design process ensured that the users were able to interact with products and services in easy-to-use, convenient, and intuitive ways. Usability may be evaluated, for example, by observing people while they use the service or by heuristic evaluation and usability standards. Also users' opinion concerning the *perceived ease of use* might be asked. The service was designed to be accessible to as many users as possible. *Accessibility* may be evaluated by using accessibility standards or by observing users while they are using the service and evaluating how people with different disabilities are able to use it. However, studying actual accessibility features, such as screen readers, was not within the scope of this project.

Finland

In Finland, usability was evaluated in a usability test with six participants: three nurses and three older people. All the users commented that the service was simple and easy to use: "This is what it (the device) is supposed to be, it does not require too much thinking and there aren't too many different options." Most of the test users (5/6) succeeded at the first or second try in making the video call. One user did not learn the right way of touching, but he was able to find the correct buttons on the screen. Some focal possibilities for errors were associated with the touch duration; the user touches the screen either too long or for too short a time.

The main usability problems were caused by lack of feedback or slow feedback from the selection made with touch gestures, and the problem of finding the correct way to touch the screen. The correct touching gesture could be supported, for example, through the shape of selection buttons—rectangular long buttons invited the user to slide their finger over the button, whereas compact round or square buttons implied a touch gesture without a slide.

It was noted that, at first, people were somewhat cautious to touch the screen, but after a few tries, they adopted the touch paradigm fairly easily (except for one user who had a habit of sliding the finger on the selection buttons). All the test users performed the touch-based interaction in their own unique way (fast/slowly, hard/lightly, by poking/sliding). Therefore, the shape of the user interface elements will greatly affect how fast people will learn to use these elements properly, e.g., regarding the duration of the touch that is needed to operate the system. When providing feedback to the user, audio-based notifications were found to be very useful, since the target user group of the service often had difficulties with their eyesight and perceptive skills.

Ireland

Overall, all 10 participants were satisfied with the usability and accessibility of the WeCare system. The users who had previous experience with technology had little or no issue in using the service. The participants who were familiar with technology adapted quickly to the service, following clear instructions and a brief coaching session during the half day that was spent with each individual. As previously mentioned, there were Internet connectivity issues relating to a small number of participants; however, this problem affects many households in rural Ireland but should be corrected by means of the two-way satellite system, which is being introduced at present. In some cases, Internet boosters were effectively used to help with Internet connection and speed. There were some compatibility issues such as screen resolution and scrolling issues, particularly with those using the Samsung Galaxy Tab.

The Netherlands

The participants were, in general, very able to use the service, but they stopped using it frequently because of little activity on the forum, difficulties in using the calendar, and little support and reactions from their social network. Because of this, they were not really satisfied and content with the service in the end. But they do consider it as a useful service for people who have little experience with ICT and are more dependent than the participants. The respondents were very enthusiastic about the layout of the site. They liked the use of colors and thought it was easily readable. They had not seen the pictograms; they just remembered the color codes. Because they had not seen the pictograms, they also did not miss them.

Spain

During the service design phase, there were some issues with usability and accessibility, but these issues were solved and reduced during the user trials, resulting in little issues at the end of the project.

Social Networks (during and after User Trials)

It is important to study both quantitative and qualitative aspects of social relationships in the aging process (Hughes et al. 2004).

Finland

It was found that the WeCare technology influenced more the *quality* of social networks rather than on their *amount*. Three families used the technology for communicating with relatives and close ones either when at home or during the respite care period. Two of these families found that it had a major impact on the quality of their social relationships with their family members. Mainly, the technology did not affect other human relationships in addition to supporting communication directly with targeted people.

Ireland

There was a clear improvement in the level of interaction that participants had with family, friends, etc., following the completion of the user trial. The majority of participants who used the Skype feature felt that their communication level with others was more than sufficient following the completion of the trial. They recognized the WeCare service as being an important means of communication, particularly with their younger family members. For the participants who used the Skype feature, they considered it as a way of meeting new people and expanding their current network. It also proved to be an effective means of reconnecting with previous networks. The service allowed the users to establish a new technique and direct method of communicating with family and friends, particularly for contacting those who live abroad. Aside from a few connectivity issues, once the users familiarized themselves with the Skype component, it became relatively easy for them to contact friends and family.

The Netherlands

Because the participants did not use the service frequently, it cannot be stated that using WeCare affected their social relations. But in the qualitative end-user evaluations, some participants stated that their children were really enthusiastic at their parents' trying out new things. For example, when the children received a call from the participant, they always asked if they were phoning via the WeCare service. One woman saved up to €8 on her telephone bill by calling via WeCare. She said she called more easily because it was free and that it was not such a pity when the call was not timed right, because she could call again any moment she liked. There were no new contacts made on the WeCare system, because two users already knew each other and they already used Skype to contact each other next to personal visits. So for them this service brought nothing new.

Spain

The participants in the pilot have enhanced the quality of the interactions in terms of frequency and strength. However, it also possible that is was not only the WeCare service itself that was responsible for this improvement. It could also have been the user involvement process; the people who participated in this process met together face to face and created a shared activity topic.

Discussion and Conclusions

We were not able to study quantitatively the relationship between using online social networking services and people's experiences of quality of life. However, based on our qualitative findings and experiences from the user trials, we found that online social networking services are able to engage people in new activities, give confidence, provide variety into users' lives, provide a possibility to meet people with similar life situations, and increase the amount and quality of social relationships. Through these factors, online social networking might very well have positive effects on people's experiences of quality of life.

Based on our findings, we cannot generalize what kind of characteristics of online social networking would apply to all older people. We can state that technological aspects of the service were found to be critical in service adoption. Although software quality and usability are common knowledge in the software business, basic things—such as a reliable Internet connection, adequate quality of sound and video, and intelligible error messages—are important, especially for older people.

One issue that cannot be emphasized enough is the simplicity of logging in to the service. If user authentication is necessary, it should be made easier than using a username and password, especially if the user has limited computer skills and experience. In one of our trials in Ireland, the researchers took care of the usernames and passwords for the first time and the service was designed in a way that later the users did not need them. We got positive experience of using touch screen computers and simple user interfaces with only a couple of icons on the screen. They were easy to use even by users with limited functional capacity after they had learned the right way of touching the screen.

In order to develop these kinds of online social networking services into viable services across Europe, more emphasis should be put on the service design. It is important to define the user requirements in close cooperation with the users and to jointly design the technology. The service should be defined and planned more thoroughly. How will the providing companies actually cooperate with each other and combine their resources to provide the service for the end users? The important questions are, for example, who does the marketing? Who establishes contacts with family and relatives? Who provides access? Who provides training, if necessary? Who provides the content? Support?

This is especially important in the case of older people who might have difficulties imagining what kind of value the technology will bring for them. They might hesitate to adopt new technology.

Basically, service designers should offer a clear and easy path to users, but also a path that could still be tailored to individual users' specific needs, such as a current technology environment (e.g., what they already understand and use) and possible functional limitations of the users (e.g., motor, cognitive, or perceptual skills).

Recommendations

Based on our experiences in the WeCare project, we articulated the following practical recommendations for developing and implementing social networking services for older people.

Organize HCD

We advocate organizing an HCD process. In such a process, potential users participate actively and creatively throughout the project's iterative cycles of research, design, and evaluation. An HCD process involves multidisciplinary teamwork in order to address diverse topics, such as user research, service design, application development, organizing user trials, business modeling, and policy making.

Furthermore, we advocate organizing codesign workshops during the project, involving relevant actors, potential customers and stakeholders, and diverse groups of users, for example, older people and people in their social networks, and informal and formal caregivers. Codesign workshops were especially valuable in helping to develop shared language and understanding.

Moreover, we advocate carefully interpreting the findings from user involvement and codesign, and articulating user requirements, based on these interactions. Please keep in mind that talking with users and stakeholders does not necessarily imply doing exactly what they say. Rather, it means listening carefully and making decisions prudently. It is critical to identify requirements that users find most important and to prioritize these.

Finally, we advocate focusing not only on those people that participated in workshops and trials but also on those that did not participate—on the wider, potential target group. This inclusive approach will help to draw more general conclusions and to better translate the findings from workshops and user trials to a wider target group. This will also help to apply the project's results in further dissemination and deployment.

Combine Face-to-Face and Online

We advocate combining *face to face* meetings and *online* tools. It may be necessary, for example, to organize meetings with people in a social network (family, friends, or neighbors) around the older people (primary users). In such meetings, people can discuss ways to request and offer support or to organize social activities. Next, online tools can enable people to engage in follow-up activities on a continuous basis. Without such meetings, people are less likely to use the online tools. Often, they need to establish communication patterns in a face-to-face manner first, before they can take these communication patterns online.

In addition, it may be necessary to organize interventions with formal caregivers or care professionals—who will also use the service. Those people need to be motivated or incentivized to participate too. And they often need to learn new working procedures in order to use the service in their work contexts. Moreover, for successful deployment of an online service, it may be necessary to make some specific people responsible for moderating (of discussions) and curating (of content) in the online service.

One can improve the match between people's needs and the service's functionality by identifying people's real needs or shared interests, and to frame or modify the service in such a manner that it better matches these needs or interests. One may, for example, find out that two people have a similar hobby, and then connect them to each other, so that this hobby can provide a point of entry for further socializing. Making such matches may raise privacy concerns, which must be dealt with carefully.

Foster Local and Existing Networks

It is recommended to create links between the people and events online, and people and events in real life. Local action, local participation, and local engagement are often necessary for the success of an online service.

Not-for-profit organizations can play a critical role in motivating and empowering people to use the online services. For example, social workers can follow these six steps: (1) find people that might benefit from using the online social networking service; (2) establish relationships and build mutual trust; (3) identify (latent) unsolved needs or problems (*pain*); (4) identify shared interests or goals (*passion*); (5) inspire and motivate people to connect to each other to engage in face-to-face interactions; and (6) help people to use online tools for online interactions.

Online social networks can only become successful if their participants experience the network as *their own*. Then they will invest in it and experience the benefits. It is therefore critical to foster—at least initially—communication and shared activities in order to get things started and to reach a critical mass.

Furthermore, it can be helpful to *use* face-to-face events to promote usage of the online services, to raise awareness about the service, to recruit participants for user trials, or to disseminate the project's findings. Moreover, it is recommended to identify *role models* within the target group and to involve them in reaching out to their peers and in promoting the service.

Develop Flexibly, with Modules (*Pick and Mix*)

The HCD approach allows for the development of different services for different target groups. In order to efficiently develop customized services, we advocate developing services based on modules and to combine these to develop different versions. This *pick and mix* approach reduces development lead time and costs, and enables one to keep up with technology trends and to anticipate emerging technologies, such as tablet computers.

Furthermore, it is critical to use—whenever possible—technologies or modules that are already available, especially those that are available in the public domain, in order to reduce development time and costs. Moreover, one can follow an *agile* development approach, focusing initially on those functionalities that are most relevant for users, such as communication and usability, and on *technical* functionalities, such as security or stability, later on, in an iterative process.

During user trials, one must pay attention to the *provisioning* of the service. In user trials, it may be necessary to install or configure specific pieces of software. This needs to be done with a minimum of inconvenience or bother for the users.

Four different versions of the WeCare service were developed in the four different countries in order to match local contexts and needs and preferences of local users. The different versions were based on one shared architecture and platform, which offered the following functions: a real-time video-communication service, tools to share news and to discuss, tools to plan and organize community events, tools to request and offer mutual support or informal care, and streams of relevant information (see Figure 25.6).

With this *pick and mix* approach, developers can pick those options that the people in their target group value, and combine these in order to develop a tailor-made version of the service.

Make the Service User Friendly

We recommend making the service as *user friendly* as possible. In the case of older people, some of them may suffer from the effects of aging, such as reduced vision or hearing, or reduced motor skills or cognitive skills—all of which may impact their abilities to

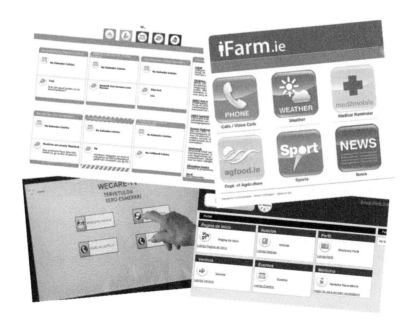

FIGURE 25.6
Screenshots of the Dutch, Irish, Finnish, and Spanish versions of the WeCare service.

effectively use the service. Based on a study by the "Web Accessibility Initiative: Ageing Education and Harmonisation (WAI-AGE)," a number of recommendations and requirements for older people have been developed—which partly coincide with the W3C guidelines for accessible content. The following recommendations are especially useful:

- Provide a simple interface and clarity about the basic functions; this is better than offering many and complex functions.
- Use a sufficiently large font size, and provide the option to change font size, for example: "change font size: A A **A**."
- Use a maximum of five to seven menu options and present these clearly, for example, as large buttons with clear titles.
- Enable people to jump between hyperlinks, using the Tab keyboard button (used by some with reduced motor skills).
- Show (most of) the content in one view so that users do not need to scroll down for relevant content.
- Make explicit *where the user* is in the website, for example, by using specific background colors for *closed* or *open* pages.
- It may be needed to organize a helpdesk, either temporarily, for example, during a user trial, or on a continuous basis.
- It may be worthwhile to enable people to personalize the user interface for each individual person.

Try-Out and Improve Business Models

It is critical to discuss viable and feasible business models from the start of the project. This is especially important if participating organizations are trying out something new that does not necessarily match with their existing service offering. Organizing meetings with potential customers and stakeholders in order to generate and evaluate ideas concerning value proposition, target groups, and revenue streams early on, and in iterative cycles, can help to develop business models that *work*. Typically business WPs are led by companies that have a lot of experience of practice. However, also researchers should be more active in business model development and show that different kinds of methods can be used to refine old business ideas and to create new ones. Also companies should be more open to use these tools and consider new business possibilities. Service concept development and definition of value proposition should not be isolated into a separate business WP, but it should be included in the service design.

In very general terms, a business model can be created (1) from a cost reduction perspective, for example, focusing on reducing costs of health care—which could be interesting for care providers or insurance companies; (2) from a marketing perspective, for example, focusing on ways to reach a specific target group—which could be interesting for home shopping or telecoms companies; or (3) from a *user pays* basis, for example, asking users to pay a monthly fee.

Since the markets for online social networking services are complex and diverse (many stakeholders, many initiatives, many target groups, many regulations, etc.), one needs to articulate precisely the service's added value. This can be done in dialogue with potential users (older people and their social networks), customers (care providers, housing companies, insurance companies), and stakeholders (local governments, policy makers).

Many business models for online services are based on *free* usage. In such cases, other revenue sources need to be found, for example, from a municipality, care provider, or not-for-profit organization—which procures the service wholesale and offers it to its citizens, its customers, or its target audience.

Project Management and Learning

Technologies are developing rapidly and people are adopting new products and services rapidly—think of social networking and tablet computers. From a project management perspective, this means that one must be able to adapt rapidly to changes. For example, one may need to update and modify the project plan every 6 months in order to allow for adaptability and flexibility.

Furthermore, one needs to carefully identify the various interests and stakes of each project partner, and to discuss whether the project is still in line with the project partners' different interests and stakes. Such discussions need to be facilitated not only at the project's start but also during its subsequent stages and iterations, because things can change in the course of the project. Finally, it is critical to be open to learning, for example, by trying out approaches and solutions, by sharing *lessons learned*, and by learning from others.

Acknowledgments

This chapter was written within the WeCare project, which was part of the European Ambient Assisted Living Programme (AAL-2009-2-026) and which received funding from TEKES (Finland), ISCIII (Spain), Enterprise Ireland (Ireland), and ZonMW (The Netherlands), and from the project partners: Caritas-Säätiö, Videra, VTT (Finland), ASSDA, I2BC (Spain), Skytek (Ireland), ANBO, Ericsson, Simac/ShareCare, and TNO (The Netherlands). The authors thank their fellow project team members for their contributions to this chapter: Carlijn Broekman (TNO), Nacho Madrid (I2BC), Fernando Rodriguez Navarro (ASSDA), Claire Reilly (Skytek), Gillian Reynolds (Skytek), Jannie Roemeling (ANBO), Marry van Baalen (ANBO), and Heini Moilanen (Caritas-Säätiö). In addition, the authors thank the other project team members for the privilege of cooperating with them and their contributions to the project: Olav Aarts (TNO), Juhani Heinilä (VTT), Veikko Ikonen (VTT), Arto Wallin (VTT), Stefan Burgers (Ericsson), Mario Goorden (Ericsson), Florin van Slingerland (Ericsson), Sin Yuk Yan (Ericsson), Rob Vermeulen (Simac/ShareCare), Paul Kiernan (Skytek), Susan Meade (Skytek), Pablo Quinones (ASSDA), Matias Itkonen (Caritas-Säätiö), Heikki Keranen (Caritas-Säätiö), Ilkka Ketola (Videra), and Mikko Puhakka (Videra).

References

Chesbrough, H.W., 2003. *Open Innovation: The New Imperative for Creating and Profiting From New Technology*. Boston: Harvard Business School Press.

Golden, J., Conroy, R.M. and Lawlor, B.A., 2009. Social support network structure in older people: Underlying dimensions and association with psychological and physical health. *Psychology, Health and Medicine*, 14(3), 280–290.

Helliwell, J.F. and Putnam, R.D., 2004. The social context of well-being. *The Royal Society*, 359(1449), 1435–1446.

Holmén, K. and Furukawa, H., 2002. Loneliness, health and social network among elderly people— A follow-up study. *Archives of Gerontology and Geriatrics*, 35(3), 261–274.

Hughes, M.E., Waite, L.J., Hawkley, L.C. and Cacioppo, J.T., 2004. A short scale for measuring loneliness in large surveys: Results from two population-based studies. *Research on Aging*, 26(6), 655–672.

Huppert, F.A., Marks, N., Clark, A.E., Siegrist, J., Stutzer, A., Vitterso, J. and Wahrendorf, M., 2009. Measuring well-being across Europe: Description of the ESS well-being module and preliminary findings. *Social Indicators Research*, 91(3), 301–315.

ISO, 1999. *ISO 13407: Human-Centred Design Processes for Interactive Systems*. Geneva, Switzerland: ISO.

Isomursu, M., Ervasti, M., Isomursu, P. and Kinnula, M., 2010. Evaluating human values in the adoption of new technology in school environment. In: *43rd Hawaii International Conference on System Sciences*, 1–10.

Seeman, T.E., 1996. Social ties and health: The benefits of social integration. *Annals of Epidemiology*, 6(5), 442–451.

Sleeswijk-Visser, F., Stappers, P.J., Van der Lugt, R., and Sanders, E.B.N., 2005. Contextmapping: Experiences from practice. *CoDesign*, 1(2), 119–149.

Steen, M., 2011. Tensions in human-centred design. *CoDesign*, 7(1), 45–60.

Steen, M., 2012. Human-centred design as a fragile encounter. *Design Issues*, 28(1), 72–80.

Steen, M., 2013. Co-design as a process of joint inquiry and imagination. *Design Issues*, 29(2), 16–28.

26

Ergonomics and Sustainable Engineering: Important Features to Develop Human Sensitivity–Based Projects

Oscar Alejandro Vásquez Bernal

CONTENTS

ABSTRACT   Today's society is now bringing in significant changes to individual behavior. A large amount of information on environmental awareness, sustainable development, eco-efficiency and sustainable production is circulating daily. Promoting conservation of natural resources and pollution reduction are needed in order to maintain a comfortable living ecosystem for people. These voices of warning encouraging preservation of our resources for the near future have changed the way engineering projects are carried out, leading to environmental awareness and human sensitivity.

A constructive, technological, and service infrastructure project requires us to think about the essence of the project, the audience it is aimed toward, and inputs needed for formulation and development, i.e., the individuals and the community they belong to. Cultural aspects, comfort, anthropometrics, lighting, and type of activity to develop, among others, are the key elements to consider when carrying out these kinds of projects. At this point, ergonomics passes into the project inputs. Ergonomic design, sustainable projects, and eco-efficient projects are issues that need to be discussed in order to raise awareness and encourage changes in our behavior.

KEY WORDS: *environmental awareness, sustainable development, eco-efficiency, sustainable production, ergonomics, engineering, ecosystems, resources, ergonomic design, sustainable projects.*

Introduction

Currently, business development and exchange of goods and services have gone beyond the physical boundaries of nations. They are needed to change the corporate vision and transform it in a prospective way to know and manage the new ground rules of doing business. Business environmental analysis has changed, and any global phenomenon affects transnational, regional, and local business decision making. This context influences development, design, and formulation of projects since the end consumers they are intended for are more aware about environmental regulations, safety, and integrity; these requirements need to be met by organizations.

This chapter conducts an analysis of human sensitivity–based project development from the perspective of design, project development, functionality, and usability for the end customer. Therefore, it requires analysis of the context of ergonomics, project management, and interaction between these concepts with regard to the development of goods and services having an impact on individuals and society; it also requires a conceptual analysis of ergonomics as an integral science, an analysis of environmental factors within business and social contexts where they interact and generate an impact. Likewise, the study of different activities developed by engineers regarding project development, design, and manufacture is required in order to ensure that products and services provided are suitable for individuals and sustainable for the environment.

Ergonomics as a Basis of Generation of Suitable Projects for Individuals

Saravia (2006) affirms that talking about ergonomics in design or ergonomics for designers in our field could have been something unusual a couple of years ago. Ergonomics was considered as an added value of products, so that the user had the possibility to get either conventional products or ergonomic ones. The trend, which remains the same, is that the latter provide a higher degree of comfort but with extra cost. However, progress in this matter has been limited because the concept of ergonomics (still vague) is highly associated with work stations (especially chairs) and a new vehicles' interiors.

According to today's trend, it is essential to consider, within the inputs, not only functional specifications, materials, and durability during the design process (and product conception) but also the design concept, which is primary in creating prototypes. Ergonomic design should be intrinsic to product design regarding the purpose intended.

Saravia (2006) states that ergonomic design elements should be included within the inputs and affirms that, excluding decorative objects or those onto which the designer intentionally wishes to stamp their personal character, the use of the term *ergonomic design* may become redundant since it becomes difficult to conceive the creation of a product or object for specific purposes (human-related activity), without considering human factors and ergonomics of the target population as well as users in order to define some determinants of design. An understanding of the importance of ergonomics for conceptual and projective design based on its own definition is as follows: "Ergonomics is a multidisciplinary applied science that aims at fitting the products, systems, and artificial environments to users' characteristics, limitations, and needs in order to optimize safety and comfort" (Asociación Española de Ergonomía [AEE] 2014). It is essential for the development of products fitting individuals.

Ergonomics focused on design develops not only the product but also the elements in the environment that determine comfort for individuals. That is why ergonomics is also focused on architectural, constructive, and productive design.

Considering people's comfort means increasing efficiency in the development of activities as it reduces fatigue as well as rest and recovery time when performing an activity that improves performance in an operations process and administrative and management activities.

Ergonomics focused on efficiency and effectiveness activities implies that the resources needed to develop an activity in a place (workstation, leisure area, and common areas) are also used efficiently and that their impact is minimal.

Ergonomic design of products includes analysis of materials, geometry, use, and functionality (designed for or adapted to a particular function or use). It must not be forgotten that after the end of a product's life cycle, the constituent materials may affect the natural environment and the area where it will be discarded as waste. This is the interaction between ergonomics as a science and environmental sustainability where humans live.

Rieradevall and Vázquez (2010) state that it is evident that most of the processes associated with design and development of products are not intended to be sustainable; therefore, they need to be *redesigned*. In order to ensure that processes associated with products have a cyclical and nonlinear approach, a perspective and knowledge of the entire process of the product from conception to disposal is required. That process is called the product life cycle. It is estimated that over 80% of environmental impacts that any product will have at all stages of its life cycle are determined by the design stage, which enhances the importance of sustainability based on the design concept.

Eco-design considers environmental impacts during all stages of design and product development for the purpose of making products that generate as little environmental impact as possible throughout their life cycles (Brezet and Van Hemel 1997). Eco-design is a good strategy to generate products, projects, and sustainable services; however, it results in a utopia for organizations and society in general. Rieradevall and Vázquez (2010) provide the following barriers and opportunities for eco-design implementation.

- The environment is not conceived as a cornerstone of competitive performance.
- Treatment strategies are still more important than prevention.
- Lack of environmental liability arising from product design activity.
- No analysis of products at an environmental level is performed. Therefore, environmental impact is unknown.
- Lack of knowledge regarding eco-design and its opportunities.
- Lack of actual demand for eco-designed products.
- Low support for managing eco-labels.

Eco-design opportunities:

- Reduction of manufacturing and distribution costs by identifying inefficient processes and using fewer natural resources.
- Promotion of innovative thinking to create new market opportunities.
- Improvement of brand image through a sensible attitude toward the environment.
- Adaptation platform to environmental regulations and anticipation of future legislation.
- Increase of value-added product: lower environmental impact throughout its life cycle and higher quality.
- Product quality improvement by increasing durability and functionality.
- Ability to access the green market.
- Possibility of access to eco-labeling systems.
- Knowledge improvement about the product and its life cycle.

Analysis of Product Life Cycle

Within reference documents, the most accurate and detailed definition for the analysis of the product life cycle was extracted from the Conama 10 working document, "Eco-Design In Managing The Life Cycle Product, 2010" (Fullana and Puig 2010). Life cycle analysis is a comparatively recent methodology and has grown rapidly to become a standard procedure for scientists and engineers to investigate and evaluate the environmental performance of a variety of processes caused by human activity.

The origins of life cycle assessment date back to the 1970s in response to the energy crisis, as a way of reducing actual energy consumption and avoiding saving in one process at the expense of increasing consumption in another. Other studies of this indicator regarding different commodities were also included, and eventually, various types of emissions were considered.

Assessment of product life cycle is a "process to evaluate the environmental burdens associated with a system (making the existence in the market possible) of a product, service or activity by identifying and quantitatively describing matter and energy used and emissions sent to the environment, and to assess the impacts associated with these uses of matter, energy, and emissions. The assessment includes the entire cycle life of the product or activity, including extraction and processing of raw materials, manufacturing, distribution, use, reuse, maintenance, recycling, final disposal, and all transportation" (Society of Environmental Toxicology and Chemistry [SETAC 2013]; subsequently amended by Nordic Life Cycle Association [NORLCA 2014]).

Life cycle assessment considers environmental impacts to be those caused by system study on ecosystems, human health, and available resources.

Economic and social impacts have recently been studied. Therefore, a multicriteria analysis is being done. Life cycle assessment turns a specific analysis into a two-variable one, for it takes into account not only information on CO_2 emissions in a factory but also an analysis of the entire chain of production, from cradle to grave (first variable), along with other impacts, such as land use, water consumption, acidification, ozone layer destruction, etc. (second variable). Assessment of these two dimensions helps prevent transfer a life cycle stage environmental impact to another or an environmental impact category to another. (More specific studies do not include this perspective and may result not in a decision to reduce impact but in a change of place.) The methodology is divided into a series of interrelated steps, such as definition of the purpose and scope of the system, life cycle inventory analysis, environmental impact assessment, and interpretation of results.

Fullana and Puig (2010) show that one of the studies developed from an ecological approach measures the carbon footprint, which consists of a life cycle assessment with regard to contribution of the system to global warming and which is being standardized internationally by the International Organization of Standardization (ISO), standard 14067, and by the World Business Council for Sustainable Development in the Greenhouse Gas Protocol of products.

The carbon footprint, the quantification of energy demand, and the water footprint are simplifications of life cycle assessment on impact categories that may have more social relevance in a particular moment and help in promoting environmental awareness and action. However, there are other categories of impact that are hidden for that product and may be more important; for example, it is more relevant to study the toxicity of a painting, the eutrophication of cheese, the acidification of a fertilizer, or the water consumption of a carton.

Life cycle assessment is used for many applications, both strategic and operational. At the strategic level, it is used to develop the product category rules of environmental product declaration programs or environmental criteria that need to be fulfilled by the products wanting to apply for a specific eco-label. It is also used to define waste management plans of governments, whether industrial, municipal, or packages (e.g., to obtain realistic and environmentally justifiable recycling rates).

It is also used by business associations at a strategic level to position their products against those of competitors. A series of life cycle assessments performed by a company over the years is an optimal way to assess environmental trends.

At an operational level, it is used by companies to do eco-design, to make an environmental statement on a product, or simply to ensure that their environmental marketing is well founded. It is also used in public procurement competitions requiring its application when describing the environmental aspect of goods or services for sale and plans of improvement offered by the company. Recently, it has often been used to calculate carbon footprints.

However, technology assessment is an application booming now and in the future, much more than others. A great amount of new processes and technologies are being developed by companies, technological institutes, and universities every day. There is no doubt that the environmental factor based on life cycle assessment will remain to be important, if not essential, which confirms its feasibility.

It is essential for groups of researchers to have knowledge of life cycle assessment. It is also important to have trained critical reviewers to avoid biased studies due to the lack of methodology or misusing of databases or software, which leads to incorrect changes and investments (Fullana and Puig 2010).

Life cycle assessment has been developed for research purposes and development. Therefore, universities and companies investing a great amount of their budget on research and development (R & D) generate new knowledge and results that may be applied for improving products and processes. The pharmaceutical industry, the food industry, and technology products invest extensively in coaching, training, and research to improve product design, manufacture, disposal, and usage after end-of-life.

Figure 26.1 shows different processes of transformation of a product applied to an industry that develops materials from concept to delivery and disposal. However, this cycle

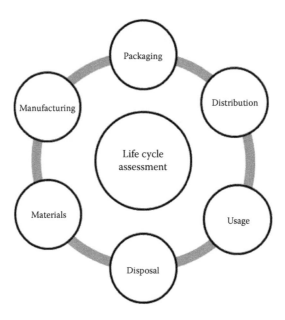

FIGURE 26.1
Life cycle assessment diagram. (Image extracted from http://www.pgbeautygroomingscience.com/break throughs-xix.html.)

also applies to companies developing processes and component parts for more complex products.

Ergonomics Focuses on Usage and User

Wever et al. (2008) defined user-centered design as a design approach that includes a user-centered stage during the entire design process. Instead of focusing on the technological possibilities and quality measurements in terms of components, the solution consists of setting users as a starting point and measuring product quality from the user's point of view, taking into account needs, wishes, characteristics, and abilities of the projected user group. The aim of adopting a user-centered design approach is to improve the quality of interaction between the user and the product.

Rooden and Kanis (2000) have also proposed a more interactive framework that includes more details about user characteristics and relationships between the product, the user, and the context. This framework includes the output of the product in terms of feedback to the user and very relevant performance in the context of design for sustainability; the side effects can be noise, heat, waste production, or energy consumption. This interactive framework is one of the few explicitly including side effects. Those effects should be minimized.

In a process, the best description of interaction between a product and process is appreciated in the system approach. Inputs are resources, raw material, information, money, workforce, and machinery; the process refers to all operations following a systematic order that transforms inputs into outputs; and outputs are transformations results that are defined as finished products (Figure 26.2).

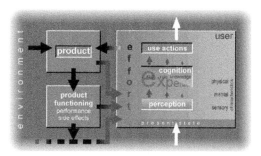

FIGURE 26.2
User–product interaction. (Rooden and Kanis 2000.)

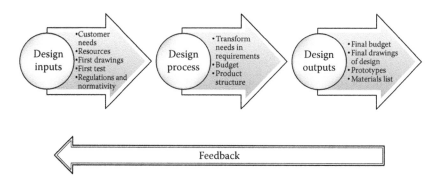

FIGURE 26.3
Design process.

Design Process

Figure 26.3 describes operations from design inputs to design outputs. It is evident that the feedback is the measurement resulting from comparing the initial needs to the final design. Adjustments, modifications, and changes can be presented during this process.

In this case, feedback is generated by the modification of the concept design before manufacture. Communication with the end customer (user) is essential because important elements of usability and functionality are defined within design aspects.

Manufacturing Process

Figure 26.4 describes the interaction between design output and manufacturing. The open system theory is applicable because the outputs of one process are inputs of others. During the manufacturing process, the feedback corresponds to compliance with quality characteristics, design characteristics, improvements, complaints, and claims regarding the finished product or service.

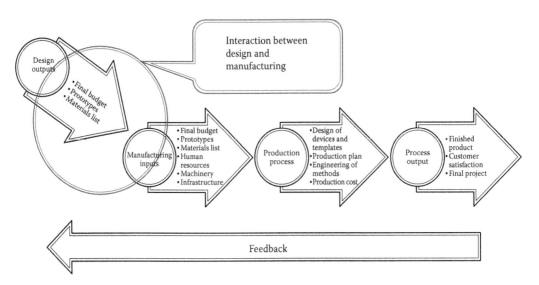

FIGURE 26.4
Interaction between design output and manufacturing.

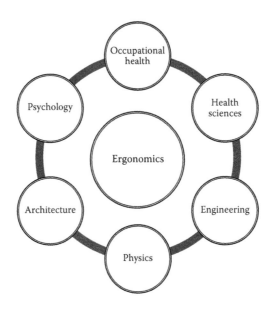

FIGURE 26.5
Interrelationship between ergonomics and applied sciences.

Once the importance of the interaction between the product and the individual product design and manufacturing is established, it is important to show the interrelation between ergonomics and applied sciences (Figure 26.5).

Ergonomics is not only a science; it also interacts with basic sciences such as physics and applies social sciences such as psychology, medicine, and architecture. The main reason that ergonomics is important is the analysis of individual behavior and performance development processes during activities. Improving physical conditions of an individual affects psychological behavior; therefore, it is important to create comfortable environments as a result of the implementation of architecture and engineering for the benefit of the individual.

Interaction between Ergonomics and Architecture

Ergonomic design applied to architecture and design of living spaces should take into consideration the quality of space to be used by the individual and the use of resources to ensure comfort in a room.

Palomera and García Izaguirre (2011) state that there is

> A relationship between architecture and environment based on ergonomics and ask a question: Is ergonomics an eco-efficiency factor in building architecture?
>
> In order to answer that question, it is important to analyze architecture as the result of a process system consisting of models of project implementation to meet the demand for living space. Each stage involves a series of actions of a mental and physical nature to solve a particular problem about the figure of a person in contact with the environment. The atmosphere surrounding the person is in a mutual interaction by the dynamics of changing needs, decision making, and planning for a better quality of life—all these through the chain of procedures for constructing a spatial configuration more suitable for handling natural resources, energy expenditure, and the consequences of activities in pursuit of objectives.
>
> Architecture's commitment of meeting space requirements is renewed in the context of sustainability. It is enough to offer benefits for one person or community, without thinking about the global consequences of doing this. Unfortunately, construction is one of the main sources of pollution, so it is very important to focus on actions, tasks, and activities involved in building. It is also important to consider that man is a person and not just a resource to meet the requirements of time and cost in design and construction programs.

Engineering and Development of Sustainable Products

The stage in which design sketches begin to create a more realistic setting, focusing on production of the product, specification review, and design of production processes, is key to realizing expectations and customer needs. Engineering has great importance because it requires communication between the designer and the engineer in order to meet the initial stages of design (design inputs), and delivers a customer's demands, fulfilling quality, cost, and time schedule for usage.

Infrastructure projects, telecommunications, and product engineering are framed within a process conceived as an open system in which environmental elements can affect the process characteristics. Checking these items in an appropriate way by applying the tools of engineering for planning, scheduling, and control will reduce uncertainty in projects.

Every project is different because the result depends on each client's need. However, there are steps that may be repeated and have worked effectively for design, planning, scheduling, and project control. Given the complexity of the projects, tools must be used for planning and controlling in such a way that a project can control several interrelated projects until the end. For that, the Project Management Institute (PMI) develops a dynamic model for planning and controlling of projects, which is framed in nine knowledge areas:

- Integration management: review of the context of the project to establish integration between processes. Process implementation approach. Creation of a team.
- Scope management: setting up the scope of the project in order to determine resources needed for development.
- Time management: determining the time required in each process, precedence, review of critical points, and establishing of controls.
- Cost management: resource planning, project budgeting, cost estimation, and budget tracking.
- Quality management: quality assurance, control processes and procedures, management indicators, and statistical quality control.
- Human resource management: recruitment, forming gangs, development, and human resource management.
- Communication management: establishing procedures for handling internal information with external teams and the project's investor and customer.

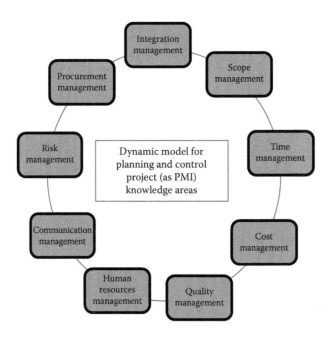

FIGURE 26.6
Dynamic model for planning and control project.

- Risk management: project analysis and planning of the potential risks facing the project, control and monitoring, and taking corrective and preventive actions for the risk.
- Procurement management: the process of purchasing and procurement, monitoring and evaluation of suppliers, contracts for the acquisition of resources needed for the project.

Each of these areas can apply tools for securing, management, and control of its threads of time and will have to be aligned with the goals and objectives of the project (strategic planning project).

In project management planning and control, these nine areas of knowledge can deliver within the time expected with budgeted costs and quality that are determined from the beginning of the project, maintaining customer satisfaction.

Figure 26.6 shows the interaction between the nine knowledge areas and systematic order of application.

A project is sustainable if it meets three key elements: quality, cost, and delivery.

- Project quality: compliance with all customer-requested features, technical specifications and performance, and specific regulations.
- Cost of the project: compliance with the budget and reduction of disposal costs and operations or processes that generate value.
- Delivery of the project: meeting delivery dates throughout all phases of the project and final delivery, reducing penalty charges, and insurance policy settlement.

Prospective Ergonomics, Technology, and Ambient Assisted Living

In order to study prospective ergonomics and ambient assisted living (AAL), an analysis of how ergonomics has changed to integrate with products that benefit people is performed. Appliances, furniture, hand tools, architecture and furniture, automobiles, and cutting-edge designs have been developed to improve and adapt to the conditions of the individual. In the application of ergonomic principles, the product suits individual needs and not otherwise.

Technology, Architecture, and Projection Image Relationship

Ziefle and Wilkowska (2010) state: "A few decades ago, the function of a room was mainly defined by its static location within an arrangement of rooms. In domestic housing, the functional roles of kitchen, bathroom, living-room and bedroom often depend on room layout and relationships between rooms." Moreover, defining elements of space—floor, ceiling, walls and openings did not exceed their primary architectural function. However, Information and Communication Technology (ICT) is becoming more important in our personal living space. The concept of *Ambient Intelligence* (AmI) and its derivative *Ambient Assisted Living* (AAL) describes the intelligent integration of ICT as well as sensors in our (living) environment, so that people become aware of their presence and context, being able to generate reactions, communications and support for people living within this environment (Raisinghani et al. 2006).

Until now, windows and doors alone linked directly inside and outside spaces. Windows had the primary function of ventilation and lighting but they also enabled communication and enabled seeing outside and inside the room. To allow technical control, a wall traditionally holds a simple light that is used to change the lighting of a room, often in a binary manner (Ziefle and Wilkowska 2010).

The analysis developed by the authors showed a strong relationship between architecture and AAL, as well as between ergonomics and AAL. The product concept and space are related by individual usability. Space and product adaptation provide a significant change in design conception.

Moreover, the interaction between people and computers has generated significant interactive spaces where elements provide simulation training aspects that can contribute to the development of applied tasks in AAL, motor activities of rehabilitation medicine, and physical therapy. Management activities for aircraft, automobiles, and other training devices show the application of simulation and human–computer interaction (HCI).

Ziefle and Wilkowska (2010) state that HCI has established itself as the subdiscipline that focuses on how to better design the interface between people and (computer) technology (Dix et al. 2003). As such, it has always had strong existing connections with cognitive psychology and the graphic/industrial design disciplines. However, until now, its major focus has been on interfaces for personal computing systems using the desktop metaphor. Only in recent years has it begun to tackle the difficult question of how to create intuitive, easy-to-use, efficient, and elegant interfaces for mobile, wearable, and ubiquitous technology.

Computers have become part of everyday life. Some are carried like jewels, being a status symbol as well as a decoration. Recently, the iPhone has shown how interface and product design can lead to success and spread technology. In this case, PDAs or smartphones were already available but overlooked by most of society. People buy iPhones and their competitor smartphones even if they intend to use them only as a phone. Similarly, it is expected that health technology will be more likely to be accepted by people who need it, as long as they are not stigmatized by technology.

The increasing demand in personal care due to demographic changes as well as the ongoing change in social structures may not be satisfied in the near future. This trend along with the desire of the elderly to stay at *home*, i.e., within their familiar environment and neighborhood rather than moving to retirement homes is leading to development of technological solutions to meet that demand (Riva 2003). AAL solutions aim not only to assist the elderly but also to provide personal care by reducing the amount of time needed for visits.

While these solutions help increase the efficiency of personal medical attention, it is also known that social contact is vital for human well-being and protects against isolation and loneliness. In the case of the elderly, daily interaction with personal care personnel and doctors may be the patient's primary source of human contact. There is an argument that such technologies should not reduce the amount of human contact but should shift or extend the social contact experience of the patient. However, assistive technologies will not be used or accepted by patients without having a full understanding of individual needs, desires, ergonomics, and usability (Ziefle and Wilkowska 2010).

Future technology and especially future interfaces, which are, by nature, centered on human beings are impossible to visualize and test without actually demonstrating what this *future* might be. For this reason, we have built the future care lab.

Conclusions and Recommendations

Human sensitivity–based project development arises from the analysis of customer needs and manufacturing processes or project management required to meet these needs. Considering ergonomic product results means user comfort without ignoring performance and usability.

Projects focused on individuals require awareness on the necessary resources for their creation, planning, and control in order to transform needs into requirements. Organizations should fulfill specifications and compliance regulations leading to protection of the user's integrity.

Organizations should tend not to develop worthless projects in terms of equity losses and implementation expenses. Professionals who plan and carry out effective monitoring control and integral management indicators are required.

Human sensitivity–based projects should be attractive for both the customer (consumer) and the stakeholders (organization, shareholders, suppliers, society involved). Effective management of such projects should be durable over time and generate the least possible impact on sustainability.

References

Asociación Española de Ergonomía (2014). Dolphin Audiovisual y Multimedia, Asturias España. Available at http://www.ergonomos.es/ergonomia.php (Retrieved March 6, 2014).

Brezet, H., and C. Van Hemel (1997). *Ecodesign. A Promising Approach to Sustainable Production and Consumption*. Paris: United Nations Publications.

Dix, A., J. Finlay, G. Abowd, and R. Beale (2003). *Human-Computer Interaction*, 3rd Edition. Prentice Hall.

Fullana Palmer, P., and R. Puig. (2010). Documento del Grupo de Trabajo de Conama 10: La inteligencia ecológica y el Ciclo de Vida. ECODES. Available at http://ecodes.org/docs/ecodiseno_CONAMA.pdf (Retieved November 10, 2010).

NORLCA (2014). The Nordic Life Cycle Association Nordic, Denmark. Availbale at http://www.norlca.org/cms/site.aspx?p=5220 (Retrieved March 6, 2014).

Palomera, J. L., and V. García Izaguirre (2011). Hacia Un Modelo Ergonómico De Construcción Ecoeficiente. Sociedad de Ergonomístas de México A.C. Available at http://www.semac.org.mx/archivos/7-7.pdf (accessed March 6, 2011).

Raisinghani, M., A. Benoit, J. Ding, M. Gomez, K. Gupta, V. Gusila, D. Power, and O. Schmedding (2006). Ambient intelligence: Changing forms of human-computer interaction and their social implications. *Journal of Digital Information* 5(4). Available at https://journals.tdl.org/jodi/index.php/jodi/article/view/149.

Rieradevall, J., and V. Vázquez (2010). Documento del Grupo de Trabajo de Conama 10: Medio Ambiente y Producto. Available at http://ECODE/ecodes.org/docs/ecodiseno_CONAMA.pdf (accessed November 10, 2010).

Riva, G. (2003). Ambient intelligence in health care. *Cyber Psychology & Behavior* 6(3), 295–300.

Rooden M. J., and H. Kanis (2000). Anticipation of Usability Problems by Practitioners *Proceedings of the Human Factors and Ergonomics Society Annual Meeting*, 44(38), 941–944. doi: 10.1177/154193120004403871.

Saravia Pinilla, M. H. (2006). *Ergonomía de Concepción Su aplicación al diseño y otros procesos proyectuales*, 1ª Edición. Bogotá: Editorial Pontificia Universidad Javeriana.

SETAC (2013). Association Management Software, *Society of Environmental Toxicology and Chemistry*. Availbale at http://www.setac.org/ (Retrieved March 6, 2014).

Wever, R., J. van Kuijk, and C. Boks (2008). User-centred design for sustainable behavior. *International Journal of Sustainable Engineer* 1(1).

Ziefle, M., and W. Wilkowska (2010). Technology acceptability for medical assistance. In *Proceedings of 4th ICST Conference on Pervasive Computing Technologies for Healthcare*. Available at http://www .humtec.rwth-aachen.de/files/05482288.pdf, doi:10.4108/CSTPERVASIVEHEAL TH20 10. 8859: http://dx.doi.org110.4108llCSTPERVASIVEHEAL TH2010. 8859 (Retrieved March 6, 2014).

Index

Page numbers followed by f and t indicate figures and tables, respectively.

Printed and bound by CPI Group (UK) Ltd, Croydon, CR0 4YY

22/10/2024

01777614-0017